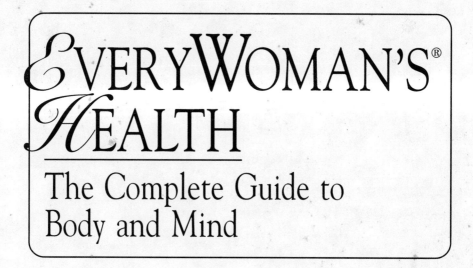

EveryWoman's®
Health

The Complete Guide to Body and Mind

*E*very **W**oman's®

*H*ealth

The Complete Guide to
Body and Mind   SIXTH EDITION

By 17 Women Doctors

JUNE JACKSON CHRISTMAS, M.D. · ELIZABETH B. CONNELL, M.D. ·
KATHRYN SCHROTENBOER COX, M.D. · FRANCES DREW, M.D. ·
BARBARA GASTEL, M.D. · ANNE GELLER, M.D. ·
TOBY OREM GRAHAM, M.D. · MARY JANE GRAY, M.D. ·
MARGARET NELSEN HARKER, M.D. · PEGGY B. HASLEY, M.D. ·
CHRISTINE E. HAYCOCK, M.D. · DOROTHY J. HICKS, M.D. ·
FRANCES M. LOVE, M.D. · HELENE MACLEAN · MAUREEN MYLANDER ·
MAXINE SCHURTER, M.D. · KATHRYN LYLE STEPHENSON, M.D. ·
LOUISE TYRER, M.D. · RUTH K. WESTHEIMER, ED.D.

Edited by Helene MacLean

Illustrated by Leonard D. Dank

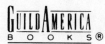

GUILD**A**MERICA
B O O K S®

DOUBLEDAY DIRECT, INC.
GARDEN CITY, NEW YORK

Book design by Robert Aulicino
Art direction by Diana Klemin

CONTRIBUTORS

Authors

JUNE JACKSON CHRISTMAS, M.D., Past President, American Public Health Association; Clinical Professor of Psychiatry, Columbia University College of Physicians & Surgeons; Professor Emeritus of Behavioral Science, City University of New York Medical School, New York City

ELIZABETH B. CONNELL, M.D., Professor, Department of Gynecology and Obstetrics, Emory University School of Medicine, Atlanta, Georgia

KATHRYN SCHROTENBOER COX, M.D., Assistant Attending Physician, Obstetrics and Gynecology, New York Hospital–Cornell Medical Center; Clinical Instructor, Cornell University Medical College, New York City

FRANCES DREW, M.D., M.P.H., Professor of Community Medicine, University of Pittsburgh School of Medicine, Pittsburgh, Pennsylvania

BARBARA GASTEL, M.D., M.P.H., Formerly of National Institute on Aging, National Institutes of Health, Bethesda, Maryland

ANNE GELLER, M.D., Chief, Smithers Alcoholism Treatment and Training Center, St. Luke's–Roosevelt Hospital Center, New York City; Associate Professor of Medicine, College of Physicians and Surgeons, Columbia University, New York City

TOBY OREM GRAHAM, M.D., Associate Professor of Medicine, University of Pittsburgh School of Medicine, Pittsburgh, Pennsylvania

MARY JANE GRAY, M.D., Professor Emeritus of Obstetrics and Gynecology, University of North Carolina Medical School, Chapel Hill

MARGARET NELSEN HARKER, M.D., Adult General Medicine, Morehead City, North Carolina; Electronics Data Systems (1979–1982), Raleigh, North Carolina; Assistant Professor of Surgery (1975–1979), University of North Carolina Medical School, Chapel Hill

PEGGY B. HASLEY, M.D., M.H.E., Assistant Professor of Medicine, University of Pittsburgh School of Medicine

5

CHRISTINE E. HAYCOCK, M.D., Professor Emeritus of Surgery, University of Medicine and Dentistry of New Jersey, New Jersey Medical School, Newark; Fellow, American College of Sports Medicine

DOROTHY J. HICKS, M.D., Professor of Obstetrics and Gynecology, University of Miami School of Medicine; Consultant, Rape Treatment Center, Jackson Memorial Hospital, Miami, Florida

GORDON LETTERMAN, M.D., Professor Emeritus of Surgery, George Washington University School of Medicine, Washington, D.C.

FRANCES M. LOVE, M.D. (late), Specialist in Occupational Medicine; Retired Southwestern Regional Medical Director, Gulf Oil Corporation

HELENE MACLEAN, Medical writer and editor; Author, *Caring for Your Parents, Relief from Chronic Arthritis Pain;* coauthor, *Recovering from a Hysterectomy, Migraine: Beating the Odds*

MAUREEN MYLANDER, Author and writer/editor, National Center for Research Resources, National Institutes of Health, Bethesda, Maryland

MAXINE SCHURTER, M.D. (late), Clinical Professor of Surgery, George Washington University School of Medicine, Washington, D.C.

KATHRYN LYLE STEPHENSON, M.D. (late), Santa Barbara Cottage Hospital, Santa Barbara, California

LOUISE TYRER, M.D., Medical Director for the Association of Reproductive Health Professionals, Washington, D.C.; Past Vice-President for Medical Affairs, Planned Parenthood Federation of America, Inc.

RUTH K. WESTHEIMER, Ed.D., Author; Psychosexual therapist; Adjunct Professor, New York University

Illustrator

LEONARD D. DANK
Consultant Medical Illustrator, St. Luke's–Roosevelt Hospital Center and Women's Hospital, New York City

CONTENTS

LIST OF ILLUSTRATIONS

A WOMAN'S BODY: STRUCTURE AND FUNCTIONS
A 16-page full-color portfolio after page 416

Part Two

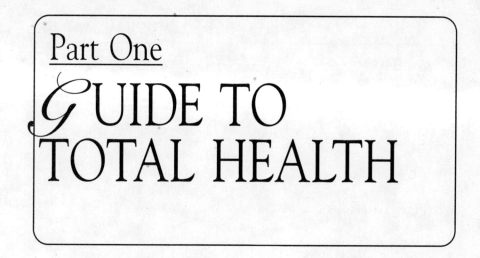

Part One

GUIDE TO TOTAL HEALTH

$\mathcal{T}$HE HEALTHY WOMAN

June Jackson Christmas, M.D.

Past President, American Public Health Association; Clinical Professor of Psychiatry, Columbia University College of Physicians & Surgeons; Professor Emeritus of Behavioral Science, City University of New York Medical School

Health is a positive state—not merely the absence of disease. Yet we often describe health in a negative way. We may consider ourselves healthy because at the moment we have no aches or pains and are not under the care of a doctor. But health is a condition of wellness, a state of physical, mental, and emotional well-being. It is too valuable to be described by what it is not. It is too important to be left entirely in the hands of others, whether they are doctors, advertisers, druggists, neighbors, or friends.

There are three things *you* can do for your health:

- Know how your body functions and be aware of the factors that affect your well-being.
- Take responsibility for making wise decisions that promote good health.
- Be an active, well-informed partner in health care.

KNOW HOW YOUR BODY FUNCTIONS

The body is a living, dynamic organism, one that is constantly replacing or repairing its old or damaged parts. It consists of many systems that are interrelated and dependent on each other for effective functioning. A weakness in one system frequently leads to malfunction in others. For example, the function of the brain and nervous system affects all parts of the body; the pituitary gland influences growth, reproduction, metabolism, and a number of other activities, including uterine contractions at childbirth.

The descriptions and illustrations that follow summarize how the systems of your body work.

THE SKELETAL MUSCULAR SYSTEM: THE FRAMEWORK

Your skeletal muscular system forms the framework of your body. It consists of bones, muscles, tendons, ligaments, and joints. The skin can also be considered part of this system in that it constitutes part of the framework. These elements give the body its shape, enable the body to move, and protect the vital organs.

The spinal column, which supports the body's weight and provides the bony corridor through which the spinal cord passes, is comprised of 33 vertebrae, some of which are fused together. Depending on their location, they differ somewhat in structure and size: 7 cervical vertebrae are at the back of the neck; 12 thoracic vertebrae support the upper back; 5 lumbar vertebrae are in the lower back; 5 fused vertebrae make up the sacrum near the base of the spine; and 4 fused vertebrae form the coccyx. The vertebrae are separated from each other by fibrous tissue and cartilage discs that act as shock absorbers.

Muscles are attached to bones by tendons. The bones are held together by ligaments of connective tissue that enable the bones to move when the muscles contract. Joints are the points at which two bones meet. They are classified as hinge, pivot, or ball-and-socket according to the kind of motion their structure allows. Joints of the skull are fixed, or nonmovable.

Muscles are composed of bundles of fibers that have the ability to contract in response to a complex system of electrochemical signals transmitted from the

SKELETAL SYSTEM

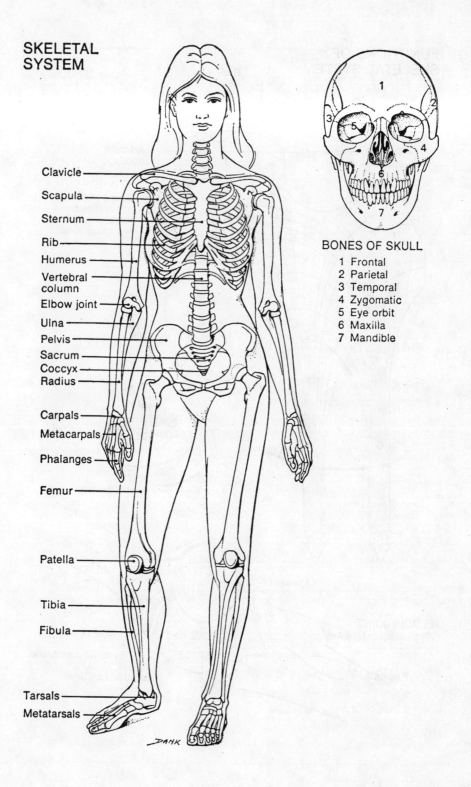

Clavicle
Scapula
Sternum
Rib
Humerus
Vertebral column
Elbow joint
Ulna
Pelvis
Sacrum
Coccyx
Radius
Carpals
Metacarpals
Phalanges
Femur
Patella
Tibia
Fibula
Tarsals
Metatarsals

DANK

BONES OF SKULL

1 Frontal
2 Parietal
3 Temporal
4 Zygomatic
5 Eye orbit
6 Maxilla
7 Mandible

FUNCTIONS OF
SKELETAL SYSTEM

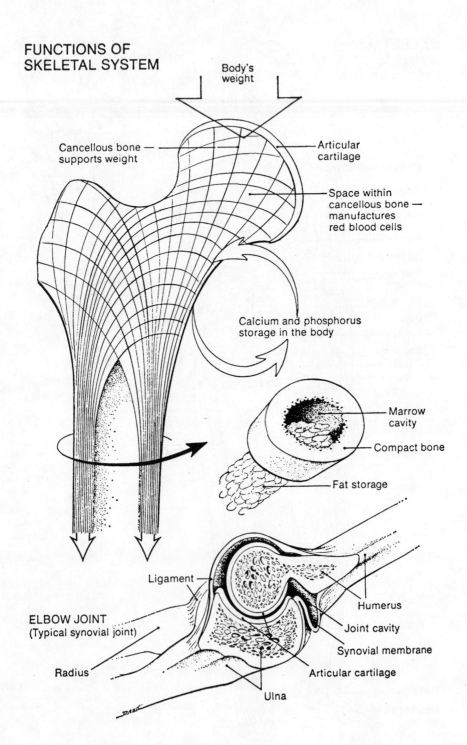

Body's
weight

Cancellous bone —
supports weight

Articular
cartilage

Space within
cancellous bone —
manufactures
red blood cells

Calcium and phosphorus
storage in the body

Marrow
cavity

Compact bone

Fat storage

Ligament

ELBOW JOINT
(Typical synovial joint)

Radius

Ulna

Humerus

Joint cavity

Synovial membrane

Articular cartilage

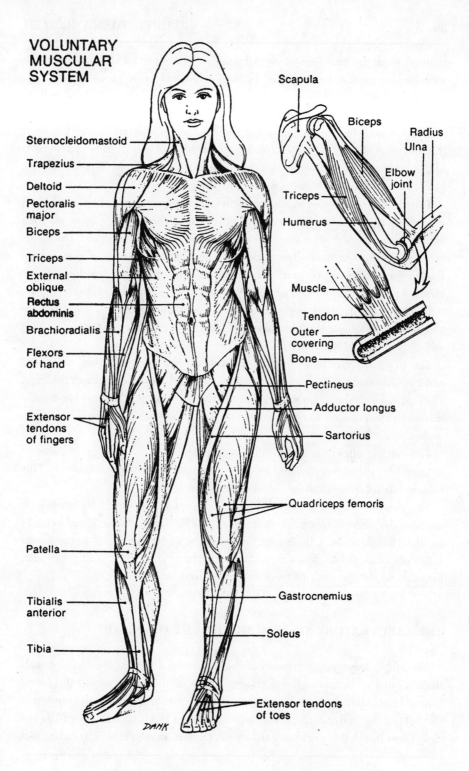

VOLUNTARY MUSCULAR SYSTEM

Sternocleidomastoid

Trapezius

Deltoid

Pectoralis major

Biceps

Triceps

External oblique

Rectus abdominis

Brachioradialis

Flexors of hand

Extensor tendons of fingers

Patella

Tibialis anterior

Tibia

Scapula

Biceps

Radius

Ulna

Triceps

Elbow joint

Humerus

Muscle

Tendon

Outer covering

Bone

Pectineus

Adductor longus

Sartorius

Quadriceps femoris

Gastrocnemius

Soleus

Extensor tendons of toes

DANK

brain through the nervous system. All muscle fibers store fuel for activity in the form of glycogen, a sugar created by the body's metabolic process.

The approximately 600 muscles of the human body make up about half its total weight. They are divided into three types. The voluntary muscles normally are controlled by the conscious mind. The involuntary muscles control the functions of internal organs, such as the caliber of the arteries and the size of the pupils, via impulses arising automatically in the brain. The cardiac, or heart, muscle (myocardium) is a third, distinct type.

The voluntary muscles move the skeletal and other parts of the body and maintain posture. When seen under a microscope, the fibers of these muscles appear to be striped; thus they are referred to as striated muscles. These are the muscles we use for walking, speaking, gesturing. The state of partial contraction in which the voluntary muscles are held is called muscle tone. Exercise and proper nutrition are necessary to maintain tone and condition. If these muscles are not used regularly, they may atrophy and become slack. They are also subject to fatigue if extended use depletes their supply of stored glycogen and causes a buildup of lactic acid.

The involuntary muscles function continually during respiration, digestion, and circulation. These muscles are not striated and are called smooth muscles. They do not atrophy when not used regularly. For example, the uterine muscle maintains the capacity to contract even if it is never used or is used only once or twice in a lifetime.

The cardiac muscle is unique in its composition. It is made up of partially striated fibers that contract and relax continuously throughout a lifetime. This muscle has its own "built-in" nerve conduction system.

The skin, the largest organ of the body, completes the body framework. It contains the sense of touch, keeps fluids in and foreign bodies out, and helps to regulate temperature. Changes in the condition of the body and in emotional states are reflected in skin temperature, moisture, and color, as may be seen, for example, in the flush of fever or embarrassment.

THE CIRCULATORY SYSTEM: MOVEMENT OF BLOOD

The circulatory system consists of the heart and a network of blood vessels throughout the body. As the pumping action of the heart moves the blood through the network, oxygen, nutrients, and other substances are distributed to all parts of the body. Perhaps the most surprising thing about the heart is not that it fails but that it works as hard and as long as it does. It weighs only about a pound. If the pathways through which the blood circulates were laid out end to end, they would cover a distance of about 75,000 miles. In order to keep approximately 5 quarts of blood circulating through these pathways, the heart pumps about 8,000 quarts of blood every 24 hours and continues to do so over a life span—on average 27,000 days, or 75 years.

The heart, essentially a muscular pump, consists of four chambers: the left and right atria and the left and right ventricles. Blood from each atrium flows into its corresponding ventricle. There is a valve between each atrium and ventricle (the tricuspid valve on the right and the mitral valve on the left) that prevents blood from flowing from the ventricle back to the atrium. The right atrium receives blood from the entire body except the lungs and contracts to pump it into the right ventricle. The right ventricle pumps blood into the pulmonary artery and then to the lungs. The left atrium receives blood from the lungs and pumps it into the left ventricle. The left ventricle pumps blood into the aorta and then to the rest of the body. There is a heart valve (pulmonic) at the junction of the right ventricle and the pulmonary artery and another (aortic) at the junction of the left ventricle and the aorta. These valves prevent the blood from flowing backward. Automatic nervous system impulses from the brain to a part of the heart called the sinoauricular node (the heart's

BLOOD FLOW IN THE HEART

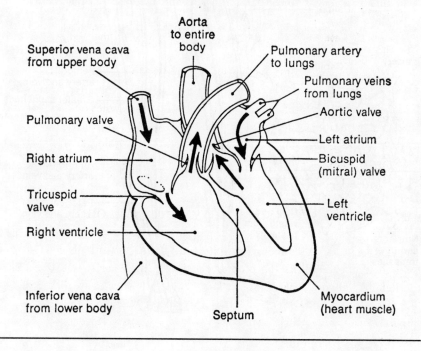

Aorta
to entire
body

Superior vena cava
from upper body

Pulmonary artery
to lungs

Pulmonary veins
from lungs

Aortic valve

Pulmonary valve

Left atrium

Right atrium

Bicuspid
(mitral) valve

Tricuspid
valve

Left
ventricle

Right ventricle

Inferior vena cava
from lower body

Septum

Myocardium
(heart muscle)

CIRCULATORY SYSTEM

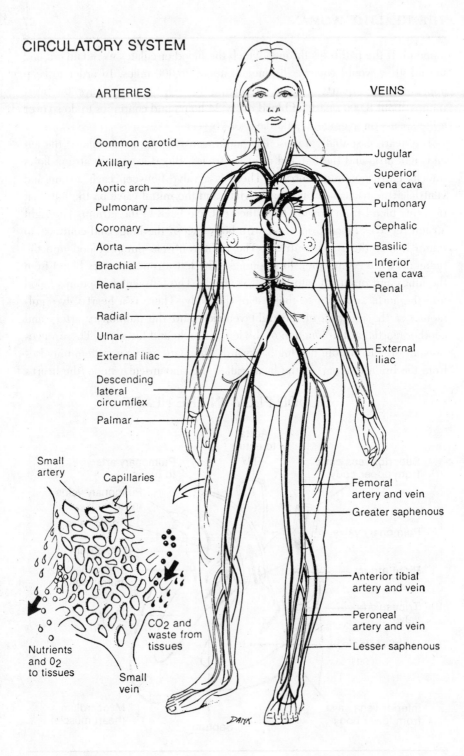

ARTERIES

Common carotid
Axillary
Aortic arch
Pulmonary
Coronary
Aorta
Brachial
Renal
Radial
Ulnar
External iliac
Descending lateral circumflex
Palmar

VEINS

Jugular
Superior vena cava
Pulmonary
Cephalic
Basilic
Inferior vena cava
Renal
External iliac
Femoral artery and vein
Greater saphenous
Anterior tibial artery and vein
Peroneal artery and vein
Lesser saphenous

Small artery
Capillaries
Nutrients and O_2 to tissues
CO_2 and waste from tissues
Small vein

DANK

pacemaker) control the rate at which the heart contracts, normally 60 to 100 times a minute when an individual is not exercising.

The pulse is caused by the flow of blood through the arteries as the heart contracts. Blood pressure in the arteries is the force exerted against the walls of these vessels as blood flows through them. As the ventricles contract, there is a spurt of blood into the arteries, and blood pressure increases. This is systolic pressure. The pressure when the ventricles are relaxed and filling with blood is diastolic pressure.

The circulatory system consists of three separate but interrelated divisions: coronary, pulmonary, and systemic. The heart has its own circulatory system made up of the coronary arteries that originate in the aorta. The pulmonary circulation carries blood from the right ventricle through the lungs via its arterial system and back via its venous system to the left atrium. In the lungs carbon dioxide is removed and oxygen is picked up. The systemic circulation carries this reoxygenated blood via its arterial system from the left ventricle throughout the body and then carries deoxygenated blood via its venous system back to the right atrium.

The arteries in this system branch into arterioles and become smaller and smaller until they become capillaries that are as fine as hairs and form a network throughout all the tissues. It is at the capillary level that oxygen and other substances seep out to the tissue cells and waste products and carbon dioxide are absorbed. The waste products are removed from the blood as it passes through the liver, kidneys, and lungs. The blood returns to the heart via the venous system, from capillaries to venules to the larger veins and finally to the right atrium.

THE RESPIRATORY SYSTEM: SUPPLY OF OXYGEN

Through the respiratory system, air moves into and out of the body. Air is inhaled through the nose and mouth; it moves into the trachea (windpipe) and its divisions (bronchi), then into the bronchioles of the lungs, and finally into the alveoli, the very thin sacs of the lung. The thin membranes of the alveoli are in contact with this air on one side and blood on the other. The oxygen in the inhaled air passes across the membranes and unites with the hemoglobin in the red blood cells. The oxygenated blood is then carried to the tissues. Carbon dioxide is transferred from the blood across the membranes to the air to be exhaled. The entire process of air moving into and out of the body and the exchange between the blood and air is called respiration.

When breathing occurs, the size of the chest cavity changes. Muscular contractions, which may be either automatic or voluntary, flatten the diaphragm and move the ribs upward to expand the chest cavity. With this expansion, air pressure around the lungs is decreased below that of the atmosphere and air enters the lungs (inhalation). Exhalation occurs because the opposite happens: the diaphragm and chest wall contract, the pressure on the lungs increases, and air is expelled.

THE DIGESTIVE SYSTEM: NOURISHMENT

Digestion is the conversion of food into energy and into the various substances that can be assimilated by the body cells. The digestive, or gastrointestinal, system includes the gastrointestinal (GI) tract and other organs related to the digestive process such as the pancreas, liver, and gall bladder. Food progresses through the body in the GI tract, a continuous hollow tube about 30 feet in length that begins at the mouth, includes the esophagus, stomach, small intestine, and large intestine (colon), and ends at the anus.

The mechanical and chemical breakdown of food begins in the mouth. Chewing grinds it into small pulpy pieces, and enzymes in the saliva, mainly ptyalin, begin the chemical conversion of some starches into sugar. The saliva also lubricates the food as it passes into the esophagus.

No chemical action takes place in the esophagus, but its rhythmic contractions (peristalsis) propel the food into the stomach. Peristaltic action continues to push the food along, helps to liquefy it, and mixes it with gastric juices.

The stomach contains glands that secrete gastric juices containing enzymes, chiefly pepsin, and hydrochloric acid, which further break down the food into a semiliquid and accelerate the digestive process. Carbohydrates pass through the stomach quickly; proteins move through more slowly because they take longer to digest. Some fats are split up in the stomach, but most are digested farther on. The only substances absorbed directly from the stomach into the blood are moderate quantities of alcohol and some other drugs. Activity in the stomach reaches its maximum about two hours after a meal. A comparatively light meal may pass through in three to four hours, while a heavy meal may take as long as six.

The end of the stomach opens into the duodenum, the first section of the small intestine. As food enters the duodenum, it is mixed with secretions from the liver, gallbladder, and pancreas. Pancreatic juices and bile from the liver or gallbladder begin to break down proteins into amino acids, convert starch and

RESPIRATORY SYSTEM

ENLARGED ALVEOLI

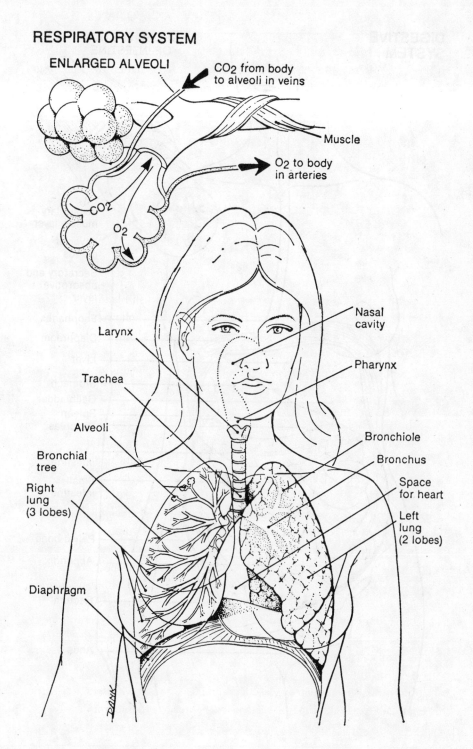

CO_2 from body
to alveoli in veins

Muscle

O_2 to body
in arteries

CO_2

O_2

Nasal
cavity

Larynx

Pharynx

Trachea

Alveoli

Bronchiole

Bronchial
tree

Bronchus

Right
lung
(3 lobes)

Space
for heart

Left
lung
(2 lobes)

Diaphragm

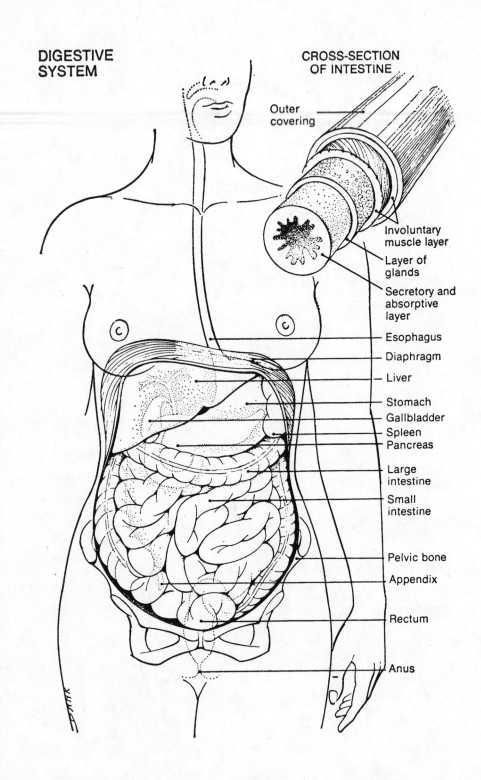

DIGESTIVE SYSTEM

CROSS-SECTION OF INTESTINE

Outer covering

Involuntary muscle layer

Layer of glands

Secretory and absorptive layer

Esophagus

Diaphragm

Liver

Stomach

Gallbladder

Spleen

Pancreas

Large intestine

Small intestine

Pelvic bone

Appendix

Rectum

Anus

FUNCTIONS OF
DIGESTIVE SYSTEM

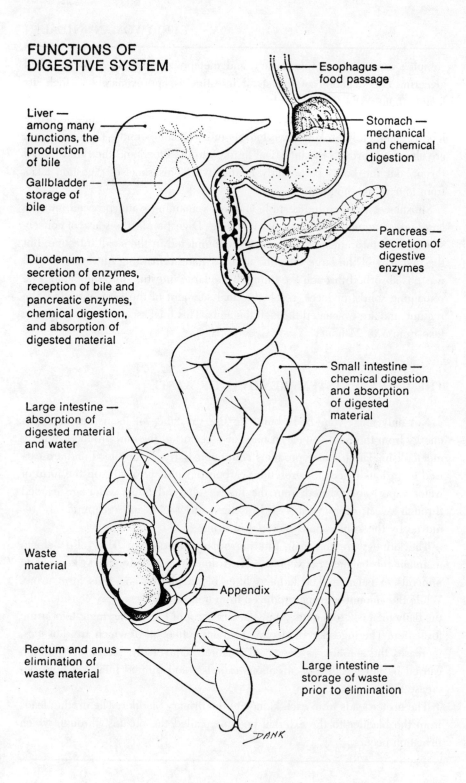

Esophagus — food passage

Liver — among many functions, the production of bile

Stomach — mechanical and chemical digestion

Gallbladder — storage of bile

Pancreas — secretion of digestive enzymes

Duodenum — secretion of enzymes, reception of bile and pancreatic enzymes, chemical digestion, and absorption of digested material

Small intestine — chemical digestion and absorption of digested material

Large intestine — absorption of digested material and water

Waste material

Appendix

Rectum and anus — elimination of waste material

Large intestine — storage of waste prior to elimination

DANK

complex sugars into simple sugars, and metabolize fats into fatty acids and glycerin. The diameter of the small intestine is approximately ½ inch, its length about 22 feet, and its total internal surface area about 100 square feet. Through the length of the small intestine these processes continue until the food is completely broken down into its nutrient compounds. These nutrients are absorbed through the intestinal lining into the blood and then transported throughout the body, particularly to the liver. This stage of digestion takes from four to five hours.

Substances that are indigestible and any remaining water proceed into the large intestine, which is about 5½ feet long. Digestion in the sense of conversion of food into nutrient compounds is completed in the small intestine, but the first part of the large intestine absorbs some remaining nutrients. Liquid waste is absorbed through the lining of the large intestine into the blood. The remaining solids, or feces, reach the final segment of the large intestine, the rectum, and are evacuated through the anus. This final aspect of digestion may take from 5 to 24 hours.

THE URINARY SYSTEM: REMOVAL OF WASTE

Not only must your body build up the substance of its tissues and gain energy from the food you eat; it must also get rid of the end products of body metabolism. These waste products continuously reach the blood and are carried to various places for excretion: carbon dioxide and water (in the form of water vapor) are exhaled from the lungs; salts and other water are exuded through sweat; other wastes such as urea, uric acid, and creatinine are removed by the kidneys and excreted in urine.

The kidneys are the main filtering organ of the body. They also help to maintain the balance between salts and fluid in the body and to keep body minerals in balance. The kidneys filter blood plasma and thus form urine. While the amount of urine produced from hour to hour can vary considerably, the daily total is 2 to 3 pints. Many factors account for the varying rate of urine formation. The ingestion of alcohol, tea, and coffee, all of which are diuretics, increases the amount, as does cold weather. Conversely, stress, perspiration caused by hot weather or strenuous exercise, and limited intake of fluid decrease the amount.

The ureter leads from each kidney to the urinary bladder. The urethra leads from the bladder to the external opening, called the meatus, through which urination occurs.

URINARY SYSTEM

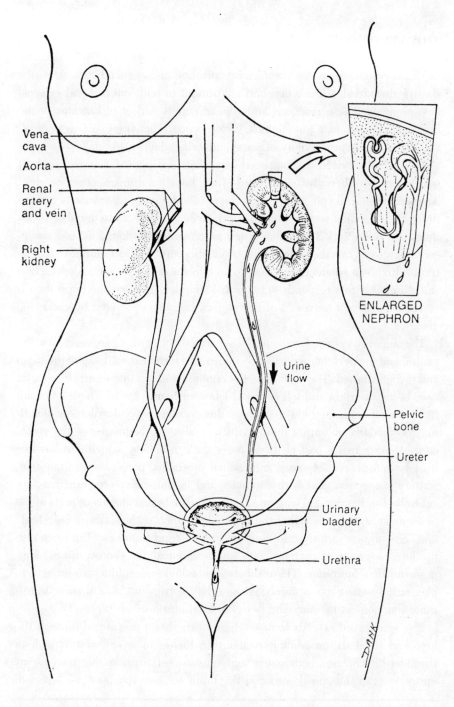

Vena cava

Aorta

Renal artery and vein

Right kidney

ENLARGED NEPHRON

Urine flow

Pelvic bone

Ureter

Urinary bladder

Urethra

THE NERVOUS SYSTEM: COMMUNICATION AND CONTROL

The nervous system is a complex organization of integrated structures that control an individual's reaction and adjustment to both internal and external environments. These reactions and adjustments include rapid actions of the body such as muscular contractions, various visceral activities such as peristalsis, and the secretory activity of some endocrine glands.

The nervous system is composed of special cells called neurons, each of which contains fibers that reach out toward, but do not touch, other neurons. An electrochemical contact between them, called a synapse, transmits the impulse. The nervous system functions primarily through a vast number of reflexes and reflex arcs. This reflex system starts with the stimulation of a receptor organ such as the skin. This stimulation initiates an impulse that is transmitted by a conduction system to an effector organ such as a skeletal or a smooth muscle that responds to the initial stimulus. This conduction system is composed solely of nerves or of nerves plus hormones secreted by endocrine glands.

The nervous system is essentially separated into two large segments: the central and the peripheral nervous systems. The former is made up of the brain and the spinal cord. The brain is in the cranium and has many parts, the major ones being the right and left occipital lobes, or hemispheres. These lobes are linked together on their lower surfaces, thus forming several structures including the medulla oblongata (bulb), which is also the beginning of the spinal cord. Another major part of the brain is the cerebellum, which also has two linked hemispheres. Memory, intellectual processes, perceptions of emotion, sensory perception, and both voluntary and involuntary motor functions are controlled and integrated with one another by the brain. The major parts of the brain make up what is called the cerebrum; hence such words as "cerebral" and "cerebration" are used to describe brain / mind functions. The brain also produces a group of proteins with analgesic capabilities many times more powerful than morphine. These substances, called endorphins, are thought to play an important role not only in the relief of pain but also in such brain / mind functions as memory and behavior modification.

The spinal cord extends from the base of the brain downward through the vertebral canal. In an adult it is about 18 inches in length and ½ inch in diameter. It contains both motor and sensory nerve tracts that traverse its entire length. The spinal cord and the brain are covered by three layers of

NERVOUS SYSTEM

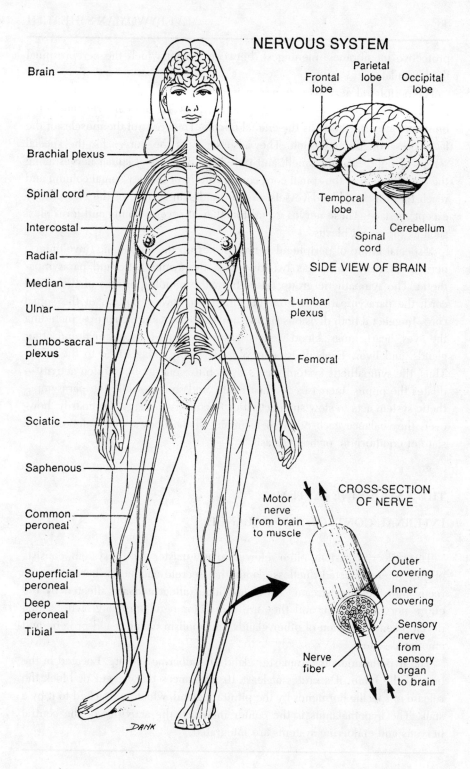

Brain

Brachial plexus

Spinal cord

Intercostal

Radial

Median

Ulnar

Lumbo-sacral plexus

Sciatic

Saphenous

Common peroneal

Superficial peroneal

Deep peroneal

Tibial

Lumbar plexus

Femoral

Frontal lobe

Parietal lobe

Occipital lobe

Temporal lobe

Spinal cord

Cerebellum

SIDE VIEW OF BRAIN

CROSS-SECTION OF NERVE

Motor nerve from brain to muscle

Outer covering

Inner covering

Sensory nerve from sensory organ to brain

Nerve fiber

DANK

protective membranes (meninges), between two of which the cerebrospinal fluid circulates.

The peripheral nervous system consists of many paired nerves that conduct impulses to and from the brain and spinal cord. Twelve of them originate in the brain and are referred to as the cranial nerves. They control the muscles of the face, eyes, tongue, and such. They also serve as the nerves for the special senses of sight, hearing, smell, and taste. The 31 pairs of spinal nerves along the entire length of the spinal cord course through the bony spinal column and reach the muscles, blood vessels, organs, and skin surface of the entire body except the face. These nerves group together at several points and form plexi such as the sacral plexus.

A special group of peripheral nerves makes up the autonomic (involuntary) nervous system, which has two divisions: the sympathetic and parasympathetic. The sympathetic group arises from the middle portions of the spinal cord; the parasympathetic, from the brain and lowest portion of the spinal cord. In general both divisions supply nerves to the same structures, including the eyes, heart, lungs, blood vessels, gastrointestinal tract, adrenal and other glands, and liver. Each division is physiologically antagonistic to the other. Thus, the sympathetic system serves to mobilize energy for sudden activity— dilates the pupils, increases the heart rate, and so on—while the parasympathetic system acts to slow such activities to conserve energy. Ordinarily, however, they balance each other to maintain all the body's vital functions in a state of equilibrium, or homeostasis.

THE ENDOCRINE SYSTEM:

INTERNAL CONTROL AND BALANCE

The endocrine system, often referred to as a master control system, consists of nine interconnected ductless glands that secrete chemicals (hormones) directly into the bloodstream. These hormones affect and are affected by the entire nervous system, and they are the major regulators of growth, sexual development, secretion of other glands, metabolism of sugar and protein, and emotional states.

The hypothalamus is the master gland of endocrine activity. Located in the base of the brain, it secretes at least 10 substances that trigger or block the release of specific hormones by the pituitary gland, which is attached to it by a stalk. The hypothalamus is the center in which the activities of the central nervous and endocrine systems are integrated.

The pituitary gland has an anterior portion and a posterior portion. The anterior pituitary secretes tropic hormones and stimulating hormones. The latter stimulate hormone secretions in several other endocrine glands. The anterior pituitary also secretes prolactin, which, among other things, initiates and maintains lactation after pregnancy, and growth hormone (GH), which is essential for cell growth and proliferation. Overproduction of GH prior to full growth causes gigantism and after full growth, acromegaly. Underproduction prior to full growth results in pituitary dwarfism. The posterior pituitary secretes vasopressin, which conserves body water. Another of its secretions (oxytocin) stimulates smooth muscles, including those of the uterus at the time of childbirth, and contributes to the ejection of breast milk.

The thyroid gland regulates the rate at which the body utilizes oxygen and food through the production of thyroxin. Underproduction of this hormone (hypothyroidism) produces cretinism in infants and the listlessness and drowsiness of myxedema in adults. Overproduction causes hyperthyroidism.

The paired parathyroid glands secrete parathyroid hormone (PTH), which controls the blood levels of calcium and phosphate in the body. Underproduction results in low levels of calcium and can cause muscle cramps, even convulsions; overproduction drains the bones of calcium and can produce kidney stones.

The islets of Langerhans, thousands of cell clusters scattered throughout the pancreas, regulate the body's use of carbohydrates through the production of insulin and glucagon. Underproduction of insulin is associated with diabetes mellitus; overproduction causes hypoglycemia (low blood sugar). Glucagon acts in the opposite way.

The paired adrenal glands have a cortex (outer portion) and a medulla (inner portion). The cortex produces steroid hormones: glucocorticoids (cortisone and several others), which control the metabolism of protein and sugar; mineralocorticoids (aldosterone), which control the balance of mineral substances and fluids; and sex hormones (androgen, mainly testosterone, and estrogen). Underproduction of both groups of corticoids produces a rare condition called Addison's disease. Overproduction causes Cushing's syndrome. Excess androgen production can induce the development of masculine secondary sex characteristics in females and young boys. Excess estrogen production has little effect on mature women. In young girls it can lead to enlargement of the breasts and early maturation of the uterus and vagina. In males it can lead to breast enlargement (gynecomastia). The medulla produces catecholamines (epinephrine, or adrenalin, and norepinephrine). These are produced also in the endings of the sympathetic nerves. They normally contribute to the maintenance of homeostasis, but they also enable the body to respond to danger,

ENDOCRINE SYSTEM

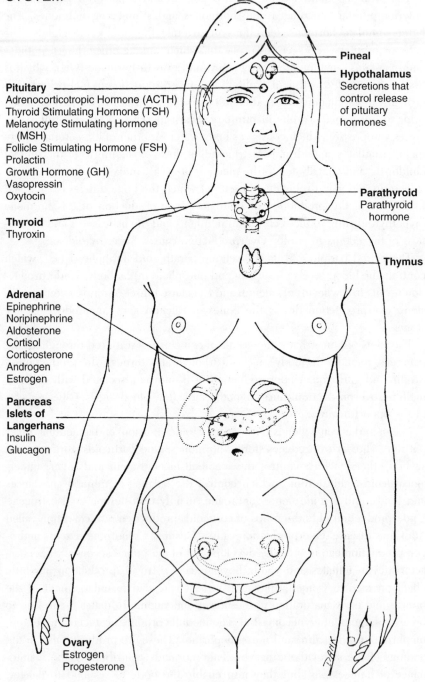

Pineal

Hypothalamus
Secretions that
control release
of pituitary
hormones

Pituitary
Adrenocorticotropic Hormone (ACTH)
Thyroid Stimulating Hormone (TSH)
Melanocyte Stimulating Hormone
  (MSH)
Follicle Stimulating Hormone (FSH)
Prolactin
Growth Hormone (GH)
Vasopressin
Oxytocin

Parathyroid
Parathyroid
hormone

Thyroid
Thyroxin

Thymus

Adrenal
Epinephrine
Noripinephrine
Aldosterone
Cortisol
Corticosterone
Androgen
Estrogen

**Pancreas
Islets of
Langerhans**
Insulin
Glucagon

Ovary
Estrogen
Progesterone

fright, anger, or sudden physical stress with an increased heart rate and faster breathing.

The male sex glands, the testes, produce sperm and the male sex hormone testosterone, which is responsible for the development of male secondary sex characteristics such as voice change and facial hair. Overproduction of testosterone produces virilism; underproduction produces eunuchism. The female sex glands, the ovaries, produce ova, or eggs. They also secrete estrogen and progesterone—hormones needed for menstruation, reproduction, feminine secondary sex characteristics, and skeletal development—plus androgens. Excessive production of these hormones occurs very rarely and then only with certain ovarian tumors. Absence of them early in life causes female eunuchism. Underproduction of them later in life causes menstrual irregularities and, ultimately, menopause.

The thymus gland appears to play a role in the body's resistance to disease, the metabolism of calcium, and the development of the skeleton and sex glands. Prior to puberty, the pineal gland secretes a hormone called melatonin, which inhibits the biochemical process of sexual maturation.

THE REPRODUCTIVE SYSTEM:

PERPETUATION OF THE SPECIES

The female reproductive system consists of internal and external sex organs. The external sex organs are called the vulva. The mons pubis (mons veneris) is a pad of fatty tissue in front of the pubic bone that from puberty on is covered with pubic hair. Two folds of fatty tissue covered with skin, the labia majora (outer lips) and the labia minora (inner lips), protect the vaginal and urethral openings that lie between them. The labia minora are sensitive to touch and sexual arousal. Just below the mons, the labia minora join to form a hood over the clitoris. The clitoris, the most sexually responsive female organ, is composed of erectile tissue that becomes engorged with blood during sexual activity. It is homologous to the penis.

Below the clitoris is the urethral meatus, the external opening of the urethra. Below that is the vaginal opening, or introitus. The hymen is a thin fold of mucous membrane across the introitus, partially blocking it. After being stretched by ordinary physical activity, insertion of tampons, or intercourse, only a ridge of tissue usually remains around the introitus. Beyond the hymen on each side of the vaginal opening is a mucus-secreting gland (Bartholin's gland). The perineum is the area between the external genitals and the anus.

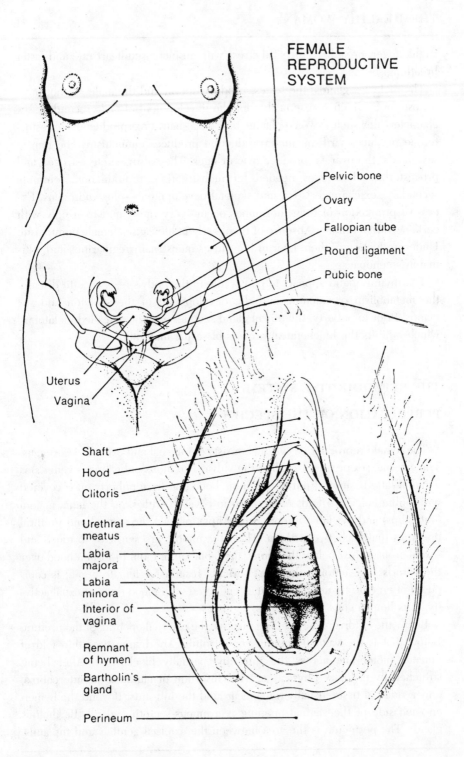

FEMALE REPRODUCTIVE SYSTEM

Pelvic bone

Ovary

Fallopian tube

Round ligament

Pubic bone

Uterus

Vagina

Shaft

Hood

Clitoris

Urethral meatus

Labia majora

Labia minora

Interior of vagina

Remnant of hymen

Bartholin's gland

Perineum

SIDE VIEW OF EXTERNAL AND INTERNAL GENITALIA

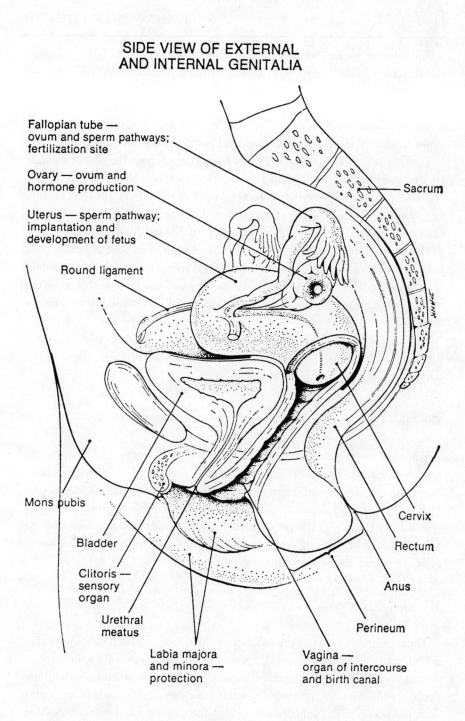

Fallopian tube — ovum and sperm pathways; fertilization site

Ovary — ovum and hormone production

Uterus — sperm pathway; implantation and development of fetus

Round ligament

Sacrum

Mons pubis

Bladder

Clitoris — sensory organ

Urethral meatus

Labia majora and minora — protection

Vagina — organ of intercourse and birth canal

Perineum

Anus

Rectum

Cervix

The internal sex organs include the vagina, the uterus, the fallopian tubes, and the ovaries. The vagina is a tubular, muscular structure covered with skin that extends from the vulva upward and backward to the uterus. The vaginal walls stretch and contract during intercourse; during childbirth, they expand greatly. Continuous secretions from the vaginal wall keep the vagina clean, maintain acidity to prevent infection, and provide lubrication for intercourse.

The uterus (womb) is a hollow, pear-shaped organ about the size of a lemon. In a nonpregnant state, its walls (myometrium) are one of the strongest muscles in the body. The cervix, the base or neck of the uterus, projects into the vagina and has a small opening (cervical os) in its center through which sperm can travel upward and through which menstrual blood flows down.

The fallopian tubes (oviducts) are paired muscular narrow canals that extend from each side of the top of the uterus to the ovaries. In an adult they are about 5 inches long. The end near the ovary is open and enlarged so that an ovum, when released from the ovary, can be "trapped" by, enter, and travel along the tube.

The ovaries, organs about the size of an almond, are located on either side of the uterus. The breasts (discussed in detail in the "Breast Care" chapter) produce milk following the birth of a baby.

The Male Reproductive System

The male reproductive system consists of the penis, urethra, scrotum, testes, and some glands. The penis contains erectile tissue that on sexual arousal is engorged with blood and becomes erect, thus facilitating sexual intercourse. The urethra is the tube in the center of the penis through which urine and semen leave the body. The prostate gland and Cowper's glands, located at the junction of the bladder and urethra, produce the seminal fluid in which sperm cells are mixed, thereby forming semen.

The Menstrual Cycle

The menstrual cycle is a dramatic example of the delicate balance and interactions maintained by your body. A series of complex feedback interactions among several organs and glands stimulate ovulation (production of the reproductive cell, the egg), prepare the uterus for pregnancy, and, if conception does not occur, make adjustments so that the process can begin again. Menstruation is the process by which tissue built up in the uterus in readiness for the implantation of a fertilized ovum is discharged through the vagina if conception does not occur.

The cycle is repeated throughout the reproductive years of a woman's life from menarche, the onset of menstruation, to menopause, the cessation of menstruation. Menarche occurs between the ages of 10 and 16 when certain secretions from the hypothalamus begin to stimulate the pituitary. Menopause occurs between the ages of 45 and 55 when ovarian follicular function ceases. Its onset is gradual.

The complete menstrual cycle takes approximately a month. That is, the time from the beginning of one menstrual period to the beginning of the next ranges from 25 to 35 days. The menstrual flow or period lasts from 2 to 7 days. The length of the cycle and of the menstrual period varies from woman to woman and in any one woman from time to time.

There are three phases in each menstrual cycle, and the primary organs involved are the hypothalamus / pituitary, ovary, and uterus.

We consider the first day of the menstrual phase to be the day menstruation begins. As estrogen and progesterone levels fall (see postovulatory phase below), the functional layers of the endometrium (the lining of the uterus) begin to shed and appear as menstrual flow. As menstruation continues, estrogen and progesterone levels drop further, and follicle-stimulating hormone (FSH) from the pituitary increases. FSH stimulates the proliferation, usually in only one ovary, of masses of cells, called follicles, that secrete estrogen. FSH also stimulates the enlargement of the ovum in a follicle. The estrogen stimulates further development of the ovum; a drop, via a negative feedback system, in FSH; and, via a positive feedback system, an increase in luteinizing hormone (LH) from the pituitary, which stimulates further follicle development and with it an increase in estrogen secretion. This additional estrogen stimulates the start of the "rebuilding" of the endometrium, which causes menstruation to end and marks the beginning of the preovulatory phase.

During the preovulatory (proliferative or follicular) phase, estrogen levels continue to increase, FSH to decrease, and LH to increase slightly. The endometrium further thickens and its glands and blood vessels increase. One of the follicles (the dominant follicle) and its ovum continue to mature, while the others shrink. Finally there is a surge of LH that triggers the dominant follicle to rupture.

Ovulation is not a phase of the menstrual cycle but an event that more or less marks the change from one phase to another. After the follicle ruptures, the ovum is expelled from it (ovulation), and the follicle is transformed into a corpus luteum (yellow body) that secretes increasing amounts of progesterone and estrogen. Some women sense a little pain with the rupturing of the follicle.

MENSTRUAL CYCLE

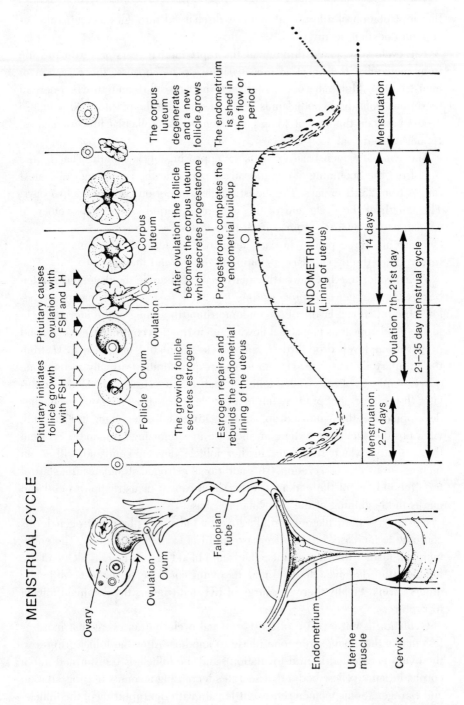

Ovary

Ovulation

Ovum

Fallopian tube

Endometrium

Uterine muscle

Cervix

Pituitary initiates follicle growth with FSH

Pituitary causes ovulation with FSH and LH

Follicle

Ovum

Ovulation

Corpus luteum

The growing follicle secretes estrogen

After ovulation the follicle becomes the corpus luteum which secretes progesterone

The corpus luteum degenerates and a new follicle grows

Estrogen repairs and rebuilds the endometrial lining of the uterus

Progesterone completes the endometrial buildup

The endometrium is shed in the flow or period

ENDOMETRIUM
(Lining of uterus)

Menstruation
2–7 days

14 days

Menstruation

Ovulation 7th–21st day

21–35 day menstrual cycle

The progesterone causes a rise in body temperature shortly after ovulation. The high level of estrogen induces temporary chemical changes in the vagina, cervical mucus, uterus, and tubes that facilitate sperm penetration of the uterus and their survival and upward movement in the uterus and tube. It also causes anatomical changes that bring the end of the tube and the ovary closer together. The ovulatory effects last for only a few days.

During the postovulatory (secretory or luteal) phase, increasingly high levels of estrogen and progesterone from the corpus luteum stimulate the endometrium to form secretory glands that prepare it for the implantation (about 7 days after conception) of a fertilized ovum if conception occurs. Some women experience breast thickening and tenderness as well as other changes such as premenstrual tension and fluid retention during the postovulatory phase.

If the ovum is not fertilized—a process that normally occurs in a fallopian tube—the corpus luteum begins to degenerate about 14 days after ovulation, and its production of progesterone and estrogen decreases. When this happens, the arteries and veins in the thickened lining of the uterus become constricted; deprived of their rich blood supply, the top layers of endometrium are shed, and menstruation occurs.

THE RELATIONSHIP BETWEEN PHYSICAL AND MENTAL HEALTH

Important relationships exist between physical health and mental health. On the one hand, an emotional state is reflected in physical responses. When you are worried or frustrated, you may have feelings of tension in your neck, a headache, or a feeling of tightness in your stomach. On the other hand, emotional or mental disorders may be caused by physical problems or diseases. Severe myxedema (thyroid malfunction) may result in mental abnormalities. Some illnesses reflect the interaction between the body and emotions, especially illnesses of the skin and the digestive, respiratory, cardiovascular, and urinary systems. These parts of the body are under the control of the involuntary nervous system. Family tensions can contribute to such disorders as dermatitis, colitis, ulcers, asthma, changes in heart rate and rhythm, hypertension, and urinary frequency. Stress on the job may contribute to arthritis or sleep disorders.

Recognition of the inextricable mind/body connection has resulted in a more widespread application of many alternative therapies, especially biofeedback and relaxation skills for treating chronic pain and stress-related ailments. Emotional health and positive thinking are known to play a critical role in the body's well-being. Researchers have discovered there is a continuous dialogue between the nervous, immune, and endocrine systems, suggesting that positive emotions may bolster the immune system and negative emotions may depress it. No one knows how these systems "converse," but they do share a common "language." They release and receive messenger molecules called peptides in response to anything out of the ordinary: anxiety, fear, bacteria, and such. Peptides can direct the flow of immune system cells called microphages, raise or lower body temperature, or make you feel pain, sadness, or joy.

TAKE RESPONSIBILITY FOR YOUR OWN HEALTH

An important aspect of health is an awareness of the sources of potential illness. Promoting your own well-being involves prevention of illness, early treatment of symptoms, and minimizing disability.

PRIMARY PREVENTION: PREVENTION OF ILLNESS

There are three levels of prevention. Primary prevention is directed toward keeping a disorder from occurring. Immunization is the classic example of primary prevention. Today primary prevention includes the vaccinations that children receive against whooping cough, diphtheria, tetanus, hepatitis B, rubella, measles, mumps, Haemophilus influenza type B, and polio. As an adult, you may have been immunized against influenza or, when you were planning to travel, against hepatitis B, meningitis, yellow fever, or other infectious diseases. Environmental health controls are another form of primary prevention: fluoridation of water to prevent dental cavities, proper sewage disposal, purification of water, and pollution control, including the elimination of hazardous air pollutants in the workplace.

The term primary prevention also refers to the choices you make in behavior and activities that may affect your health. Do you smoke? Do you abuse other substances such as caffeine or alcohol? How much sleep do you usually get? Do you eat a nourishing breakfast? Do you practice daily oral hygiene? Do you use seat belts? Would you be in better shape if you lost about 20 pounds? Do you get enough exercise? Do you protect your skin and eyes against harmful exposure to the sun? Do you protect yourself against sexually transmissible diseases?

Clearly, eating a well-balanced diet, not smoking, and drinking in moderation if at all are activities that have a major effect on your health and are within your power to control. Also, although you may not be able to eliminate stress in your life, you can take a good look at how you handle it. Are you quick to rely on sleeping pills in order to get a good night's sleep, to seek (and to receive) tranquilizers because some of the problems of everyday living seem to be too difficult? Some women become dependent on alcohol, the most serious drug abuse problem in our country. Others smoke or eat too much. If any of these habits continues, you may be placing yourself at a greater risk of hypertension; of heart, liver, or lung disease; or of cancer.

In recent years more and more women have been learning to deal with stress in ways that are not self-destructive: setting aside money for a weekly massage or enrollment in a dance class; setting aside time for an hour of breathing exercises and meditation or for the pure pleasure of soaking in a warm tub fragrant with carefully selected aromatic oils. One of the most important steps you can take in reducing stress in your life is to recognize your responsibility to *yourself* in the midst of dealing with your many responsibilities to others—a demanding boss, an ailing parent, a willful offspring—not to mention the day-in, day-out demands of running a household. Within your busy life, you owe it to yourself to plan a regular schedule of self-indulgence, even if it is only one hour on Tuesdays and Thursdays or half an hour four times a week. Scheduling time for yourself is much more productive than grabbing a minute here or an hour there because when the time is scheduled, you have the added pleasure of looking forward to it. (See "Alternative Therapies.")

SECONDARY PREVENTION:

EARLY DIAGNOSIS AND TREATMENT

Secondary prevention refers to early diagnosis, detection, and treatment of a disease in order to reduce its consequences, duration, and severity. Breast self-examination, an annual visit to a gynecologist for professional breast examination, a mammography as recommended, a Pap smear to detect signs of cervical cancer, blood pressure measurements to keep track of hypertension risk, blood analysis for signs of anemia or dangerous cholesterol levels, and eye examinations to check on the onset of glaucoma are among the things you can do to facilitate secondary prevention. Where there is a family history of colon cancer, a colonoscopy at regular intervals is mandatory for early diagnosis.

TERTIARY PREVENTION: REHABILITATION

Finally, there is a third level of prevention—rehabilitation. Rehabilitation is directed toward minimizing disability, deterioration, or the limitations that might result from a stroke or a serious accident. If help is sought early in the course of a chronic illness such as arthritis, rehabilitation can prevent further deterioration and improve the chances for social, psychological, and physical adjustment.

BE AN ACTIVE, WELL-INFORMED PARTNER
IN HEALTH CARE

In order to take greater responsibility for your own health and well-being, it is important to become as knowledgeable as possible about the various approaches to health care.

HOLISTIC HEALTH

There is an increasing interest in looking at people as whole human beings living in their community, family, workplace, and social environments, rather than as isolated organs or systems.

Concern with the whole person is the essential element of effective health care. It does not compartmentalize you into the various parts of your body or even according to the kinds of specialists that you might see. Because there is an overemphasis on specialization in medical care, interest has recently been expressed in a return to the family physician, to the primary care physician, to that person who can deal with the individual on many levels. Doctors sensitive to all the circumstances of their patients' lives not only concern themselves with procedures and prescriptions but also ask relevant questions about whether a spouse is smoking or whether the workplace environment might be causing the respiratory distress and headaches ascribable to the sick building syndrome. (See "Health Safeguards for Working Women.") Many doctors are also recommending alternative therapies instead of prescribing medications as the best way to handle some health problems.

SELF-CARE

Self-care is directed toward reducing overreliance on medical services. Self-care as a concept may be considered to be enlightened self-interest. This means that you do a regular monthly breast examination so that you are able to detect any suspicious findings and bring them to the attention of your health care provider. It also means modifying your behavior to achieve a health-promoting life-style.

Taking full advantage of the benefits of self-care involves the ability to make informed decisions. To get the right answers, you have to ask the right questions. Make use of library facilities. Send for free literature offered by respected volunteer organizations such as the American Heart Association, the American Cancer Society, the Arthritis Foundation, and the like. Know when medical intervention is required. Although the body has wonderful curative abilities and many ailments and disorders will respond to home remedies, rest, and tender loving care, there are also many that will not. Your knowledge of when to turn to a doctor for professional diagnosis and treatment is part of enlightened health care.

Like so many aspects of life in the United States, the self-care concept has been widely exploited by quacks and promoters of questionable remedies. Manuals of self-knowledge and health care flood the bookshops, presenting a challenge to you as a discriminating reader. Can you differentiate between sound practical advice and a simple-minded panacea for a complicated problem that requires professional expertise and advanced diagnostic tools?

One of the most popular approaches to self-care has been the development of self-help groups. You are probably aware of Weight Watchers, Overeaters Anonymous, and Alcoholics Anonymous. Now there are self-help and support groups for people coping with diabetes, hypertension, muscular dystrophy, or chronic depression, as well as with aging parents or a mentally ill child. Self-help groups have been organized to provide information, to clarify the role of medical care in dealing with problems, and to help people through serious physical and emotional problems or through life crises such as bereavement and loneliness.

The benefit of self-help groups comes from the fact that when you are with someone who has some of the same problems you have, you tend to share positive experiences as well as burdens and to generalize or universalize your experiences. In doing this, you gain some insight and understanding. Self-help groups provide both the knowledge and the emotional support offered by membership in any group. According to the dictionary, the term networking did not enter the language until 1966, but since time immemorial, women have been giving each other mutual help within the family, the clan, and the community. Whether they are trying to find a new babysitter or a new job, networking is increasingly the way in which women are solving some of their more urgent problems.

Some self-help groups have led to the establishment of clinical services for women, including medical services provided by women health practitioners, counseling programs, and educational and consciousness-raising discussion groups. These are consistent with the increased participation of consumers in making decisions.

Increased awareness of health care among consumers may lead to changes and reform in the ways in which all services are organized and provided. The consumer movement has caused consternation, resentment, and anger among many people in medicine whose attitudes and approaches had never before been questioned by the people who used their services. This is particularly true of physicians who have occupied a sacrosanct position. The desire for change, especially by women whose emotional and intellectual needs have not been met, is very much related to becoming an equal participant in the health care partnership.

HEALTH SERVICES

Citizen participation in health service now extends to the establishment of alternative health care services, particularly those in which potential patients carry on health care activities themselves. In some instances women's groups have banded together for education—to understand how their bodies function; to learn what to expect during an examination by a gynecologist, during childbirth, during sexual intercourse; to become informed regarding all aspects of sexuality and reproduction about which women as patients have been kept ignorant. Other groups seek to ensure less sexist behavior on the part of physicians, generally males, or to demand their rights as patients to accept or not accept a doctor's recommendation for medication as the only solution to a health problem or for proceeding with a radical mastectomy or a hysterectomy before other options are seriously evaluated. Still others are concerned with abortion rights and reproductive freedom.

Even if you feel that the medical care you personally receive is adequate, you might consider that active participation in a women's health group (to whatever degree seems best for you) can have an effect in the long run on the health care system. Your participation will help to influence those within the medical community to be more attuned to the needs of the individual patient. Your participation can help to demonstrate that the patient can be an equal in a process that depends on the persons on both sides of the relationship. The progress of treatment and rehabilitation can be influenced by your attitude, knowledge, and involvement in the health care partnership. Already there have been many influential forces. The patients' rights movement, the women's movement, the public's increased concern with elitism in medical practice, and the demands for more citizen participation in the affairs of hospitals, clinics, and health centers have already affected the attitudes of health care providers.

This exchange of information gives those in the field of health care a better sense of what helps you accept their guidance and follow their recommendations. This issue has sometimes been referred to as "patient compliance," a misnomer. Ideally it should be a more active process in which a knowledgeable person (1) understands her role in the process of becoming or staying well, (2) asks pertinent questions, and (3) knows to whom to turn for further information or help. Unfortunately, when knowledge and understanding are lacking, you may find yourself misunderstanding directions, confused about what the problem is, and reluctant to follow instructions.

Alternative health services may be effective in dealing with such issues, but there is a need for real reform in the way health care is organized and provided. Health care should emphasize health rather than sickness, partnership rather than hierarchy, and quality health care as the right of all women—and of all people.

NUTRITION, WEIGHT, BODY IMAGE, AND EATING DISORDERS

Toby Orem Graham, M.D.

Associate Professor of Medicine, University of Pittsburgh School of Medicine, Pittsburgh, Pennsylvania

Helene MacLean

Medical Writer and Editor; Author, *Caring for Your Parents*, *Relief from Chronic Arthritis Pain*; Coauthor, *Recovering from a Hysterectomy*, *Migraine: Beating the Odds*

We are what we eat! Our food choices affect our health, energy, appearance, and disposition. Eating the right amounts and kinds of foods supplies us with energy and stamina for work and play, provides for our growth, maintains our bodies in good health, and helps to keep us mentally alert. That is what nutrition is all about. It is unfortunate, but too often true, that many women become interested in nutrition only because of some specific circumstance: when they are pregnant or breast-feeding, or are overweight and want to diet, or have children with a weight problem, or develop symptoms stemming from inadequate nutrition such as fatigue resulting from iron-deficiency anemia. It is also unfortunate that, over the last 50 years, Americans have been receiving many mixed messages about what to eat to maintain good health. The only advice that has remained unchanged—and alas, too often unheeded—is *eat less fat*. Although most surveys indicate that American women are more aware than ever of the need to count calories and to exercise every day, overweight is increasing nationwide. Even women who know the essentials of good nutrition find themselves fighting a losing battle not only with their own tendency to nibble their way through days when there's no time for sitting down to a proper meal, but also with spouses who insist on meals with lots of meat and no vegetables and with offspring whose ideas about what to eat come from television promotion of junk food.

If a grounding in the importance of nutritional principles is to counteract the many social forces that prevail against it, nutrition education must begin early. As with other health-threatening habits, prevention rather than treatment should be the goal. But the federal government allocates practically no money to the states to promote nutrition education in the schools. Practically no insurance company or health maintenance organization reimburses the cost of medical nutritional counseling, nor are preventive nutrition programs part of any of the health care bills being considered by Congress.

Equally unfortunate for the country's health is the fact that most doctors-to-be are taught very little about nutrition as an important aspect of preventive patient care. Dr. Marion Nestle, chair of the department of nutrition at New York University, believes that "the source of the problem is money. The bottom line is that you don't get reimbursed for teaching patients about nutrition. The government won't pay you, and you can't charge patients."

But money has also been the motivating factor in getting some doctors to inform themselves in this area because they are becoming aware of the fact that their patients are spending considerable sums for the guidance of qualified nutritionists. These certified practitioners, who are fast joining the growing ranks of alternative therapists, answer the needs of many women for individualized meal planning at certain critical times—during the weeks of recovery from major surgery; at the sudden onset of a chronic gastrointestinal disorder; during the metabolic changes following menopause—and can teach them how to provide nourishing, attractive meals for family members dealing with different kinds of health problems.

RETHINKING OUR NUTRITIONAL NEEDS

In 1992, following the expenditure of a great deal of time and money in research and debate, the government issued a new educational device for teaching Americans how best to achieve healthful nutrition. Abandoning the once-sacred model of *four food groups of equal weight*—meat, poultry, fish;

grains; dairy products; fruits and vegetables—the USDA now recommends the *pyramid of five groups of food,* as shown on page 59.

While the pyramid promotes a drastic change in the eating habits of most American families, an even more drastic change was recommended in 1991 by the 3,000 doctors who make up the Washington-based Physicians Committee for Responsible Medicine. Their proposal is based on a radical redefinition of the four food groups as (1) fruits, (2) grains, (3) vegetables, and (4) legumes, consisting of beans, peanut butter, and soybeans. Meat and dairy products are optional, with smaller servings than the government's proposals. The rationale for this profound change is one on which most health professionals agree: that the eating habits of the Western world—high in animal fat and protein and low in fiber—has put all of us at higher risk for obesity, cancer, and heart disease.

Considering current eating patterns, however, it is unlikely that most of us would conform willingly to a diet in which only 2 or 3 ounces of meat, poultry, or fish is the daily allowance. Even the government's new recommendations may be hard to follow unless a conscious effort is made in the interests of healthful living. Even at a glance, it is obvious that the Food Guide Pyramid sets the goal of greatly increasing the consumption of grains, vegetables, and fruits while also cutting down on the intake of protein and dairy products and keeping fats and sweets at a minimum. There is general agreement among medical professionals and nutritionists that this eating plan provides all the essential nutrients at the same time that it combats obesity and other health problems that presently plague many Americans.

In order to plan meals that conform to new nutritional goals, it is essential to know what is meant by a "serving." Differences of opinion may abound among your family and friends; differences also exist between the federal government's recommendations and the recommendations of the Physicians Committee for Responsible Medicine. This 300,000-member organization has asserted that the government's plan continues to maintain that, in the interests of good health, meat and dairy products should have a place in the menu—no more than about 3 ounces of each per day whereas the Physicians Committee makes these products optional. Here are their specific suggestions:

FOOD GROUP	SERVINGS PER DAY	SIZE OF SERVINGS
Whole grains	5 or more	1/2 cup hot cereal, cooked rice, cooked pasta, or kasha; 1 ounce dried cereal; 1 bread slice
Vegetables	3 or more	1 cup raw; 1/2 cup cooked; 1/2 cup juice
Legumes	2 to 3	1/2 cup cooked beans or lentils; 4 ounces tofu

Fruits   3 or more   1 medium piece of fruit; ½ cup cooked fruit; ½ cup fruit
                                juice
Meats, fish, and dairy products optional

BACK TO BASICS: THE NUTRIENT CONTENT
OF FOOD

Nutrients are the chemical components of food that supply the body with materials that can be transformed into heat, activity, and other forms of energy; that build, maintain, and repair body tissues; and that regulate all body processes. These chemical components are grouped into five classes—protein, carbohydrates, fats, vitamins, and minerals—plus two other essentials, water and fiber.

PROTEIN

Protein is the basic substance of all living cells and is therefore vital in the diet for cellular growth, replacement, and repair. Protein is composed of combinations of amino acids, which are organic compounds containing nitrogen and hydrogen. The material needed for different types of body cells, including enzymes, hormones, red blood cells, and antibodies, is provided by different combinations of the amino acids. The protein derived from such animal foods as meat, fish, eggs, and dairy products contains all of the amino acids we need to construct proteins in our body (essential amino acids) and is therefore known as complete protein. The protein derived from plant foods such as nuts, legumes, and grains usually lacks some essential amino acids in the amounts needed and is therefore incomplete. However, complete protein can be obtained by eating plant foods if they are combined to complement one another, that is, to supply in combination all the required amino acids. Examples of such complementary foods are dried beans with corn, peanuts with wheat, and soybean products with rice. These combinations are the basis for healthful vegetarianism, and they also form an essential part of a nutritious diet in parts of the world where meat and fish are either unavailable or too expensive for the majority of the population.

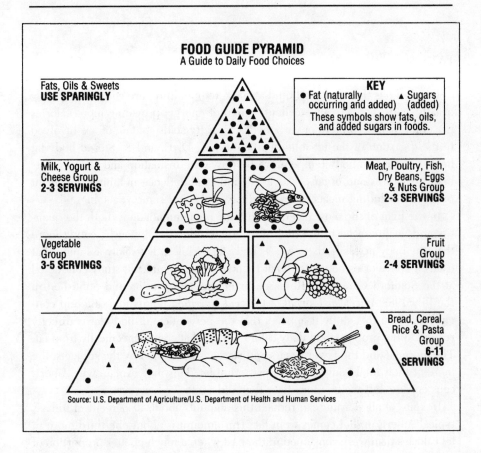

FOOD GUIDE PYRAMID
A Guide to Daily Food Choices

Fats, Oils & Sweets
USE SPARINGLY

KEY
● Fat (naturally   ▲ Sugars
occurring and added)   (added)
These symbols show fats, oils,
and added sugars in foods.

Milk, Yogurt &
Cheese Group
2-3 SERVINGS

Meat, Poultry, Fish,
Dry Beans, Eggs
& Nuts Group
2-3 SERVINGS

Vegetable
Group
3-5 SERVINGS

Fruit
Group
2-4 SERVINGS

Bread, Cereal,
Rice & Pasta
Group
**6-11
SERVINGS**

Source: U.S. Department of Agriculture/U.S. Department of Health and Human Services

CARBOHYDRATES

Carbohydrates, the sugars and starches, supply most of the body's energy needs. They are also necessary for protein digestion and certain brain functions. Simple carbohydrates such as sugar are rapidly absorbed into the bloodstream unchanged to provide energy immediately. Complex carbohydrates (the starch in potatoes, whole-grain bread, brown rice, and pasta) are converted by digestion into a form that can be stored for later use. Their presence in adequate amounts allows the body to preserve protein, which also supplies energy, primarily for body building and maintenance functions. Carbohydrates are obtained from fruits, vegetables, and grains.

FATS

Fats and oils (fats that are liquid at room temperature) are composed mainly of fatty acids. Fats are an excellent source of energy, providing more calories per gram than do protein or carbohydrates. Fatty acids contain or are involved in the digestion of the fat-soluble vitamins—A, D, E, and K. Stored body fat helps to maintain body temperature by providing insulation and also protects body structures and organs. Fats are found in abundance in animal and plant products, including meats, dairy products, nuts, and some vegetables.

In the light of the most recent nutritional recommendations, both the quantity and quality of fat in the diet must be considered. Obviously, eating more than the body needs leads to excess body fat. While it is usually assumed that calories are calories no matter what their source, a significant study conducted at the Stanford Center for Research in Disease Prevention and published in the July 1988 *American Journal of Clinical Nutrition* points to a different conclusion. From this study it appears that the percentage of body fat is directly related to the proportion of daily caloric intake that comes specifically from fat. The more fat and the fewer sugars and starches consumed by the subjects, the more of their total body weight consisted of fat. This may explain why Americans eat less but weigh more than they did 50 to 75 years ago.

In spite of all warnings to reduce this amount, about 40 percent of today's typical American diet comes from fat. This amount is about one-third more in fat calories than were consumed in the past when a much greater proportion of starchy foods were part of the normal diet. This conclusion is consistent with an extensive study of the Chinese diet. On a pound-for-pound basis, the Chinese consume 20 percent more calories than Americans, but they derive only 15 percent of their calories from fat. Because their diet is rich in starchy and fibrous carbohydrates that offer protection against clogged arteries, both heart disease and clinical overweight are quite rare among the Chinese.

In warning that the dietary fat intake of Americans is far above the upper limit of 30 percent recommended by the American Heart Association and the American Cancer Society, the surgeon general's *Report on Nutrition and Health* issued in 1988 points to the substantial epidemiological evidence that there is an association between this excess of fat in the diet and the increased risk for breast and colon cancer as well as gallbladder disease.

Cholesterol

The *type* of fat consumed is equally important. Fatty acids differ in their chemical structure. If one additional hydrogen atom can be incorporated into the carbon chain, the fatty acid is called an unsaturated fat. If the hydrogen cannot be incorporated, it is a saturated fat. If two or more hydrogen ions can be added, it is known as a polyunsaturated fat. The polyunsaturates are almost exclusively vegetable in origin: corn oil, safflower oil, soybean oil, and the like. Practically all animal fats are saturated. The fats found in milk and cream substitutes as well as those that are in solid white shortenings derived from palm oil or coconut oil are also saturated. Excess consumption of saturated fats is known to raise the amount of cholesterol, a lipid, in the bloodstream. The relationship between excessively high blood cholesterol levels and arterial disease (atherosclerosis) has been firmly established.

Cholesterol is a waxy type of animal compound present in all animal tissues and essential to many body processes. It is manufactured by the body and stored in the liver. Cholesterol also comes from the food we eat, and a high level in the blood (called serum cholesterol) is a danger to health because it encourages the formation of fatty plaque in the arterial walls, causing them to narrow and lose their elasticity.

Because cholesterol is a fatty substance, fatty proteins are required to transport it to the liver for storage or eventual secretion. These proteins, known as high density lipids (HDLs), perform a beneficial function in removing cholesterol from the arterial walls. Low density lipids (LDLs) have the opposite effect, adding to the amount of accumulated cholesterol instead of diminishing it. Thus, the *nature* of the fats in the diet plays a critical role.

It is generally agreed that the level of cholesterol should be approximately 200 milligrams per deciliter of blood, and that a measurement above 225 is considered somewhat risky. It has recently been recommended by members of the National Heart, Lung and Blood Institute of the National Institutes of Health that when your cholesterol level is measured, you should find out the proportion of "good" cholesterol, or HDL. The institute's panel advised that levels of HDL cholesterol *below* 35 milligrams per 100 milliliters of blood represent a high risk of developing heart disease even when total cholesterol levels are below 200. When the measurement appears to be suspect in terms of the patient's general health and dietary precautions, the test should be done again, preferably by a different laboratory. Lab technicians can and do make mistakes.

Because blood cholesterol levels tend to increase with age and arterial health is diminished not only by a natural loss of elasticity but more dangerously by clogged walls, any measures that decrease cholesterol are important. The usual recommendations include weight control, reduction of salt intake, increased exercise, abstention from smoking, cutting down on alcoholic beverages, and above all, attention to diet.

Cholesterol and Diet

One of the major pieces of dietary advice in the surgeon general's comprehensive *Report on Nutrition and Health* was that most people should reduce total fat in the diet but particularly saturated fats, defined as animal or vegetable fats that remain solid at room temperature. Especially to be avoided are butter, untrimmed meat, coconut oil, and palm oil.

The American Heart Association has recommended that fats should make up no more than 25 percent of the total daily caloric intake, an amount that can be measured as 2 tablespoons of polyunsaturated fats.

Here are some guidelines:

- Choose turkey, chicken, and fish rather than beef, pork, or lamb.
- Bacon, sausages, and cold cuts should be eaten only occasionally.
- Remove the skin from chicken and turkey to reduce the fat.
- Substitute yogurt for sour cream, and yogurt spread for cream cheese.
- Barley, oatmeal, rice, pasta, and bulgur are low in fat and should be a regular part of everyone's diet.
- Examine the color of ground meat. The lighter it is, the more fat it contains.
- Avoid egg yolks, butter, cream, and vegetable shortening.
- Trim all fat from beef and poultry; skim off all fat from stews and soups.
- Examine labels on packaged breakfast cereals, crackers, and snack foods and avoid those containing oils derived from palm and coconut.
- Eat more low-fat dairy products such as low-fat cheeses, skim milk, and buttermilk.
- Eat fatty ocean fish and shellfish in moderation.
- Olive oil and peanut oil are the preferred vegetable oils for cooking and salad dressings.

The following menus, each of which adds up to less than 2,100 calories, should be helpful in showing you how to plan satisfying meals that are low in fat:

LOW-FAT DIETS GRAM BY GRAM

30 Percent Menu
(Desirable diet)

BREAKFAST

40% Bran Flakes, 1 ounce	90	0.4 gram
Milk, 1 percent, ½ cup	50	1.5 grams
Orange juice, 6 ounces	83	0 grams
Coffee, decaffeinated	0	0 grams
Milk, 1 percent, 1 tablespoon	6	0.2 gram

LUNCH

Minestrone soup, 1 cup	80	3 grams
Tuna, 3 ounces	111	4.7 grams
Mayonnaise, 2 tablespoons	200	22 grams
Lettuce, tomato	7	0 grams
Whole-wheat bread, 2 slices	140	2 grams

SNACK

Swiss cheese, 1 ounce	105	8 grams
Apple, 1	80	0.2 gram

DINNER

Spaghetti, 2 cups, plus 6 ounces tomato sauce and 3 ounces cooked lean ground beef	619	13.6 grams
Grated Parmesan cheese, 1 tablespoon	25	2 grams
French bread, 1 slice	100	1 gram
Butter, 1 pat, and garlic	50	4 grams
Green salad	14	0.1 gram
Oil and vinegar dressing, 1 tablespoon	63	7 grams
Frozen fruit-flavored yogurt, 8 ounces	210	2 grams

20 Percent Menu
(Most desirable diet)

BREAKFAST

Cheerios, 1 ounce	110	2 grams
Raisins, 2 tablespoons	52	0.1 gram
Banana, ½ cup	70	0.5 gram
Milk, 1 percent, ½ cup	50	1.5 grams
Orange juice, 6 ounces	83	0 grams

LUNCH

Split-pea soup, 1 bowl	240	5 grams
Turkey breast, 3 ounces, with lettuce and mustard	106	3 grams
Rye bread, 2 slices	130	2 grams

SNACK

Pear, 1	100	1 gram
Toasted corn tortilla with skim-milk mozzarella cheese, 1 ounce	145	6 grams

DINNER

Spaghetti, 2 cups, plus 6 ounces tomato and mushroom sauce	432	5 grams
Grated Parmesan cheese, 2 tablespoons	50	4 grams
Spinach salad, 1 cup, plus ½ cup orange sections	38	0.1 gram
Oil and vinegar dressing, 1 tablespoon	63	7 grams
French bread, 2 slices	200	2 grams
Parmesan cheese and garlic, 1 tablespoon	30	2 grams
Sherbet, ⅔ cup	181	2.7 grams

SOURCE: Center for Science in the Public Interest

VITAMINS

Vitamins, sometimes referred to as micronutrients, are organic substances that are present in foods and are needed in very small amounts (a few micrograms or milligrams) to enable specific metabolic reactions to occur. Each vitamin has a specific function. Because only small amounts of vitamins are needed to trigger and control these reactions and because they are used again and again, only small amounts are needed daily for replenishment. Although some vitamins can be synthesized by humans, all vitamins should be supplied in essential amounts by the food we eat each day (see Table 1).

A woman in normal health who is eating properly prepared and adequately balanced meals does not need supplemental vitamins (see Table 2). However, although nutritionists agree that people need two to three servings of fruit daily and three to five servings of vegetables, an extensive survey has shown that on any given day, more than half the American population does not consume a single serving of fruit, fruit juice, or vegetables. (No, ketchup is *not* a vegetable.)

TABLE 1

RECOMMENDED DAILY DIETARY ALLOWANCES (RDA) FOR VITAMINS AND MINERALS[a]

		Fat-Soluble Vitamins			Water-Soluble Vitamins							Minerals					
	AGE (years)	VITAMIN A (µg RE)	VITAMIN D (µg)	VITAMIN E (mg α-TE)	VITAMIN C (mg)	THIAMIN (mg)	RIBO-FLAVIN (mg)	NIACIN (mg NE)	VITAMIN B-6 (mg)	FOLACIN (µg)	VITAMIN B-12 (µg)	CALCIUM (mg)	PHOS-PHORUS (mg)	MAG-NESIUM (mg)	IRON (mg)	ZINC (mg)	IODINE (µg)
Females	11–14	800	10	8	50	1.1	1.3	15	1.8	400	3.0	1200	1200	300	18	15	150
	15–18	800	10	8	60	1.1	1.3	14	2.0	400	3.0	1200	1200	300	18	15	150
	19–22	800	7.5	8	60	1.1	1.3	14	1.6	190	2.0	1200	800	280	18	12	150
	23–50	800	5	8	60	1.0	1.2	13	1.6	190	2.0	800[b]	800	280	18	12	150
	51+	800	5	8	60	1.0	1.2	13	1.6	190	2.0	800	800	280	15	12	150
Pregnant		+200	+5	+2	+20	+0.4	+0.3	+2	+0.6	+400	+1.0	+400	+400	+150	+10[c]	+5	+25
Lactating		+400	+5	+3	+40	+0.5	+0.5	+5	+0.5	+100	+1.0	+400	+400	+150	h	+10	+50

[a] The allowances are intended to provide for individual variations among most normal persons as they live in the United States under usual environmental stresses. Diets should be based on a variety of common foods in order to provide other nutrients for which human requirements have been less well defined.

[b] Until age 25, the calcium allowance should be 1200 mg.

[c] The increased requirement during pregnancy cannot be met by the iron content of habitual American diets nor by the existing iron stores of many women; therefore the use of 30–60 mg of supplemental iron is recommended. Iron needs during lactation are not substantially different from those of nonpregnant women, but continued supplementation of the mother for 2–3 months after parturition is advisable in order to replenish stores depleted by pregnancy.

SOURCE: *Recommended Daily Dietary Allowances, Revised 1989*, adapted from the National Academy of Sciences–National Research Council, Washington, DC.

TABLE 2 A GUIDE TO THE VITAMINS

Vitamin	Best Sources
A	Liver; eggs, cheese, butter, fortified margarine and milk; yellow, orange, and dark green vegetables (e.g., carrots, broccoli, squash, spinach)
B$_1$ (thiamin)	Pork (especially ham), liver, oysters; whole grain and enriched cereals, pasta, and bread, wheat germ; brewers yeast; green peas
B$_2$ (riboflavin)	Liver, meat; milk; dark green vegetables; whole grain and enriched cereals, pasta, and bread; mushrooms
B$_3$ (niacin)	Liver, poultry, meat, tuna; whole grain and enriched cereals, pasta, and bread; nuts, dried beans, and peas; made in body from amino acid tryptophan
B$_6$ (pyridoxine)	Whole grain (but not enriched) cereals and bread; liver; avocados, spinach, green beans; bananas
B$_{12}$ (cobalamin)	Liver, kidneys, meat, fish, oysters; eggs; milk
Folic acid (folacin)	Liver, kidneys; dark green leafy vegetables; wheat germ; brewers yeast
Pantothenic acid	Liver, kidneys; whole grain bread and cereal; nuts; eggs; dark green vegetables; yeast
Biotin	Egg yolk; liver, kidneys; dark green vegetables, green beans; made in intestinal tract
C (ascorbic acid)	Many fruits and vegetables, including citrus, tomato, strawberries, melon, green pepper, potato, dark green vegetables
D	Milk; egg yolk; liver, tuna, salmon; made on skin in sunlight
E	Vegetable oils; margarine; whole grain cereal and bread, wheat germ; liver; dried beans; green leafy vegetables
K	Green leafy vegetables; vegetables in cabbage family; milk; made in intestinal tract

Main Roles	Deficiency Symptoms
Formation and maintenance of skin and mucous membranes, bone growth, vision, reproduction, teeth	Night blindness, rough skin and mucous membranes, no bone growth, cracked or decayed teeth, drying of eyes
Release of energy from carbohydrates, synthesis of nerve-regulating substance	Beriberi, mental confusion, muscular weakness, swelling of heart, leg cramps
Release of energy to cells from carbohydrates, proteins, and fats; maintenance of mucous membranes	Skin disorders, especially around nose and lips; cracks at mouth corners; eyes very sensitive to light
Works with thiamin and riboflavin in energy-producing reactions in cells	Pellagra; skin disorders, especially parts exposed to sun; smooth tongue; diarrhea; mental confusion; irritability
Absorption and metabolism of proteins, use of fats, formation of red blood cells	Skin disorders, cracks at mouth corners, smooth tongue, convulsions, dizziness, nausea, anemia, kidney stones
Building of genetic material, formation of red blood cells, functioning of nervous system	Pernicious anemia, anemia, degeneration of peripheral nerves
Assists in forming body proteins and genetic material, formation of hemoglobin	Anemia with large red blood cells, smooth tongue, diarrhea
Metabolism of carbohydrates, proteins, and fats; formation of hormones and nerve-regulating substances	Not known except experimentally in man: vomiting, abdominal pain, fatigue, sleep problems
Formation of fatty acids, release of energy from carbohydrates	Not known except experimentally in man: fatigue, depression, nausea, pains, loss of appetite
Maintenance of health of bones, teeth, blood vessels; formation of collagen, which supports body structure; antioxidant	Scurvy; gums bleed; muscles degenerate; wounds don't heal; skin rough, brown, and dry; teeth loosen
Essential for normal bone growth and maintenance of strong bones	Rickets (in children): retarded growth, bowed legs, malformed teeth, protruding abdomen; osteomalacia (in adults): bones soften, deform, and fracture easily, muscular twitching and spasms
Formation of red blood cells, muscle, and other tissues; prevents oxidation of vitamin A and fats	Breakdown of red blood cells; symptoms in animals (reproductive failure, liver degeneration, muscular dystrophy, etc.) not seen in man
Essential for normal blood clotting	Hemorrhage (especially in newborns)

VITAMIN SUPPLEMENTS:
A CLOSER LOOK AT HEALTH CLAIMS

In 1994, Congress passed legislation regulating many of the previously misleading health claims made by the manufacturers of vitamins and other dietary supplements. The legislation represents a compromise between the FDA's attempts to bar all health claims unless they were backed by "significant scientific agreement" and the $4-billion-dollar industry's lobbying campaign against all regulations. Spokespersons for the industry claimed that half of all Americans use its products at least occasionally. (This aspect of consumerism is unique in the Western world.)

In essence, the law now requires a strict standard of proof when product labels or advertisements make claims about cures or disease prevention, but it permits claims about how vitamins and supplements can help promote good health. Thus an elixir may not be presented as a cure for arthritis without substantial proof, but calcium supplements can be said to be helpful in preventing the damage of osteoporosis. However, the bill makes it more difficult for the FDA to take dangerous products off the market. Previously when the agency found that a product was apparently causing injury or harm, it could be removed from the market. Now the agency has to prove that *significant* harm has been caused before it can act. The legislation also requires that manufacturers of vitamins, minerals, herbal products, and amino acids refrain for four years from making health claims for these products while a presidential commission reviews the validity of these claims for future promotion.

Following passage of the legislation, a *New York Times* editorial made the following observation: "Now that Congress has acted, nutritional honesty will need to be enforced by a vigilant FDA and by the scepticism of consumers." In other words, when you're in a health food store looking for a quick fix, *Caveat emptor!*

Women over 55 or 60 years of age may need vitamin supplements not only because their diets are inadequate but also because, as some clinicians believe, their gastrointestinal absorption mechanisms are impaired. Women on special or restricted diets should discuss the advisability of vitamin supplements with their doctors. When a situation exists that increases tissue requirements for vitamins, such as hyperthyroidism, pregnancy, lactation, or postoperative convalescence, or when there is disturbance in vitamin absorption as occurs in hypothyroidism, the doctor usually prescribes any necessary vitamin supplements. In addition, some women who regularly take certain medications such as Dilantin, isoniazid, antibiotics, and oral contraceptives may need supplemental vitamins.

A diet deficient in necessary vitamin content leads to clinically identifiable deficiency states that can be successfully treated with therapeutic doses of the appropriate vitamins or minerals. For example, here are some troublesome symptoms and the nutritional deficiencies that cause them*:

- **VITAMIN A** Dry or rough, thickened skin.
- **VITAMIN C** Bleeding gums, poor wound healing.
- **VITAMIN B6** Sores in the mouth, cracks at the corner of the mouth, flaky skin.
- **VITAMIN B12** Darkening of the skin, loss of hair pigment.
- **RIBOFLAVIN** Oily skin, sores in the mouth, cracks at the corner of the mouth.
- **NIACIN** Dark plaques in areas exposed to the sun, sores in the mouth and around the rectum.
- **ZINC** Sores on arms or legs, hair loss.

The efficacy of small doses of vitamins in deficiency diseases led to the hypothesis that large doses might cure other diseases, sharpen natural functions, and prevent illness. The use of vitamins in doses many times the RDA for the cure or prevention of disease is termed *megavitamin therapy.* In 1968 the Nobelist Dr. Linus Pauling created the designation *orthomolecular medicine* to describe it. It is based on the theory that various cells need different amounts of vitamins and minerals.

The most widely accepted use of megavitamins has been Dr. Pauling's recommendation that the common cold can be prevented and treated with large doses of vitamin C. Other conditions for which much larger than standard doses of dietary supplements appear to be of demonstrable value include:

- **Niacin** to lower blood cholesterol levels.
- **Vitamin A** for treating severe acne and for correcting a deficiency caused by HIV infection.
- **Vitamin E** to prevent blood clotting following major surgery.

Because megadoses of any dietary supplement can result in serious complications, they should never be self-administered. Monitoring by a physician is mandatory.

* Source: Journal of the American Academy of Dermatology

Here are some additional facts and fables about vitamin and mineral supplements.

- While some nutrients are lost in shipping, storing, and processing, far more are lost in the kitchen because of inappropriate refrigeration and overcooking.
- Women whose eating patterns do not meet all nutritional needs because they are constantly on one or another trendy diet should accept the fact that pills and capsules cannot take the place of food on a permanent basis.
- Supplements are in order for the many Americans who consume significantly less than the recommended levels of vitamins A, B_6, and C as well as calcium, iron, and magnesium.
- Women concerned about the advantages of organically grown food—and there *are* advantages—should be aware that the vitamin content of food is a function of its genes and not of the soil in which it is grown.
- On stress and vitamins: megadoses are needed only for the major stress of surgery, serious burns, fractures, or advanced cancer and not for the stresses of daily life.
- On supplements of vitamin A: if your diet is rich in beta carotene, a nutrient transformed by the body into vitamin A, you are at lower risk for lung and colon cancer. (One medium-sized carrot supplies a full four days' worth of beta carotene.)
- Pregnant women should not take any vitamin A supplements without a physician's advice because excessive doses are highly toxic and can cause malformations of the fetus.
- Too much vitamin B_6 can lead to numbness and irreversible damage to peripheral nerves.

High doses of vitamin C have been recommended by Nobel laureate Linus Pauling and others for the prevention and treatment of the common cold. While there is some evidence that chronic vitamin C supplementation results in a slight decrease in the duration and severity of cold symptoms, there is no evidence that large supplements are more effective than more modest supplements (50–100 mg / day). *However, there is considerable cause for concern about potential harmful consequences of high doses of vitamin C,* which (1) acidify the urine and may lead to the development of kidney stones in people with gout, (2) are metabolized to oxalate and may contribute to the development of calcium oxalate kidney stones, (3) may condition the body so that a reduction of vitamin C intake to normal levels may cause abnormally low blood levels of vitamin C, (4) interfere with the guaiac test for blood in the stool (a test that is widely used in screening people for colon and rectal cancer), making it falsely negative, and (5) may result in scurvy when infants born to mothers who took high doses of vitamin C during pregnancy are placed on formula containing normal levels of vitamin C.

Terminology in vitamin science is confusing because over the years some vitamins have been assigned letters, some have been given names, and some are referred to by both a letter and a name. Names are used on food packages. Vitamins can be divided into two main groups—fat soluble and water soluble.

The fat-soluble vitamins are A, D, E, and K. Because dietary excesses can be stored in the body, they are not absolutely necessary in the diet every day, and evidence of deficiencies is slow to develop.

The water-soluble vitamins are the so-called B complex vitamins and vitamin C. (Two additional substances, choline and inositol, are sometimes considered B vitamins, but they are actually not vitamins.) Each B vitamin is unique, and there is now no functional justification for continuing to refer to them as a group. Dietary excesses of water-soluble vitamins can be stored only in limited amounts. Ascorbic acid can be stored for longer periods. Therefore, they must be supplied every day, and deficiencies can develop rapidly.

MINERALS

The minerals important in human nutrition can be classified into three categories: those that the body stores in large quantities (sodium, potassium, calcium, magnesium, phosphorus); the trace minerals whose importance is known (iron, zinc, copper, iodine, fluoride, selenium, chromium); and other trace minerals (cobalt, molybdenum, manganese, cadmium, arsenic, nickel) whose role in human nutrition is uncertain (see Table 1).

Many minerals are widely available in foods. Moreover, they are easy to provide as supplements. Because of these facts and because it is difficult to assess body stores, it is not surprising that overload syndromes occur more frequently for minerals than for vitamins. Sodium (Na), potassium (K), calcium (Ca), iron (Fe), and fluoride (F) are most commonly involved in overload syndromes.

Sodium as salt or NaCl can be harmful even under common conditions of use. Sodium and chloride, along with potassium, are the regulators for the passage of nutrients in and out of cells. Although the process is complicated, the most important factor is balance. Too much or too little salt upsets this balance. While the average daily intake of salt is between 8 and 12 grams, the amount needed to stay healthy is less than 200 milligrams a day. One teaspoon

TABLE 3

SODIUM CONTENT OF VARIOUS CONDIMENTS

Product	Portion	Representative Na Content (mg)
Baking powder	1 tsp	339
Baking soda	1 tsp	821
Ketchup	1 tsp	156
Meat tenderizer	1 tsp	1,750
Monosodium glutamate	1 tsp	492
Mustard, prepared	1 tsp	65
Pickle, dill	one	928
Pickle, sweet	one	128
Salt	1 tsp	1,938
Sauce, A-1	1 tbsp	275
barbecue	1 tbsp	130
soy	1 tbsp	1,029
Worcestershire	1 tbsp	206
Butter, regular	1 tbsp	116
Margarine	1 tbsp	140
Salad dressing, bottled	1 tbsp	109–224

of salt contains 2 grams of sodium. It is the sodium that concerns us most: in excess, sodium can cause fluid retention and contributes to hypertension in susceptible individuals.

In Western societies an adult with free access to salt may consume from 2.3 to 6.9 grams (100–300 mEq) of sodium per day, or from 8 to 12 grams of salt, and much more is added in the form of condiments, fats, and salad dressings. Some of the most commonly used products are listed in Table 3.

In food preparation a number of compounds are added in addition to salt (NaCl). Those that increase the sodium content of most prepared foods are listed below as they appear on package labels:

- Monosodium glutamate (MSG)*—in packaged and frozen foods
- Baking powder—in breads and cakes
- Baking soda (sodium bicarbonate)—in breads and cakes
- Brine—in processed foods (e.g., pickles)
- Disodium phosphate—in cereals and cheeses
- Sodium alginate or caseinate—as thickener and binder

* MSG is also a well-known headache trigger for many people who suffer from migraine. If you are in this category, make a habit of reading all processed food labels carefully. You may be surprised at how pervasive an ingredient it is.

TABLE 4

**NATURAL LOW-SODIUM SEASONINGS THAT CAN
SUBSTITUTE FOR SALT**

Uses	Alternate Seasonings
General cooking	Lemon juice, garlic, onion, and yogurt are the most useful; pepper and chili powder are good if tolerated
Meat	Lemon, garlic, onion, pepper, oregano, curry powder, rosemary, thyme, paprika, ginger
Fish and poultry	Lemon, garlic, onion, pepper, ginger, oregano, paprika, parsley, sesame seed, savory, tarragon, thyme
Egg dishes	Pepper (red or black), basil, marjoram, onion, oregano, tarragon, thyme
Vegetables	Pepper, basil (especially on tomatoes), dill, thyme, oregano, chervil, rosemary, yogurt (especially on potatoes)
Soups	Garlic, onion, pepper, bay leaf, basil, thyme

- Sodium benzoate or nitrite—as preservative
- Sodium hydroxide—to soften skins of fruits and olives
- Sodium propionate—to inhibit mold in cheeses
- Sodium sulfate—as preservative in dried fruit
- Sodium citrate—as buffer for canned and bottled citrus drinks

Because of a growing demand by consumers for salt-free processed foods, the availability of canned and frozen soups and vegetables in this category has increased, simplifying meal planning for millions of concerned women. Low-sodium additions to food that give zest and appeal to foods prepared and served without salt are listed in Table 4. Commercially available salt substitutes and packaged salt containing as much as one-third less sodium than the usual product can now be found on supermarket shelves. If significant amounts of these salt substitutes are used, they may contribute a major supplementary source of potassium and provide that potassium in a form that is ten times cheaper than potassium chloride solutions or powders. Many cookbooks and government pamphlets are available in local libraries for those who require low-sodium diets.

Potassium (K), the major mineral within the body's cells, along with sodium and calcium, regulates the passage of nutrients into and out of cells. It also regulates the heart and may provide protection against stroke. Good sources of potassium are meat, fish, citrus fruits, dairy products, nuts, leafy green vegetables, potatoes, bananas, and watermelon. Those taking diuretics for high blood pressure, heart failure, or fluid retention lose significant amounts of potassium in the urine and often require additional potassium as a supplement or in the diet.

Calcium circulating in the bloodstream helps blood to clot, is required for muscle contraction and relaxation, and helps to regulate nerve activity. The most important muscle of all, the heart, contracts and relaxes in large measure because of an adequate and controlled level of calcium. Combined with phosphorus as calcium phosphate, it forms the hard material of bones and teeth. Calcium in bone is absorbed and replaced continually to maintain the proper

TABLE 5

FOODS THAT ARE GOOD SOURCES OF CALCIUM

	Serving Size	*Calcium Content* (milligrams)	*Calories*
Skim milk	1 cup	302	86
Low-fat milk (2%)	1 cup	297	121
Whole milk	1 cup	291	150
Buttermilk	1 cup	285	99
Low-fat yogurt:			
Plain	1 cup	415	144
Fruited	1 cup	314	225
Low-fat cottage			
cheese	1 cup	138	164
Swiss cheese	1 ounce	272	107
Cheddar cheese	1 ounce	204	114
American cheese	1 ounce	174	106
Ice cream	1 cup	176	296
Frozen yogurt	1 cup	200	290
Sardines (with bones)	3 ounces	372	175
Salmon (canned)	3 ounces	285	188
Shrimp	1 cup	147	148
Oysters	1 cup	226	158
Bean curd (tofu)	4 ounces	154	86
Bok choy	1 cup	116	11
Collard greens	1 cup	357	63
Dandelion greens	1 cup	147	35
Kale	1 cup	206	43
Mustard greens	1 cup	193	32
Turnip greens	1 cup	267	29
Broccoli	1 cup	136	40

Certain dark green leafy vegetables are rich in calcium but also contain oxalic acid, which binds with calcium and blocks its absorption. These include spinach, Swiss chard, sorrel, parsley, and beet greens.

level in the blood. Calcium absorbed from the teeth, however, cannot be replaced. Therefore, broken bones heal but teeth cannot repair themselves. (See Table 5 for foods high in calcium.) Vitamin D is essential in the diet for the proper metabolism of calcium from food sources. Important sources are milk, milk products, and egg yolk.

Self-medication with calcium supplements can have undesirable effects. Three or four times the recommended daily amount can lead to the formation of kidney stones and might also interfere with iron absorption. In some cases excess calcium can be deposited in soft tissues and be confused with cancer. Excess supplements can also cause constipation and may increase the release of excess stomach acid, possibly heightening the risk of ulcers. (Women who show signs of osteoporosis should discuss methods of calcium replacement with their doctor.)

Other minerals required by the body include magnesium and phosphorus. Some foods rich in the former are meats, seafood, green vegetables, dairy products, and cereals. Phosphorus is found in all foods, but some of its major dietary sources are milk, grains, and cereals.

Trace minerals of importance in human nutrition include iron (Fe), zinc (Zn), iodine (I), and fluoride (F).

Iron is the constituent of hemoglobin that enables the red blood cells to transport oxygen to all parts of the body. Only 15 milligrams of dietary iron are needed each day to replace the red blood cells that are destroyed in the body's processes. During menstruation a woman needs an additional 3 milligrams to compensate for the blood loss. These daily requirements are easily obtained in a diet containing such foods as eggs, lean meat, liver, peanut butter, molasses, kidney beans, raisins, and green leafy vegetables. In those cases when heavy menstrual bleeding over a period of months results in iron-deficiency anemia, a prescribed supplement is indicated.

Zinc is a cofactor for nearly 100 of the body's essential enzymes. Eye tissues, especially those involved in dark adaptation, contain high concentrations of zinc. Zinc also speeds the healing of wounds and is necessary for the proper functioning of the immune system. (If it is insufficient, disease-fighting cells called T-lymphocytes may be inadequately produced.) The average zinc content of the diet in adults ranges from 10 to 15 milligrams per day and is just adequate to provide the RDA. During growth, pregnancy, and lactation, an additional 5 to 10 milligrams per day are required. Muscle meats and seafood, especially oysters, are rich in zinc. Conditions that compromise the body's zinc supply include excessive alcohol intake, cirrhosis of the liver, and gastrointestinal diseases, especially Crohn's disease.

Iodine is required to prevent thyroid goiter in adults. The RDA is 150 milligrams per day, and the requirement during pregnancy and lactation is somewhat higher. Seafood is an excellent and consistent source. Iodized table salt, which contains 76 milligrams of iodine per gram of salt, is the usual supplement for dietary iodine in the United States. One teaspoon of iodized salt contains 260 milligrams of iodine and 2 grams of sodium.

Fluoride is concentrated in bones and teeth and results in increased resistance to tooth decay. The recommended daily intake is 1.5 to 4.0 milligrams for adults, 2.0 to 2.5 milligrams for children, and 0.1 to 1.0 milligrams for infants. These recommendations are based on prevention of dental caries, not on total body requirement. Water is the major source of fluoride, and it is recommended that water supplies contain at least 1 milligram per liter, a level that will ensure adequate fluoride intake to decrease the incidence of caries. Foods naturally high in fluoride include ocean fish and tea.

TABLE 6

FIBER IN FOODS

Portion	Fiber (in grams)
Apple, 1 small	3.1
Banana, 1 medium	1.8
Beans, green, $\frac{1}{2}$ cup	1.2
Beets, cooked, $\frac{2}{3}$ cup	2.1
Bran, 1 cup	2.3
Bread, rye, 1 slice	2.0
Bread, whole wheat, 1 slice	2.4
Bulgur, dry, $\frac{1}{3}$ cup	5.6
Carrots, cooked, $\frac{3}{4}$ cup	2.1
Celery, raw, $2\frac{1}{2}$ stalks	3.0
Grapefruit, $\frac{1}{2}$	2.6
Grape-Nuts, $\frac{1}{3}$ cup	5.0
Orange, 1 small	1.8
Pear, 1 medium	2.8
Peas, green, $\frac{1}{2}$ cup	3.8
Potatoes, cooked, $\frac{2}{3}$ cup	3.1
Rice, brown, cooked, 1 cup	1.1
Rice, white, cooked, 1 cup	.4
Rolled oats, dry, $\frac{1}{2}$ cup	4.5
Shredded wheat biscuit, 1	.3
Strawberries, fresh, $\frac{1}{2}$ cup	2.6

WATER AND FIBER

Two substances that are technically not nutrients but are essential to healthy function and structure are water and fiber. Water, the most abundant substance in our bodies, carries all nutrients and wastes to and from our cells and regulates body temperature. Fiber (cellulose in plant food) speeds and stimulates the digestive process and the elimination of unused and indigestible foods. The fiber content of foods is usually described on the basis of crude fiber, the residue of food after sequential acid and alkali treatment. A high-fiber diet increases stool bulk, produces more frequent stools, and decreases transit time through the intestine. There is compelling evidence that high-fiber diets reduce the likelihood of diverticulosis, irritable bowel syndrome, and colon cancer. Table 5 lists total dietary fiber per average serving and can be used as a guide to design a high-fiber diet. In addition, many nonprescription psyllium preparations such as Metamucil, which add bulk to the diet, are available.

BALANCED NUTRITION

Nutrients work together. Each nutrient has specific functions, several may be necessary for a particular function, and one may affect how another operates in the body. For example, vitamin A cannot be absorbed unless the right amount of vitamin D is present. A sudden increase in the amount of phosphorus without a proportionate increase in calcium makes the unchanged amount of calcium inadequate for the body's needs. An extra supply of one nutrient cannot make up for the deficiency of another. Therefore good nutrition means balanced nutrition, with all the necessary nutrients supplied in the right proportions.

VEGETARIAN DIETS

More than 10 million Americans now call themselves vegetarians, and the ranks continue to grow. A large number eat fish, a smaller number also eat chicken, and most eat dairy products that strict vegetarians (called vegans) do not. Some women who eliminate meat from their diet do so out of strong convictions about unnecessary cruelty to animals; others are convinced of the health benefits of abstaining from red meat.

A properly planned vegetarian diet contains all the necessary nutrients. Proteins are supplied by combining complementary proteins, especially legumes, with grains or with nuts and seeds. The most frequently used legumes fall into two categories: peas (lentils, split peas, chick peas, black-eyed peas) and beans (kidney, lima, navy, pinto, fava, and soy, also used as tofu). Dairy products, such as eggs, milk, yogurt, and cheese, need not be combined with other nutrients to supply protein. Many delicious ethnic dishes that originated with cooks who had to economize while providing proper nourishment for their families have become great favorites with vegetarians: mushroom and barley soup, meatless pasta dishes, grape leaves stuffed with rice and pine nuts, scallion and bean sprout omelets, and the like. Augmented with fruit and vegetables, such meals can be comparatively inexpensive and rich in vitamins, minerals, and fiber, high in complex carbohydrates, and very low in fats.

While there is no conclusive evidence that a vegetarian diet can cure various ailments (there are many such claims, ranging from relief for arthritis sufferers to prevention of vaginal infections), obvious health benefits abound. Here are a few:

- Lower blood levels of cholesterol and triglycerides
- Lower risk of heart attack
- Less likelihood of high blood pressure
- Lower prevalence of serious overweight
- Lower prevalence of breast and colon cancer

FOOD LABELING REFORM

After a decade of trying to find middle ground between the federal government's desire to provide useful nutritional information for the consumer and the food industry's fondness for meaningless comparatives ("less fat," "more fiber," "lower cholesterol"), the Nutrition Labeling and Education Act was finally passed into law in 1994. It mandated the first significant change in food labeling since the mid-1970s when voluntary nutrition labeling was first introduced, and it was a triumph for accuracy.

The chief difference between the old food labels and the current ones is that the information panel not only lists percentages of certain ingredients but also tells you how a particular food fits into your overall daily nutritional requirements. The percentages given for "daily value" of the essential ingredients are based on a 2,000-calorie diet. The guideline to follow is simple: if the daily value of a particular nutrient is less than 5 percent, it's too low to take into account; if the daily value of fat is 50 percent, that's half of your daily value. The estimates of the number of servings in the total contents are based on a more-or-less realistic definition of a serving: for Hershey's Kisses, 8 pieces; for potato chips, 20. Especially useful is the information about how many calories per serving and, of this total number, how many calories are from fat.

The 1994 labeling law permits only seven claims linking specific nutrients and physical conditions, but these may be subjected to closer scrutiny and modification with the passage of time and the accumulation of new information: excessive fat and cancer; calcium to diminish the likelihood of osteoporosis; saturated fat and cholesterol as contributors to heart disease; fiber to diminish the likelihood of certain cancers; fruits, vegetables, and grains with fiber to lessen the possibility of heart disease; the link between high sodium intake and hypertension; and fruits and vegetables to lower the probability of certain cancers.

Obviously all labels needn't be scanned every time you go marketing, but it makes sense to check out processed foods for fat content if you're watching your weight or to be sure that food additives don't include MSG, sulfites, or other substances that are likely to trigger a headache or an allergic response. And if one of your goals is improving nutritional standards for yourself (and your family), the label information is much more reliable and less ambiguous than the hype contained in TV commercials. You might be surprised at the extent of the difference in the nutrients supplied by various breakfast cereals. After you've done your own evaluation, you can stay with one or two brands that best fulfill your requirements. If children's tastes must be considered, it's cheaper (and healthier) to let them add their own raisins, slivered almonds, brown sugar, or chopped dates than to pay for the packager's trimmings.

FOOD ADDITIVES

The FDA defines food additives as "substances added directly to food, or substances which may reasonably be expected to become components of food through surface contact with equipment or packaging materials, or even substances that may otherwise affect food without becoming part of it."

Most intentional additives, such as spices, herbs, flavorings, and oil extracts, are added for flavor. Some, such as monosodium glutamate, are flavor enhancers. Foods lose quality or become unsafe to eat because of chemical changes within the food or because bacteria or molds develop. Antioxidants, such as butylated-hydroxy anisole (BHA), prevent fats from becoming rancid and are added to oils, salad dressings, fried foods, potato chips, margarines, and baked goods or cake mixes that contain shortening. Ascorbic acid (vitamin C) is added to keep peeled and cut fruits from turning brown. Sugar, the oldest additive, is used to prevent molds from growing in bread, baked goods, cheese, syrup, candy, and jams and jellies. Additives such as salt, sodium nitrate, and sodium nitrite are used to cure meat, thus preventing harmful bacteria from developing.

Mineral and vitamin additives are used to enrich the nutritive value of foods, most commonly bread and flour. Milk is enriched with vitamin D, while margarine, skim milk, and nonfat dry milk are enriched with vitamin A. Potassium iodide is added to table salt to prevent thyroid goiter, and fluoride is added to water because of its preventive action against tooth decay.

While food colors were once derived from plants, 90 percent of all colors now in use are synthetic and are obvious in such foods as ice cream, soft drinks, pudding mixes, and gelatin desserts. Many of the synthetic dyes used to color foods, especially dyes prepared from aromatic compounds, were banned several years ago as a result of toxicity tests.

Sodium nitrite, sodium nitrate, which is converted to nitrite in the body, and sodium chloride (table salt) have been used for centuries to keep meat from spoiling. Before the advent of refrigeration and freezing, salting was the only way to keep meat. The formation of botulism toxin, the most deadly of all food poisons, can be prevented by the sodium nitrite in the salting mixture used to cure meats. In addition, sodium nitrite prevents fat from becoming rancid, produces the popular cured flavor, and gives the meat a pleasant pink color. These substances are added to all cured and smoked meats (bacon, bologna, ham, frankfurter, corned beef, and so forth).

During the last decade there has been a great deal of research on factors in food and the environment that might cause cancer. Among the compounds found to produce cancer in rats were nitrite and its precursor, nitrate. Although cancers occurred only when the intake of either was high, the results cast suspicion on the safety of cured meats. Harmful compounds are more easily formed at a high temperature. For instance, nitrosamines, which are derivatives of nitrate and nitrite, are carcinogenic agents formed when bacon, which has been cured with nitrate or nitrite, is cooked. The nitrosamines then are present in the bacon and also are released into the air. As a result, neither nitrate nor nitrite is used now in many cured meats such as bacon, and when they are used, the amount has been reduced to the minimum needed to pre-serve the product.

The leading food additive used in the United States is sugar. The prejudice against sugar is conspicuous in the supermarket, where an increasing number of foods are labeled "natural," "no sugar added," or "in natural juice." The concern about sugar stems not only from a preoccupation with overweight and tooth decay but also from an accumulation of evidence that for some women, sugar is a powerful mood-altering substance that can undermine emotional stability.

The concern about excess sugar in food has prompted the development of artificial, non-nutritive sweeteners, such as saccharin and aspartame, which taste sweet because they stimulate taste receptors in the same way but which cannot be oxidized by the body to yield energy.

Aspartame (NutraSweet), a synthetic combination of two amino acids, is now available in the United States for use as a sweetener in breakfast cereals, powdered beverages, gelatins, puddings, fillings, whipped toppings, and chew-ing gum. It is also available under the trade name Equal as a tablet or powder for table use. It is 180 times as sweet as sugar (sucrose), and the amount of aspartame equivalent in sweetness to 1 teaspoonful of sugar (16 calories) con-tains only 0.1 calorie. Studies in rats indicate that, unlike sugar (sucrose), aspartame does not promote dental caries. Aspartame was kept off the market for many years because one study suggested that rats fed aspartame might have a higher incidence of brain tumors. Other studies did not show a higher inci-dence, and the U.S. Food and Drug Administration has concluded with "rea-sonable certainty" that aspartame does not cause brain tumors. Its long-term safety remains to be determined.

THE IMPORTANCE OF BREAKFAST

Too many working women skip breakfast and then gobble down the wrong foods after they've checked in with the boss. Take-out breakfasts from fast-food establishments are very high in fat, salt, sugar, and cholesterol—typically eggs, croissants, doughnuts, sweet rolls, fried ham, sausages, or bacon. Commercial bran muffins are likely to be high in sugar and saturated fats. Fruited yogurt contains 140 calories of heavily sugared preserves and 140 calories of yogurt. Watch out for bagels with cream cheese and for commercial granola, usually high in fat and sugar. Nondairy creamers are a bad idea because they're made of corn syrup and coconut oil.

If you can possibly take the time to do so, have breakfast at home. Prepare a dish of hot cereal in the microwave oven. Blend yogurt, buttermilk, or lique-fied powdered milk with bananas, peaches, or fruit juice.

If you don't have to hurry, sit down to a proper breakfast of fresh fruit or juice and whole grain cereal or whole wheat toast or prepare something un-traditional such as brown rice with yogurt and raisins or a chicken sandwich on whole wheat pita bread. Remember that eating a good breakfast means eating less and spending less on lunch; breakfast can supply nutrients such as vita-mins C and D and calcium and iron that may be missing in other meals of the day; and eating a nourishing breakfast can reduce impatience and irritability and improve late-morning concentration span.

FAST FOODS

Because many of us eat more than half our meals away from home, fast-food chains have thrived and the industry continues to grow. Women are attracted to the foods they offer because they are filling, inexpensive, attractive to chil-dren, and sometimes even taste quite good. While not synonymous with "junk," which provides little or no nutrients other than sugar and calories, fast foods are not nutritionally balanced. For the number of calories they provide, fast-food meals oversupply us with fats and salt while undersupplying us with vitamins. The meals at fast-food chains may be low in sugar, but the beverages (soft drinks and shakes) and desserts are not. In terms of food groups, these meals are severely deficient in vegetables (except potatoes) and fruit. However, in response to a growing demand, some chains are offering salads in addition to their usual menus. But the salads are likely to have their "freshness" preserved with sulfites and may not contain a sufficient variety of fresh greens. In any case, fast-food meals should not be eaten regularly and, on days when they are, they should be augmented at other times of the day with a good assortment of fresh fruit, vegetables, and grains.

A word about those french fries, which are always a nutritional boobytrap. Potatoes when baked or steamed are an excellent food because in proportion to their calories they provide relatively large amounts of protein, vitamins, and minerals. But when fried in deep fat, they become a high-fat, high-calorie food, and when doused with salt and ketchup, their sodium content is very high.

NUTRITIONAL NEEDS AT SPECIAL AGES AND STAGES

The general information presented on calorie requirements and balanced nutrition applies to the healthy woman aged 23 to 50 who is not pregnant and not lactating. Older women and those who are pregnant or lactating have special nutritional needs.

NUTRITION IN PREGNANCY

Pregnancy is a unique and special time in the life of a woman. All women want their babies to be healthy. The main reason some babies die or are not healthy is that they weigh 2,500 grams (5.5 pounds) or less at birth. While smoking and excessive alcohol consumption are two leading causes of the low birth weight problem, the major cause is inadequate maternal nutrition during the pregnancy and even before conception.

Adequate nutrition is needed not only to provide the caloric energy and the essential nutrients required by the growing fetus but also to sustain the many physiologic and metabolic changes that occur in the mother. A healthy, well-nourished woman who is not underweight during pregnancy requires about 300 extra calories each day over the nonpregnant diet of approximately 2,100 calories. These ideally should be provided from food in the following ratios: 50 to 60 percent from complex carbohydrates, 15 to 20 percent from protein (animal and vegetable), and 25 to 30 percent from fat. Such a 2,400 to 2,500 calorie daily diet will provide all her energy needs.

Equally important, however, is attention to other essential nutrients and the variety of sources that supply them. It is also preferable to eat smaller meals more frequently than to stick with the three "square meals" that may cause a certain amount of discomfort as the pregnancy progresses.

Here are some guidelines for daily essentials:

- *Protein and iron:* 4 servings chosen from lean meat; poultry; organ meats such as liver, kidney, sweetbreads; fish; eggs; nuts; and for vegetarians, legumes combined with whole grains.
- *Calcium and protein:* 4 servings chosen from low-fat milk, buttermilk, yogurt, cottage cheese, farmer cheese, low-fat hard cheeses, ice cream.
- *Vitamins A and C:* 5 servings chosen from green leafy vegetables, carrots,

tomatoes, citrus and other fruits, red and green peppers, potatoes (white and sweet).

- *B vitamins:* 4 servings chosen from whole grains and enriched grains in brown rice, pasta, breads, muffins, oatmeal and other cereals (preferably cooked and sweetened with fruit juice rather than packaged products processed with too much salt, sugar, and saturated fats).
- *Lots of fluids:* water, natural fruit juices, 3 cups of tea or coffee (preferably decaffeinated), salt-free seltzer (an alcoholic beverage only on special occasions).

Of the essential nutrients, protein is most important because it is vital to the formation and growth of the fetal brain, which is more fully developed at birth than the rest of the body. A healthy woman needs approximately 76 grams of protein each day, particularly in the last three months of pregnancy. This is 30 grams more than an acceptable nonpregnant daily protein diet of 46 grams. A quart of milk contains 32 grams of protein. Vegetarian diets are often deficient in certain types of amino acids, and special care must be taken to eat the complementary foods to get complete proteins.

Another essential nutrient is iron, used by the body to make the needed additional maternal hemoglobin that carries oxygen to all the tissues, including the fetus. Because many women have insufficient stored iron and no diet can supply the increased amounts necessary, ferrous sulfate is often prescribed— one 5-grain tablet a day is sufficient—starting as early in pregnancy as possible and continuing for about a month after birth. Daily folic acid is often prescribed too, to prevent both folate deficiency and a rare kind of anemia called megaloblastic anemia. Accumulating evidence suggests that supplements of other vitamins are also important during pregnancy. These supplements can be critical if the daily diet is not sufficiently varied and nutritious enough to contain the amounts of vitamins A, C, D, and several of the B vitamins that are required to meet the needs both of the mother-to-be and the growing fetus. This safeguard is especially important for those vegetarians who don't eat dairy products. Whatever the nature of your diet, do not supplement it with megadoses of vitamins before getting your doctor's opinion.

Because individual eating habits vary so much and because only 20 to 30 percent of women in the United States begin pregnancy in a good nutritional state, it is crucial for every pregnant woman to discuss her nutritional needs with her health care provider early in her pregnancy or even before pregnancy if possible. Women with poor or marginal diets, adolescents, underweight women, and women carrying twins, for example, need more calories and protein than the amounts noted above.

As pregnancy continues, the most convenient way to assess nutritional status is by observing weight changes from week to week. This should be about 2 to 4 pounds of tissue, not fluid (edema), during the first trimester, and then a little less than 1 pound a week thereafter for a total gain of around 27 pounds. Such a gain suggests good nutritional intake. Lesser gains usually indicate inadequate nutrition and the possibility of a resultant low birth weight baby. Most obese women also should gain this amount. Slightly greater gains ordinarily are not a problem for the baby or mother.

In the past salt restriction was invariably suggested if not demanded. We now know that salt restriction is unnecessary and unwise except when pregnant women have certain chronic diseases such as congestive heart failure or high blood pressure, which are often treated by restricting salt. One problem with excessive salt is that it tends to be associated with empty calorie foods such as potato chips, which may replace foods containing other essential nutrients.

NUTRITION WHEN BREAST-FEEDING

Proper nutrition is essential for successful breast-feeding. The energy and nutritional costs to the nursing mother are high. Compared to her pre-pregnancy needs, she needs as much as an extra 1,000 calories per day for the first three months and more from the fourth month on if breast-feeding continues. She needs an extra 20 grams of protein daily. Needs for vitamins A and C are modestly increased. The high calcium content of breast milk requires an extra 400 milligrams per day in the diet. The extra calcium, vitamin A, and protein can be supplied by drinking an extra 1¼ pints of milk each day; the extra vitamin C can be supplied by two additional servings of citrus fruit or tomatoes.

During a normal full-term pregnancy, about 3 kilograms of nutrients (fat and protein) are stored in the body. These provide 200 to 300 calories of energy a day for three months. Women who breast-feed their babies lose most of this extra tissue by six months unless they maintain a very high intake of food. Women who do not breast-feed but wish to lose weight must restrict their caloric intake or increase their activity to get rid of the additional fat gained during pregnancy. Regular eating and drinking habits and responding to thirst usually assure an appropriate amount of fluid.

NUTRITION FOR THE OLDER WOMAN

Older women who live alone are at special risk of being undernourished or poorly nourished because they can't be bothered preparing proper meals for themselves, or because they snack and then have no appetite, or because they smoke too much, drink too much, and get too little exercise.

If mealtime is a chore rather than a pleasure, alter your mealtime habits. Instead of the standard three "squares" a day, have two meals—a late breakfast or brunch and an early dinner when you are most hungry—or if you're an early riser, have four smaller meals arranged somewhat as follows: at 7 A.M.—fruit juice or a piece of fresh fruit and a hot cereal with milk; "elevenses"—a boiled or coddled egg, whole wheat toast with margarine or a muffin with peanut butter, and tea or coffee; lunch at 2—tuna or salmon salad with watercress, sliced tomato, shredded carrot, stewed fruit, tea or coffee; dinner at 6— steamed vegetables and pasta, yogurt with fresh fruit; before bedtime—crisp rye crackers and hot cocoa.

If you find you're not very hungry most of the time, the best thing to do for working up an appetite is to schedule some form of exercise on a regular basis, such as swimming at the local "Y," joining an exercise class especially designed for older women (seek out a t'ai chi class if possible), finding a senior folk dance group, taking a brisk 2-mile walk every day with a friend, and you'll find that food takes on a new importance. If foot problems have been the excuse for not walking, have the problems investigated by a podiatrist who may recommend more comfortable footwear fitted with orthotics.

Food should appeal to the eye too. Make meals that look appetizing by including colorful vegetables and garnishing with a parsley sprig. If your sense of taste has become less acute, and food seems bland and unappealing, don't add large and potentially harmful amounts of salt and sugar to your meals. Use lemon, herbs, and spices to enhance flavor. Books about "cooking for one" can give you new ideas for attractive meals. When possible, invite a friend, a relative, or a congenial neighbor for dinner and use this as an occasion to try out a new recipe.

Fruits, vegetables, and grains high in fiber are especially important to help counter several common problems among the elderly, especially constipation and diverticular disease.

Excess phosphorus tends to enhance the loss of bone as we get older, yet the typical American diet contains proportionately more phosphorus than calcium in foods such as meats, soft drinks, snacks, and cheeses, especially processed cheeses that contain phosphorus in the form of phosphates used as additives. Snack foods that are just as tasty include unsalted nuts, pumpkin seeds toasted in a little bit of olive oil flavored with garlic, yogurt with fresh fruit, and whole grain crackers with some homemade applesauce dressed up with cinnamon, nutmeg, and a few slivers of candied ginger instead of sugar.

Many older women require special diets for their chronic health problems. For example, if you have heart disease or high blood pressure, you may need to restrict your intake of salt. Diet is the main way to control many cases of diabetes that begin in the later years of life. Women taking blood pressure medication often require foods rich in potassium. Some medications may interfere with nutrients in food and thereby create the need for dietary supplements. Supplements in no matter what category should not be taken without discussing them with your primary care doctor who prescribed the medication rather than with a salesperson in a health food store.

In addition to the many special diet cookbooks to be found in public libraries and bookshops, such diets are also available on request from the American Diabetes Association, the American Heart Association, and the American Cancer Society (see the "Directory of Health Information" for addresses).

Geriatric specialists point out that many older women suffering from memory loss, depression, and apathy may be assumed by family members and sometimes even by doctors to be showing signs of senile dementia when, in fact, the symptoms are attributable to nutritional deficiencies. (And when these deficiencies are combined with overmedication with tranquilizers, the results can be quite distressing.) If in fact faulty and insufficient diet accounts for the symptoms, they are likely to vanish when dietary essentials are provided.

When illness and disability occur, shopping for and preparing nutritious foods can become difficult. Check your phone book for agencies that deliver meals and that can refer you to group meal programs and homemaker services. For information about community facilities and all your entitlements as a senior citizen, get in touch with your local area agency on aging.

WEIGHT

While it may be true that in the abstract, there is a physiologically "desirable" weight for each of us, the weight that we "desire" depends on many factors: the dictates of our doctor, the dictates of fashion, the demands of a spouse or companion, peer pressure, what feels "comfortable," how we order

our priorities in terms of expending psychological effort. Too many young
women are smoking because they're afraid of getting "fat" if they stop, by
which they mean they might have to wear a size 10 instead of a size 8. In an
article in *Cosmopolitan* (1/85), Jane Fonda revealed that she had been bingeing
and purging as often as 20 times a day between the ages of 12 and 35 when she
decided to overcome this eating disorder known as bulimia. Many health experts now believe that the chronic unhappiness of repeated, unsuccessful efforts at weight control may in itself shorten life.

TABLE 7

FEDERAL GUIDELINES FOR "HEALTHY" WEIGHT: 1990

Height	19 to 34 years	35 years plus
5'0"	97–128 lbs.	108–138 lbs.
5'3"	107–141	119–152
5'6"	118–155	130–167
5'9"	129–169	142–183
6'0"	140–184	155–199

(Ranges are given to account for individual differences in body fat, muscle, and bones. The higher
weights generally apply to men and the lower ones to women. Note that the guidelines are based
on the assumption that people over 35 can be heavier than young adults without risk to their
health.) Issued by the U.S. Departments of Agriculture and Health and Human Services. These
guidelines have not been superseded as of 1995.

OVERWEIGHT

With the complete revision of its guidelines for weight in 1990, the government stressed health as a goal rather than desire. In doing so, it shifted the
emphasis from how your body looks to how good it feels. This shift is based on
research indicating that as women grow older, their health is by no means
endangered if they wear a size 16 instead of a size 12. They are far more likely
to feel the ill effects of crash dieting or of yo-yo weight loss and gain than of
being slightly overweight. This conclusion has been seriously challenged by
the findings of a 14-year study of nearly 116,000 women published in the
Journal of the American Medical Association in February 1995. These findings
indicate that women who gain 10 to 40 pounds in midlife, an amount considered acceptable and even desirable under current guidelines, have a significantly increased risk of suffering a heart attack. In view of these conflicting

attitudes to weight gain, each woman must decide for herself how she will order her priorities.

OBESITY

Except in very obvious cases, it is difficult to draw the line between overweight and obesity. A September 1993 article in the *New England Journal of Medicine* defined a typically obese woman as 5 feet 3 inches and weighing 200 pounds. In the article a 34-year-old woman who is 5 feet 4 inches and weighs 257 pounds stated the most painful issue she has to deal with: "Society is disgusted by me, and I deal with this shame every day."

In general, controlling obesity is difficult and frustrating. The statistics on treatment leave no doubt that treatment rarely produces a permanent and sustained weight reduction. While any method of weight reduction (and there are more than 17,000 such methods published to date) will produce some degree of weight loss in almost all motivated obese women, maintenance of the reduced body weight occurs in something less than 10 percent. After reviewing most studies on obesity and treatment programs, one must conclude that one of the surest ways to reduce the prevalence of obesity is to prevent its occurrence!

In typical cases of overweight, the goals of treatment are basically to decrease calorie intake and to increase calorie expenditure through a daily exercise program. *Motivation* is the fundamental factor for the success of any weight reduction program. The obese woman must *want* to lose weight and must make her peace with the fact that *keeping* the weight off is a lifetime endeavor.

Basically, the major areas of treatment for significant weight loss are diet, exercise, drugs, and group therapy such as behavior modification or participation in one of the recently established nutrition and weight management centers to be found at many prestigious medical facilities. These centers are staffed by a team of physicians, psychologists, exercise physiologists, cooking instructors, dieticians, and stress management experts. Before discussing these it should be pointed out that:

- Very thin isn't as "in" as it used to be. Fashion models now weigh about 8 pounds more than they did 15 years ago.
- Women with visibly extra pounds aren't the pariahs they used to be. Very attractive distinctly overweight models appear regularly on television ads promoting extra-large pantyhose and plus-size clothes.

- Women spend more than $20 billion on diets and diet products, mostly without permanent success.
- More and more young women are risking impaired growth and maturity by substituting soft drinks for milk, which results in fragile bones.
- The risks of being overweight are exaggerated, while the risks of constant dieting are largely ignored.
- There is an increase in the number of young women on college campuses suffering from serious eating disorders.
- Years of yo-yo dieting can induce strong self-dislike.
- Brisk walking for one hour a day can result in a loss of 25 pounds a year as well as an improvement in physical fitness.
- We are not all the same metabolically. No one should try to stay on a diet of less than 1,500 calories a day, especially because such a diet would be impossible to maintain over a lifetime.

DIETING

Trendy diets aren't following each other with the speed they once did. One of the reasons is that it has become increasingly apparent that they don't work over the long term. Another is that many women are reordering their priorities: between going to work, taking care of children without a husband to help, wanting to be physically fit rather than faddish, and making good health an important consideration, they are less likely to fall for "miracle" ways of losing weight.

The large variety of diets as well as the transience of their popularity indicates that none can guarantee long-term success. Of course, any diet that results in a negative calorie balance, meaning that fewer calories are consumed than are burned for energy, will allow the obese woman to lose weight. However, no single diet is good for everyone, and there is no real evidence that any particular dietary mixture accelerates the rate of weight loss. The main reasons for the failure of these fashionable diets are that they do little to educate the woman with a serious and chronic weight problem in the basic and sound nutritional principles necessary to achieve and maintain the weight that is best for her, nor do they address either the underlying emotional issues or behavior patterns that cause overeating. Dr. George Blackburn, an associate professor at Harvard University and director of the school's Center for the Study of Nutrition and Medicine at Deaconess Hospital in Boston, points out that "weight loss research is in worse shape than cancer research." Referring to the fact that there was a 25 percent increase in obesity between 1980 and 1990, he says, "It is clear that the monolithic low-calorie, low-fat approach does not work. We have to address the stress, life-style, genetic and environmental-related components of weight control."

REGULATING THE DIET INDUSTRY

With the recognition that chronic dieting and not fatness as such can be a great danger to health, the government's health agencies that establish body size, weight, and diet guidelines have turned their attention to diet products that promote unrealistic body ideals for women. Congressional hearings were held on the diet industry in 1990 that explored the misleading claims of weight loss products and diet programs. Testimony was taken from former NutriSystem dieters who claimed that their health problems had resulted from the rapid weight loss they had experienced. Among the results of these hearings was the removal of a fraudulent product from the market as well as the enjoining of the manufacturers of the Optifast liquid diet from making false claims about the safety and long-term effectiveness of its product.

In 1991, New York City passed the first law of its kind in the nation—the Truth in Diet Law—following undercover investigations revealing that popular weight-loss programs, including Optifast, Medifast, NutriSystem, and Diet Center, were covering up the health risks of rapid weight loss and were engaging in deceptive advertising, high-pressure sales tactics, and quackery.

EXERCISE

Physical activity is an important factor in determining caloric needs and, clearly, inactivity promotes obesity. Obese adults, by and large, are less active than normal weight individuals. Not only do they spend less time in physical activity, but even when they participate, their time is spent less vigorously.

While exercise can be an important factor in any weight reduction program, the use of exercise in the treatment of obesity is surrounded by faddism. Despite the advertisements of reducing salons, there is no evidence to support the claims that by mechanical means you can selectively remove fat from one part of the body. In studies done with tennis players, the greater amount of exercise in the playing arm was not accompanied by any decrease in fat deposits in that arm.

Without a reduction in calorie consumption, exercise is not an effective way to reduce weight because it takes far too much activity to burn up a significant number of calories. Would you walk 3 to 4 miles for a piece of cake? That's the distance it takes to burn up the energy in the cake's calories.

It is important to point out, however, that exercise is often accompanied by a reduction in excessive food intake, apparently by reducing appetite. Not only can exercise decrease food intake, but it can also decrease body fat. Studies involving college students have shown that a program of mild to moderate jogging or walking on a treadmill reduced body fat, increased lean body mass, and decreased body weight without other dietary control.

With grossly obese patients, although it is harder to achieve effective levels of exercise, more weight is lost through exercise than in patients of normal weight. In a study of 12 massively obese patients all maintained on the same liquid formula diet, 6 had an exercise program and 6 did not. In the 6 who exercised, the rate of fat loss and weight loss was clearly increased.

In summary, exercise in combination with diet produces greater weight loss than diet alone. If you are trying to lose weight, drive less and walk more. On public transportation signal for a stop before you reach home and walk the rest of the way. Climb stairs instead of pushing the elevator button, especially when you must negotiate three or fewer flights. Walking daily is the easiest form of exercise, and 1 mile a day costs your body more than 500 calories a week. In a year that's 8 pounds walked away. By reducing food intake by 100 calories each day, you will take off another 10 pounds.

DRUGS

Drugs are not an effective treatment of obesity and many, in fact, are harmful. Used not only to suppress appetite but supposedly to break down fat, their effectiveness, if any, is short term. And there are inherent side effects and potential dangers associated with the use of thyroid hormone, amphetamines, diuretics, and starch blockers.

GROUP THERAPY

A number of successful weight reduction organizations administer their programs in a group setting. Weight Watchers and Overeaters Anonymous are the best-known self-help organizations for the obese. In general, the cost to the individual is modest and less than that of standard medical therapies. Studies evaluating the effectiveness of group treatment compared to standard medical treatment in achieving weight loss suggest that patients in group programs stay in treatment longer and are more successful in losing weight. Presumably, this is because people with a similar problem reinforce and encourage one another.

UNDERWEIGHT

While most women who are concerned about their weight want to lose, or at least not add, pounds, some want to gain weight. Usually the reason is to have a better figure, occasionally to be "healthier," though in general an underweight person who achieves ideal body weight will not be healthier. However, women who are 10 or more percent below ideal body weight when they become pregnant are more likely to have low birth weight babies. The approach to gaining weight is the opposite, of course, to that used for losing weight. Caloric intake must exceed caloric expenditure. In theory at least, a pound will be gained for every 3,500 calories of intake in excess of expenditure. Women who have been underweight for a long time rarely have a disease that makes them underweight, though some may have a "genetic predisposition" to being slim or lean. Many of them smoke and get too little sleep and too little exercise. Almost all of them simply do not eat enough. To eat more and gain weight, they usually need to reorganize their eating styles: three meals a day (some suggest that six smaller meals are better) of proper quality. If you want to gain weight without stuffing yourself with the wrong foods, here are some suggestions:

- Instead of eating foods high in animal fats such as heavy cream, cold cuts, and hard cheeses, choose high-fat vegetable foods such as peanut butter, avocado, nuts, and olive oil salad dressing.
- Eat plenty of high-calorie vegetables, especially potatoes, corn, winter squash, peas, and beans.
- Have servings of pasta, rice, cracked wheat, kasha, or whole grain bread at *every* meal.
- Cut down on coffee, tea, and cola drinks, and drink milk instead.

A change in exercise activity usually is necessary too. Some exercise is essential to develop abdominal muscle tone, to enhance digestion, and to assure that the weight gained will be pleasingly distributed and not just "blubber." Moderate exercise may stimulate appetite. We do not recommend any other appetite enhancers or high-calorie preparations. Stopping smoking will help you gain weight. None of this will be easy, because you almost certainly will be attempting to alter long-standing eating and exercise patterns.

FINDING A QUALIFIED NUTRITIONIST

Trying to find a qualified nutrition counselor is no simple matter. In 1991 New York State passed a law setting standards for the certification of dieticians and nutritionists. The certification, based on certain educational requirements and the ability to pass a statewide examination, is observed in only 28 states. And even in these states, anyone from a health food store employee to a fraudulent "holistic herbalist" can present himself or herself as a nutritionist or a dietician. Thus, one of the key qualifications to look for is certification. Another credential to look for, especially if you live in a state that does not require certification, is the designation "registered dietician." There are currently about 46,000 professionals in this category who have undergraduate and often graduate training in nutrition and who are likely to be members of the American Dietetic Association, which requires passing an examination for registration. While many primary care doctors are well qualified to provide guidelines for special diets for a patient with diabetes or lactose intolerance, they are not likely to have the time or the inclination to guide and support a patient through the detailed regimen of analyzing eating habits bite by bite and making practical suggestions every step of the way so that the goal of losing 20 pounds can be achieved and maintained over a long period.

When choosing a nutritionist with the required qualifications, it's a good idea to have an exploratory consultation. Here are some of the considerations to watch for: If the first recommendation is an expensive supplement of vitamins and minerals sold to you on the premises, you're in the presence of a quack and should leave. Hair analysis as a way of detecting dietary deficiencies or excesses is practically useless. Any promise of a quick cure of a chronic condition through dietary changes should be viewed with suspicion. A competent nutrition counselor should present you with a detailed plan *after* finding out as much as possible about your eating habits, state of health, life-style, and family circumstances. Be sure to ask specific questions about fees, payment plans, frequency of consultation, telephone availability, and the like.

THE BODY IMAGE PROBLEM
AND THE BEAUTY SHRINK

Never mind fat; never mind overweight. The fact is that 75 percent of women are dissatisfied with their bodies and 75 percent of men are satisfied with theirs. And this dissatisfaction is just as profound among women in the normal weight range as it is among women who are borderline overweight. For women who are always "dieting," the result of the ritual of getting on the scale every morning determines their mood for the rest of the day. Sometimes the dissatisfaction leads to cosmetic surgery for breast augmentation or to liposuction. Sometimes it leads to pathological eating disorders. If you have a preteen daughter, are you underfeeding her so she won't grow up to be obese? Do you discourage her from thinking that her Barbie doll is a role model?

In the United States many women say they fear being fat more than they fear dying, and when asked what would make them happiest, losing weight gets more votes than any other accomplishment. Females of all ages torment themselves about the disparity between what they see in the mirror (those disfiguring lumps and bumps!) and the perfection, beauty, blondness, fitness, smoothness, thinness they see on TV and in the pages of fashion magazines. Who created this standard of physical perfection anyway, and why do so many American women submit to it in spite of their claims of independence?

A significant development has occurred recently as a result of the negative self-perception that bedevils the many women who are convinced they are fat and unattractive (no matter what *anybody* else says). This development is the growth of the number of therapists (informally called "beauty shrinks") who treat the syndrome currently known as an "image disorder." Under the guidance of these therapists and under the banner of self-acceptance, patients go to body image classes; they undergo short-term one-to-one cognitive therapy with the goal of learning to focus on their assets as a human being rather than to obsess about their heavy thighs or flat chest. At a California spa, workshops specialize in "beautyspeak." Janet Wolfe, a Manhattan therapist, uses tapes, imagery exercises, and a simple pie chart in which body shape is a very small segment of the total assets on which a woman should base her sense of self-worth.

Dr. Thomas F. Cash, a professor of psychology at Old Dominion University in Virginia and a leading authority on body images, points out that "beauty is no guarantee of a positive body image, nor is homeliness a decree for a nega-tive one. Body image is subjective and intertwined with all the feelings about the self."

If you think you might be suffering from a distorted image perception that interferes with your happiness and that casts a blight on your interpersonal relationships, you can seek out an accredited psychotherapist who specializes in treating your problem before it leads to a serious eating disorder.

EATING DISORDERS

Negative body images are a major component of eating disorders. While most American females confess to being unhappy about their weight, for some it becomes an obsession that results in anorexia and bulimia.

ANOREXIA NERVOSA

Anorexia nervosa, which afflicts adolescent and young women, is the relent-less pursuit of thinness through self-starvation. Basically, anorexia nervosa is a psychiatric disorder with the main issue a struggle for control and a sense of identity. Many young women affected with this disorder try to make them-selves over and to be "perfect" in the eyes of others, usually of parents with extremely high expectations. Even when they are less than ideal body weight for their age, height, and body frame, they see themselves as fat when looking in a mirror.

The outstanding characteristic of this disorder is reduced calorie intake. Not only is the amount of food rigidly restricted, but the pattern of eating becomes disorganized in bizarre ways. In contrast to the ordinary dieter, who makes the supreme sacrifice each time she rejects an ice cream sundae or suffers every time she declines her hostess' offer of chocolate cake, the anorectic will insist that she is not hungry, does not need to eat, and that not wanting to eat is "normal." In contrast to her emaciated appearance, she is overly active, often exercising religiously for many hours each day or increasing her participation in sports. She is an overachiever, and her parents will describe her as "a real perfectionist." Secondary amenorrhea, the cessation of menstrual periods, may occur not only as a result of psychological stress but especially because of too little body fat in relation to total weight. The cessation of menstruation is nature's way of saying, "This body would not be able to carry a baby."

In advanced stages of emaciation, true loss of appetite may result from severe nutritional deficiency, similar to the complete lack of interest in food that occurs in the late stages of starvation during a famine. If such becomes the case, hospitalization may be recommended. Before such an advanced stage of the illness is reached, it is essential that the condition be approached by psychotherapists who specialize in the treatment of eating disorders. Therapy usually involves the family as well as the young woman herself.

BULIMIA

Bulimia is characterized by compulsively eating large amounts of food very quickly and then getting rid of it by vomiting or using strong laxatives. These episodes of "bingeing and purging" may occur as often as a dozen times a day.

The health risks can be devastating, and where signs of the disorder exist, treatment should be sought as promptly as possible. All specialists agree that early treatment of this disorder is essential to recovery because the aberration not only can become a lifelong pattern but can do irreversible bodily harm if permitted to continue.

Since many bulimics are likely to suffer from depression and obsessive-compulsive disorders, psychotherapy may be combined with Prozac. This drug was approved by the FDA in 1994 for treating bulimia because it effectively helps the body produce and maintain adequate levels of serotonin, the natural substance that regulates moods.

BINGE EATING

Unlike bulimia, binge eating is not followed by purging but by profound feelings of guilt, shame, and distress. This eating disorder, which is far more prevalent than either anorexia or bulimia, is presumed to account for the large number of seriously obese women who repeatedly try to lose weight and fail.

Research conducted by Dr. Robert L. Spitzer, a psychiatrist at the New York State Psychiatric Institute, indicates that binge-eating disorder affects 30 percent of women participating in hospital-based reduction programs, 10 to 15 percent of participants in Weight Watchers, and 70 percent of the members of Overeaters Anonymous. Basically the disorder is a form of compulsive eating or eating gone out of control. It should not be confused with occasionally consuming a whole box of cookies or a quart of ice cream at one sitting, or with "grazing" one's way through the day by eating small amounts of this and that from morning to night.

The diagnostic criteria for the disorder include eating relatively large amounts of food in a short time until one feels uncomfortably stuffed. The binges must occur at least twice a week for six months and be accompanied by "marked distress" over the behavior. There must be no purging or abuse of diet pills to try to avoid gaining weight.

Women suffering from this disorder say that once a binge starts, they can't control how much or what they eat. In addition, their binges have three or more of these characteristics:

- Eating much faster than usual.
- Eating huge amounts when not hungry.
- Eating until uncomfortably full.
- Eating throughout the day without regard for normal mealtimes.
- Eating alone because of shame at the amounts consumed.
- Feeling ashamed, disgusted, or very guilty after overeating.

It is generally agreed that women who suffer from this disorder won't be helped by "going on a diet," no matter what they've been led to believe by TV advertising. Specialists who have been studying this disorder have found that it can be brought under control by treating the underlying depression and anxiety with medication, trying to identify and avoid "trigger" situations, and working with a nutritionist to develop a personalized regimen of meals that reduce underlying feelings of deprivation and emotional "emptiness." Regular counseling and participation in a support group can counteract feelings of guilt and isolation. (See "Directory of Health Information.")

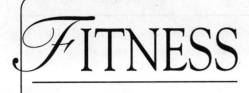

FITNESS

Christine E. Haycock, M.D.

Professor Emeritus of Surgery, University of Medicine and Dentistry of New Jersey, New Jersey Medical School, Newark, New Jersey; Fellow, American College of Sports Medicine

Serious interest in physical fitness and a more than casual involvement in sports for women have become increasingly widespread since the late 1960s. Even before this period, health authorities were placing more and more emphasis on the relationship between physical fitness and improved health. And for the rapidly growing ranks of women who were self-supporting or who were the sole support of their families, good health had become more than a matter of good looks: it was a top priority for compelling economic reasons.

Since the 1970s, ads for sturdy hiking boots and sneakers for women have displaced those for "spectator" sports shoes, and jogging clothes have joined "dressy" dresses in the wardrobe. Across the United States, the athletic achievements of Martina Navratilova, Chris Evert, Steffi Graf, Nancy Lopez, and Evelyn Ashford—not to mention Monica Seles and Lindsay Davenport—are inspiring women of all ages, competitive or not, to set themselves the goal of good health through fitness. Young and old alike are hiking, playing tennis, dancing, swimming, and playing team sports. Women in wheelchairs and those with less serious physical disabilities are no longer immobilized and isolated. They are enjoying the physical and emotional benefits of competitive sports, and their high profiles in the media are an inspiration to disabled young girls, who no longer languish in their beds. Women have discovered that the bicycle is a blessing, for exercise, convenient door-to-door travel, economy, and environmental protection. More and more women are joining physical fitness classes at the Y, spending their vacations at health spas, and banding together to organize community sports programs. And everywhere—in city streets, local gyms, athletic clubs, suburban roads—women of all ages are *walking*. In 1991 walking surpassed swimming as the nation's favorite form of exercise. Jogging has been abandoned by many women, especially those over 30, because of the wear and tear on the joints, particularly on the knees, and brisk walking with or without weights has become the favored activity for fitness maintenance.

Much publicity has been given to the aspect of the women's movement that has focused on giving equal access to athletic facilities to school children of both sexes, on allowing young girls to participate in traditional male sports, and on breaking down sexist barriers to achievement for girls who would prefer to pitch in Little League than go to social dancing class. What is sometimes not emphasized is how physical activity relates to changing the overall stereotype of the female as nonphysical, helpless, and weak. Increased attention to physical activity can allow a young girl to develop the habit of thinking in terms of physical fitness, to acquire an awareness of the capabilities of her body, and to experience the satisfaction that can be derived from achieving competence in any area.

NEW GUIDELINES GIVE YOU MORE OPTIONS

It is true that more and more girls are participating in gymnastics and competitive sports (including football!), and young women continue to enroll in extremely demanding body-building programs. Some working women take an occasional exercise class at the local "Y" or rearrange their schedules so that they can fit in a dance class or go swimming after five. But in spite of the fact that most women accept the fact that "exercise is good for you," millions of American women are essentially sedentary and have never made even moderate physical activity a *regular and consistent* feature of their lives. The excuses offered by the countless women in this category include lack of time, lack of money for health club membership, physical limitations, and in a significant number of cases, a dislike of vigorous, exhausting physical effort. Well, here's good news for women who don't like to work up a sweat in the interest of fitness. According to a message delivered in 1995 in the *Journal of the American Medical Association* by a prestigious panel of experts in preventive medicine and exercise physiology, fitness can be achieved by incorporating 30 minutes of moderate activity into your normal daily routine *every day*. This means walking up several flights of stairs instead of using an elevator; walking to and from nearby shops instead of using the car, and balancing moderately heavy purchases in each hand; playing golf without a cart; playing an active game of catch with the children or an active game of fetch with the dog; doing yard work yourself instead of paying your son or the neighbor's son to do it.

The Centers for Disease Control and the American College of Sports Medicine endorsed the panel's findings that the substantial protective health benefits associated with physical fitness can be achieved without working up a sweat. The panelists defined fitness as the ability to perform demanding physical activities such as shoveling snow or walking uphill for half a mile without becoming fatigued or out of breath. They concluded: "An active life-style does not require a regimented vigorous exercise program. Instead, small changes that increase daily physical activity will enable individuals to reduce their risk of chronic disease and may contribute to enhanced quality of life." Of course if you're one of a minority of women dedicated to muscle building or competitive sports, and you enjoy the euphoria that follows working out to the max, you've earned the many benefits resulting from your self-discipline and dedication. But if you spend more time watching TV than is good for your body and mind, or you play bridge with your friends rather than table tennis, or you use the food processor for every kitchen chore rather than chopping food by hand or vigorously kneading dough the old-fashioned way, review your options in terms of healthier choices. You can fight fat, osteoporosis, heart problems, and depression and make a major difference in your well-being through small changes in your daily activities.

BENEFITS OF PHYSICAL FITNESS

The benefits of exercise are not confined to any particular age group, and it is beyond doubt that exercise is a more critical health factor for women than for men because women are more likely to suffer from obesity and from the disabilities resulting from osteoporosis. Recent studies have provided evidence that a suitably designed exercise program for postmenopausal women, combined with supplemental calcium and estrogen and progesterone when indicated, can retard the development of bone-thinning osteoporosis. This devastating condition is responsible for most of the large numbers of hip and spinal fractures, resulting from even minor falls, in elderly women and appears related to changes in calcium metabolism and low estrogen hormone levels in this group.

We also now know that women who do weight lifting will not develop the bulging muscles seen in their male counterparts because they have much less of the male hormone testosterone. Exercise using weights or resistance apparatus is a valuable tool for women to develop the upper limb strength they otherwise may lack.

Exercise contributes to the physiological improvement of the body by increasing muscle strength, flexibility of the joints, and cardiovascular endurance. (The American Heart Association recognizes inactivity as the fourth major risk factor for heart disease along with overweight, hypertension, and smoking.) Exercise, along with suitable diet, also heightens muscle tone and reduces the amount of fat in the body. Exercise that strengthens the muscles can also improve cardiac and respiratory function and circulation. The heart muscle is strengthened, and the reduction of the general proportion of fat in the body aids in lowering blood pressure and lessening the amount of cholesterol. Healthier muscle tone makes it possible to perform daily tasks at home or in the office with much less fatigue.

An improvement in flexibility enables women to bend and stoop and reach without undue risk of muscle strains and pulls. Women tend to be more flexible than men because they generally have looser joints. Because of this flexibility and because their muscles are smaller, they can bend their backs and touch their toes more easily than most men. Flexibility exercises involve stretching muscles and maintaining the mobility of joints. These are the exercises that have traditionally been encouraged more for women than for men, not only because they are consistent with the female physique but also because they do not produce the muscular development that was assumed would result from other types of exercises. This supposition is gradually changing: men are working to develop more flexibility, while women are lifting weights to become stronger.

Endurance is the ability to persist in an exercise: for example, to engage in long distance running, to play a game for an extended period of time, or, in nonsports terms, to be able to complete or remain at a task that requires physical exertion. Endurance depends in part on cardiovascular function, the ability of the heart to pump blood efficiently through the lungs and the circulatory system, thereby supplying plenty of oxygen to muscles. Cardiovascular endurance can be measured by how far a woman can run, how long she can exercise on her bicycle, or how far she can swim in a specified time, all depending on her age.

One of the most highly publicized aspects of jogging has been its role in improving cardiovascular endurance. It is believed that vigorous exercise increases the rate of circulation, makes the body more efficient at delivering oxygen to the heart and other body tissue, widens the coronary arteries, and perhaps increases the level of high density lipoprotein, a substance thought to remove cholesterol from the arteries. Even mild exercise, such as brisk walking several times a week, wards off cardiovascular disease, as well as hypertension. Whatever else research proves about the relationship between a strong heart and regular exercise, it unambiguously indicates that the *absence* of exercise and a sedentary life-style go hand in hand with cardiovascular disease.

In addition to muscle strength, flexibility, and endurance, there are secondary aspects of physical improvement through exercise: power, agility, and speed. *Power* determines how far you can throw an object, how far you can jump, or how much you can lift or push. *Agility* enables you to change direction quickly as you chase a tennis ball, skip a rope, or climb a ladder. *Speed* enables you to win the race, chase a ball, or run after a child. These three assets are obviously critical for excellence in a particular sport, and although they are not critical for general physical fitness, they certainly do contribute to the ability to do everyday activities that anyone might be called on to perform.

Exercise affects other body processes as well. It enhances the digestive function: it is a reliable and effective aid to normal bowel movements and thereby reduces the incidence of conditions and complaints resulting from constipation. Doing exercises that produce muscle fatigue also helps us to sleep. Exercise reduces muscle tension caused by stress and is, therefore, an invaluable and comparatively simple way to achieve relaxation. Women who are experiencing anxiety, depression, and other emotional disorders benefit from exercise programs that provide an outward release from their repressed frustrations and tensions. Because exercise improves you by conditioning your body, it helps make you aware of your good health, which produces a general feeling of well-being and personal contentment.

Strenuous exercise programs such as jogging, gymnastics, and other highly competitive sports may produce amenorrhea (absence of menstrual periods). When the menstrual cycle is turned off, temporary infertility is the inevitable result. The body has its own reasons for this connection. Women athletes who train very hard (and ballerinas too) are usually abnormally thin. When the ratio of body fat to lean muscle mass is diminished, the body's survival is threatened. To keep the body alive, and because it is not strong enough to carry a pregnancy, the estrogen supply is turned off, which in turn results in a cessation of the menstrual cycle. However, it should never be assumed that exercise is the cause of disruption or cessation of the menstrual cycle unless all other causes, particularly anorectic behavior in adolescents, have been ruled out.

When strenuous exercise does prove to be the cause, the amenorrhea is likely to be temporary, and menstruation returns when stressful training has been reduced. As for the effect of exercise on menstruation itself, women who engage regularly in physical activity such as brisk walking or daily jogging report less premenstrual tension, less discomfort, shorter periods, and less bleeding.

Nor does strenuous exercise have adverse effects on a later pregnancy. Indeed, pregnant women may also benefit from proper exercise programs by improving their muscle tone for delivery. The results of an advanced study published recently in the *Journal of the American Medical Association* indicated that only when pregnant women were pushed to exercise at maximum level did the heart rate of the fetus appear to be affected. While the American College of Obstetricians and Gynecologists recommends that pregnant women should not exceed a pulse rate of 140 beats per minute when exercising, the new study points out that even at pulse rates of 150 per minute, the fetal heart rate remains unaffected. This applies primarily to well-trained athletes. Most pregnant women who exercise should probably not exceed the 140 per minute pulse rate. Thus, the long-term results of a woman's participation in sports and exercise are usually beneficial for her health and well-being at all stages of her life.

YOUR BODY'S ENERGY

When we work or play, we need energy. That energy is produced by our bodies from fuel in the form of the foods we eat. (The importance of proper diet is emphasized in the chapter on nutrition.) Here it should be pointed out that many firmly held opinions about the right food and drink for high energy have been discredited. Muscle cells depend mainly on carbohydrates for fuel: thus, a high protein diet is a poor choice. Most Americans consume about twice as much protein as their bodies need, and they would be in better condition if they ate more foods containing the slow-burning starches found in grains, beans, breads, and pastas made with unrefined flour. The fast-burning carbohydrates, especially the sugars found in candy bars, are effective for a quick energy spurt, but they are burned up too quickly to provide a steady source of fuel.

An essential component for all energy production is oxygen. Oxygen is obtained from the air through our lungs. It is absorbed into the bloodstream and carried by our red cells (in hemoglobin) to all parts of the body. In addition, our hormones—thyroid, parathyroid, and insulin—play necessary roles in en-

TABLE 1

CALORIES BURNED PER HOUR IN VARIOUS ACTIVITIES
(BODY WEIGHT, 125 LB)

Daily Activities

Chopping wood	367	House painting	176
Class-work, lecture	84	Housework	203
Cleaning windows	207	Kneeling	60
Conversing	92	Making bed	196
Dancing (moderate)	209	Mowing grass	
(vigorous)	284	(power, self-propelled)	203
(fox trot)	222	(power, not self-propelled)	222
(rhumba)	347	Office work	150
(square)	342	Personal toilet	95
(waltz)	257	Resting in bed	59
Dressing or showering	160	Sawing wood	391
Driving	150	Shining shoes	149
Eating	70	Shoveling snow	389
Farm chores or carpentry	193	Sleeping	59
Floor (mopping)	227	Standing (no activity)	71
(sweeping)	183	(light activity)	122
Gardening	178	Watching television	60
Gardening and weeding	295	Working in yard	177
Hoeing, raking, and planting	235	Writing	92

ergy production and availability for use. For example, a woman with an over- or underactive thyroid gland will have difficulty exercising. An underactive gland slows down all of her metabolic processes to reduce the role of energy production, while an overactive thyroid speeds up the body processes to the degree that energy is used up even when she is not exercising.

Energy is measured in the form of calories. We know that the body requires a certain number of calories per day in order to maintain itself and to carry on normal activities. The number of calories consumed during exercise is variable. Vigorous activity such as jogging, jumping rope, or bicycling obviously will consume more calories than team sports such as softball, and these in turn more calories than less active sports such as golf or bowling.

THE FIRST STEP: A PHYSICAL EXAMINATION

Before embarking on an active exercise program of any kind, a woman of any age who has been leading a sedentary life or who has been exercising only

TABLE 2

EXERCISE AND CALORIE EXPENDITURE (BODY WEIGHT, 150 LB)

Activity (for one hour)	Calories
Bicycling 6 mph	240
Bicycling 12 mph	410
Cross-country skiing	700
Jogging 5½ mph	740
Jogging 7 mph	920
Jumping rope	750
Running in place	650
Running 10 mph	1,280
Swimming 25 yds / min	275
Swimming 50 yds / min	500
Tennis—singles	400
Walking 2 mph	240
Walking 3 mph	320
Walking 4½ mph	440

SOURCE: Exercise and Your Heart; *NIH Publication No. 83-1677*
Note: A lighter person will burn fewer calories and a heavier one will burn more. For example, a 100-pound person would burn about one-third fewer calories than shown in the chart, and a 200-pound person would burn about one-third more calories. Exercising *harder* or *faster* for a given activity will only slightly increase the calories spent. A better way to burn more calories, says NIH, is to exercise *longer* and cover more distance.

mildly or sporadically should have a thorough physical examination. It is worth noting that until the introduction of the specialty known as sports medicine, medical schools did not teach doctors-to-be about the negative effects of exercise. This is therefore an area that most doctors know very little about.

A checkup is especially important for women who suffer from hypertension, backaches, or bursitis, or who have had major surgery or a reset limb. Also health problems may exist that a woman is not aware of. For this reason, in addition to the routine general physical, she should have a Pap smear, a chemical analysis of the blood that includes a blood count and a basic thyroid screening test, a cardiac evaluation, and a pulmonary evaluation.

Mild cases of iron deficiency anemia are common, due in some cases to poor dietary habits but more often to the fact that some women lose more iron during menstruation than they get in their diets. An anemic woman is handicapped in exercises requiring endurance or strenuous exertion. When the oxygen-carrying capacity in the bloodstream is reduced, the ability to produce energy is also reduced. Iron deficiency anemia is quickly corrected by taking iron tablets daily.

An electrocardiogram can reveal certain malfunctions of the heart, and if the woman is over 35, a stress cardiac test may be done. In this test electrocardio-graph leads are attached to the subject's chest while she runs on a treadmill. The result gives a good indication of the heart's reaction to the extra stress of exercise.

Where special conditions such as heart disease, hypertension, diabetes, or pregnancy exist, medical monitoring is a must, but this does not mean you cannot participate. Quite the contrary, exercise can be very beneficial and actually lead to physical improvement. Asthma is a case in point. Many world-class athletes have asthma: Jackie Joyner-Kersee, the Olympic long jump and heptathlon gold medalist; Karen Smith, a four-time Olympian in the javelin throw; and Nancy Hogshead, a swimmer who won three gold medals in 1984. It has become obvious that exercise is especially helpful to people with asthma because it increases the efficiency of the body's use of oxygen. Medically ap-proved programs and sensible precautions make it possible for women with asthma to engage in exercise, spurred on by role models undeterred by their ailment.

SUITABLE CLOTHES AND PROPER EQUIPMENT

Clothing and equipment for the exercise of your choice should be selected carefully. Clothing in general should be loose-fitting, have a high cotton con-tent for absorbency, and have an open weave to permit sweat to evaporate. These characteristics are especially important in both underclothing and uni-forms worn in warm climates or for indoor sports. Underpants should have soft inside seams and should not rub, bind, rise up, or cause overheating. Leotards and tights are unsuitable wear for intense exercise, and rubber suits or pants are especially ill-advised because they do not allow body heat to be dissipated and therefore prevent the body from cooling off naturally. In outer garments a higher percentage of synthetic materials is acceptable, but they should be lined with cotton.

Studies indicate that the considerable force involved in breast motion during vigorous exercise can result in chafing, sore breasts, and irritated, bleeding nipples. A properly made bra restricts this abrasive motion and prevents chaf-ing or discomfort caused by bra straps that slip off the shoulders. While a small-breasted woman seldom has problems related to her bra, large-breasted women often do. A bra that is well made and correctly fitted will not slip up over the breast no matter how strenuous the exercise. Bras specifically de-signed for wear by women engaged in active sports are available.

Shoes and socks should always be selected with care because improperly fitted footwear will result in blisters, foot strains, and sprains. It should not be assumed that one type of footwear is suitable for all purposes. Sports experts make the following recommendations:

- For brisk walking, shoes should be lightweight, well-cushioned, especially under the toes, and have flexible patterned soles, uppers of "breathable" material, and a reinforced area at the toe to protect against stubbing.
- For running, shoes should have soles that curve upward front and back and a heel that is slightly raised.
- For tennis, shoes should be sturdy, with flat soles, a reinforced front, and hard squared-off edges. On clay courts, shoes should be soled in open-treaded rubber to accommodate sliding; on hard courts, rubbed or patterned polyurethane soles are recommended.

Shoes for active sports should be bought in a store with an experienced, knowledgeable staff. The size of the shoe is irrelevant and the fit all-important. Shoes should feel right in the store because they are made of materials that can't be "broken in," nor will they stretch when you get them home. It is not appropriate to buy men's shoes even though they may feel more "comfortable" at first try. Women's feet have higher arches and narrower heels, and their footwear is designed to take these differences into account. It is also advisable to shop for shoes at the end of the day (and especially at the end of a warm day) when the feet are largest.

In caring for sports shoes, wear them only for the purpose for which they were bought and not for casual street wear. If they get wet, dry them away from direct sun and heat.

In addition to absorbing moisture, socks should be thicker at points of greatest stress so that they provide added cushioning. They should be roomy enough to enable the toes to wiggle easily but not so large that they bunch into wrinkles and folds inside the shoe. Socks should be changed at least once a day or more often if feet perspire heavily.

Foot care is critical to the enjoyment of an active life. To prevent blisters, calluses, and in-grown toenails, the following procedures are recommended:

- Wash your feet with soap and lukewarm water every day and dry them thoroughly, especially between the toes.
- If your feet perspire heavily, sprinkle them each day with cornstarch or medicated foot powder.
- For protection against fungal infections, use an antifungal powder or spray.

- About twice a week, soak your feet in warm soapy water for 10 minutes and, after drying them, rub away dried or thickened skin surfaces with a pumice stone.
- Cut toenails straight across.
- Do not cut corns away with a razor blade. Treat yourself to a visit to a podiatrist for treatment of corns and discard the ill-fitting footwear responsible for causing the corns.

Equipment such as tennis racquets and golf clubs should be chosen with the advice of a professional or at least with the help of a knowledgeable clerk in a well-equipped sporting goods store. Equipment that is the wrong size or weight or is poorly made may lead to injuries such as tennis elbow (an inflammation of the tendons in the elbow).

INJURIES AND AILMENTS

Injuries to women in sports are basically no different from those sustained by men. Injuries seemed more prevalent among women when they first began their active involvement in sports in large numbers, but their vulnerability was due primarily to poor physical fitness before beginning to participate, lack of conditioning, and poor training and coaching. Inadequate preparation caused more accidents not only among women playing on teams but among individuals who jogged, played tennis, or went skiing before they knew how to handle themselves and their equipment.

Even though it now appears that women in general are no more susceptible to injury than men, it is still true that any individual in poor condition beginning a new activity is especially vulnerable. If no other help is available, read a good book on the sport that interests you. A knowledgeable friend can be a good guide. It is often worth the expense of joining a sports club or taking a few private or group lessons before dashing off into a disaster on the tennis court or ski slope.

In general, most injuries sustained by women involve the lower limbs. Ankle and knee strains and sprains are especially common, and shin splints (pain in the anterior shin area of the lower leg) and chondromalacia (cartilage inflammation of the knees) occur more frequently in women than in men.

Women do not suffer severe injuries to the breast, and the idea that a blow to the breast will cause cancer has no foundation in fact. Injuries to the reproductive organs of the nonpregnant female are rare. After the first trimester of pregnancy, when the uterus rises up out of the protective bony pelvis, there is a danger of injury as a result of a severe blow. Therefore, after the third month, a pregnant woman should avoid sports in which there is any possibility of a blow to the abdomen, but other activities, such as swimming, dancing, or tennis, may be continued as long as she desires. Certainly a woman's menstrual period is no reason to discontinue any sport, even swimming.

Whatever exercise or sport you choose, be alert to signals from your body indicating that you should stop at once to rest, and if the symptoms continue, have them evaluated by a doctor. Watch out especially for sharp pains, marked shortness of breath, dizziness or lightheadedness, chest pressure, and pressure in the throat.

In addition to these potentially life-threatening signals, there are other health hazards and discomforts you can guard against.

- The muscle inflammation and soreness that are likely to result from sustained vigorous exercise can be minimized by taking 800 international units of vitamin E every day. This recommendation is the result of studies conducted by the Department of Agriculture's Human Nutrition Research Center.
- Ozone can inflame lung tissue and cause harmful changes in breathing passages. To minimize the effect of air pollution on breathing when you're distance walking, running, or bicycling outdoors, the American Lung Association makes the following recommendations: (1) Watch the calendar; ozone smog tends to be worst from May to September. (2) Watch the clock; since sunlight is necessary for ozone formation, the highest levels usually occur during the afternoon. (3) Watch the news; pollution levels are usually announced or printed with weather reports.
- Of course drowning is the chief hazard faced by swimmers, but there is also a long list of potential skin, eye, ear, and intestinal problems as well as upper respiratory infections to guard against. *To prevent swimmer's ear* (infection caused by the retention of polluted water in the ear canal), some physicians recommend the use of earplugs. If you find these uncomfortable or you think it dangerous not to be able to hear while you're in the water, be sure to dry the ear canal thoroughly as soon as you get out. If this is not done, the ear canal becomes a soggy breeding ground for fungi and bacteria. The first signs of infection are itchiness and a hearing blockage. To keep the condition from worsening, ear specialists recommend homemade or commercial eardrops. You can make your own drops by combining equal parts of rubbing alcohol and vinegar. Put the solution into a medicine dropper and insert the drops by tilting your head so that

the ear is up. After the drops have been inserted, shake the earlobe so that the drops go all the way into the canal. If this treatment doesn't eliminate the infection, consult your doctor about antibiotic treatment. *To prevent eye inflammation* from chlorine in the water, wear wraparound goggles. *To reduce risk of intestinal infection* be sure not to swallow any water, and *to reduce the risk of sinus infection,* wear a nose clip. *To avoid muscle strain* in the neck and upper back, look down and not forward, and when you're doing the breaststroke, keep your back as flat as possible.

- *Proper protection against the cold* enables you to continue your outdoor fitness activities throughout the winter. Dressing in layers is the secret for comfort and warmth. The fabric next to the skin should be a synthetic that keeps the skin dry and the body heat in. The middle layer should be a garment made of fleece or wool to provide insulation. The outer layer should be a wind- and water-resistant shell that permits the body to breathe, allowing perspiration and excess heat to escape. Other protective measures include sunscreen and sunglasses (especially for skiers), covering for the head and ears, thermal socks and thermal gloves, and footwear with skidproof soles to avoid falling on icy surfaces.
- Bicyclists and Rollerbladers *should always wear a helmet.*
- Rollerbladers also *should always wear knee and wrist guards.*

DEVELOPING A FITNESS PROGRAM
TO CONDITION YOUR BODY

You can develop your own fitness program to suit your available time, your activity preferences, and available facilities. It might consist of an exercise routine or sports activity alone or a combination of exercises and any other vigorous activity, such as jogging, swimming, or whatever you like to do. However, there are certain requirements that your program should meet. First, it should include activities to develop all the components of fitness—flexibility, strength, and cardiovascular endurance. Second, it must be done regularly. Third, it must include adequate warm-up and cool-down periods. Fourth, it must involve a high enough level of exertion of long enough duration to achieve its intended benefits.

If you decide that the best way to pursue a fitness program is to join a health club, investigate your options carefully. Take a close look at the facilities from the point of view of cleanliness, equipment availability, and trained supervision. Before you sign a contract, be sure that you understand exactly what facilities will be available to you and the hours you are permitted to use them. A health club associated with a reputable community organization is preferable to one that might turn out to be a fly-by-night enterprise.

If you work for a company that has initiated an employee fitness program or if you belong to a union that has a special membership arrangement with a health club, be sure to investigate the advantages of participation. Following the lead of Japan and Scandinavia, many corporations in this country now permit employees to work out on company time, thereby achieving big savings in health insurance costs, cutting down absenteeism, and increasing production by raising employee morale.

An increasing number of women whose main job is running a household and caring for children are following an exercise program at home. This alternative is less boring if one or two friends or neighbors get together on a regular basis and also share the cost of some of the home equipment, which can range from a few dollars for a jump rope to several thousand for a well-equipped home gym. In comparison shopping, keep in mind that price is not necessarily an indication of sturdiness. This is especially true of exercise bicycles. Also, a rowing machine or a ski machine provides a more complete workout than a bicycle does.

Special attention should be given to the hazards of unsupervised exercise at home, especially neglecting to do the necessary warm-ups, wearing the wrong shoes, and doing aerobic dance routines on a nonresilient floor.

In many communities it is possible to find a "mobile" health club that makes house calls for women on tight schedules, for those who wish to avoid the embarrassment of performing in public, or for those who want more personalized attention than is possible at a conventional health club. Prices vary depending on the number of sessions per week and the length of each session. Find out whether a package deal is substantially cheaper, but avoid making a long-term commitment until you learn whether the "trainer" is congenial as well as competent.

Whatever arrangements are made, it should be noted that different types of activities develop different components of fitness. Sports also vary in the aspect of fitness they develop. For example, softball is good for strength but not for endurance. Jogging and bike riding are excellent for endurance and for strengthening pelvic and leg muscles but do not increase flexibility or exercise the arms. Walking contributes to muscle strength and grace of motion while also improving blood circulation in the legs and reducing foot tiredness. When done frequently and briskly, it can equal the physical fitness achieved by jogging with less risk of injury. Further, it can be done almost anywhere and anytime over a variety of interesting routes.

A special note for walkers, runners, and cyclists: to avoid attacks, especially sexual attacks, the following rules should be observed:

- Don't go into areas that are completely deserted.
- Don't take shortcuts through unknown territory.
- Avoid being out before dawn or after dark.
- Don't run with unknown men and, if possible, use the buddy system.
- Be alert and figure out an escape route if you sense trouble.
- Know where the phones are.
- Change direction suddenly if it seems sensible to do so.
- Don't carry mace or a weapon that can be taken away from you and used against you.
- The best defense against unexpected attacks is running or cycling in groups.

Yoga is excellent for flexibility and relaxation but does little for strength and endurance. Dancing, particularly aerobic dancing, develops all components and uses all parts of the body. Swimming is considered by many experts to be the perfect exercise because it involves all the muscles, relieves tension, and conditions the cardiovascular system. It is often prescribed for back or joint problems or injuries incurred in jogging or racquet sports. The backstroke is particularly helpful for those who suffer from chronic backaches, and it is ideal for people with arthritis. In addition to providing a feeling of relaxation and exhilaration, it is much less boring than jogging, and working women can usually find a conveniently located pool where they can swim during their lunch hour or before or after work.

Swimmers should be alert to such risks as swimmer's ear and leg or foot cramps resulting from overexertion, cold, or insufficient warm-up. To be on the safe side:

- Don't swim alone for long distances in a lake or any body of water where no lifeguard can see you.
- Don't take a sudden dive into very cold water.
- Don't swim when overly tired or after a heavy meal or after alcohol consumption.

When you've chosen the activity most congenial to you, be sure to combine it with other activities to achieve a total conditioning program.

Maintaining a regular routine may be the hardest part of conditioning. Plan the time you intend to devote to it and stick to your schedule. Studies have

TABLE 3

ACTIVITIES RATED ACCORDING TO PHYSICAL FITNESS BENEFITS (FLEXIBILITY, STRENGTH, CARDIOVASCULAR ENDURANCE)

	Flexibility	Upper Body Strength	Lower Body Strength	Cardio-vascular Endurance	RATING 1 Poor 2 Fair 3 Average 4 Good 5 Excellent
Walking, slowly			x		1
briskly			x	x	2
Running			x	x	3
Running program*	x	x	x	x	5
Bicycling			x	x	3
Swimming (all basic strokes)	x	x	x	x	5
Kayaking		x			2
Canoeing		x			2
Sailing, small boats	x	x	x		3
large boats					1
Rowing	x	x			2
Horseback riding			x	x	3
Karate (martial arts)	x	x	x	x	5
Bowling		x	x		1
Ballet	x		x		4
Folk dance			x	x	3
Square dance			x	x	3
Modern dance	x	x	x	x	5
Aerobic dance	x	x	x	x	5
Gymnastics	x	x	x	x	5
Backpacking		x	x		2
Golf, walking		x	x		2
cart		x			1
Snow skiing, Alpine	x		x	x	4
Nordic	x	x	x	x	5
Water skiing		x	x		3
Mountain climbing	x	x	x	x	5
Yoga	x				2
Weight lifting		x	x		2
Tennis, singles	x	x	x	x	4
doubles	x	x	x		3
Badminton	x	x	x	x	4
Racquetball	x	x	x	x	5
Field hockey	x	x	x	x	4
Basketball	x	x	x	x	4
Soccer	x	x	x	x	5
Softball	x	x	x	x	3
Volleyball	x	x	x	x	4

*Running combined with upper body flexibility and strength exercises.

SOURCE: *Total Woman's Fitness Guide*, © 1979 by Gail Shierman and Christine Haycock. World Publications, Inc., Mountain View, California. Reprinted with permission.

shown that effective results will not be derived from less than three periods of activity each week. If you find it hard to carry out an exercise routine at home or on your own, try to interest your neighbors or friends in forming a group. Exercises done with a group are generally more pleasurable than those done alone. Some women are too self-conscious to join a group until they have achieved some competence, but eventually they find that the social benefits of the group include many psychological advantages. Join the local Y, see if a local university has an open sports program, or find a community center with exercise classes. Health clubs can be good, but check with members to find out whether the privileges are worth the price. You should also check on the staff to find out whether they are properly trained in the use of the equipment and in handling any medical emergencies that might arise. Find out if the club requires a physical examination prior to admission and what types of exercise programs it has. Don't commit yourself to a year's membership until you have visited the premises as a guest once or twice. Unless you participate regularly in its programs, you will probably waste money. On the other hand, if investing the money in a membership will discipline you into regular participation, it might be money well spent.

Remember that you cannot plunge into vigorous activity directly. If you are just beginning your routine, you must work into it gradually. Even after you are in condition to sustain strenuous activity, your body needs a warm-up and cool-down period of moderate exertion to avoid undue stress. Ten minutes of some of the stretching exercises described below would provide the necessary transition.

The question of how long each period of activity should be depends on the kind of activity. The most fitness benefit is derived from activity that maintains the heart beat at 70 percent of its maximum rate for 30 minutes, producing what is called the "training effect." For the average woman the maximum is about 180 to 190 beats per minute. If you can maintain your rate at about 125 to 135, you will be achieving fitness. You can measure your heart rate by counting the pulse at the neck (carotid artery) or wrist (radial artery). The less stress your activity places on the heart and muscles, the longer you have to do it to achieve fitness. Movements that bring the pulse up to achieve a training effect are commonly called "aerobic" exercises. For example, running produces a steady stress that can sustain the 70 percent heart rate, so that 30 minutes of running is sufficient exercise for one period of activity. Sports that produce less or more sporadic stress have to be done longer to achieve the same results.

CONCLUSION

If heavy effort and serious commitment to body building are anathema to you, the alternative is *not* minimal physical activity, which leads to overweight, huffing and puffing after climbing a flight of stairs, and a general lack of stamina. Specialists have concluded that an adequate level of fitness can be achieved by changing your sedentary routine to include 30 minutes of sustained physical activity *every day*. In addition to previous suggestions, here are some choices:

- If you're too self-conscious to join a dance class or a yoga group, invite two or three friends to join you in hiring a private exercise instructor to come to the house three times a week.
- Buy a tai chi video and learn this ancient discipline, which seems to require minimum effort and is the favorite form of exercise practiced daily in China by all ages, including the very old.
- Take the dog for a 10-minute walk every day.
- Take your next vacation at a spa that offers various levels of physical activity, and remember the routines so that you can practice them on your own when you get home.
- Walk home from the supermarket with a five-pound shopping bag of groceries in each hand.
- Walk up the three flights of stairs to your workplace instead of taking the elevator.

And do yourself the favor of lowering your risk of osteoporosis and heart attack, controlling your weight, diminishing your anxiety, and enjoying a newly found sense of emotional and physical health.

*S*EXUAL HEALTH

Ruth K. Westheimer, Ed.D.

Author; Psychosexual therapist; Adjunct Professor, New York University

W e have come a long way from the days—not too long ago—when most people believed, and preached, that the female child was born without any sexual urges and that she remained like this (unless corrupted by a seducing male) until holy matrimony, when she would be taught and sexually "awakened" by a loving husband. So much harm was wrought in the name of this sexual purity that young girls and women believed they were abnormal because they had sexual feelings. We know now that sexual feelings and pleasures begin—for both boys and girls—soon after birth and for some even *in utero*. These feelings and the desire to satisfy them through sexual pleasure continue for most persons through childhood and into adolescence, adulthood, and old age.

INFANCY AND CHILDHOOD

We know, through observations as parents and babysitters, as well as through research, that infants play with and explore their own bodies and the limited world of the crib. Female babies can often be seen rubbing their genital area when unencumbered by a diaper. Male infants often have erections that they rub and play with in obvious pleasure (some have had erections before they were born). Even orgasms can occur among infants and may be fairly common during the first few years of life, for both boys and girls. Infants and toddlers of both sexes may deliberately induce pleasurable sexual sensations by rubbing against clothing and toys—and later blankets and pillows—as well as by rubbing their legs together or sliding down banisters and the like. It isn't long before these little geniuses discover the value of their hands and fingers in very creative ways to achieve sexual pleasure.

Many parents, despite the pleasure that their child may be having, are bothered by this behavior (sometimes because they erroneously believe it is harmful, sometimes because of religious beliefs, and sometimes merely because they are embarrassed about expressions of sexual pleasure), and they try to make the baby stop. Some parents will slap the child's hand and firmly say, "No! That's bad for you!" (as if the infant were capable of understanding). Others will try to divert the infant's or child's attention to something else by offering a toy or food. There are parents who carry this to an extreme by bundling their child under blankets and fastening the blankets with diaper pins in such a manner that he or she cannot touch this source of pleasure. And there are some who threaten to "cut it off" should they notice their three- or four-year-old son masturbating. I do not mean to suggest that I want children masturbating on public streets, but it does seem that too many parents are excessively concerned about this.

I share the belief of many of my colleagues that impressions made on and associations made by even a very young child can have a lasting effect on the child's emotional development and may carry through to the adult years. Try to imagine what must go through the innocent mind of a child who is giving himself or herself pleasure only to learn that such pleasure is bad, dirty, wrong, and forbidden. Fortunately for some children, there are those parents who, instead of overreacting, wait until the child is old enough to understand that genital touching may feel good but should be done only in private.

Many parents are so uncomfortable about discussions of sex with or in the presence of their children that they impart a message loud and clear—although unintentional—that sex is so forbidden one should not even know about it, let alone discuss it. In a sense these parents may even believe that prohibition alone, of both sexual behavior and knowledge, is the extent of the moral teachings in raising a "good" child. These parents should think about the "forbidden fruit" concept and avoid making sex unreasonably mysterious and attractive through total prohibition and avoidance of the subject. Parents who shy away from talking about sex because they don't want to give their children "ideas" are advised by Dr. John E. Schowalter, chief of child psychiatry at the Yale Child Studies Center, "not to worry about putting sex in their child's head" because "it's there already." Some parents abrogate their responsibility in the area of sex education by assuming that the schools will teach all their child has to know and that all they have to preach is abstinence. Others militantly oppose sex education in the public schools, thereby exposing their children to the disastrous consequences of misinformation from their peers or total ignorance. Parents need to recognize that there are many more facets to sex education than merely teaching about reproductive mechanisms and preaching "Just say no." Discussion in classrooms and with parents should stress the complexities and responsibilities involved in sexual behavior as an interpersonal activity involving human values, not merely a physiological exercise that provides self-satisfaction.

Children receive many messages about sex from sources other than their parents and their schools: from their peers (the main source of misinformation); from religious leaders more likely to stress abstinence than facts; and especially from the media. Unfortunately, mixed messages concerning sex and sexual values are prevalent in American culture. From the moment that little girls begin watching TV, they see other little girls flirting with little boys in commercials and shows; they see and hear an emphasis on sexy hair, sexy makeup, and sexy clothes—even for the preadolescent—with the main contradictory message being "Be sexy, but don't have sex."

ADOLESCENCE

The sexual activity of teenagers has become a matter of major concern nationwide. At the same time that politicians are arguing about family values, welfare programs, and abortion, and parents are wrangling about who should be responsible for the sexual education of their children and about the distribution of condoms in secondary schools, a significant number of Americans consider that the consequences of the mindless sexual behavior of boys and girls is more devastating to American society than drugs or crime.

Whatever one's point of view about whether teenagers should be sexually active, the need for detailed, explicit sex education in the schools is a social responsibility that is taken more seriously in other Western countries than it is in the United States. Of course sex education should not be separated from interpersonal relationships on all levels, and this aspect of sex education should be part of the curriculum too. But as far as young people are concerned, they perceive "family values" from the way the members of their own family behave with them and with each other, and not by what they are told in school. Nor can the government legislate how adolescents behave in bed with each other unless a system of rewards and punishments becomes the law of the land.

To those who provide care and counsel to America's teenagers, the issue is not something as vague as "values" but the increase in sexual activity resulting in a sharp rise in AIDS and early pregnancies. Every year, more than one million teenagers, one in nine girls aged 15 to 18, become pregnant. For these experts, the most effective prevention programs are those that combine sex education and the distribution of condoms with lessons in how to resist social and peer pressure. A 14-year-old in California is being taught the strategies for saying "No" to sex by her health instructor. If her boyfriend tells her she's going to be dumped for someone more accommodating, she continues to say "No." If he says she's a big baby, or she's scared, or she's stuck-up, she learns to say, "Stop pressuring me. I'm not into that now. I'm into education." This 14-year-old is one of a growing number of teenagers and college students who want to prepare for success, who don't want to be young single mothers or to deal with the expense of a safe abortion.

In some parts of the country, the concerted effort of community leaders, both secular and religious, to promote the positive values of abstinence has led to state-funded billboard campaigns and the formation of chastity clubs. In California, a program adopted by several other states doesn't preach abstinence but rather promotes the practical reasons for it. Each year, thousands of girls learn that even with the use of a condom, it's possible to get genital herpes or genital warts; that a teenage boy can't support a baby on his lunch money, and above all, that there are more fulfilling ways to prove one's feminine appeal and one's manliness.

Of course, the onset of puberty is a very troublesome time for boys and girls—but especially for girls. While boys usually receive support from other boys (concerning not only the legitimacy of sexual feelings but also acting upon them through intercourse or at the least through masturbation), the contradictory messages just described not only continue for girls but may even become more troublesome. If an adolescent boy walks around in his underwear, even though his mother is present, little is said unless a sister or other female is present, but if a daughter does the same, there is usually an admonishment about the propriety of it, lest her father see her in a near-nude state. Often the affection formerly expressed by a father through touching and hugging and kissing suddenly turns into a more distant and formal relationship. That this growing distance may support the incest taboo is very likely, but it seems to apply much more, in many families, to daughters than to sons.

The growing sexual feelings of adolescent girls become a source of concern for them because the message from conservative members of adult society seems to be chastity until marriage and then a passionate—with fireworks exploding—orgasmic life with a loving husband. This model not only violates the bodily urges of adolescent females but is sharply contradicted by the media, in particular contemporary rock and rap groups. Rental movies have provided the adolescents of today a private viewing of the most vivid depictions of every aspect of sexuality and sensual pleasure, often in the most desirable of terms even for the young. And young people seem to manage to buy their way into theaters showing films that are rated "R" or "Parental Guidance Advised."

Several important changes in our society should be mentioned because of their effect on teenage sexual activity. "Society doesn't get really uptight about teenage boys being sexual," says Dr. Lillian Rubin, a psychologist at the Institute for Social Change at the University of California in Berkeley. "What's new among boys is that they're having their first sexual experience at younger and younger ages and they expect girls to do the same." Related to this is that, for many young males, virginity as a precondition for marrying a "nice girl" does not seem as important as it did in previous generations. Perhaps even more important, in many households single parents are dating at the same time that they're trying to impose traditional morality on their adolescent offspring. This can easily lead to inconsistencies that undermine parental authority. Dr. Hirsch Silverman, a well-known New Jersey family therapist, says that even the best-educated parents no longer "know how to deal with their children's sexual activity."

Another area in early adolescence that is much neglected is the appropriate preparation of a young girl for her menarche—her first menstrual period. I believe that parents often communicate (or, for that matter, do not communicate) certain attitudes about menstruation that have an impact on a young girl's self-image. Such parental messages can also affect young boys' attitudes toward their sisters and other girls. When a girl has her first menses, it is a sign that she is biologically prepared for the creation of human life. This should be a wonderful time in her life—a time to celebrate. In some cultures, there is a community or tribal party and gifts are given to mark this rite of passage. In our society, wouldn't it be much better if we could have a meaningful coming-of-age party with gifts to the celebrant, who has become a young woman, instead of the vacuous sweet 16 parties that are still given—the closest thing we have to acknowledging that a girl has become a young woman? The time spent in anticipation of the menarche could be wisely used not only for sexual information from the parents to the daughter but also for the necessary discussions of the morality and responsibility related to the act and consequences of intercourse.

ADULTHOOD

Until the fear of AIDS became a reality, most adult women in the United States had their patterns of sexual behavior determined by their upbringing: essentially, their moral and religious education as well as the extent of their personal experiences with sexual partners. Thus, some women were "swinging singles," while others were divorced with multiple lovers. Some chose celibacy, while others worked at landing "Mr. Right." In any case, women had choices—and the decisions were often based on their passions and desires. Fear of disease had been all but eliminated by the 1980s, and even guilt was a rapidly diminishing constraint.

In the 1960s and 1970s, many women who were not married developed their own interpretations of moral standards and values, which were often at odds with their religious and parental upbringing but which seemed to work for them. Freedom from fear of pregnancy and disease gave many women the opportunity for extensive experimentation but brought with it a questioning of the meaning of sex in the larger fabric of one's life. The relevant and highly personal moral issues that concerned so many women paled with the rise of AIDS in the 1980s, when a new code of behavior was required by the ever-present threat of AIDS for all but the long-term monogamous, the celibate, and lesbians. (Homosexual women still have to deal with various societal problems, but they have always enjoyed a sex life free of the anxiety about pregnancy and the fear of sexually transmitted diseases.)

Through December 1994, the Centers for Disease Control reported 58,428 cases of AIDS among females aged 13 and up. Cases have increased in this category from 7 percent of *all* cases in 1985 to 18 percent in 1994. Sexual contact with an HIV-infected male is the most rapidly increasing means of transmission for females of all ages. Since a man infected with the AIDS virus can remain healthy for years, he can spread the virus unknowingly. You should keep in mind that a sexual partner may not tell you about all his past and present sexual activities. If he has been an IV drug user or has had even one encounter with a homosexual man, he puts you at even greater risk. (For a more detailed discussion of AIDS and other STDs, see the chapter titled "Sexually Transmissible Diseases.")

There are no easy answers for the single woman who wants a full sex life.

But it is certain that "safe sex" rather than maximum pleasure must become one of her guiding principles.

HOMOSEXUALITY AND BISEXUALITY

It is unlikely that any survey of how many American women define themselves as lesbians will provide an accurate answer. After all, there is no general agreement on whether homosexuality is a matter of self-identification, physical desire, romantic obsession, behavior, or some combination of these factors. In terms of acknowledged behavior, same-sex relationships cover a broad range of the spectrum, from what used to be called "Boston marriages" to the loving connection between Eleanor Roosevelt and Lorena Hickok. How much "sex" was involved in these connections is anyone's guess and is in fact considered irrelevant. Also many women who might be defined by the homosexual community as lesbians would never label themselves in that way, especially if they are women living in small towns. As for African American women, they are more likely to define themselves not in terms of sexual orientation but in terms of racial identity.

If homosexual interpersonal connections resist easy definition, the question of sexuality has recently been complicated by the emergence of a growing and highly vocal bisexual community. In an extensive survey on sexuality in the United States conducted in 1994 by University of Chicago researchers, the number of bisexuals ranged from 1.5 million to 7.5 million over age 18, depending on how the term was defined. The results of this survey are supported by other investigations indicating that the sexual preferences of bisexuals are far more fluid than formerly assumed. It would also appear that many members of a generation raised on erotically charged images designed to appeal to both sexes reject being labeled either gay or straight. Marjorie Garber, Harvard professor of English and author of *Vice Versa*, a book published in 1995 that examines bisexuality in literature and society, has this to say: "There are periods of bisexual chic, and we're in a moment when it's visible again."

Bisexuals have become highly visible and highly vocal on talk shows and elsewhere in their attempt to achieve greater acceptance. Those who are male feel they are mistakenly scapegoated as the source for the spread of AIDS. Many women who define themselves as bisexual are viewed by the committed lesbian community as opportunists who are looking for a nurturing relationship with another woman after the breakup of a marriage.

Whatever the motivation for bisexual behavior, the woman-woman relationship can be the source of comfort and pleasure. But the sexual relationship between a straight woman and a bisexual man can be the source of perpetual anxiety. There are instances where a straight woman is aware of the bisexual proclivities of her spouse but tries to work out an arrangement that seems satisfactory to both. Yet it is the woman who is obviously putting her life on the line; if she feels she is a slave of love, she might consider liberating herself from the potential perils of HIV infection by consulting a psychotherapist.

SEX AND HEALTH CARE

There's little doubt that the joy of sex, for many women, has been greatly diminished by the barrage of negative media attention given to date rape, incest, child molestation, sexual harassment, and, of course, sexually transmitted diseases. But women still have a right—and a need—for sexual fulfillment. For women whose sex lives are unsatisfactory or nonexistent, the unsatisfied needs may become transformed into physical symptoms: headaches, backaches, digestive problems, sleeplessness, and depression. But complaints to many doctors are often treated as trivial, and rarely will a physician investigate the possibility of a psychosexual origin to a problem. While doctors are very good when it comes to the physical components of female problems, all too many are insensitive to or embarrassed by the psychosexual components or origins of problems. And the absence of cutaneous stimulation—the skin-to-skin contact and stroking that we all need and desire—is rarely considered a valid medical problem.

DOES "SEX IN AMERICA" GET THE NUMBERS RIGHT?

According to the numbers presented in what was claimed to be the most definitive study to date of America's sexual behavior when it was published in 1994, marital fidelity is not only alive and well (85 percent of married women and more than 75 percent of married men said they were faithful to their spouses), but also (big surprise!) married people are more sexually active than their single counterparts (41 percent say they have sex twice a week or more compared with 23 percent of singles). But unmarried couples who live together have the most sex of all, with 56 percent reporting that they have sex at least twice a week.

The survey, which was based on a random selection of approximately 3,500 men and women aged 18 to 59, was the end result of the government's attempt in 1987 to accumulate information about sexual practices that would be helpful in the fight against AIDS. It was stymied in 1991 when Jesse Helms convinced the Senate to block federal funds for the project, which he defined as a plot to promote homosexuality. Private foundations came through with the necessary money for the survey to go forward, and the accumulated information was made public in a hefty 700-page report entitled "The Social Organization of Sexuality." These findings were distilled by several writers in the book *Sex in America: A Definitive Survey.*

The term "definitive" is always highly misleading in connection with any survey, especially one that deals with the most intimate details of a person's life. There was considerable disbelief in gay and lesbian circles about the reliability of responses indicating that only 2.8 percent of the men and 1.4 percent of the women identified themselves as homosexual or bisexual. A *New York Times* editorial as well as other newspaper and magazine articles nationwide were astonished by the fidelity figures, and observed that, sexually speaking, "This is a nation of squares." (But how do the fidelity figures square with the unexamined divorce statistics?) The *Times* writer also comments, "There is no better way to measure one's own sex life than to compare it with the well-documented (as opposed to barroom boasts and locker room anecdotes) sex lives of others."

"Well-documented?" "Definitive?" Whatever the findings of this survey, the random sampling of 3,500 individuals is comparatively small for a country of this size and diversity. And there is a great deal of justification for questioning many of the findings. Do corporate executives on a business trip consider time out with a prostitute or a call girl "marital infidelity"? Does a conventional married woman acknowledge an extramarital affair when questioned by a stranger if she's never been able to talk about it to her closest friend, or to her minister, or even admit it to herself? What about incest? What about the private lives of Americans as reflected not in tabloid "trash" and TV but in the novels and short stories of John Updike?

As for the responses to the many questions put to the participants in the survey, each reader can decide on their authenticity from her own experience.

ADULT SEXUAL DYSFUNCTIONS

One of the most frequent questions women ask of sex therapists is "How normal is my sex life?" The woman who asks this question may be referring to her frequency of sex, type of sexual behavior, intensity of feelings or kinds of responses during sex, or many other aspects of her sexuality. Of course, "normal" sex—between two consenting adults—cannot be easily defined. Even statistical descriptions from surveys only describe what may be a statistical norm or average and do not take into account the fact that women vary in their libidinal drive, upbringing, and beliefs about the appropriateness of different aspects of sexual behavior. Perhaps the only important and relevant question for a woman to ask (assuming she really likes her partner) is "Am I satisfied with all aspects of my sexual desire, performance, and response?" If the answer is yes to all three parts of the question, then she is having a "normal" and satisfying sex life *for her.* If she has some dissatisfaction, then there may be a problem or a sexual dysfunction *for her.* What are some possible problems? The most common sexual dysfunctions are difficulties in orgasm, painful intercourse, and lack of sexual interest.

ORGASM DIFFICULTIES

Perhaps the most common concern among women regarding their sexual performance is orgasm. Do women need orgasms? This simple question needs a two-part answer. First, we know that once a woman is sexually aroused, the flow of blood to the labia, clitoris, and other parts of the genitals creates a tension that is best relieved through orgasm. Frequent sexual excitement without orgasmic relief has resulted, for some women, in various aches and pains as well as nervous tension.

Second, while it is true that women can conceive without experiencing orgasm and that they can feel sexual pleasure, excitement, and satisfaction without orgasm, they are clearly missing out on a bonus of nature. Many sex therapists support the view of those scientists who point out that the process of evolution (or God) has created a magnificent human male and female body whose every part, system, and response has a reason to exist. The female, as well as the male, has the ability to have this marvelous sensual experience we call an orgasm.

Some people, professionals and lay alike, have unfairly labeled a woman's nonorgasmic condition as an affliction. A woman who has not yet learned to create the conditions or to receive sufficient stimulation to allow the orgasm reflex to occur might be called frigid by an insensitive, impatient spouse or lover. On the other hand, some husbands and partners put an unfair amount of pressure on women, even out of loving consideration, to make sure they have an orgasm every time. The reality and complexities of the female physiology and situational factors such as stress may at times work against the likelihood of an orgasm.

Some women are not certain whether they are having orgasms or just good sensations. Orgasms are very subjective—consistently mild for some women while overpowering for others. If a woman has a partner who gives her sufficient physical stimulation, or if she gives herself sufficient stimulation, then she will be quite aware of the sensation of not reaching orgasm—usually a sense that she is still sexually aroused. She might achieve orgasm and still want more, but she usually knows that she has had an orgasm. If the mild sensations are of concern to you, speak to a sex therapist about this.

A woman who knows that she consistently does not have orgasms may be considered to be, *at present*, nonorgasmic. Being nonorgasmic is not a permanent condition and certainly is not a sickness. It merely means that the right conditions or stimulations have not been met to reach the optimal sexual response we call orgasm.

Orgasmic difficulties may be broadly classified into two types. In one, the problem is due to the inability of a partner to bring a woman to orgasm. In the other, no matter how sexually skilled the partner is, the woman just cannot reach orgasm. To treat the problem, it is necessary for sex therapists to understand the conditions under which orgasms may or may not occur. A woman may be orgasmic with self-stimulation but not with her partner; orgasmic with one partner but not another; or not orgasmic by herself or with the help of her partner. Since these situations require somewhat different corrective approaches, a woman has to know which situation applies to her.

There is another type of orgasmic problem that is sometimes seen. There are some women who do not know that there may be a "flat" moment preceding the orgasmic response when it seems as if nothing is going to happen. Many women say that they don't experience this at all. But other women, when they have this flat moment sometimes think, "Nothing is going to happen, so I might as well forget about it." They then turn themselves off and their lack of faith becomes a self-fulfilling prophecy. However, if a woman who experiences this flat moment keeps up the stimulation to get past this point, she may very well have her orgasm.

If a woman is able to reach orgasm through self-stimulation or if she reached orgasm with a previous partner but not with her present mate, this does not mean that she is subconsciously rejecting her present lover. It may indicate an inability to communicate what kinds of physical pressures and movements she needs to reach an orgasm. The problem does not necessarily point to any sexual diffidence on the part of the man. After all, he can't guess what's on her mind.

In order to get a clearer understanding of what is producing an orgasmic problem, a woman must consider the relationship she has with her husband or partner. All the sex therapy and advice in the world won't help those women who basically don't like the person they are having sex with. If they really don't, then they should see a marriage counselor, pastoral counselor, or other professional to resolve an interpersonal problem.

One special kind of orgasmic difficulty is caused mainly by the mass media and folk myths. That is the idea that only young women are sexually attractive and that, when a woman gets older, she replaces her interest in sex with sitting in a rocking chair or baking or obsessive concern for her grandchildren. It is merely a cultural stereotype that an older woman (or man) loses interest in sex. Not even the removal of the uterus or menopause or the empty nest syndrome results in significant decreases in sexual desire. You have to *will* yourself to lose interest by believing in these myths. "Hot flashes," which often accompany menopause, are sometimes used as an excuse by women who don't want to have sex with their husbands for other reasons. It is as if they were saying to themselves, "See, my body is now telling me that my sexual life is over." Hot flashes do signal hormonal changes during menopause, but they definitely do not mean the end of sexuality. On the contrary, many women feel freed from the concerns of becoming pregnant and raising children, who by now are grown. For them, menopause is a time to renew intimacy in their marriage, which may have been buried for decades. Husband and wife can now behave like newlyweds if they so desire. Sexiness is mainly in the head, and often a change in attitude is needed before women can experience a desired change in orgasmic response. For some women, sex is better than ever when they get older. Although the orgasmic response may be a little weaker, it can still be very enjoyable and satisfying for women into their eighties and nineties. The Reverend Andrew Greeley, a sociologist, priest, novelist, and professor at the University of Chicago, issued a report concluding that men and women who engage in frequent sex after 60 have the happiest marriages and live the most exciting lives.

Another concern some women have about orgasms stems from their disappointment that they have orgasms only when the clitoral area is stimulated and not when their partner is thrusting during coitus. These women are bothered by what they believe to be true: that an orgasm resulting from clitoral stimulation is less "mature" than one that is vaginally induced. This incorrect notion is mainly the result of a controversial aspect of Freud's thinking. It was his belief that women have two types of orgasms: vaginal and clitoral. He also believed that vaginal orgasm was an indication that a woman had reached the genital stage and that women who could have only clitoral orgasms probably had not successfully resolved the conflicts of the phallic stage. Modern sex researchers such as Masters and Johnson claim there is no scientific evidence for such differentiation of women's orgasms. There are merely differences in the techniques that bring on orgasm in women and variation in the intensities of orgasmic response to different techniques under differing circumstances. Furthermore, the belief that vaginal orgasm exists and is superior to or more mature than clitoral orgasm may itself create conflicts in women who do not regularly achieve orgasm through vaginal intercourse but need manual stimulation through masturbation during or after intercourse.

There are some women who come to sex therapists because they are concerned about not being able to find their "G spot." What is it? Some sex therapists claim there is a spot in women's bodies—about two inches inside and on the upper side of the vagina, between the pubic bone and the cervix—which, if sufficiently stimulated by a finger or some other means of rubbing, will bring on a very intense orgasm and secretion equivalent to an ejaculation. This spot was first identified by the German gynecologist Ernest Gräfenberg. At present there is no scientific research or consensus supporting this assertion, but writers have noted that different areas of the vagina may be intensely erotic for different women and that urinary secretions, perhaps mistaken for an ejaculate, occasionally accompany orgasmic responses in some women. Certainly women should not feel that they are inadequate or have a physiological problem because they cannot find a G spot.

PAINFUL INTERCOURSE

Women who complain of painful intercourse are usually referring to pain from one of two separate causes. One condition of pain in the vaginal area is the result of attempts at penetration. This pain may be caused by penetration not only of a penis but also of a finger or even a tampon. The other main condition of pain occurs after penetration of the penis.

What do I mean by pain, and how much discomfort should a woman accept during the act of intercourse? The only safe answer I can give is that *any discomfort* a woman feels during intercourse, whether she calls it pain or not, should be considered as such and dealt with. Slight pain doesn't mean that the woman has a problem—it may simply be caused by the position of the penis entering the vagina. On the other hand, any discomfort or pain, even when innocuous, detracts from the pleasure of the sexual act and may have harmful psychological consequences. Even a subconscious aversion to sex because of minor pain can lead to a broken relationship, something more difficult to mend than most medical or physical problems.

Of course, in the absence of an obvious simple cause for pain or discomfort, a woman should see her gynecologist as soon as possible. Use your common sense. Do not downplay the problem as just one more of the aches and pains of life. It is true that some young women having intercourse for the first few times can experience slight discomfort or painful pressure upon penetration. However, if there is more than just slight discomfort or if the slight discomfort lasts more than a reasonable number of coital acts, she must see a gynecologist.

Probably the most commonly felt pain upon and immediately following penetration occurs when a woman has not been sufficiently aroused to generate good lubrication in the vagina. Sometimes a woman does not naturally produce sufficient lubrication. If the pain seems to be due just to this, then a sexual lubricant such as K-Y jelly can be used. Petroleum-based gels should not be used when one is using a condom or diaphragm because they can cause deterioration of the contraceptive material. If the use of a lubricant does not prevent painful penetration, then a visit to a gynecologist is in order.

What about the situation where the man cannot penetrate with his penis? He may be able to get a finger in but not the penis. It may be that his penis is unusually wide, and the couple may have to try a different position. Research has shown that the vagina is very elastic and can usually accommodate all penis sizes. Sometimes the problem lies in the woman's *perception* that the penis is too large. If she grew up conditioned to think of the penis as huge, dangerous, or disgusting, perhaps because of a childhood experience, she might involuntarily contract the vaginal muscle before penetration as a way of keeping it out. The resulting pain would have nothing to do with lack of lubrication or insufficient love for the man, but would result instead from a deeply rooted fear of the penis. This type of problem must be treated by a clinical psychologist or psychiatrist.

LACK OF SEXUAL INTEREST

Several years ago I analyzed the letters that came to the different "Dr. Ruth" radio and TV shows and newspaper columns. One of the interesting findings was that almost one-fourth (24 percent) of all the people who said that they had a sexual dysfunction problem also mentioned a lack of sexual desire—and this was equally divided between men and women.

In the past, medical people apparently didn't take much notice of this problem because it was assumed that all men have a naturally strong libido, or urge to have sex, and that women have to be aroused during loving foreplay. Modern studies have found, however, that sexual desire is the natural outcome of *interest* in sex. Sexual desire, just like interest, may precede any kind of physical or psychological stimulation. In the vernacular, people use the term "horny" to mean a state of strong and sustained sexual desire. "Horniness" is the inner sexual feeling that doesn't need erotic stimulation and is the basic sensation upon which further sexual stimulation builds. Sexual desire, then, is not something that someone gives you; it is worked upon and acted upon through sensuous and other kinds of stimulation and erotic behavior you engage in even when you are by yourself. Horniness is the feeling women have that makes them want to have sex with their husbands as soon as they get home or that urges them to go call someone listed in their address book for an intimate dinner and what follows.

The sex manuals of yesteryear were certainly well intentioned and romantic in orientation but not very knowledgeable about the workings of sexual desire. The great work of Masters and Johnson and then of the sex educator and therapist Helen Singer Kaplan revolutionized our thinking about sex based on scientific research. (It should be noted that it was not until the work of Masters and Johnson was published that the medical profession began to take an interest in human sexuality. The *first* course for medical students in this subject was taught in 1968 at the Harvard Medical School.)

We now know that all too many men and women deprive themselves of the pleasures of a loving sexual relationship, even within marriage, because they are just not interested in sex—that is, they prefer not to do anything about sex, not even to think about it. In a sense, lack of interest in sex is the most extreme form of lack of sexual desire. Most people with this problem appear to have *some* interest in sex, but no real passions, urges, or strong positive feelings about it.

What do I mean by female lack of sexual desire? Some people think this describes a woman who experiences no orgasm or even sexual excitement after stimulation from a sexual partner or through masturbation. But that is *not* what I mean because lack of desire exists before the arousal stage, before the sexual interaction. It is, in its most extreme form, no desire to do anything at all about having sex.

Do not confuse lack of orgasmic response with lack of sexual desire. The lack of desire is, in varying degrees, the lack of interest—a problem of the mind, not the genitalia. When you have no interest at all, you don't even put yourself in the position where you have to behave sexually. When you have some interest but very little desire, you may act very passively and wait until your partner takes the initiative. Some people have suggested that the lack of desire is the result of the way some women have been brought up in our Western culture—that is, they have been taught to suppress their sexual feelings until aroused by a man. The paradox is that some women who complain of lack of sexual desire can easily reach orgasm, while other women who have a great deal of sexual interest and desire may be nonorgasmic. Where is it written that sex is simple to understand?

I have seen a number of cases in which women—some of them married for many years—married because it was the right time and because the men seemed like potentially good husbands and fathers. Or they were in marriages of convenience or arranged marriages. These women knew that they were expected to have intercourse, and even though they had no desire for sex, they knew there would be conflict if they didn't carry out their part of the marital contract. So they went through the motions without ever enjoying it. This does not mean that they did not care for or love their husbands but that the element of passion was missing. Many of these women realized that something was wrong, but they did not want to risk their marriages by confronting their feelings.

Their sexual performance may have been perfectly adequate. They lubricated, engaged in the pelvic motions, felt no pain or discomfort, and most conceived and became perfectly good mothers as well as wives. Except for this lack of desire, they may even have been ideal wives. These are the cases where we hear the woman saying, "Sex? I can take it or leave it." She has no aversion to sex but no desire or real interest in her human capacity for eroticism.

In some cases, this lack of desire is what we call situational. It occurs most often in the woman who professes to have no real desire for sex but can respond and even have an orgasm upon stimulation. If the husband initiates the sex, she is responsive, but if he doesn't, she is just as content. We call this case situational because some outside factor is interfering with the innate desire for sex. If the situation were altered to remove the intruding factor, she would more readily perceive that she does indeed have a desire for sex, perhaps even a very strong desire. One intruding factor that is fairly common is unrecognized anger that a woman has for her husband and that she takes to bed with her. The anger serves as a kind of colonial bundling board to keep the husband away. If her husband does not take the initiative and leap over this figurative board, they do not have sex. If you took the same woman and put her into bed with the man of her erotic dreams, she would be an aggressive tigress. If you are that potential tigress, think about what you may be bringing to bed with you before you accept the belief that you have a very low libido.

There are many other situations that can result in lowered or even blocked libido, sexual desire, or performance:

- **Stress from work, parenting, money shortages, and other problems**
- **Fear of becoming pregnant**
- **Lack of erotic and sensual practice**
  Not enough practice in pleasuring the body
- **Fear of sexual fantasizing and revealing the subconscious**
  Homosexual, incestuous, and other forbidden images come to mind
- **Problems with your partner**
  Poor hygiene, weight gain, sexual illiteracy, anger
- **Medications, alcohol, and other drugs**
  Over-the-counter medications like cold preparations, liquor, opiates, "downers," and others
- **Changing male and female roles**
  Coping with the more assertive woman, equality in marriage, and the elimination of the double standard
- **Aversion to genitalia**
  Unconscious thoughts about the vagina or penis being dirty, smelly, or dangerous
- **Sexual abuse as a child or adult**
  Incest, rape, sexual molestation, or psychosexual abuse
- **Poor self-image**
  Growing up with verbal abuse by parents: "We hope you will be lucky enough to find some man who will marry you."
- **Boredom**
  You've done it all. "Is that all there is, my friend?"

Let me make clear that it is not a case of either you do or you don't have desire. It is a matter of degree. Look at it as a scale of 1 to 10. How can you measure whether you are a 10 or an 8 or a 1? You can't! It's only a relative indicator that you can try to measure by how often and how intensely you think about sex and act upon those thoughts. I don't believe that there are people who have no desire for sex. There are those who have developed a negative desire—something that therapy could turn around to provide the person with the potential for a satisfying sex life. The first thing for such people is the recognition that their lack of sexual desire is something they probably have control over.

Can you move up your sexual desire quotient from a 3 to a 7? I believe you can by heightening your desires through developing more erotic attitudes along with healthy self-esteem.

To make matters more complicated, people vary in their desire for variety in sexual activity. Some people with a low desire for sex may still have a high desire for variety, while others with a very high desire for sex may be very much monogamous and monotonous in bed. Sex is never simple to understand! Ultimately, you have to evaluate your own desires and their impact on your love life. You'll know if you want to make it better.

TREATMENT OF SEXUAL DYSFUNCTIONS

While overcoming orgasmic difficulties may require the help of a competent sex therapist, and understanding or treating painful intercourse usually needs the services of a sex therapist or gynecologist, lack of desire is something most people can handle themselves unless it is deeply rooted in childhood trauma. In that case, you should see a clinical psychologist or psychiatrist. But in many cases, particularly where sexual boredom has set in, a little imagination, practice, and a willingness to try can do wonders. Sexually bored people generally have good emotional relations with a sexual partner but have developed a lack of sexual interest that they may interpret as a loss of libido. However, where the diminishing of sexual desire is not the result of organic difficulties or the effects of medications, it has very likely resulted from boredom with sexual activity due to long-term repetition of time, place, and techniques for sexual episodes. This can result in a loss of the excitement of anticipating sexual activity. Routinization may lead to predictability and, for many, boredom.

The treatment for sexual boredom depends, first of all, upon both partners recognizing that routinization is probably the cause of the problem and that all five senses—smell, touch, taste, sight, and hearing—are usually involved in a successful sexual act. They should also recognize that solutions depend on altering as many as possible of the sensory components surrounding the sexual act. Thus, using scented body oils, massages, and syrups that are licked from the skin, viewing erotic movies, and even verbalizing fantasies are just a few of the wide variety of activities that may help overcome boredom. What else can be tried? There are the usual strategies of going to a motel, having candlelight dinners, wearing sexy underwear, having a massage, and so forth. But there are other, lesser known or at least less often considered things you may do.

MIRRORS

One useful strategy is to use a mirror. If you don't already own one, you should buy a handheld mirror about 6 to 9 inches across. (If it has an enlarging mirror on the reverse side, all the better.) With this mirror you can more closely examine your sexual parts and become more familiar with those parts of your anatomy which give you erotic pleasure. Learn to make this association of imagery and sensation, which can be very helpful for later use in fantasy to enhance arousal and response. So lie back comfortably, propped up by pillows, and examine your genitals and other parts of your body with the mirror as you touch them. Become as familiar with the look of your genitals as you are with the back of your hand. And, if practical, why not hang a mirror above your bed or cover the wall along one side of the bed?

PORTABLE VIDEO CAMERAS

You can use a VCR in the same way that you might use a mirror. Get to know and appreciate your body as it might be seen through the eyes of your spouse or lover. Discover your best features. Study your facial and body gestures. Practice the kind of look that you want to project to your love partner. If you are not satisfied with the way you look or sound when you are turned on, change it. It is within your control. Become the film star, the hero or heroine you imagine yourself to be. There is nothing wrong with a little bit of acting.

Learn to become comfortable with your own image and the different poses, gestures, and facial expressions that make you appear more seductive and alluring. You may even find that making these very personal videos is a definite turn-on. A little bit of narcissism is good for the ego. Later on, you might consider using the video camera for an erotic turn-on when you are with your spouse or lover. Try to be an exquisite director of romantic and sensual films for your own very private viewing.

BODY MAPPING

Which part of your body is erogenous? Practically every part of the body, even the belly button, may produce erotic sensations when touched—from stroking the hair to touching and sucking the toes. It all depends upon who is doing it, how, when, and where. It is very important to get to know your own body's likes and be able to communicate them. Therefore, you should touch and stimulate yourself, within practical limits, on all parts of your body, with your bare hands, with oils, massagers, vibrators, and such. Later your partner should help touch and stimulate you in the erogenous areas you have discovered and in other places you couldn't successfully reach. It doesn't matter if you believe you are the only one in the world who enjoys a certain kind of stimulation. It's your body. Only you know the sensations you feel, so learn as much as you can about that wonderful body of yours.

Think of your entire body as a mapmaker thinks of the planet Earth. You, and later your partner, will begin to map the different types and degrees of erotic sensations you get from exploring every inch of your body. And just as mapmakers have kept refining maps over the years after more exploration, you should keep on exploring your own body, at times with the help of others, to know every inch of the erotic road. You might want to chart and rate the intensity of the erotic sensations for each part of your body: for example, the inner thigh might rate a 5, the back of the neck a 4, the nipples a 10, and so on. Later, when you are working to bring yourself to orgasm through self-stimulation or teaching your partner how to bring you to greater orgasms, start with lower levels of stimulation and proceed upward until all the 10 areas are stimulated.

VIBRATORS AND MASSAGERS

How can you best map out your body? I think that the best way is to use a vibrator. I do not mean using a vibrator to excite the clitoris and bring on an orgasm (although it is great for that too), but rather using it to become more aware of how your skin sensitivity varies in each part of the body. The use of a vibrator, in this case, merely multiplies the effect of touching lightly in each area. For instance, if you were to touch the area just below your armpit with your fingers and gently rub in a circular motion, you would probably experience a very pleasant, somewhat erotic sensation. If you tried the same thing with a vibrator, you would notice how much more you feel the sensation. And if a sexy partner were to use the vibrator on you in the same spot, you would probably experience the sensation even more pleasurably.

Which vibrator should you use out of all the types on the market? The most useful and versatile type is, luckily, the easiest one to buy. They are usually just called massagers, and you can find them in most department stores and in the mail order catalogs of the larger chains. They look a little like the portable electric mixers you hold in your hand when you beat a cake batter. Instead of the metal mixing attachments, however, there are small attachments for massaging the scalp, face, or small areas of the body. Make sure there is an attachment that is about 1½ inches in diameter with a convex surface for broader areas of skin or an attachment that is about ¾ inch long and shaped like a skinny egg for more precise identification of tiny places on the body that arouse you.

Two other types of massagers that are readily available in department stores and through the major mail order catalogs are the Swedish-type hand massager and the wand type. The wand has a cylindrical handle about 12 inches long and a vibrating knob on the end that looks like a doorknob or a slightly flattened tennis ball. It can be used in a number of ways for erotic arousal and increasing your body's sensual awareness.

The Swedish type (sometimes called the back-of-the-hand massager) has been around the longest and has been used by professional masseurs for many years. Sometimes barbers use them to relax the face and neck muscles of a customer after a haircut and shave. They are not too easy to use on yourself, except on the front of the body. Their greatest value lies in the fact that the vibrations of the motor are transferred to your fingertips. The vibrating effect of your fingers magnifies the sensitivity that the massaged skin feels, and most people prefer to be massaged by human fingertips rather than something artificial. I think you should try them all and see which you like best. You may find that each device has its good and bad points for different parts of the body.

A recently developed type of vibrator called the Eroscillator is more highly specialized and is, I believe, the best for stimulation of the labia and clitoris. The Eroscillator is small, only 7 inches in length, and shaped like an electric toothbrush with an oscillating head and a variable speed motor. While it cannot be used for wider massaging and muscle relaxation, it is so effective at narrowly focused stimulation of sensitive parts of the body that you might want to experiment with it. You might especially want one when you exercise to stimulate the clitoris.

There is one other common type of vibrator, but most women do not get much out of them. This is the type, shaped like an erect penis, that you might see in a sleazy porno store window. They seem to be more the product of male fantasy than a design for effective use by women. While they might turn some people on, they are not generally considered to be as effective as any of the models described above.

A word of caution: If you buy a massager from a reputable store or mail order service, the instruction booklet will probably contain a paragraph warning you not to use the vibrator or massager on areas of the body that are swollen or on the calf of your leg if you have any pain there. It is wise to observe these precautions because pain or swelling may conceal a blood clot that could break loose and harm you. If you have any questions about massaging any pains or swellings, consult your physician.

Some of the devices we have discussed are good for mapping out the most sensitive areas of your body—especially the portable mixer lookalike—while others are best used to increase your appreciation of your body's sensitivity to touch and pleasure. They can help you get accustomed to allowing and welcoming more bodily pleasure—a total body pleasure that can be erotic and not merely genital.

More than the finest mechanical devices on the market, you need the skills to get your body to relax. Relaxation, both mental and physical, reduces pleasure-destroying stress. I believe that massage, done by yourself or better yet with the help of a partner, is a very convenient and enjoyable way of relaxing. It helps prepare your mind and body for increased enjoyment of the sexual act. Learning how to achieve relaxation through breathing exercises can also be helpful.

Once you have bought one or more of these massagers, you will want to know how best to use it. First, you need to set aside a time for privacy when you are not going to be interrupted. Make the room as comfortable and as warm as you can. Splash on a little scented oil or massaging oil or whatever you might use to pamper yourself. Why not? You deserve it—this is *your* body you want to give more pleasure to. Take about 15 to 20 minutes a few times a week for these sessions. They will get better as you make them routine.

Make sure that negative thinking and stress factors don't interfere with your pleasure. Don't think that these exercises are only for people who have problems. All women can benefit from them, even those who have the most fantastic orgasms in the world. Everyone's appreciation of their sexuality is enhanced by increased sensitivity to the total body.

As these exercises help you become more sensitive and more relaxed, you will be better able to communicate this information to your partner, and your sexual relationship will benefit. What I am suggesting is not therapy as such; it is a technique for enhancing appreciation of your body—something you will want to do for the rest of your life and to encourage others to do for themselves. It is done for the pleasure and relaxation of your body, not as foreplay to an orgasm.

Later you may want to use similar techniques of sensual massage for accelerating and enhancing an orgasm, but first you should learn to please and pleasure your body without sexual climax always being the implicit goal. Later, when you apply what you have learned about yourself to specifically sexual and orgasmic goals, you can educate your partner about your body, your likes and dislikes. Ignore the old myth that men have an instinctive ability to please the women they really love. This is pure nonsense. Each woman is different, and each woman's body must be learned by a man who begins a sexual relationship. Without instructions from the woman, he will fumble and grope, hit and miss, until maybe, *maybe*, he stumbles onto her likes and dislikes.

And the same is true for each woman. Your knowledge of what your male partner likes and where his body is sensitive depends to a large degree on his learning about his *own* body. Each partner in a relationship must take responsibility for his or her own pleasure and responsiveness. So let the education process begin!

I suggest you consider experimenting with some other methods that can also enhance your sensual appreciation by enabling you to relax and stimulate your entire body. The first of these you can buy fairly inexpensively and install in your bathroom, even if you live in an apartment.

SHOWER MASSAGERS

The shower massager is a replacement for the conventional shower head. Yet these gadgets are quite different from ordinary shower heads. First, the head usually has an adjustable pulsator that allows the water to flow over your body in pulses rather than in a steady stream. This action, similar to certain types of massagers, can have a very soothing and sensual effect on the body. You can also vary the intensity of the steady stream from a fine needlelike spray to a heavy downpour.

Some shower massagers have a head that is attached to a portable handle. You simply unclip the massager and move the water spray to any part of your body. The warm pulsations can be aimed within an inch or two of, or directly at, your most intimate parts if you desire. Try adjusting the spray to a fine sensual mist and directing it at your genitals and other areas of your body. You are sure to learn about new sensations that your body is capable of responding to. Some people use these gadgets in the shower to reach orgasm by self-stimulation. That is fine, but first just use it for total body stimulation and relaxation and to learn more about your body's sensuality.

WHIRLPOOLS

There is a wide range of whirlpools. You can get a simple device inserted into your current bathtub to create jets of circulating air through the water. Or you can buy a larger bathtub already equipped with these jets. The larger hot-tub-size whirlpools, usually called spas, can accommodate from three to six people. They are usually installed indoors, where they take the place of the regular bathtub. They allow you to place various parts of your body right in front of the jets so that you get a powerful water massage. This can be very erotic depending on which part of the body is stimulated. Household whirlpools were developed from the kinds that athletes and patients with muscular problems have used for many years in clinics, clubhouses, and hospitals for the rehabilitation of injured or strained muscles. They have many beneficial effects on the body and they certainly do feel good. Why not double the sensuality and therapy of a whirlpool by sharing the experience with a loved one?

GETTING OLDER

One of the most prevalent sexual myths is that men and women lose their sexual drive and ability to perform as they get older. Total nonsense! For some women orgasms may become even more intense as they get on in years, while for others the intensity may remain the same or decline a bit. But certainly if you were orgasmic, you will still be able to bring on this wonderful sensation by yourself or with the help of others. And even if you have never had orgasms, it is never too late to begin!

I recommend that the older woman place a greater emphasis on lubrication, which frequently diminishes with age. If a younger woman does not lubricate sufficiently when she wants to have sex, it is usually because she has not been sufficiently stimulated and is not ready for intercourse. But when an older woman does not lubricate, it may mean that the physiology of aging just doesn't permit her to lubricate as much as she needs. It doesn't mean that her libido has changed or that she is not desirous of sex.

The treatment for reduced lubrication involves two things: first, an increase in erotic stimulation and even a little fantasy, and second, the use of a good lubricant such as K-Y jelly. Even for masturbation, I recommend that older women use a good lubricant, and it is always a good idea to use it during intercourse to avoid any pain.

Another problem I sometimes see in the older woman is not really her own problem but one that is imposed upon her by TV, movies, advertising, and so forth. The media put so much emphasis upon youth and the so-called beautiful people that they make many older women think that they are no longer attractive, especially sexually, to their husbands or any other men. But we are only as old or as attractive as we feel. Frequent and satisfying sexual activities will make you feel and be more desirable because they put you in touch with your capacity for desire and pleasure. Inactivity is the enemy for people of all ages. The more active you become with desirable interests, the more desirable and interesting you will be.

There are some women, however, who experience a loss of sexual desire due to hormonal changes. Women who notice a sharp drop in their libido should discuss this with a physician. If it turns out that your loss of desire is partly or mainly psychological, then you may want to do some of the activities suggested earlier in this chapter and get some of the mechanical aids to increase erotic stimulation or even have a consultation with a sex therapist for other suggestions.

Any hormonal causes of a loss of desire that your physician discovers should, of course, be treated medically. But this assumes that you have a comfortable relationship with your physician and can freely discuss your lack of sexual desire. Many women do not find it easy to discuss this topic. If you are one of them, what can you do? When you go to your physician, don't wait for her or him to begin the discussion of sex, particularly if your physician is a male. Even though you may have some difficulty talking about sex, keep in mind that your physician, especially if he comes from the same background as yours, probably has the same hang-ups about discussing sex comfortably as other people do. Many older physicians have had little training in human sexuality at medical school, so *you* will have to ask the right questions. If your physician cannot give you a satisfactory answer to your sex questions, he or she should refer you to someone. So don't wait for your physician to take the initiative in asking you about any changes in your sex drive—you bring up the subject. Just as I often say, *Don't complain,* now I say, *Don't wait!*

Remember, coping with stress, being more erotically oriented, pleasuring your body, learning to turn yourself on, and masturbating are not activities just for young people. They are some of the ways, along with love and commitment and caring, for all of us to have more satisfying sexual enjoyment for the rest of our lives.

USING YOUR PC

No, I don't mean using your personal computer. I mean your pubococcygeal muscle, sometimes called the PC muscle or even the "love" muscle by some writers. It is the main muscle in the pelvic area, and the more firmly toned it is, the more a woman is able to avoid urinary stress and other problems in the pelvic area. Research on this muscle has also shown that women seem to enjoy sex more and seem more likely to have orgasms when it is in good shape. I think that women should exercise this important muscle as they do other muscles in their bodies in order to stay fit. Certainly, as for all other exercise programs, you should check with your physician first to see if you have any problems that might interfere.

It is fairly easy to identify the PC muscle. It is the one you use when you want to cut off the flow of urine at will. Another way you can identify this muscle is to lie on your back and place one of your fingers about 2 inches inside your vagina. Then contract the muscles in your vaginal area just as if you wanted to stop the flow of urine. You will feel the pubococcygeal muscle tighten around your finger. Hold it there, tightly, for a few seconds. Then relax. These two motions of tightening and relaxing are essentially all you have to do to strengthen this important muscle. It will come in handy when you and your partner want to experiment with somewhat different sensations during intercourse. Try this exercise once or twice a day for a few minutes at a time. Each time you tighten the muscle, hold it tight for 5 or 6 seconds, then slowly and completely relax it. After a few seconds, repeat the contracting and relaxing of the muscle. After a few weeks you might want to hold the contraction for about 10 seconds or more. I can't promise that toning up this muscle will increase your likelihood to have orgasms or the frequency or intensity of orgasms, but at least you can use this new strength for an interesting variation during intercourse.

During coitus when you are on top, instead of moving your body up and down or forward and back, sit still and contract the PC muscle around the penis as if you were drawing the penis deeper into the vagina. After a few seconds, slowly relax and repeat the cycle. You should soon get into a rhythm of contraction and relaxation that approximates the increasing movement in most instances of intercourse. (Knowledge of this skill was brought back by many servicemen who had experienced it with Asian women, who seem to be better trained at sexual pleasuring than most women in Western culture.) You can increase the speed of these contractions until the man ejaculates. While doing this, he can stimulate your clitoris with his fingers or with a vibrator to bring you to orgasm.

A side benefit of these exercises and of this particular sexual position is that when your partner is unusually tired or seems to have more difficulty getting an erection than when he was younger, you can sit on top of him, stuff his penis inside you, and stimulate his penis to erection with these contractions. Many men report that this experience is fantastic.

EMPTY NEST SYNDROME

The portrayal of women—and to a lesser degree their husbands—as becoming depressed after their youngest child goes off to college or marries has been part of the popular mythology since the early 1970s. It is assumed that the parents' relationship changes, diminishes, because many or most couples have little communication in their marriage except around issues concerning their children. There also is the popular belief that unless the marriage is a very good one—usually assumed to be a minority of marriages—the situation precipitates crises and problems, often manifested in a loss of sexual desire resulting from depression. Proponents of the empty nest concept sometimes point out its temporal association with menopause and note the assumption that menopause also causes depression and anxiety about advancing years.

Researchers have repeatedly contradicted the popular assumptions about the empty nest syndrome as well as the psychological consequences of menopause. Studies of women from all socioeconomic classes who were primarily homemakers until the youngest child left home report they feel only brief sadness at separation from the child, usually quickly followed by feelings of relief that they are no longer tied down by the needs of the children. In another study of aging, women whose children had grown up and left home were more likely to report happy marriages than women who still had dependent children at home. This study also reported that the psychosexual life of post-middle-aged persons was far more joyous than popular myths had assumed. Recently the feminist writer Germaine Greer wrote an excellent book on the subject of menopause titled *The Change: Women, Aging and the Menopause*. In it she advocates that as women grow older, they should not look upon menopause as the end of fruitful life or as a signal to work hard at trying to look youthful through cosmetic surgery and inappropriate clothing and behavior. Instead, she would have women enjoy the experience of living fully in the joy of the present, no matter what their age, instead of bemoaning a youth long gone. Many other women writers have confronted the aging process in books that emphasize the advantages of a positive outlook. Your local library can direct you to books by Betty Friedan, Gail Sheehy, and others who are shedding a new light on the pleasures of growing older.

While depression is not inevitable at this stage of life, if it occurs it should be taken as a warning signal that there may be a problem in the marriage or elsewhere in a woman's life. Unless the causes are obvious, depression is a serious condition that should be addressed by an appropriate physician, counselor, or therapist.

A FINAL WORD

I believe that most sex educators and therapists would agree that the best sex can result from a lifelong process of learning. People change and grow, and the relationships between love, affection, sensuality, and eroticism change at different ages and time periods. If you allow yourself the right to have maximum erotic pleasure, if you are open to new ideas and erotic growth, and if you are willing to work at this learning process, sex can become better and better as you get older. And the older you become, the better lover you can be. Continue to learn and continue to love!

CONTRACEPTION AND ABORTION

Elizabeth B. Connell, M.D.

Professor, Department of Gynecology and Obstetrics, Emory
University School of Medicine, Atlanta, Georgia

Despite the many developments in all forms of birth control, sterilization, and abortion procedures, the benefits of these advances in family planning are not uniformly available in the United States, not to mention other parts of the world. Society has placed varying degrees of emphasis on the importance of these techniques. In some areas their use has been facilitated, even encouraged; in others such services have been totally discouraged; and in still others they are impossible to obtain without breaking the law.

When the *New York Times* gave comprehensive coverage in 1992 to the problems encountered by women seeking abortions, experts agreed that the percentage of women with no access to abortion was steadily increasing as the pool of hospitals, clinics, and doctors willing to perform the procedure continued to decrease. Since that time, things have become progressively worse. Fewer doctors are being trained to perform abortions, while others have become unwilling to be the targets of protesters, bomb threats and actual firebombing, murder, and continuous harassment and threats against themselves and their families. Even in large urban areas the directors of abortion clinics say that their most serious problem is recruiting doctors. Confirmation of the fact that this problem was continuing and growing worse was provided in a

1995 report by the Alan Guttmacher Institute (AGI), a nonprofit organization that does research on reproductive issues. In the years since 1988, the number of doctors available to perform abortions had fallen by 8 percent, and the percentage of obstetric and gynecology residency programs requiring first trimester abortion training had declined by 12 percent, half of what it was in 1985.

Soon after the report appeared, and coincidental with the rejection of the nomination of Dr. Henry W. Foster, Jr., to be surgeon general because he had performed a small number of abortions in his 30-year career as an obstetrician-gynecologist, the highest echelons of the medical profession decided the time had come for a more adequate fulfillment of its professional and legal responsibilities to women. Among these responsibilities was the need to increase the number of doctors properly trained to treat women who had aborted spontaneously or to perform an abortion as a life-saving measure. To achieve this goal, the Accreditation Council for Graduate Medical Education voted unanimously that, with certain exceptions, abortion skills had to be included in the training programs of prospective gynecologists and obstetricians in the teaching hospitals that employed them as residents. These new education requirements are the first to mention "abortion," replacing the previous standard that said residents were to receive clinical experience in "family planning." Although the requirements exempt institutions with moral or religious objections to abortion, such institutions must arrange for the required training at some other accredited teaching facility. Teaching hospitals that refuse to comply with this new program can be denied the accreditation required for federal reimbursement for the services provided by residents to patients.

In announcing its support for this new directive, the American Medical Association was quoted in the *New York Times* (2/15/95) as saying, "Abortion is a legal medical procedure. For the safety of patients, it is essential that physicians providing abortion services are trained and competent. Therefore the A.M.A. believes this requirement is necessary for the health and well-being of patients." In spite of this development, many women seeking an abortion still often have to travel a considerable distance or even to another state to locate a suitable facility.

From a purely economic point of view, it is clear that effective contraception has every advantage over unwanted pregnancy. This is equally true of the health implications. When one views the medical problems wrought by large numbers of unwanted pregnancies in terms of illegal abortion, increased infant and maternal illness and death, and the increase in psychological problems (in both parents and children), there are compelling reasons for making contraceptives freely available to all those who need and wish to use them. Most women who want the most up-to-date information about contraception can usually find it through a health provider in their own community. This is critical, since women's ability to have the number of children they want and at a time that they want them is central to the quality of their lives and the well-being of their families. Unfortunately, most politicians who have made a political issue of "family values" rarely acknowledge the role of family planning in promoting these values.

RISK-BENEFIT RATIO

The question is often asked, "What is the best method of family planning?" At the present time there is no single "best" method, and there will be none until the "ideal contraceptive" is discovered, which will probably never happen. The attributes of the ideal contraceptive are that it be totally safe, effective, and reversible; that it be inexpensive, easy to distribute, and easy to use; and that its use be unrelated to the actual time of sexual relations. Since no such contraceptive is yet available, we must continue to deal with what is known as the risk-benefit ratio. The results of a report presented by the Guttmacher Institute in 1991 indicate that, contrary to popular opinion, using birth control is safer and healthier for the majority of women than not using it.

Among the significant findings of the report was the fact that, on average, women who have used the pill at some time are less likely to develop cancer and die as a result before age 55 than women who have never used the pill. Using contraception, including the pill, saves 120 to 150 lives per 100,000 women, and it also prevents about 1,500 hospitalizations per 100,000 women each year. The report also presents compelling evidence that the protective effects of oral contraceptives—which include lowering the risk of endometrial and ovarian cancer, endometriosis, pelvic inflammatory disease, benign breast disease, and ectopic pregnancy, as well as eliminating the hazards of pregnancy and/or abortion—far outweigh the danger of serious side effects. As for the conflicting statistics about breast cancer and the pill, the Guttmacher Institute's study points out that while women in their thirties and early forties who have used the pill for many years may have an increased risk of breast cancer, there are fewer breast cancers among long-term users of the pill who are in their late forties and early fifties than among women in that age group who have never used the pill at all. Also, the use of barrier methods such as the condom or the diaphragm, as well as spermicides, lowers the risk of developing cervical cancer and pelvic inflammatory disease. According to Dr. Jacqueline

Forrest, vice-president for research at the institute, "The riskiest thing to do for your health if you are sexually active, is to use no method of contraception."

Since this study, a number of new contraceptive methods have become available. They are discussed in detail in the pages that follow.

Unfortunately, leaving aside the easy availability of the condom for both sexes, a 1995 study by the Kaiser Family Foundation of Menlo Park, California, has found that 70 percent of the men surveyed thought that "men are not responsible enough to make birth control choices" and about the same number of women agreed.

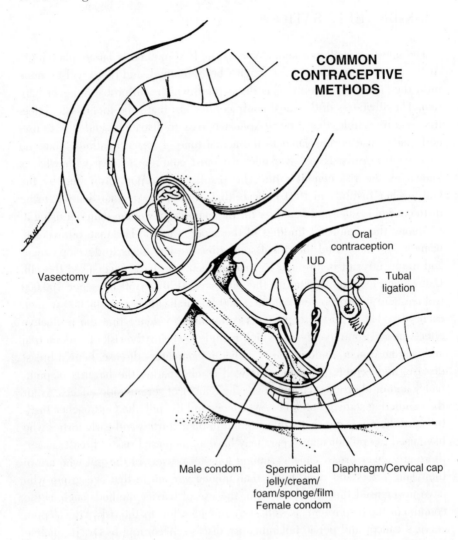

**COMMON
CONTRACEPTIVE
METHODS**

Oral
contraception

IUD

Vasectomy

Tubal
ligation

Male condom   Spermicidal   Diaphragm/Cervical cap
                     jelly/cream/
                     foam/sponge/film
                     Female condom

SELECTION OF METHODS

A woman should carefully consider several factors when deciding which birth control method to use, after discussing all the options with her health care provider. First of all, medical factors must be considered. It has been shown that the risk of death for any woman in good health up to the age of 35 is lower using any of the currently available methods than becoming pregnant and carrying a child to term. After the age of 35, any method is much safer than becoming pregnant and having a baby, except for women who take oral contraceptives and smoke. In the current climate of great anxiety about the side effects of pills, IUDs, Norplant, and DMPA, these two facts are often ignored. These comparisons are valid in developed countries where health care is excellent; they are infinitely more important in developing countries. In areas of the world where health care is minimal or absent, the risks associated with pregnancy, illegal abortion, and childbirth far outweigh any possible danger associated with contraceptive use. When a woman is not in perfect health, it is necessary to look at the specific contraindications to the use of any particular form of family planning. These will be considered under the various methods.

In addition to purely physical factors, emotional, behavioral, and psychological factors must also be taken into consideration when selecting a contraceptive technique. Even though you may be perfectly capable of using a particular method from a purely medical point of view, if you have a distaste for that method or harbor undue concern or anxiety about its use, then it is not the method for you. If you know that you cannot remember to take pills properly or use a barrier method each time you have intercourse, or if you find the use of implants or DMPA unacceptable, you must take this into account.

Certain social and economic factors also come into play, including the cost of the contraceptive method, the availability of health care for the initiation of the technique and for the follow-up required, and numerous religious and cultural attitudes.

It must also be recognized that the method that is "best" for a particular woman may change a number of times during her lifetime. For example, a teenager or a college student who has sexual relations only infrequently should probably not take oral contraceptives but should use a male or female barrier method. However, if she is sexually active, she may well turn to the use of oral contraceptives. Barring any difficulties and if she does not smoke, she may continue with this method up to the time of her menopause. She also has the option of using an IUD, or she may consider being injected every three months with Depo-Provera DMPA, a recently approved contraceptive drug. A young woman who wishes to postpone starting a family for several years may choose the subdermal contraceptive implant, which is effective for five years. Once she has had a child, she may select an intrauterine device but only if she is in a mutually monogamous situation. As she approaches her perimenopausal years, she has several options. She may continue with the pill, have an intrauterine device inserted, use Norplant or DMPA, go back to a barrier method, or if she and her partner are convinced that they do not want any more children, consider sterilization of either one as a possible alternative.

It should be added that many women who rely on other methods to prevent pregnancy should use female condoms in addition for protection against sexually transmissible diseases—not only the AIDS virus but also genital warts, chlamydia, herpes, hepatitis, and others. The female condom is described in this chapter as the barrier methods of contraception.

HORMONAL METHODS—FEMALE: "THE PILL"

Women through the centuries have swallowed all sorts of concoctions made of plant and animal materials in their attempts to prevent or terminate unwanted pregnancies. During the Middle Ages thousands of women died of mercury, strychnine, or lead poisoning when they used these agents to try to control their fertility. With the discovery of oral contraceptives, women for the first time had a technique that, if taken as directed, was virtually 100 percent effective.

The combined oral contraceptives (estrogen plus progestin) have been in use since 1960, and the mini-pill (progestin alone) for more than 20 years. These agents have been more widely studied than any medication in medical history.

The OCs of today are radically different from their predecessors. Although the specific hormones are essentially the same or similar, the dosages and formulations have undergone tremendous changes. There are two major types of OCs available in the United States today. One is the combined pill made in two different forms: estrogen and progestin in the same dose throughout the treatment cycle and the newer form, the multiphasic pill, with varying doses in different parts of the cycle to reduce the total hormone dose to the lowest possible levels consistent with effectiveness. The other, the minipill, contains only the progestin and is taken daily.

The combined estrogen and progestin pills prevent pregnancy by stopping ovulation, the monthly release of an egg by an ovary. Their use as a contraceptive method is based on the fact that during pregnancy these hormones, made by the ovaries and placenta, block the production of the hormones that are responsible for ovulation, thus preventing the establishment of an additional pregnancy. In the case of the minipill, the mechanism is somewhat more complicated. Studies have shown that not all women who use these pills stop ovulating. The mechanism (or mechanisms) of action in this instance appears to be the effects of the hormone on the cervical mucus, the lining of the uterus, the fallopian tubes, and other anatomical changes. While similar effects also occur with the combined pills, their effectiveness is achieved mainly by the blocking of ovulation.

POTENTIAL SIDE EFFECTS

Not long after widespread use of the pill began, early studies began to suggest that certain complications were occurring in a small number of women. However, because of the complexity of our daily lives, it is very difficult to relate a particular adverse reaction to a particular medication. Given the number of drugs in common use, the various food additives, the multiple pollutants in our environment, not to mention the innumerable variables of individual responses, it takes wide usage of a particular drug over a considerable period of time to be able to make an accurate assessment of possible adverse side effects. It is important to note that many of the earlier fears were overstated and some actually unfounded. This was particularly true as the hormonal doses were radically decreased.

Cardiovascular

The first side effects reported were related to the cardiovascular system. The first risk that was described in both British and American studies was the development of thromboembolic disease—the formation of blood clots, usually in the deep veins of the legs, some of which could break off and travel to the lungs or the brain, producing serious damage and occasionally death. This complication was found to be related to the estrogen component, and its frequency has progressively decreased as the dosage of estrogen in the pill has been reduced from 100 to 150 micrograms to 30 to 35 micrograms or less.

The next cardiovascular risk to be identified was stroke. Once again, the chances of having a stroke have decreased as the dosages of estrogen and, more importantly, progestin have been reduced.

The complication of heart attack is rare before the age of 35; prior to that age there is virtually no difference in the rate of heart attack between users and nonusers of the pill. It is essential to note that the risk of heart attack associated with the use of oral contraceptives is almost entirely limited to those women over 35 who smoke, particularly those who smoke heavily, and especially in those who have additional risk factors such as high blood pressure, diabetes, obesity, elevated blood cholesterol or low-density lipoproteins (LDL), or lowered high-density lipoproteins (HDL).

Women who have major surgery, particularly pelvic or abdominal surgery, also have been found to have a four- to sixfold increase in thromboembolic complications. Pills should be stopped at least four weeks prior to major elective surgery and another contraceptive prescribed. The alternative contraceptive should be continued after surgery until the woman is fully ambulatory. The same rules hold true for women who are immobilized—for example, because of serious fractures—for a long period of time.

Metabolic

A number of metabolic changes have been observed in women taking oral contraceptives, related primarily to sugar and fat metabolism. These changes are primarily due to the progestin component. They lead to the elevation of blood sugar as seen in diabetics and to a pattern in blood lipids similar to those found in people with cardiovascular diseases. With the new low-dose pills, however, these alterations are either minimal or entirely absent. What this means from a clinical point of view, however, has yet to be determined.

A very few women have a profound elevation in their blood pressure when they first start taking oral contraceptives. This hypertension disappears promptly when the pill is stopped. A certain number of other women develop a mild increase of blood pressure as they continue to take oral contraceptives. However, their blood pressure usually remains within normal limits and usually returns to pretreatment levels after stopping the pill.

Where liver, kidney, or gallbladder malfunction is present, it might be advised to discontinue or not begin the birth control pill in favor of some other form of contraception.

Fetal

A number of years ago, it was alleged that oral contraceptives caused fetal damage. However, there have been many studies to determine whether oral contraceptives taken early in pregnancy have any adverse effect on an unborn baby. It is important to note that current studies do not show any relationship between nongenital fetal damage and use of OCs.

Tumors and Cancers

British and American studies have both shown that there is a 50 percent lower incidence of benign and malignant ovarian tumors in women taking the combined pill. In addition, it exerts a similar protective effect against endometrial cancer. Even more important, this protection against both ovarian and endometrial cancers occurs once a woman has taken the pill for at least one year and lasts for over 15 years after she stops. Studies to determine if there is an increase in cervical dysplasia and cancer attributable to the pill remain inconclusive. Some researchers report an increase in cervical cancer in women who use the pill for more than five years. No such findings have been reported by the Centers for Disease Control and Health Promotion. As is the case with all women, since cervical cancer can be detected in its earliest stages, an annual Pap test should be done. Also, a pelvic exam can screen for STDs, now believed to be the major cause of cervical cancer.

Although there has been a great deal of negative publicity about the relationship between the use of the pill and breast cancer, there are no data confirming a causative connection. One of the most reliable studies, conducted under the auspices of the Centers for Disease Control, concluded that regular use of the pill results in a slight increase in breast cancers diagnosed before age 35, no increased risk between ages 35 and 44, and a lowered risk for ages 45 to 54. All of the larger, more recent well-controlled studies have failed to show any association even in women considered to be at high risk because of factors such as a family history of this disease. Moreover, there is a significant reduction in the number of women who develop two very common benign conditions—fibroadenomas and fibrocystic disorder.

Drug Interactions

Studies have shown that interactions may occur between certain drugs. In the case of the pill, several drugs can reduce the pill's contraceptive effectiveness and also may result in bleeding between periods. Many women no longer have a primary care doctor who has a computerized record of all their medications. In such cases, when a woman using the pill is handed a prescription for a drug she has never taken before, it is extremely important that she ask the doctor how this medication will affect the performance of the pill. Although rarely necessary, she may have to make a temporary switch to a higher dose pill or to a different contraceptive method. The most important of these agents include barbiturates (phenobarbital), phenytoin (Dilantin), and certain antibiotics, especially isoniazid, rifampin, and possibly tetracycline. Women who have to take these products on a long-term basis should be given a 50-microgram oral contraceptive.

CONTRAINDICATIONS

At the present time the U.S. Food and Drug Administration (FDA) lists a number of absolute contraindications to the use of the pill. The list is based on proven major adverse side effects, as in the case of the cardiovascular disorders, and on conditions for which a relationship is suspected but not necessarily proven.

1. Known cardiovascular conditions or a past history of these conditions, including thrombophlebitis and thromboembolic disorders (formation of blood clots and embolisms), cerebrovascular disease (stroke), myocardial infarction (type of heart attack), or coronary artery disease.
2. Markedly impaired liver function.
3. Known or suspected carcinoma of the breast.
4. Known or suspected estrogen-dependent neoplasia (abnormal tissue growth).
5. Undiagnosed abnormal genital bleeding.
6. Known or suspected pregnancy.

As we have mentioned, more and more evidence is being accumulated showing that the combination of increasing age and heavy smoking raises the risks of heart attack and stroke considerably higher than either age or smoking alone. In fact, current data indicate that the two factors have a synergistic effect—one in the presence of the other increases the risk that each could produce separately, and their combined effect is greater than the sum of their effects simply added together.

Therefore women over 35, particularly those with additional risk factors, should not take the pill if they smoke or should not smoke if they take the pill. Obviously, as a general health measure, women should be encouraged not to smoke whether they take the pill or not. Indeed, it has been suggested, not entirely facetiously, that, given the differences in relative risks, pills should be put in vending machines and cigarettes placed on prescription!

There is increasing concern about the use of Accutane for severe acne because it is clearly associated with fetal damage. Women using this drug should not become pregnant and should always be protected by a highly effective method of contraception such as the pill.

MINOR ADVERSE SIDE EFFECTS

There are a number of side effects, most of which disappear by the end of the third cycle, that are annoying but not serious or life-threatening. Among the most frequent of these are alterations in the menstrual flow, most often a decrease (a change that is considered to be desirable by many women and prevents iron deficiency anemia). There may also be irregular spotting and bleeding between periods, heavier bleeding at the time of the menses, and, on occasion, a total absence of menses. Breast tenderness may be observed, and there is often an increase in the amount of vaginal discharge. Nausea with occasional vomiting occurs but is usually seen early. Weight gain is noted by some women, but this is much more apt to be related to changes in food intake than to the pill. Pigmentation over the forehead and cheeks, the same type seen in pregnancy, may also occur with use of oral contraceptives and often does not go away after stopping use of the pill.

BENEFICIAL SIDE EFFECTS

Too often only the potential adverse side effects of the pill are presented by all forms of media. The beneficial side effects of the pill are only rarely discussed in the same context, which is most unfortunate since it is the considered opinion of the medical profession that the advantages of using the pill far outweigh the disadvantages. Even when new evidence refutes earlier indications of risks, this is either not reported or is underreported.

A number of salutary changes have been noted, such as decreases in breast, ovarian, and uterine tumors. In addition, certain very common benign breast tumors, fibroadenomas, and fibrocystic disorder are less common in women who use OCs. Women whose cycles are extremely irregular or who have heavy menstrual bleeding resulting in anemia may be virtually assured that these problems will be solved by the use of oral contraceptives. Premenstrual syndrome (PMS) and menstrual discomfort are also often relieved, and acne frequently diminishes markedly. Of major importance is the fact that women who take the pill have fewer ectopic pregnancies and ovarian retention cysts as well as less risk of developing rheumatoid arthritis and pelvic inflammatory disease (PID), toxic shock syndrome, uterine fibroids, osteoporosis, and endometriosis.

INJECTABLES

An injectable intraceptive, Depo-Provera is now approved by the FDA. It is a long-acting hormonal preparation given by injection to block ovulation. This contraceptive method benefits all women but particularly women who, because of medical, social, or psychological reasons, cannot cope with the demands of pill-taking or the use of barrier methods. Moreover, when health care personnel and facilities are limited, a technique that requires a single act of motivation on the part of the patient and infrequent professional follow-up is obviously highly desirable.

Depo-Provera is a synthetic form of the natural hormone progesterone. It prevents pregnancy by inhibiting ovulation. It is administered every three months by injection into the buttocks or into the muscle at the back of the arm and is 99 percent effective. Since it contains no estrogen, it has none of the undesirable side effects associated with this hormone. Before it was approved by the FDA in 1992, it had already been available for more than 20 years in more than 90 countries worldwide and used by more than 30 million women.

Among the advantages of using Depo-Provera are the following: It is effective and safe for most women. It is effective for three months and can be discontinued at any time. It reduces some of the discomforts of PMS, as well as menstrual cramps. Some studies indicate that it reduces the risk of pelvic inflammatory disease and endometrial cancer.

There are also disadvantages: It offers no protection against sexually transmitted diseases. There is no way of discontinuing its contraceptive effectiveness during the three-month period following injection. In some cases it may take as long as two years to reestablish fertility, although ultimate fertility is not changed. Weight gain and irregular bleeding are possible side effects, particularly early in use. The majority of those who continue to use Depo-Provera stop having menstrual periods, a fact found to be attractive to teenagers once they know that this does not mean that they are pregnant or sick.

Women who do not intend to become pregnant in the near future and would like to be relieved of the responsibility of remembering to take their oral contraceptive on the indicated days now have the option of trying out another type of birth control that they need think about no more often than four times a year. Use of this agent, like any other, should be discussed in detail with one's doctor. Unfortunately, it along with breast implants and Norplant, has become a target for personal injury attorneys claiming autoimmune damage in the absence of scientific evidence.

IMPLANTS

Following many years of research here and abroad in attempts to create a safe and effective implantable contraceptive, the FDA gave its approval in 1990 to Norplant, which uses implants that provide contraception for up to five years. Six matchstick-size capsules containing progestin are implanted under the skin of the woman's upper arm in a procedure requiring local anesthesia. The capsules slowly release the hormone over a five-year period and can be renewed if desired. Fertility is restored when they are removed. The capsules or rods are made of a blend of silicone and plastic; the incision through which they are implanted is no larger than 1/4 inch deep and is usually closed with a single stitch or an adhesive strip. In the event of any complications, the implants are removed. Both procedures are done on an outpatient basis. It is important that the insertion be done by someone well trained in the procedure. Removal may be difficult if the insertion was not done properly. The implant has many attractions for women who do not wish to begin a family or who don't want any more children even though they are many years away from the menopause. It has a low failure rate, and in a recent study of teenage mothers seeking an effective contraceptive, Norplant was their preference over the pill by a significant margin.

Among the advantages of Norplant is that it may reduce the risk of pelvic inflammatory disease and endometrial cancer; it decreases anemia and has no unpleasant estrogen-related side effects; it releases the user from the responsibility of having to remember her pill days. As for the high cost of the product and the implantation procedure, Medicaid and other third-party health insurance cover some of the expenses. Where this coverage is not available, it should be taken into account that the total cost is probably no greater than a five years' supply of oral contraceptives. As with the other hormonal methods, Norplant should not be used by women who have breast cancer, liver dysfunction, phlebitis, or unexplained irregular vaginal bleeding. Unfortunately, the use of this highly effective method of contraception is now sharply reduced because of escalating numbers of lawsuits. Many of these allege the causation of autoimmune diseases or symptoms, despite the fact that there are no scientific data to support this.

THE "MORNING AFTER" PILL

According to a 1995 survey supervised by the Kaiser Family Foundation of Menlo Park, California, most gynecologists know about morning-after pills that can prevent pregnancy, but they seldom prescribe them because they wait for women to ask. And a related survey indicates that most women don't ask about the pills because they don't know anything about them. Many doctors have been aware of this method (more appropriately called emergency contraception to indicate one-time use) for at least 20 years, and it has been prescribed on college campuses for some time. It has just recently been approved by the FDA, but no company has yet been willing to bring it to the market for fear of litigation. It remains largely unknown to women in their thirties and to teenagers and their social workers.

When the pills are used properly within 72 hours of unprotected mid-cycle intercourse, they prevent at least 98 percent of the pregnancies that might otherwise occur. Some authorities estimate that the general availability of emergency contraception could conservatively reduce unintended pregnancies by 1.7 annually and abortions by about 8,000. And what a great relief to a woman who realizes after the fact that she had completely unprotected sex the night before or is at risk of pregnancy because a condom broke or her diaphragm or cervical cap was dislodged or, at worst, because of rape.

Although there are several treatment options, including high doses of estrogen, the regimen currently favored in the United States uses one of the oral contraceptive pills, Ovral, containing a high dose of progestin. Two tablets are taken within 72 hours of unprotected sex, then two more 12 hours after the first dose, once a prior pregnancy has been ruled out. The pills probably act by preventing the fertilized egg from implanting itself in the lining of the uterus. Far less likely, the release of the egg from the ovary is stopped, or fertilization of the released egg by the sperm is disrupted.

Because many women experience extreme nausea after taking the treatment, it is advisable to ask for an oral or suppository antinauseant or to ask for extra pills in the event that vomiting occurs. The nausea and severe cramps usually subside the day after treatment is completed. Other possible side effects include breast tenderness, headache, and dizziness. A gynecological checkup should be scheduled three weeks after treatment. If menstruation hasn't occurred within that time, a pregnancy test should be performed and a therapeutic abortion offered, if positive.

INTRAUTERINE DEVICES

We know that the use of intrauterine devices goes back to the dawn of history. Among the earliest were the pebbles placed in the uterus of a camel to keep her from getting pregnant on long trips across the desert. Metal devices have also been used by women in the past. However, because of concerns about infection, their use flourished briefly and then was abandoned.

In the 1970s and '80s, IUDs once again regained their popularity, being used by 2 to 3 million American women. Unfortunately, because of growing problems related to litigation and product liability insurance, all but one IUD (Progestasert) were taken off the market. Fortunately for women for whom IUDs are the method of choice, the best of the copper-bearing IUDs, the Copper T-380A or ParaGard, was introduced in mid-1988. Currently, the Copper T-380 and Progestasert are the only IUDs available in the United States. Both are T-shaped and have plastic strings attached to the tails. According to the *PDR (Physician's Desk Reference) Family Guide to Women's Health*, the Copper-T "has the best track record of any contraceptive product. Your odds of becoming pregnant during the first year of use are only 1 in 500." The ParaGard remains effective for 10 years and acts to prevent fertilization.

An intrauterine device is inserted through the cervix into the uterus by a trained specialist with the use of special instruments. Following insertion, it is quite common to have cramping and spotting, but this usually disappears after a few hours or days. IUDs may be inserted at any time, but it is easier to do so around the time of ovulation because the cervix is dilated slightly, if there is no chance of the woman's being pregnant.

The Progestasert—a hormone-bearing device—contains progesterone, which it releases daily, causing the cervical mucus to thicken and prevent the sperm from traveling any farther. While it is effective, it has the disadvantage of having to be changed each year.

A woman who wants an IUD needs to be evaluated carefully. She needs to have a thorough medical evaluation including a pelvic examination, Pap smear, and any other indicated studies. Most important is an investigation of her personal history. A woman who has a sexually transmitted disease, who has a large number of sexual partners, or who is monogamous but unsure that her spouse or partner is the same is not a good candidate for an IUD. Recurrent pelvic infections, problems with blood clotting, and very heavy periods or severe menstrual cramps are reasons for choosing some other contraceptive method. When careful evaluation indicates the woman is a suitable candidate for an IUD, an insertion may be carried out. The cervix is cleansed, and a tube containing the collapsed IUD is inserted through the cervix. When the tube is removed, the IUD unfolds in place. The strings that extend through the cervical opening should be used to check after each menstrual period that the IUD remains in its proper position. If the string is longer or shorter than usual or if it can no longer be felt, the doctor should be consulted promptly to find out whether the IUD has shifted to an improper place or if it has been expelled.

It is currently believed that the IUD is not the method of choice for most women who have not yet had a child.

ADVERSE SIDE EFFECTS

Women who are considering an IUD should recognize that use of an IUD carries with it the risk of certain adverse effects.

Initial Discomfort

For the first few days after insertion, women often experience cramps and bleeding. During the first few periods that follow, there may be heavier bleeding than usual, and the periods may last longer. Since increased bleeding for as long as three months can result in anemia, iron supplements should be considered.

Expulsion

Any IUD may be expelled, most often during the first menses or the first three months of use. Although in most cases the expulsion is noted, some women are unaware that this has happened. Signs of expulsion are

- return of cramps and abdominal pain;
- disappearance of strings or strings that have become longer than before;
- visibility or palpability of the tip of the IUD;
- signs of pregnancy.

Perforation of the Uterus

One of the most compelling reasons for a medical checkup when the strings cannot be felt is the possibility that the IUD has perforated the wall of the uterus or cervix or has become embedded in the uterine wall. Although most perforations occur at the time of insertion, on occasion they may be noted later. Prompt location with special instruments and, if necessary, with ultrasound, enables the doctor to remove it and take any additional measures that are necessary.

Pelvic Inflammatory Disease

(For a detailed discussion of PID, see "Gynecologic Problems and Treatment.")

It is now well documented that the incidence of PID is highest among women who have multiple sex partners or whose partner(s) have multiple sexual partners and in those who have had this disease before. The notion that the IUD in and of itself is the cause of PID was proved false by a recent study conducted by the World Health Organization. Of approximately 23,000 IUD users, only 81 cases developed PID, with the risk six times higher during the first three weeks after insertion. Administering an antibiotic at the time of insertion may lower the risk, although this remains unproven.

Intrauterine Pregnancy

If a pregnancy develops in the uterus even though the IUD is in place, there is a 50 percent chance that a miscarriage will occur. The possibility of a miscarriage is reduced by half if the IUD is removed as soon as the diagnosis of pregnancy is made. If this is not done, there is an increased risk of infection, stillbirth, and premature delivery. However, it is important to note that there is no risk of direct damage to the fetus if a pregnancy goes to term with the IUD still in place.

Ectopic Pregnancy

Recent research indicates that one in every five users of Progestasert has an ectopic pregnancy every year, but only one in 60 women using a copper IUD will have a similar experience. This latter group also has far fewer ectopic pregnancies than women who use no contraception.

Effects on Fertility

In most instances a contraceptive method other than an IUD should be the choice of a woman who has not yet had a child but who is planning to become pregnant at some time in the future. However, there are occasional situations where the IUD is still the method of choice for such women when they are in a mutually monogamous, uninfected relationship and have contraindications to other birth control methods. In addition, use of the ParaGard is the most cost-effective method available today.

Malignancy

Considerable concern has been expressed about whether or not the continued presence of an IUD can stimulate malignancy. Careful prolonged study of thousands of women wearing IUDs, some of them for many years, has failed to show a connection between the presence of this device and the subsequent development of a malignancy of the cervix or the uterus.

BARRIER CONTRACEPTIVES

Barrier contraceptives, such as the condom and the diaphragm combined with spermicides, were virtually discarded in favor of the pill and IUD because the newer methods were more effective, easier to use, and didn't require application with each act of intercourse. The older methods were considered messy, unromantic, a nuisance, and the cause of diminished pleasure, whereas the pill and IUD could provide close to 100 percent assurance against unwanted pregnancy with ease and unobtrusiveness. More recently, however, several factors have caused a partial reversal in attitudes.

The earliest return to the diaphragm and other barrier methods resulted from objections to the pill by many feminists and health advocates on the following grounds: that it introduced chemicals into the body whose long-term effects might not be known for decades, that the pill was an invasive factor contraindicated by a respect for the body's natural functioning, and that it was an ongoing expensive procedure whose end result was the enrichment of the pharmaceutical companies. Particularly among educated women, ironically enough, the slogan was "If the diaphragm was good enough for mother, it's good enough for me."

As for the male latex condom, it has now emerged as the major and only FDA-approved form of protection against the transmission of AIDS as well as herpes, hepatitis, gonorrhea, and other sexually transmissible diseases. In addition, studies have shown that the various spermicides (foams, jellies, creams, film suppositories, foaming tablets), diaphragms, cervical caps, and the contraceptive sponge (no longer on the market), when used properly and consistently with each act of sexual intercourse, actually have a far higher rate of effectiveness than thought by the general public and, in fact, by many physicians. The key to this, of course, is absolute adherence to proper and consistent usage. Each barrier method has its own special instructions for use on the package, which must be followed carefully if these levels of effectiveness are to be attained.

A major compelling advantage of barrier methods is the fact that there are no health risks associated with them except for rare cases of allergic response or local irritation. The most vexing problem is the rate of unwanted pregnancies when these methods are used. A woman who relies on them through all the years of her childbearing capability may have an average of two or three unwanted pregnancies. However, from a statistical point of view, if they are terminated early by suction abortion, the combined health risks she faces are extremely low.

DIAPHRAGM

It has been shown recently that, despite widespread opinions to the contrary, the diaphragm can be used effectively by women who are young and inexperienced and who, for these and other reasons, would hardly be considered ideal candidates for the use of any sex-related method. In one study, when such a group was properly instructed and constantly encouraged, they had a failure rate of less than 2 percent, which is in the general range of pills and intrauterine devices.

To fit properly, the size and type of diaphragm must be determined by the anatomy of the individual woman. If a diaphragm is too small, it may not stay in place and may slip off the cervix; if it is too large, it may press on the urethra and cause a urinary tract infection. It must always be used with a spermicidal agent and be left in place for approximately six hours but no more than 24 hours. If intercourse occurs again during this time, more spermicide must be inserted. Because of the possibility of developing toxic shock syndrome, diaphragms should not be left in for more than six hours after the last act of intercourse and should not be used during menses.

CERVICAL CAP

The cervical cap was used in the U.S. but disappeared with the emergence of the pill and IUD. It has been used with spermicide by many women, especially by those in self-help groups, and was approved by the FDA in 1988. It is popular because it is smaller than a diaphragm and may be left in place for 48 hours without having to add additional spermicide. The device, which is made of plastic, looks like a thimble. It fits over the cervix and is held in place by suction. When used correctly and combined with a spermicide, it has an effectiveness rate of approximately 94 to 95 percent. Not every woman who wants to use a cap can be fitted, and some women find insertion and removal more difficult than with the diaphragm. Reported risks include vaginal or cervical infections, and abnormal Pap test results but no increase in cervical cancer.

VAGINAL SPONGE

A barrier method formerly available over the counter was a small disposable sponge made of polyurethane and permeated with a spermicide. The sponge did not need to be fitted by a physician, and one of its chief attractions was that it allowed for more spontaneous sexual activity than the diaphragm. Its effectiveness was based on its action as a barrier, the inactivation of sperm by the spermicide, and the absorption by the sponge of the ejaculated semen. The sponge could be inserted hours before intercourse and kept in place for 24 hours, during which time intercourse could take place repeatedly without any further preparation. It had approximately the same effectiveness as the diaphragm and the cervical cap. The sponge was removed from the market by its manufacturers not because of health risks, but because FDA-mandated improvements in its production proved to be too costly.

CONDOM—WORN BY THE MALE

While condoms have been used in one form or another since the time of the ancient Egyptians, it is only in recent years that they have been used not only for contraception but also as protection against the transmission of sexually transmissible diseases (STDs), including HIV. In 1977, when the Supreme Court declared anti-condom laws unconstitutional, condoms came out of the druggists' hidden stock. They are now openly displayed and sold in vending machines nationwide. They are also available free and on request in many high schools nationwide.

According to a recent study by the National Center for Health Statistics, the condom remains the device most commonly used in the first sexual encounter. Today sales to women make up 40 percent or more of the total; condoms are advertised in women's magazines and displayed in drugstores next to feminine hygiene products. They are now being made in a variety of colors and are being manufactured out of materials that are thinner and therefore interfere less with sensation. Various textures are being used to increase the pleasurable sensations accompanying their use. Lubricants and spermicides are being applied to the condom for easier and more effective use; however, extra lubricant may increase the risk of slippage during withdrawal.

It is important that the condom be put on before any contact is made with the vulva and that ½ inch be left free at the end of the penis to catch the seminal fluid unless the condom is made with a reservoir at the tip. The penis and condom should be removed together from the vagina shortly after ejaculation, holding onto the rim of the condom so that no spillage occurs. Furthermore, in the training of potential users, efforts are being made to involve the female in applying the condom to eliminate the serious objection many men have when they are forced to stop in the middle of foreplay to put one on. When putting on the condom is made part of foreplay, this sense of interruption is dispelled and the acceptability of the condom is proportionately increased.

Condom use should be recommended to all women who are at risk for STDs. This is true even for those who are using a highly effective contraceptive method such as the pill, Depo-Provera, or Norplant because they provide no protection against the transmission of STDs, including HIV.

CONDOM—WORN BY THE FEMALE

Approved by the FDA in 1993, the female condom, named Reality, is a disposable birth control device made of polyurethane, which is stronger and less likely to tear than the latex used for most male condoms. The device is a sheath with a diaphragm-like ring at each end. The ring at the closed end is inserted into the vagina like a diaphragm and holds the sheath in place over the cervix. Because the ring at the other end remains outside the vagina, it provides additional protection by forming a barrier between the labia and the base of the penis.

This female condom requires no fitting because it comes in one size only, and it can be inserted at any time before intercourse. While it is more expensive than a male condom, it has the unique advantage of giving women complete control over a barrier method of contraception that also provides maximum protection against sexually transmissible diseases.

BARRIER METHODS IN COMBINATION

It is now being increasingly appreciated that the combination of a male and a female method such as, for example, condom plus spermicide, has a very high rate of effectiveness with a failure rate of approximately 1 percent. The lack of any serious side effects of the various barrier methods makes them extremely attractive for those individuals who have sexual relations very infrequently, who have contraindications to the pill and the IUD, and who are looking for maximum safety in the use of a form of contraception as well as for protection against AIDS and other STDs.

NATURAL FAMILY PLANNING—
PERIODIC ABSTINENCE

New attention is also being paid to methods of natural family planning—previously called rhythm and now often called fertility observation or ovulation detection and periodic abstinence—largely because these techniques are the only ones acceptable to the Roman Catholic church and other groups. They are all based on the premise that sexual intercourse must be avoided during that time span of each menstrual cycle when ovulation is occurring. Calculations of "safe" and "unsafe" days for intercourse can be made in different ways, all based on the fact that the unsafe days usually begin several days before ovulation and continue for three to five days thereafter.

The four recognized methods of natural planning are the ovulation method, the temperature method, and the cervical mucus method, and the symptothermal method. (1) In the *ovulation method,* a precise record is compiled of the length of the menstrual cycle for one year. In typical cases, ovulation occurs 14 days before menstruation begins. Therefore, taking into account the four- to five-day life span of the sperm and the 24-hour life span of the egg, the unsafe days can be calculated. (2) *The temperature method:* Body temperature rises slightly following ovulation and stays elevated until the next onset of menstruation. A woman must take her temperature every morning before she gets out of bed. She must abstain from intercourse each month until three days after the temperature rise. (3) *The cervical mucus method:* In the course of the menstrual cycle, the consistency of the mucus varies greatly. At the time of ovulation it is clear, thin, copious, and watery. At all other times it is thick, gray, and sparse. (4) *The symptothermal method:* This is a combination of the temperature method plus the detection of a number of physical changes associated with ovulation. The advantages of these methods are that they are economical and eliminate the need for prescriptions, chemicals, and mechanical intrusion. But all of these methods are especially unreliable if the menstrual cycles are short, and they suffer from the disadvantage of moderate to severe curtailment of the frequency of sexual relations. Furthermore, if a woman's cycles are grossly irregular, it is extremely difficult to predict the actual time of ovulation, and therefore the number of days she must abstain from sexual intercourse is increased proportionately.

Although if natural family planning is rigorously followed, it can be successful in 9 out of 10 cases, the usual success rate is more likely to be 50 to 80 percent or even less.

FEMALE STERILIZATION

Voluntary sterilization, male plus female, continues to be the most widely used method of birth control in the United States. The latest survey indicates that it accounts for 42 percent of the methods used, compared to 28.5 percent for the pill and 17.7 percent for condoms. More than half of all women electing to use this method are over 35 years of age. They do not want to have any more children and do not wish to continue using the pill, an IUD, a barrier contraceptive, or other methods for the many remaining years of fertility during which they might have an unwanted pregnancy.

TUBAL LIGATION

Sterilization of women has been made much easier in recent years by the development of new instruments and new techniques replacing the previously used laparotomy—the surgical opening of the abdomen—after which the fallopian tubes can be occluded or blocked in any number of ways, by tying, cutting, or clipping. It makes no difference how it is done, provided that a segment of each tube is blocked. The tubes can also be occluded using the vaginal route (colpotomy) and, still experimentally, via the uterine route (hysteroscopy). Tissue adhesives can be introduced using the hysteroscope. Alternatively, silicone plugs may be placed into the tubal openings. All of these are research studies, and the latter technique is theoretically reversible, but sufficient work has not yet been done to see if pregnancies will result after removal.

With the development of the laparoscope and other more sophisticated forms of equipment, the entire scene changed radically. Procedures may now be done at any time during a woman's reproductive life, whereas they were previously done mainly after a delivery. Moreover, a steadily larger percentage of these procedures are now being carried out in hospital and free-standing outpatient clinics and often under local rather than general anesthesia. Many patients come in, have their procedures done, and go home the same day or, at most, stay one night in the hospital.

Most recently, the mini-lap procedure has been developed. This method is even simpler than the laparoscopic techniques. A small incision is made near the top of the pubic hair and the tubes are grasped under direct vision and ligated. The entire procedure takes only a few minutes, and after a few hours' rest the patient is able to go home.

Tubal sterilization is also remarkably safe, with a fatality rate in the United States reported to be as low as 4 per 100,000, much lower than the rate associated with pregnancy. But a 1996 article from the U.S. Collaborative Review of Sterilization has shown that sterilization may no longer be considered permanent. Failures range from 1–5 percent, are most common in younger women and increase with time.

LAPAROSCOPIC TUBAL STERILIZATION

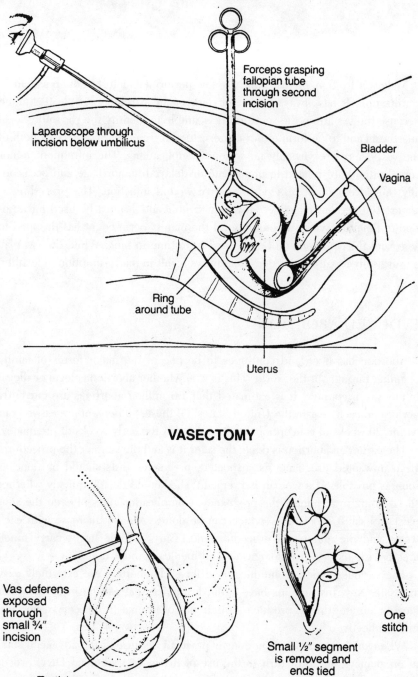

Forceps grasping fallopian tube through second incision

Laparoscope through incision below umbilicus

Bladder

Vagina

Ring around tube

Uterus

VASECTOMY

Vas deferens exposed through small ¾" incision

Testicle

Small ½" segment is removed and ends tied

One stitch

MALE STERILIZATION

Male sterilization, or vasectomy, is now performed almost as often as female sterilization. It has always been and remains an extremely simple technique because the vas are in the scrotum. It is simple to identify the vas under local anesthesia and to perform either cauterization or removal of a piece of both of the vas. There are virtually no serious complications. The infrequent minor complications are related to immediate or delayed hemorrhage and occasionally the development of a postoperative wound infection. The procedure is almost 100 percent effective. However, contraception must be used for a period of time following vasectomy until the man's sperm count has dropped to zero, and the count should be checked from time to time. While the vas may be surgically repaired, this does not always result in the resumption of fertility.

INDUCED ABORTION

Abortion has been and continues to be one of the major forms of family planning throughout the world. This is true whether abortion is legal or illegal in any given country. It is estimated that 1.6 million abortions are currently performed each year in the United States. Of these, 99 percent are carried out within 20 weeks of conception, most of them in the early weeks of pregnancy.

The earlier an abortion is done, the safer it is and the simpler the procedure. If an unwanted pregnancy is suspected, pregnancy tests should be done as soon as possible. If a woman is pregnant, she should decide quickly whether she is going to terminate the pregnancy. Complication rates of even the simplest and safest procedures, which can be done vaginally, increase with each week, and the abdominal procedures necessary at later stages carry much greater risk and are psychologically and medically more traumatic.

The various suction techniques used for early abortion are extremely easy and safe. New instruments have been developed that can be inserted under local or no anesthesia, produce a minimum of trauma to the cervix, and are highly effective.

When suction abortion is no longer practical because of the advanced state of pregnancy, one must turn to the use of the more traditional D&C procedures. And, once pregnancy has advanced well into the second trimester, an entirely different approach must be used. The uterus may be emptied by the induction of labor, using one or more chemical agents such as prostaglandins, saline, or glucose, or the fetal material can be removed by surgical procedure, a hysterotomy or hysterectomy. In addition, the prior insertion of laminaria into the cervix may speed up the induction of labor.

MENSTRUAL EXTRACTION

Menstrual extraction is a term usually applied to abortions done within six weeks of the last menstrual period. It is also commonly referred to as menstrual regulation, endometrial aspiration, endometrial extraction, preemptive abortion, and a variety of other terms. The original menstrual regulation was carried out simply to cut down on the length of time a menstrual period took. It removed all of the tissue at one time so that it did not flow out over a period of several days. The same name and the same technique were subsequently applied to the termination of early pregnancy, usually before a positive diagnosis was made. The term has been maintained for several reasons. First, in those areas of the world where abortion is illegal, these procedures are carried out as therapy for the delayed onset of menses. Because pregnancy is not diagnosed, there can be no legal consequences. Secondly, women who find themselves in these situations very often do not wish to know whether or not they were pregnant.

DILATATION AND EVACUATION (D&E)

As more experience has been gained in doing early abortions, dilatation and evacuation (suction abortion, suction curettage, vacuum curettage) has come to be used for the majority of abortions done during the first 14 or 15 weeks of gestation. The instrument most frequently used is a suction curette (vacurette) made out of a soft material and inserted into the uterine cavity after dilatation of the cervix. This reduces the possibility of perforation of the uterus. The procedure is usually done under local anesthesia, the woman being given a tranquilizer or a short-acting intravenous barbiturate.

The advantages of these procedures are that they are relatively easy to do, the complication rates are very low, the amount of blood lost is minimal, and the effectiveness in totally removing the pregnancy is very high. The procedures can usually be done in less than one minute in early pregnan-

DILATATION AND EVACUATION
(SUCTION ABORTION)

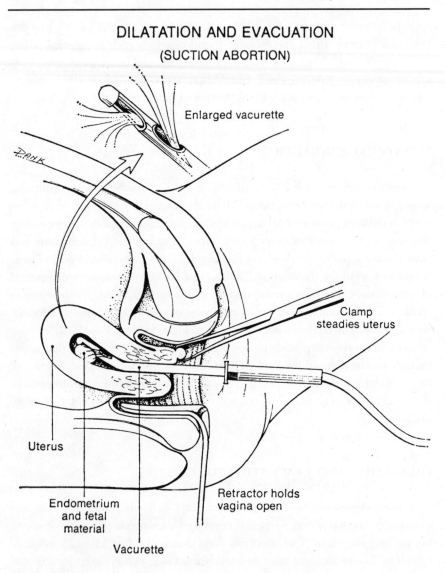

Enlarged vacurette

Clamp
steadies uterus

Uterus

Endometrium
and fetal
material

Retractor holds
vagina open

Vacurette

cies but require somewhat more time when the pregnancies are more advanced.

Patients recover rapidly from these procedures; they usually return to their
homes within a matter of hours and resume their normal activities almost
immediately. Complications, which are rare, include perforation of the uterus,
excessive bleeding, postoperative infection, and, on occasion, leaving some
tissue behind requiring a repeat procedure.

DILATATION AND CURETTAGE (D&C)

This procedure has been carried out for the diagnosis and treatment of uterine conditions for many years and is also used for first and early (sometimes later) second-trimester abortions. In most instances it is carried out under general anesthesia. However, dilatation and curettage can also be done using paracervical block, backed up with tranquilizers, sedatives, and other drugs.

Before doing the curettage, it is necessary to dilate the cervix in order to introduce the curette. This may be done by progressively enlarging the size of the endocervical canal using metal dilators. It may also be done by inserting laminaria (a form of seaweed) and leaving it for several hours, usually overnight, to absorb water and swell. This technique allows for the gradual dilatation of the cervix. Studies are currently under way to see whether this gradual dilatation may produce less long-term damage such as premature delivery and spontaneous abortion than the more rapid dilatation with metal dilators.

Once the cervix has been dilated, a surgical curette, usually made of metal, is introduced into the uterus through the cervical canal. The entire surface of the uterine cavity is then scraped with the curette, removing all the fetal and placental tissues.

In this procedure the complications are also rare. They include perforation of the uterus, excessive bleeding, and the development of postoperative infection.

INTRA-AMNIOTIC INFUSION

Intra-amniotic infusion is the procedure most commonly used for abortions too far advanced for the earlier methods. Abortion is induced by the introduction of various fluids into the amniotic sac. Preparations that have been used are hypertonic saline, hypertonic glucose, urea, and prostaglandins. These techniques are indicated when the pregnancy has advanced too far to do a D&E or D&C. The skin is sterilized, a local anesthetic is injected, a needle is put through the abdominal wall into the amniotic cavity, amniotic fluid is withdrawn, and then the solution is introduced into the cavity. Contractions generally begin 12 to 24 hours later, and the patient then proceeds to deliver the dead fetus and the placenta. Very very rarely is the infant born alive.

There are a number of complications that have been noticed with these techniques. With the use of saline, patients may develop abdominal pain, vomiting, hypertension, and a rapid heart rate. In rare instances they may develop problems with blood clotting. Patients receiving prostaglandins often have the side effects of lowering of blood pressure, nausea and vomiting, and diarrhea. Inasmuch as these are surgical procedures, there is always the risk of hemorrhage. Incomplete evacuation of the uterus, delayed hemorrhage, and infection may also occur, although not frequently.

HYSTEROTOMY AND HYSTERECTOMY

Hysterotomy (the surgical opening of the uterus) is also employed as a form of abortion but only in late pregnancy. The abdomen and the wall of the uterus are opened surgically, and the fetus and the placenta are removed. The uterine wall is sewed back together. On rare occasions the uterus and the fetus may be removed by hysterectomy, usually because of some uterine abnormality.

These two surgical techniques are much more complicated and therefore have a higher rate of complications than the simpler techniques described earlier.

NONSURGICAL METHODS

The drug RU 486, known as the "abortion pill," was developed in France in 1980, and since 1981, 250,000 women in 20 countries have used it. In 1990 the American Medical Association, whose 290,000 members represent almost half of the physicians in the United States, voted to endorse the testing and possible use of RU 486 in this country. Members pointed out not only that the pill appeared to be safer and cheaper than surgical abortion but that it might also prove useful in treating brain tumors, breast and endometrial cancer, endometriosis, premenstrual syndrome, induction of labor, Cushing's syndrome, and Addison's disease and as a contraceptive.

In 1994, following years of violent protest by anti-choice forces against the introduction of the pill into this country, the French company, Roussel-Uclaf, which makes and distributes it in Europe, turned over to the Population Council the rights to the drug mifepristone, the chemical name for RU 486. The council, a nonprofit research organization located in New York City, selected a total of 20 Planned Parenthood clinics and hospital clinics nationwide to begin testing the safety and effectiveness of the drug with 2,100 volunteers. For purpose of the trials, volunteers had to be within the first nine weeks of pregnancy and have no underlying health problems.

The testing procedure begins with counseling and a thorough medical examination that includes a sonogram to confirm the stage of the pregnancy. Women found to be suitable candidates are then given three mifepristone pills, which block the body's hormones and prevent the continued development of the embryo. Two days later they return to take two pills of misoprostol, a prostaglandin that causes contractions, cramping, bleeding, and tissue loss. During the required four-hour observation period that follows, 70 percent of the women abort, but the others do not respond quite that quickly. While some women have very little pain, there are those who spend several days in varying degrees of discomfort, with cramps and bleeding similar to the experience of a miscarriage. A follow-up visit is required after two weeks. In 4 or 5 percent of the participating women, the pills do not work, either leaving a continuing pregnancy or causing an incomplete abortion. In such cases a surgical abortion is scheduled after the follow-up visit. Ongoing monitoring is part of the procedure for all trial participants.

Doctors and women's rights advocates point out that mifepristone is safer than a surgical abortion because it eliminates the risk of anesthesia or perforation of the uterus. Also, it allows for confidentiality and avoids the harassment and actual danger of going to an abortion clinic.

By the end of 1995, and in spite of continuing opposition of anti-choice groups, hundreds of women in various parts of the country had already used the abortion pills. In the meantime, because the studies have had a very slow start in some parts of the country, they are likely to continue into 1996. When they are complete, the Population Council will seek FDA approval so that a manufacturer and distributor of the drug can be chosen.

An Experimental Alternative to RU 486

In October 1994 the *Journal of the American Medical Association* contained a report by two researchers on the 90 percent effectiveness of inducing abortion with a combination of two drugs already on the market and approved by the FDA for other purposes.

The first drug is methotrexate, used to treat cancer, psoriasis, arthritis, and to terminate ectopic pregnancies; the second is an anti-ulcer drug called misoprostol. The two drugs are available by prescription for this purpose for a total of less than 10 dollars. The drug combination is effective only before the ninth week of pregnancy. It works in the following way: the woman is given an injection of methotrexate, which inhibits tissue growth and destabilizes the lining of the uterus; four days later misoprostol tablets are inserted into her vagina. She goes home, and in typical cases, following severe cramping, the embryo is expelled within three days. Clinical trials of this procedure involving hundreds of women are being conducted in three American cities.

By the time the report appeared, a New York gynecologist had already used the drug combination on 126 women, and only five required follow-up surgery to complete the abortion.

In the same report the author acknowledged a political motive: "My goal is to show the medical community that there is a safe, simple, effective, legal technique of terminating pregnancies that is private and inexpensive."

In August 1995 the *New England Journal of Medicine* published the results of a new study, concluding that this procedure was safe and effective when performed in early pregnancy. Researchers pointed out that this method provides a welcome alternative to RU 486, which may not be approved by the FDA for several years. Family planners pointed out that this two-drug combination enables trained providers to offer women medical abortions in the privacy of their offices without having to confront picket lines or face potential violence.

COUNSELING

Effective counseling is one of the most important aspects of abortion services, and any facility that does not provide it must be viewed as inadequate. A counselor can explain and answer questions about a procedure to reduce fears and clear up any misunderstanding about what is about to happen. Since it is almost inevitable that the woman will have some feelings of guilt and anxiety, the counselor can support the decision to have the abortion and offer the woman a chance to express these feelings.

Given current knowledge about contraception and its easy availability, the question of why the pregnancy occurred can be explored. Perhaps the woman did not know enough about contraceptive methods, a situation that the counselor can remedy easily. Bringing out into the open more complex reasons that led to an unwanted pregnancy—social factors, personal relationships, or even just lack of forethought—may not eliminate the reasons, but awareness of them may help her to avoid another unwanted pregnancy. Whatever her explanation, a discussion of future contraception is essential, even though the abortion

procedure is safe and most women overcome the psychological trauma associated with it. In fact, postpartum depression or the depression following a
miscarriage is far more common than deep distress after an abortion.

It is becoming increasingly apparent through surveys that a majority of men
want some type of counseling when an abortion is to terminate a pregnancy for
which they are responsible. While some clinics are hostile to men, and many
women want to preserve total autonomy in every aspect of their decision, more
and more family planning centers have inaugurated counseling for both partners. A spouse who indicates that he intends to interfere with this autonomy
should be informed that in a series of decisions beginning in 1976 and most
recently in 1992 (Planned Parenthood vs. Casey et al.) the Supreme Court has
ruled that a woman's right to an abortion is not contingent on her husband's
permission, nor is she required to notify him of her intentions.

In addition to the personal and public health implications of unplanned
pregnancies, from a purely economic point of view, it is clear that effective
contraception has every advantage over unwanted pregnancy. This is equally
true of the health implications. When one views the medical problems wrought
by large numbers of unwanted pregnancies in terms of illegal abortion, increased infant and maternal illness and death, and the increase in psychological and social problems, it is clear that there are compelling reasons for making
contraceptives freely available to all those who need and wish to use them.

$\mathscr{P}$REGNANCY AND CHILDBIRTH

Kathryn Schrotenboer Cox, M.D.

Assistant Attending Physician, Obstetrics and Gynecology, New York Hospital-Cornell Medical Center; Clinical Instructor, Cornell University Medical College

The birth of a first child is a major milestone in a woman's life: it marks the end of one stage and the beginning of a new one. Whether to have a child or not is a decision that must be weighed carefully. It is not uncommon today for a couple to decide that for them the burdens outweigh the rewards. On the other hand, a couple who waits until they know they are ready for the responsibilities of a child often finds that the commitment that results from such a decision increases their enjoyment of parenthood. A conscious decision that now is the right time for you to have a baby will help you to see beyond the problems and permit you to focus on the joys of pregnancy and parenthood.

Having a baby before finishing high school can create difficult, and often lifetime, psychosocial and financial problems. Many women fear that having a first baby after age 35 will increase the risks. Older women face somewhat greater risks because they are more likely than younger ones to have a chronic disease such as diabetes or hypertension. The risks relate to these maternal risks and also to increased fetal genetic risks. However, most healthy older women do well in pregnancy, and those with diseases who get specialized clinical care generally do well also. Many genetic conditions can and should be diagnosed prior to birth, as noted later in this chapter.

If you plan to delay your first pregnancy for some time, you can do several things to help assure future fertility and good health. Find out from a doctor whether you ovulate regularly and, if not, be evaluated and treated. Also, you should have periodic pelvic examinations and Pap tests; get immunized, if necessary, against measles, rubella, and chicken pox; get family genetic histories assembled and be evaluated for personal genetic diseases or traits; keep your body in good shape by exercising regularly; stop smoking altogether; minimize alcohol intake; and get good medical care promptly when necessary. A complete dental checkup is advisable, especially if X-rays might be required for necessary repairs. One session with a qualified nutritionist for a review of your eating habits can help you plan more balanced meals. (Essential dietary supplements during early pregnancy are discussed later in this chapter.)

About three months before trying to conceive:

- If there is even the slightest possibility of having contracted HIV through intravenous drug use, blood transfusions prior to testing for the HIV virus, or sexual contact with a bisexual man or an intravenous drug user, arrange to be tested for HIV.
- If you've been on the pill, stop taking it so that ovulation and your periods can return to their normal cycle.
- If you've been using an IUD, have it removed.
- If your method of contraception is the Norplant system, have the capsules removed by a health care provider trained in the technique for doing so.
- If you haven't done so already, stop smoking and stop drinking.

One month before trying to conceive:

- Stop taking all over-the-counter medications, including aspirin, cough medicine, and high doses of vitamins.
- Have a session with your doctor about any and all your prescription medications and their potentially harmful effects on the fetus-to-be.
- If you have a cat, ask someone else to change the cat litter so that you're not exposed to the dangers of toxoplasmosis during pregnancy.

GENETIC DISEASES

If there is any history of congenital malformation, mental retardation, or known genetic disorders in your family, you should see a qualified genetic counselor *before you become pregnant.* Make an effort to collect as much material about affected family members as you can to facilitate counseling. More than 5,000 birth defects have been identified, and although some are relatively uncommon, in the aggregate they occur in 7 percent of all births and are the leading cause of death in the first year of life. Some birth defects are caused by specific environmental circumstances, such as air and water pollutants that affect fetal health; others result from substance abuse by the mother or from the father's damaged sperm; but the largest number involve hereditary factors.

Genetic counseling is concerned with *all* birth defects. If there is a history of such disorders as Tay-Sachs disease, sickle cell anemia, or cystic fibrosis (among others) in your family, genetic counselors can provide risk figures, medical explanations, and the information on which to base personal decisions. Even if there is no family history, certain population groups are more likely than others to have these diseases and blood testing for carrier status can be done. Comprehensive genetic service centers are usually connected with the obstetric and pediatric departments of major medical centers. The local March of Dimes chapter can provide reliable referral or you can consult the National Society of Genetic Counselors, which has 1,300 members nationwide. If now or at some future time you need the comfort of a support group, the Alliance of Genetic Support Groups (1-800-336-GENE) is a coalition of voluntary organizations and professionals representing practically every category of genetic and birth disorder. (See the "Directory of Health Information" for details.)

CONCEPTION AND EARLY DEVELOPMENT

The reproductive process begins as your body hormones make the necessary changes to ripen an egg (ovum) in one of your ovaries. If you have a 28-day menstrual cycle, this will take place in the first 14 days of the cycle. As the egg ripens, it moves to the outer surface of the ovary. On about the fourteenth day ovulation occurs—a surge of hormones causes the egg to burst forth from the ovary. In a woman with a shorter or longer cycle, the day of ovulation will be sooner or later, as described below.

The menstrual cycle may be divided into two parts by ovulation. From the first day of the menstrual period to ovulation is the preovulatory (also called the proliferative or follicular) phase. From ovulation until the next menstrual period is the postovulatory (also called the secretory or luteal) phase. Regardless of the length of the menstrual cycle, the postovulatory phase lasts approximately 14 days. The variation in women with shorter or longer cycles takes place in the first part of the cycle. For example, in a woman with a 21-day cycle, the first part of the cycle lasts 7 days, ovulation takes place on the seventh day, and the second part of the cycle lasts 14 days. In a woman with a 35-day cycle, the preovulatory phase lasts 21 days, ovulation occurs on the twenty-first day, and the postovulatory phase lasts 14 days.

During sexual intercourse semen is deposited in the vagina, usually near the cervix. The sperm move first through the cervical canal and then through the uterus to the fallopian tubes. The sperm are best able to fertilize an egg in the first 48 hours after intercourse, although there are reports of sperm living as long as a week before fertilization.

After ovulation the egg begins traveling down the fallopian tube toward the uterus. The sperm usually meet the egg in the outer third of the fallopian tube where one sperm penetrates the egg to fertilize it. The egg is generally fertilized within 4 to 20 hours after ovulation, but there are exceptions to this as well. After the egg has been fertilized, no other sperm can enter it. The egg and the sperm each contribute to the child half of its genetic material.

Each egg carries an X chromosome. Half of the sperm carry Y chromosomes and the other half carry X chromosomes. If an X-bearing sperm fertilizes the egg, the resulting child is female (XX). If, instead, a Y-bearing sperm fertilizes the egg, the resulting child is male (XY). Therefore, the sex of the child is predetermined by the sperm. The anatomical differences develop early in gestation when something called the H-Y antigen, present only in XY embryos, stimulates the gonads to become testicles, which start producing hormones in proportions that cause the embryo to develop as a male. In the absence of the H-Y antigen the embryonic gonads will not become testicles and the resultant infant will be female.

Recent laboratory studies have shown that there are biochemical differences between X-bearing and the Y-bearing sperm. These differences may allow either the X or Y sperm to survive longer or move faster in certain environments. Books and articles have been written that suggest using acid or alkaline douches or changing the position, frequency, or timing of intercourse help alter the odds of having a boy or a girl. Unfortunately, the reproductive tract is

FEMALE GENITAL TRACT
OVULATION, FERTILIZATION AND IMPLANTATION

CROSS-SECTION OF UTERUS

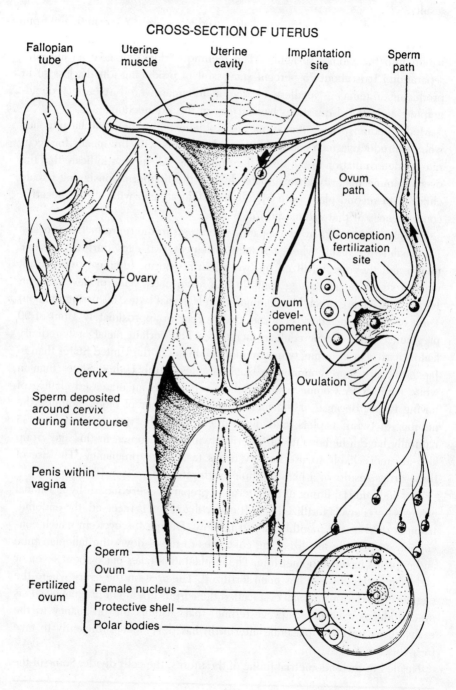

more complex than the test tube, and many studies have given conflicting results.

There is a laboratory technique that is used to separate Y sperm (male) from X sperm, and the desired sex sperm can then be injected via artificial insemination into the woman's vagina. (The technique does not give an absolute separation.) It is about 75 percent successful in producing a male, less so in producing a female. Needless to say, many unanswered scientific, demographic, and ethical questions have arisen in this connection.

Medical ethicists are anticipating the problems that society will have to face when reproductive technology will provide parents with the means for accurate predetermination of the sex of their offspring. All surveys indicate that the overwhelming majority favor a male child as the firstborn, consigning female children to second place both literally and figuratively, with all the negative consequences of that ordinal position.

Twinning may occur by two separate alterations in the reproductive process. Fraternal twins result when a woman produces two eggs during the same month and they are fertilized by two different sperm. Identical twins result when a single fertilized egg splits in half at an early stage of development. Identical twins are much less common than fraternal twins, occurring in about 1 out of 250 pregnancies. Fraternal twins occur in approximately 1 out of 90 pregnancies, but the percentage increases when certain racial or hereditary factors exist. For example, twins are more common in the United States than in Japan and are more common in black families in the United States than in white families. A woman who herself is a twin has an increased chance of having twins. Because of the increase in the number of older mothers, the number of twins, triplets, and quadruplets is on the rise. Women over 35 naturally have a higher rate of fraternal twins, and women in this age group also are more likely to use fertility drugs to achieve pregnancy. The use of these drugs results in a high multiple birth rate.

The endometrial lining of the uterus is prepared every month by hormonal changes to receive a fertilized egg. If no fertilized egg is received, the endometrium is shed as the monthly menstrual flow. During the cycle in which conception occurs, the fertilized egg continues to travel down the fallopian tube and implants in the endometrium. The implantation takes place about seven or eight days after the egg has been fertilized. The area on the ovary where the egg developed forms a small cyst (called the corpus luteum of pregnancy). This cyst produces a hormone (progesterone) that sustains the pregnancy in the early weeks until the placenta (afterbirth) has developed sufficiently to take over this function.

Nestled in the endometrial lining of the uterus, the cells divide. Some of the

UTERINE-FETAL RELATIONSHIP

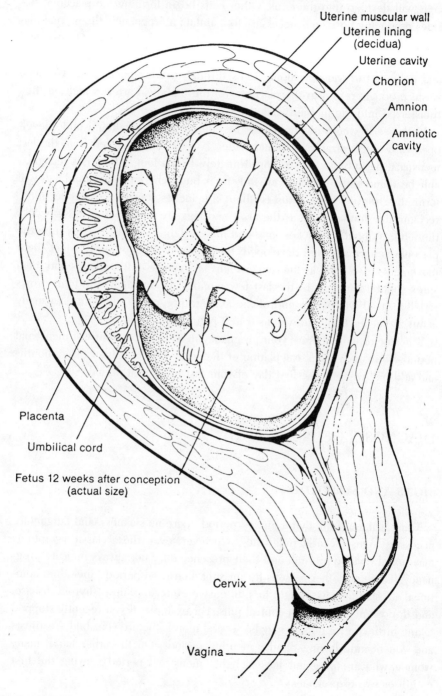

Uterine muscular wall

Uterine lining
(decidua)

Uterine cavity

Chorion

Amnion

Amniotic
cavity

Placenta

Umbilical cord

Fetus 12 weeks after conception
(actual size)

Cervix

Vagina

cells will develop into the fetus. Other cells begin forming the placenta. Besides producing hormones necessary to maintain a pregnancy, the normal placenta acts as an organ of exchange between mother and fetus. Oxygen and nutrients are removed from the mother's blood, absorbed by the fetal blood, and delivered to the developing fetus through the umbilical vein. The fetal waste products return to the placenta via the umbilical arteries and are then transferred into the mother's bloodstream.

In the early weeks of pregnancy the embryo is too small and underdeveloped to be recognizable as human. After 7 weeks have elapsed from the last menstrual period, the fetus is approximately 1 inch long. There is a recognizable head and body, but there are only thick buds where the arms and legs will form. By 10 weeks the fetus is about 2½ inches long and is taking more recognizable human form as the arms and legs are lengthening. At 14 weeks the fetus is about 4½ inches long and may weigh 3 ounces. By this time the placenta is normally well developed. By 18 weeks the mother may feel slight movements. At 28 weeks the fetus weighs an average of 2½ pounds and measures about 14 inches. In the last few months of pregnancy, the fetus grows rapidly. At 40 weeks, the end of the average pregnancy, the fetus is usually about 20 inches long and weighs 6 to 9 pounds.

Your doctor will measure your pregnancy in weeks from your last menstrual period. To make a quick calculation of the "due date," subtract three months and add one week to the first day of your last menstrual period.

DIAGNOSIS OF PREGNANCY

SIGNS AND SYMPTOMS

Many women think that a missed period, morning sickness, and fatigue are necessary signs of early pregnancy. However, even these classic symptoms may not always be present, and their presence does not always indicate pregnancy. There are other reasons for missing menstrual periods, including emotional stress, excessive weight loss, intensive exercise, illness, thyroid disease, and the recent use of birth control pills. For example, if you recently stopped taking birth control pills, it may be several months before your body readjusts and you resume having regular monthly periods. On the other hand, many women who are pregnant have a light "menstrual period" during the first month or two of pregnancy.

Nausea or inability to tolerate certain foods or tobacco smoke is common during early pregnancy. Often the nausea can be relieved by eating a few crackers in the morning before getting out of bed. Sometimes, however, vomiting is such a problem that medication is required to control it.

Breast tenderness is a reliable sign of pregnancy. The feeling of soreness usually starts about the time of the missed menstrual period or a week or two later. But because the feeling also occurs premenstrually, it is possible to be fooled by this sign. Some women begin producing excessive saliva; others experience fatigue. Some are constipated; others have diarrhea. Still others experience a large increase in appetite. Every person is slightly different. You may experience all of these symptoms or you may experience none of them.

PREGNANCY TESTS

There are several different tests that can tell you whether or not you are pregnant. Some are more accurate than others, and in recent years home pregnancy tests provide reliable results, but only if instructions are followed very carefully.

All pregnancy tests are based on the detection in the blood or urine of the hormone called human chorionic gonadotropin (HCG). The levels of secretion of HCG double every two days in the first trimester.

Tests have been developed in which antibodies are used to detect HCG in the woman's blood or urine. The blood test, called radioimmunoassay or RIA, can detect HCG as early as seven days after ovulation and fertilization, or about one week before a missed period. Urine pregnancy tests, which were previously less accurate than blood pregnancy tests, have been improved to the point where they are almost as sensitive as the blood tests. However, urine pregnancy tests cannot be relied on to detect pregnancy until almost two weeks following conception or a few days before the missed period. While these tests are highly accurate, a lower than normal amount of HCG in the blood or urine may produce a false-negative result, and the test should therefore be repeated after a week if a pregnancy is suspected. An ectopic pregnancy or an impending miscarriage may result in lower than normal HCG values. (Higher than normal HCG levels are produced by a multiple pregnancy or some other anomaly that should be investigated further.)

Pregnancy tests are offered free of charge or at low cost by some family planning clinics. Your local health department or the county medical society can supply information of this kind.

HOME PREGNANCY TESTS

Many of these tests are essentially the same as the urine pregnancy tests performed professionally in clinics and in doctors' offices. The test kits are available in most drugstores and can be bought without a doctor's prescription. Instructions on how to take the test and how to read the results must be followed with extreme care.

If the results of the home test are positive, you still must see your doctor for confirmation of the pregnancy. Some false positives occur, usually because the directions were not followed carefully. If the results are negative, you may still be pregnant. The test should be repeated in about 10 days if your period still has not begun. If the result is negative the second time around, pregnancy has probably not occurred, but a doctor should be consulted to find out why menstruation has been interrupted.

WHO WILL DELIVER YOUR BABY?

In the United States babies are delivered every day by obstetrician-gynecologists, family practitioners, nurse-midwives, and lay midwives. Depending on the state in which you live and the size of your community, some or all of these choices may be available to you. Whichever type of professional you select, the most important thing is to find someone with whom you are comfortable and in whom you have confidence. If you have a special problem such as heart disease, hypertension, or hyperthyroidism, you should be cared for by an appropriate specialist as well.

OBSTETRICIAN-GYNECOLOGIST

To become an obstetrician-gynecologist, a physician who has already received a medical degree must spend a minimum of four years in an approved residency program working in the field of obstetrics and gynecology under the supervision of specialists in that field. After completing this training, most become certified in obstetrics and gynecology by passing written and oral examinations given by the American Board of Obstetrics and Gynecology. Obstetrician-gynecologists and residents in obstetrics and gynecology deliver approximately 70 percent of the babies born in the United States. At the present time approximately one out of every six obstetrician-gynecologists in the United States is a woman. This percentage is increasing as more women are graduating from medical schools and selecting a career in this specialty.

Obstetricians vary in their attitudes toward childbirth as well as such specifics as medications during labor, breast feeding, role of the father, episiotomy, rooming-in, and length of hospital stay. If any of these things are important to you, discuss them with your obstetrician early in pregnancy.

FAMILY PRACTITIONER

Many babies are delivered by family practitioners, particularly in rural areas or small towns where such a doctor may be the only one available. Many women enjoy having the family doctor, who takes care of the entire family for all medical problems, care for them during pregnancy, labor, and delivery. Many family practitioners have had some advanced training in obstetrics. A family doctor trained in obstetrics can handle a normal pregnancy and childbirth, but he or she may refer you to an obstetrician or other specialist if you have serious complications at any time during pregnancy.

NURSE-MIDWIFE

Certified nurse-midwives deliver approximately 2.3 percent of the babies born in the United States. These midwives are registered nurses (RNs) who have had an additional one or two years of training in obstetrics. Almost all are women. There are approximately 3,000 certified nurse-midwives in clinical practice in all 50 states. The profession continues to grow, with up to 250 new practitioners certified annually.

According to the American College of Nurse-Midwives, the nurse-midwife's management of labor and delivery may differ from that of some physicians. Nurse-midwives are less likely to use fetal monitors or use forceps. They often prefer deliveries in a bed instead of on a delivery table. An episiotomy, an incision to enlarge the vaginal opening prior to delivery, is often not done by nurse-midwives. Many offer family planning and postpartum checkups. Typically, they try to encourage breast feeding and rooming-in. (Of course, many physicians are willing to deliver your baby and care for you in this manner.)

Because nurse-midwives generally have fewer patients than either obstetricians or family practitioners, they may have more time to spend with each patient during prenatal visits or during labor. Nurse-midwives handle uncomplicated pregnancies quite satisfactorily. However, if complications arise, the patient may have to be transferred to the care of a physician.

The licensing of medical personnel varies from state to state, and a few states still have very restrictive laws regarding nurse-midwives. By law in most states there must be an obstetrician available to the midwife in case of emergency. Most midwives today practice with obstetricians or use obstetricians as consultants. If you would like to know whether there are any nurse-midwives practicing in your area, contact the American College of Nurse-Midwives.

LAY MIDWIFE

Lay midwives are people without nursing degrees who are trained to deliver babies. As a group, lay midwives are the most willing to perform home deliveries. Many states recognize only nurse-midwives and do not allow lay midwives to practice. Some states that permit lay midwives to practice have little or no regulation. Because of this wide variation in regulation by states, the level of training required of a lay midwife also varies enormously. Before you select a lay midwife, you should inquire thoroughly into the level of his or her training.

WHERE WILL YOU HAVE YOUR BABY?

The choice of where to have your baby should be made only after you have weighed the advantages and disadvantages of each option. A major circumstance affecting the choice of many women is the 1995 decision by health maintenance organizations to cover only 24 hours of hospital care after a normal birth. Public and professional outcry against what have been called "drive-through deliveries" has resulted in state-by-state rulings to extend the hospital stay of new mothers to a minimum of two days. Many health authorities, however, feel that at least three to four days are required for complete screenings of the newborns to detect genetic diseases, to adjust both mother and baby to possible complications of breast feeding, not to mention the problems that might arise because of inadequate care at home. Several physicians' groups, including the American College of Obstetricians and Gynecologists, have called for curtailment of early discharge until more hard research is collected on the various safety issues involved.

In view of this recent development, the expectant mother should find out whether her state has passed a bill affecting the length of her hospital stay after delivery, especially if this is her first pregnancy.

HOSPITAL DELIVERY

Approximately 99 percent of all babies born in the United States today are born in hospitals. The birth of a baby is a normal physiological process and is usually uncomplicated. However, when complications do occur, they often happen very quickly and with little or no warning. Labor may be progressing well when vaginal bleeding begins and the baby's heartbeat starts to slow. Even a healthy mother with an uncomplicated pregnancy and a normal labor and delivery may have a baby that has difficulty breathing and needs to be given oxygen and receive immediate pediatric care. Similarly, a woman with a totally uncomplicated labor and delivery may have a postpartum hemorrhage 10 minutes later. While these complications are not common, they can be catastrophic if proper medical care, including needed blood, oxygen, or medications, is not available. Most women opt for a hospital birth to have the assurance that necessary treatment is immediately available if any complications do occur. In the past, hospitals were criticized for providing an overly clinical and "cold" environment. Happily, in many hospitals this has changed, with homelike "birthing rooms" and rooming-in arrangements available when requested.

HOSPITAL DELIVERY BY A NURSE-MIDWIFE

A significant development since 1975 is the revolution that has occurred not only in the training of nurse-midwives, but also in the increasingly important role they have been playing in providing obstetrical and gynecological services to a rapidly growing number of women in this country and even more in Europe. The current qualifications of these health professionals and their standing in the medical community has led more and more middle class, well-educated women to choose them to attend the delivery of their babies, most often in a hospital, with a doctor available as a consultant in the event of an unanticipated complication. Under normal circumstances, these deliveries oc-

cur vaginally, without induction of labor, fetal monitoring, or the use of forceps. Since 1985, the number of babies delivered by certified nurse-midwives
in hospitals has doubled.

There are approximately 4,000 certified practitioners in the United States
today, with an estimated 350 new certifications conferred every year by the
American College of Nurse-Midwives. In the United States, as of 1995, there
are 46 educational programs accredited by this parent organization. The usual
candidate is a registered nurse who has completed training in obstetrics and
gynecology and is required to pass a national examination. Certified nurse-
midwives are licensed to practice in all 50 states, with California having the
largest number, followed by New York, Florida, Pennsylvania, and Illinois.

A pregnant woman who finds the philosophical approach of nurse-midwifery
congenial and who wants to find out more about this option can write for
information and referral to the American College of Nurse-Midwives, 818
Connecticut Avenue NW, Suite 900, Washington, DC 20006.

CHILDBEARING CENTER DELIVERY

Another option is an independent licensed childbearing center staffed by
certified nurse-midwives. These centers are usually located in a suitably converted private dwelling where the mother-to-be goes for prenatal care and
delivery after she has been evaluated by a physician who rules out the likelihood of complications. There are approximately 135 freestanding childbearing
centers in 38 states, with 100 additional ones expected to open soon. An increasing number of states have enacted licensing requirements for the centers.
Licensing is required for insurance coverage.

An important aspect of the appeal of this lying-in arrangement is the considerable saving it represents. On average, with all services included, delivery in a
childbearing center costs about half of a hospital delivery. Typical services
include a preparation-for-parenthood program consisting of 10 to 14 weekly
sessions of 2 hours each; prenatal care provided by a licensed nurse-midwife
who also attends the mother during labor and birth; the services as necessary
of a backup team of obstetricians, pediatricians, and nurse assistants; facilities
for a 12-hour stay by the family after the baby is born; a complete examination
of the baby by a pediatrician; home visits by public health nurses within 24
hours as well as on the third and fifth days; a checkup of the mother at the
center a week after delivery and a final checkup 5 to 6 weeks later.

If you are interested in having your baby at such a center, be sure to investigate the arrangements for transfer to a hospital in case of an emergency. Information about a childbearing facility in your area is available from the National Association of Childbearing Centers, 3123 Gottschall Road, Perkiomonville, PA 18074, phone: (215) 234-8068.

HOME DELIVERY

Some women choose to have their babies at home. They share the intimate joyous experience of birth with their families and friends rather than with doctors and nurses in masks and gowns. Labor and delivery are normal processes, not diseases. This choice may also be made by women for whom it has always been a family tradition. For others, it eliminates the need to make arrangements for the care of their very young children in their absence.

If you are considering home delivery, discuss it thoroughly with the person who is overseeing your prenatal care and delivery (your clinician, whether it be physician, nurse-midwife, or lay midwife). During the course of your prenatal care, the clinician can tell you if any condition indicates a likelihood of complication. In such a case you may be advised that hospital delivery would be much safer.

Even if it is assumed that delivery will be normal, arrangements must be made for emergency transportation and additional medical aid in case of unexpected difficulty. Even if arrangements have been made, there is still a risk that complications may develop too quickly to be treated adequately. In many European countries home delivery is safer than in the United States because of an extensive system of back-up ambulances and emergency teams that can be dispatched at a moment's notice. Here comparable systems have been developed in only a few communities.

PREGNANT PATIENTS' RIGHTS

In 1990 George Washington University Medical Center in Washington, D.C., became the first hospital to establish a policy to ensure that ethically difficult decisions on how to treat a severely ill pregnant woman and her fetus would be made by the woman, her family, and her doctors and not by the courts. In addition, the hospital announced that "respect for patient autonomy compels us to accede to the treatment decisions of a pregnant patient, including her unwillingness to abide by medical recommendations." These stipulations, as well as others of great consequence, were the result of a legal decision involving a suit against the hospital in which neither the pregnant patient nor her family was consulted about undertaking a procedure that proved fatal. In overturning the judicial order that resulted in the hospital's action, the highest court in the District of Columbia declared that "the right of bodily integrity is not extinguished simply because someone is ill, or even at death's door." Many groups, including the National Women's Health Network, have been urging the general formulation of a comprehensive statement of pregnant women's rights. As of 1995, the American Hospital Association has not provided such a "bill of rights," although it has promulgated a general "patients' rights" statement in wide use nationwide. It is hoped that other hospitals will follow the lead of George Washington University Medical Center. Until this occurs, medical ethicists and the courts will continue to make decisions uncongenial in many cases to the wishes of the people concerned.

HEALTH CARE DURING NORMAL PREGNANCY

As soon as you think or know you are pregnant, you should begin your prenatal care. Early visits to your doctor or other health care provider are important to identify any problems or potential problems. If you are healthy, such visits will probably occur only once a month. Toward the end of pregnancy your visits will probably be weekly.

The first visit is likely to be the longest. It should include a medical history, family history, and a physical examination. If you have a full-time job and intend working through most of your pregnancy, your doctor should be told about the nature of your work, the environmental risks, whether you're expected to stand all day, and other circumstances that might affect your well-being and that of the fetus. Your personal habits will be reviewed in terms of smoking, alcohol consumption, daily food intake, coffee dependency, and the like, because anything that might reduce the blood supply to the fetus puts its healthy development at risk. Blood tests will be taken to determine your blood type, whether you are Rh-negative or Rh-positive, and whether you are anemic. Other tests will be taken to see if you have syphilis, gonorrhea, or a urinary tract infection. You may also be tested for immunity to German measles and toxoplasmosis. Because ongoing research indicates that there is a direct connection between sperm damaged by exposure to toxic chemicals in the workplace and birth defects, you may also be asked about the father's working environment, alcohol consumption, drug use, and the like. As for AIDS testing,

1995 was the first year that the federal Centers for Disease Control recommended that HIV testing should be part of prenatal care for *all* pregnant women in the United States, even those with little risk of contracting the virus. The agency made the recommendation because of strong evidence that infected women can protect their unborn children by taking the drug AZT during pregnancy. Test results would remain confidential between the woman and her doctor unless otherwise required by state laws.

If you are healthy and your pregnancy is uncomplicated, subsequent visits will include an examination of the size of the uterus, a measurement of your blood pressure and weight change, and perhaps a urine test. Blood tests may be repeated later in pregnancy. Other tests frequently performed during pregnancy include blood APF screening at 14 to 18 weeks (to see if your baby is at increased risk for spinal defects or chromosome abnormalities), ultrasound, and screening for gestational diabetes. Although these checkups are simple, they can detect many of the problems that can occur during pregnancy. At the beginning of the third trimester, your doctor may review the demands of your job and will recommend when you should begin your maternity leave.

Now that you are pregnant, you will undoubtedly want to learn as much as possible about the process that you are about to experience. Recently there has been an increase in the availability of preparation-for-childbirth classes. These classes may be given in hospitals, doctors' offices, prenatal clinics, community meeting places, or private homes. The classes sponsored by nurse-midwife associations are usually very good. Most courses of this kind include the father-to-be during the sessions, especially if one of the "natural" childbirth methods is your choice.

EMOTIONAL AND PHYSICAL CHANGES

For many women pregnancy is a pleasant, happy time; it may also be a time of psychological stress and mixed emotions. Much of what a woman expects of pregnancy is a result of what she has heard over the years from her mother, sisters, friends, and relatives. A woman who has heard repeatedly of the horrors and terrible pain of labor may face childbirth with fear and apprehension. A woman who has grown up in a neighborhood where many families have five or six children may assume it must be easy.

Though often a time of closeness between a husband and wife, pregnancy can also be a time of friction in a marriage. Men's attitudes toward childbirth vary as much as women's. Some men cannot relate to the pregnancy at all, while others feel every wave of nausea and every contraction personally. The important thing to remember is that these attitudes don't make them better or worse as husbands or as fathers.

Of course your appearance will change. The radiant glow that accompanies pregnancy may be attributable not only to the state of excitement and elation but also to the hormones of pregnancy that affect your skin. (In this connection, either avoid exposure to the sun or, if you insist on sunbathing, be sure to use a sunblock with a sun protection factor—SPF—of at least 15. Your sunglasses should be the kind that are chemically treated to filter out the ultraviolet rays of the sun as protection against premature cataract formation.) Don't be upset by the spidery veins that may suddenly appear on your legs. They are caused by blood vessel changes. Red stretch marks that appear on the abdomen and breasts may turn white after delivery but will not disappear.

DIET

A woman who is seriously underweight or a teenager who hasn't finished growing herself is much more likely to have a low-birth-weight baby than a woman of normal weight. And in a significant number of cases, low birth weight is accompanied by birth defects.

If a woman is healthy and has good eating habits, it may be unnecessary for her to make any major diet changes during pregnancy. Many women are surprised that there is not a great increase in the amount of food required during pregnancy. Although a pregnant woman's caloric intake may not be greatly increased, it is important that the calories be obtained from foods that will provide the proper protein, vitamins, and minerals for her baby's development. If you have not been eating a well-balanced diet, it is essential that you correct that once you become pregnant. Your baby is totally dependent on you to supply it with the necessary nutrients for proper growth and development. You are feeding your baby! Also, in reviewing your diet, find out whether it contains enough foods to supply you with essential amounts of folic acid, the nutrient that prevents several serious birth defects. Foods rich in folic acid include citrus fruits, dark leafy vegetables, broccoli, dried beans, and peas. As for your calcium, for detailed advice on proper nutrition and weight gain during pregnancy, see chapter on "Nutrition, Weight, Body Image, and Eating Disorders."

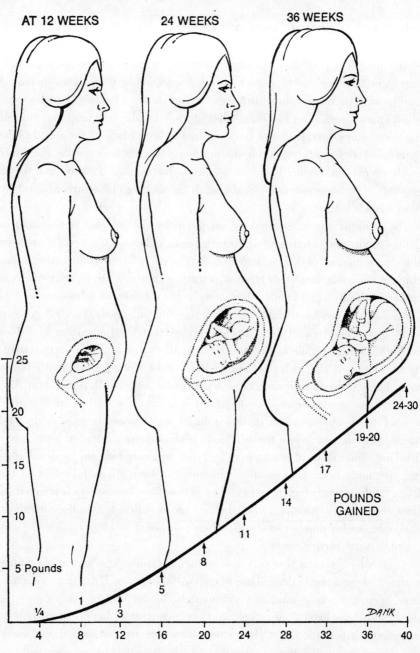

WEIGHT GAIN DURING PREGNANCY

AT 12 WEEKS   24 WEEKS   36 WEEKS

25

20

15

10

5 Pounds

24-30

19-20

17

14

11

8

5

3

1

¼

POUNDS
GAINED

DANK

4   8   12   16   20   24   28   32   36   40

Weeks after last normal menstrual period

SMOKING, ALCOHOL, AND DRUGS

Any time is a good time to stop smoking, but pregnancy is an especially important time for you to stop. In women who smoke there is an increased likelihood of premature, low-birth-weight, and stillborn babies. Complications of pregnancy, including bleeding, placenta previa, and premature rupture of the membranes, are also more frequent in smokers. Many of these complications are thought to be caused by higher levels of carbon monoxide and lower levels of oxygen in the blood of women who smoke. Nicotine and small amounts of carbon monoxide circulating in the mother's bloodstream also may have adverse effects.

The harmful effects of smoking on the baby do not end at the time of delivery. Nicotine is transmitted through breast milk, and some of the undesirable consequences of this are known to produce a mild irritability. Also, bronchitis, pneumonia, and other types of respiratory distress are more common in children who live in a family where one or more family members smoke.

Alcohol also has been shown to affect the fetus adversely. In 1995 government researchers issued the distressing news that the percentage of babies born with health problems because their mothers drank alcohol during pregnancy increased sixfold from 1979 to 1993. Babies of alcoholic mothers are more likely to have birth defects such as mental and growth retardation. The fetal alcohol syndrome (FAS) consists of a small baby with a smaller than normal head, characteristic distorted facial appearance, heart defects, and mental retardation. While these serious problems are associated with heavy drinking, some medical researchers feel that no alcohol should be drunk during pregnancy because even small amounts can have a harmful effect on the fetus. (Only recently has there been any research on how sperm is affected by the father's heavy drinking.) Also, the caffeine in coffee, tea, many soft drinks, chocolate, and a number of drugs, when consumed in large quantities, may possibly cause birth defects.

Studies have shown that very few women go through an entire pregnancy without taking a single drug. This, of course, includes such things as vitamins, iron, or an occasional aspirin. Unfortunately, in our society many drugs are used more from habit than actual need—a decongestant for every stuffy nose or a sleeping pill that is not always necessary. Pregnant women should avoid the use of any medications that are not truly essential, because virtually no drug has been proven to be 100 percent safe for the unborn. Drugs taken by a woman during pregnancy can cross the placenta and reach the fetus, and unfortunately, most pregnant women use as many as four drugs during the early months, when the fetus is at greatest risk.

At least 80 percent of the drugs on the market have never been tested for safety during pregnancy because of FDA restrictions and the potential dangers of such testing. However, the following drugs are known to be potentially harmful: aspirin taken near the end of pregnancy (acetaminophen is a better choice); such antibiotics as tetracycline, streptomycin, and the sulfas (penicillin, ampicillin, and the cephalosporins are safer); the anticonvulsant Dilantin; the anticoagulant Warfarin; some high blood pressure medications; and excessive amounts of vitamins C, D, K, and of calcium and copper. Studies have also shown that Accutane, the drug widely prescribed for acne, if used during the first three months of pregnancy, puts the mother at 25 times the normal risk of having a baby with a major malformation. In addition, the FDA has issued warnings on Valium and Librium, which may cause cleft lip and palate or other defects in a small percentage of babies if taken by the mother during the first three months of pregnancy. Lithium, a drug used in certain psychiatric conditions, is thought to cause a significant increase in congenital cardiovascular malformation if taken during early pregnancy. (Additional information on drugs to be avoided during pregnancy can be found in the chapter on "Plain Talk about Medications.")

A pregnant woman must be concerned about other substances besides drugs. Chemicals, pesticides, and other toxic sprays may be absorbed into the mother's bloodstream. Because the effects of such substances on the fetus are unknown, it is best to limit contact with them. Any live-virus vaccines should also be avoided.

ACTIVITY

Keeping active during your pregnancy is very important. A 1988 study indicates that participation in a physical fitness program designed especially for pregnant women had no negative effects on either mother or fetus. These mothers-to-be had shorter second stages of labor, perhaps because of increased cardiovascular fitness and increased ability to postpone fatigue. A 1990 study published in the *American Journal of Obstetrics and Gynecology* presents reassuring evidence that vigorous exercise by *women who are already in good shape* does not harm a developing embryo during the first 10 weeks of pregnancy. Various studies continue to present statistics indicating that women who usually exercise should continue to do so during pregnancy and those who don't should begin. The standard advice offered by the American College of Obstetricians and Gynecologists is that pregnant women should engage in moderate activity three times a week. They should avoid any undue twisting of joints and jarring motions and should not exercise while lying flat on their back because this position may impede blood flow to the fetus.

If your pregnancy is proceeding normally, most of the activities you enjoyed before can be continued. Your guiding principle should be *moderation*. Walking is one of the best exercises for a pregnant woman. If there are no complications, exercising in water guaranteed to be unpolluted can continue up to the due date. Deep breathing exercises of the type recommended for stress management should be performed during the last month of pregnancy. This relaxation skill can be very helpful in minimizing labor pains.

Do not do any exercise that raises your pulse rate above 160. Avoid saunas, hot tubs, steam rooms, or excessive heat in any form. Abstain from exercise in hot, humid weather, and if you must exert yourself to the point of heavy sweating, be sure to increase your liquid intake. Avoid workouts involving bouncy movements such as jumping rope and hard games of tennis requiring abrupt changes in direction. Other sports to be given up during pregnancy include horseback riding, downhill skiing, and scuba diving.

Anyone with a chronic condition such as diabetes, high blood pressure, or cardiac impairment should ask the doctor for advice about an exercise schedule.

Many women wonder if they should travel while they are pregnant. This question usually can be answered with a bit of common sense. It would normally be wise not to travel to any part of the world where primitive public sanitation conditions prevail or where there is an epidemic. In general, the greatest risk in traveling is that you could develop a complication in a place where it would be difficult to obtain adequate medical care. Because complications are fewest during the middle three months, that is the safest time to travel. During the first three months there is always a possibility of a spontaneous abortion (miscarriage); during the last three there is a chance of premature labor or of ruptured membranes.

Continuing or starting to work during pregnancy is a matter of great concern to a growing number of women. They ask how long they can work. The answer depends on a realistic assessment of workplace hazards for the mother-to-be and the fetus, the financial situation of the household, the physical and emotional demands of the job, the company's pregnancy benefit policies, whether the pregnancy is complicated in some way, how much energy the woman uses getting to and from work and doing things at home, and other factors. A healthy woman with a normal pregnancy whose energy expenditure on the job and at other times is not more than minimally fatiguing can work until she is at least 36 weeks pregnant, maybe longer.

According to a study that was reported in 1990 in the *New England Journal of Medicine,* demanding and stressful work and long hours don't have an adverse effect on the outcome of a pregnancy. Researchers at the National Institutes of Health compared 1,293 physicians who became pregnant during their residencies with 1,494 wives of their male colleagues. The latter group of women also held full-time jobs but of a much less demanding nature. The female residents worked an average of more than 70 hours a week, and many kept working until a few days before delivery. The women in both groups had the same rates of miscarriage, stillbirths, and early deliveries, and these rates were comparable to those of the general population. From the study it would appear that the negative effects of highly demanding work are less significant than such socioeconomic factors as inadequate diet, poor prenatal care, and substance abuse.

Physically, a woman can return to work, if there have been no complications of great consequence, two weeks after delivery. However, specialists on early childhood development feel that the early weeks and months are important times for mother and baby to be together. Many women do not return to work until six weeks to three months after delivery, and many more choose to stay home longer or work on a part-time basis if these arrangements can be made. Thanks to fax machines and other technological advances, more women with preschool-age children are able to work at home, thus freeing themselves of the burden of finding affordable and acceptable child care. Every woman should know her employer's benefits and maternity policies and discuss her particular situation with her physician or other care provider (see the chapter on "Health Safeguards for Working Women").

Many factors contribute to the change in sexual relations that most couples experience during pregnancy. A woman may feel extremely attractive during pregnancy, or she may feel that she is totally undesirable. A man's feeling about the attractiveness of his pregnant lover may be just as variable. Some couples find that pregnancy is a time of increased sexual intimacy. Others find that their previously good sexual relationship has deteriorated. Some men express anxiety about possible trauma to the developing fetus during intercourse. Women often experience uterine cramping after orgasm, which may lead to fear of inducing abortion in early pregnancy or inducing labor later on. The pregnant woman's expanding shape may cause difficulty in finding comfortable positions.

Certain conditions may cause your doctor or nurse-midwife to recommend limitation of sexual relations during pregnancy. Among these conditions are a history of several early or mid-trimester spontaneous abortions or of premature labor, multiple pregnancy, polyhydramnios (excess amniotic fluid causing overdistention of the uterus), low-lying placenta, or placenta previa. Sexual relations should be discontinued if you have been told that your cervix has started to dilate, if your membranes have ruptured, or if you are having vaginal bleeding.

If the pregnancy is uncomplicated, many physicians feel that sexual relations can be continued throughout pregnancy. Because of the dilation of the cervix that may occur during the last month of pregnancy, some physicians routinely recommend discontinuance of sexual intercourse a month before the baby is due. Some recent studies have questioned the safety of intercourse in uncomplicated pregnancies, pointing to a small number of spontaneous abortions, infections, and premature deliveries occurring after sexual intercourse. More definitive studies need to be done in this area. In spite of the questions raised by these studies, the evidence doesn't seem conclusive enough to recommend limitation of sexual relations during the first eight months of a normal pregnancy.

COMPLICATIONS OF PREGNANCY

Although most pregnancies are uneventful and result in the birth of a normal healthy baby, complications sometimes arise. These complications include bleeding and spontaneous abortion, premature labor, ectopic pregnancy, preeclampsia and eclampsia, chronic and genetic disease, infections, Rh disease, intrauterine fetal death, and hydatidiform mole.

BLEEDING AND SPONTANEOUS ABORTION (MISCARRIAGE)

It is calculated that 15 to 20 percent of known pregnancies end in miscarriage (technically called spontaneous abortion) and that in 60 percent of all miscarriages the fetus is either anatomically or genetically abnormal. Thus, the phenomenon of spontaneous abortion can be viewed as a process of natural selection, because a healthy fetus is not easily dislodged. Most miscarriages occur during the first three months, and the increase in occurrence is attributed to many factors: the rising rate of sexually transmissible diseases, complications arising from the use of IUDs, and the postponement of pregnancy by more and more women into their late thirties, when eggs are likely to develop chromosomal abnormalities.

Although the occurrence of a bloody vaginal discharge reminiscent of menstruation once or twice in early pregnancy is not uncommon, it is sufficient reason to contact your doctor promptly. Until consultation and examination, limit physical activity as much as possible and avoid sexual intercourse. Often the bleeding stops spontaneously and is no further a problem. In cases like these, usually no cause for the bleeding is found.

The bleeding, however, may be evidence of a threatened abortion—an indication that a spontaneous abortion (miscarriage) may occur. By definition, pregnancies that end before the completion of the twentieth week of gestation are called abortions. If the bleeding is heavy, persists for a number of days or weeks, and is accompanied by cramping pain, it is even more suggestive of a threatened abortion. An abortion may be, of course, either spontaneous or induced. A threatened abortion becomes an inevitable abortion if the cervix dilates and the membranes rupture. This progresses to a complete or an incomplete abortion according to whether or not all the tissue comes out of the uterus spontaneously. Any tissue or suspected tissue appearing with vaginal bleeding should be kept and shown to your physician. Any tissue remaining in the uterus must be removed by a D&C. Sometimes an abortion occurs without any bleeding or other symptoms. This is most commonly diagnosed when the uterus stops growing in early pregnancy and is confirmed by an ultrasound examination that reveals a shriveled sac instead of a live fetus. This is a missed abortion, and a D&C is performed to remove the abnormal tissue.

A spontaneous abortion can be a very upsetting experience. It is important to realize that spontaneous abortions are very common and usually cannot be prevented. Furthermore, recent studies on the aborted tissue have shown that many of these pregnancies were not developing normally. Less commonly, a spontaneous abortion may occur when not enough progesterone is produced in early pregnancy to support the pregnancy. This can be tested and treated in subsequent pregnancies. Thus, spontaneous abortions help to assure that most pregnancies that reach the sixth month will result in normal, healthy babies. Having one spontaneous abortion does not mean that you will experience difficulty with your next pregnancy, nor does it mean that there is anything wrong with you or your partner. However, if a woman has had one miscarriage or more than one, there is a 25 to 40 percent likelihood that she will have another. After the second one, she should have a complete workup.

BLEEDING IN LATER PREGNANCY

One relatively uncommon problem that causes bleeding in later pregnancy is placenta previa. The placenta normally attaches to the side or the top of the uterine cavity. In placenta previa it attaches instead to the lowest part of the uterus and covers all or part of the cervix, thus possibly blocking the baby's exit through the birth canal. Bed rest will decrease the likelihood of bleeding, although extensive bleeding may nevertheless occur. The baby must be delivered by cesarean section if the placenta is blocking the entire cervix.

Another cause of bleeding in pregnancy is separation of a portion of the placenta from the uterine wall (placental abruption). If the detached portion is large, labor may begin. If the placenta detaches completely, the fetus will be unable to receive oxygen and nutrients from the mother and will die. Fortunately, the amount of separation is often small enough to allow the pregnancy to proceed normally.

If you have any bleeding during pregnancy, you should contact your physician. Keep in mind that not all bleeding during pregnancy means that something is wrong. Some women bleed during the first few months of pregnancy at the time they would have had their menstrual period. Sometimes an irritation on the cervix can cause bleeding after intercourse. During the last few weeks of pregnancy, many women have some spotting after a vaginal examination. Also, a small amount of bleeding sometimes occurs near the end of pregnancy as the cervix begins to dilate.

ECTOPIC PREGNANCY

In some pregnancies the fertilized egg does not implant in the uterus but in an ectopic (abnormal) location. By far the most common type of ectopic pregnancy is the tubal pregnancy. Other types include abdominal, ovarian, and cervical pregnancy.

Some women with an ectopic pregnancy exhibit all of the normal symptoms of pregnancy; others have none because of the lower hormone levels associated with ectopic pregnancies. Spotting is quite common in tubal pregnancies. As the embryo grows and pushes on the walls of the fallopian tube, pain can develop. Because the diameter of the tube is small, the pregnancy may rupture through the side of the fallopian tube, causing extensive intra-abdominal bleeding. In some cases the first sign of an ectopic pregnancy is a fainting spell caused by this sudden loss of blood internally. Ectopic pregnancies almost always cause symptoms that differ from those of a normal pregnancy before 12 weeks. Occasionally such pregnancies wither away, the woman remains well, and they are never diagnosed. They almost never result in a live birth.

The chances of developing an ectopic pregnancy are greater among women over 35 and among those who have had a history of pelvic infections, an infection after an abortion, an ectopic pregnancy in the past, or who use intrauterine contraceptive devices (see chapter on contraception for the relationship between IUDs and ectopic pregnancy). However, ectopic pregnancies often occur in the absence of any of these factors, and they are one of the four major causes of death during pregnancy, the other three being toxemia, infection, and hemorrhaging. It is a matter of concern that extrauterine pregnancies have increased dramatically in recent decades. Some authorities attribute this rise to the increase in cases of gonorrhea, chlamydia, and inadequately treated pelvic inflammatory disease.

In many cases an early tubal pregnancy may be removed and the fallopian tube repaired. This surgery may be performed either by laparoscopy or by laparotomy. If the tube is irreparably damaged, it may have to be removed. However, if the other tube is normal, future pregnancies are possible. If both fallopian tubes have been removed, pregnancy is possible with the aid of an infertility technique such as IVF (see chapter on "Infertility"). As more women are learning to recognize the symptoms of a possible ectopic pregnancy and seek earlier care, and with the development of more sophisticated diagnostic techniques such as laparoscopy and sonography, more surgery is being done before the tube is irreparably damaged. This, coupled with improved surgical techniques, means that it is becoming less and less necessary to remove the tube. On occasion methotrexate, a drug originally used for cancer chemotherapy, can be used to dissolve an ectopic pregnancy.

PRE-ECLAMPSIA AND ECLAMPSIA

(FORMERLY CALLED TOXEMIA OF PREGNANCY)

An abnormal elevation of blood pressure developing during the latter half of pregnancy (gestational hypertension) may occur in up to 5 percent of all pregnancies. A mild increase in blood pressure without any other symptoms is common. Though bleeding during pregnancy and placental abruption are more common in women with gestational hypertension, in most cases there is no ill effect. If the increase in blood pressure is significant, bed rest may be recommended in an attempt to reduce complications.

However, a rise in blood pressure accompanied by edema (fluid retention), protein in the urine, and abnormal blood testing indicates the onset of a condition called pre-eclampsia. Rapid weight gain caused by the fluid retention, severe headaches, and visual disturbances may occur. Pre-eclampsia is more common with first pregnancies. When mild, it can be treated by bed rest. Severe cases may require medications to lower the blood pressure and to prevent seizures. In its most severe form pre-eclampsia can be life threatening to both mother and baby, and delivery may be necessary even if the infant is premature. Severe pre-eclampsia is rare and with proper treatment is usually not a problem after delivery.

Eclampsia is an intensification of the symptoms designated as pre-eclampsia and is also characterized by convulsions. Eclampsia may develop from untreated pre-eclampsia, or it may occur without preliminary milder symptoms. No matter when in pregnancy eclampsia occurs, the pregnancy must be terminated after appropriate anticonvulsive-antihypertensive medication has been given. In women without chronic high blood pressure or kidney disease, pre-eclampsia or eclampsia usually does not recur during subsequent pregnancies.

CHRONIC DISEASES

Because of medical advances, successful pregnancy is now possible for women who in past years might not have been able to have children. This includes women under treatment for diabetes, high blood pressure, heart disease, epilepsy, and many other diseases. However, because proper treatment during pregnancy may be quite complicated, a woman with any of these problems should consult a doctor before she becomes pregnant.

If you have a mild form of diabetes, which is controlled by diet or by constant amounts of insulin, your diabetes probably will not prevent you from conceiving. It is very important that your diabetes be under good control before you conceive. Oral diabetic medications cannot be used in pregnancy, so the diabetes must be controlled by diet or insulin. Pregnancy is not always easy for a diabetic woman. Blood sugar levels must be followed closely and the insulin dosage adjusted frequently during pregnancy. Hospitalization is often necessary, especially late in pregnancy, and additional tests are done to assess the well-being of the fetus. If your diabetes has been difficult to control or if it has affected your kidneys or vision, pregnancy could seriously worsen your diabetes and threaten your life. Some women develop diabetes during pregnancy. Many physicians now perform screening tests for diabetes on all women during pregnancy. If this test is *not* done routinely by your doctor, you should ask to have it performed.

Diabetic mothers have an increased chance of needing a cesarean section, because babies born to diabetic mothers may be large, sometimes over 10 pounds. Also, many babies of diabetic mothers are delivered early to avoid fetal complications during the last few weeks of pregnancy. A baby of a diabetic mother may have hypoglycemia (low blood sugar) for the first day or two of life, but this can usually be treated by prompt feeding or intravenous feeding of sugar solutions.

Medication for high blood pressure may have to be adjusted during pregnancy. Some drugs are safer than others during pregnancy, and you should be on the safest possible drugs in the lowest dosage that will control your blood pressure. Some complications, such as bleeding and separation of the placenta, are more common in patients with high blood pressure. Babies born to mothers with severe high blood pressure may be smaller than average.

There are many changes in your heart and circulatory system during pregnancy. Some, but not all, heart problems may be worsened.

Pregnancy may be complicated by epilepsy. The risk of having a baby with a serious congenital defect is three to four times higher in epileptic women. Many of these birth defects, including cardiac anomalies, facial anomalies, and cleft lip and palate, are thought to be caused by the drugs used to control epilepsy, yet studies have shown that epileptic mothers who did not take medications during pregnancy also had an increased incidence of birth defects. Occasionally these defects may be diagnosed prior to birth by ultrasound. However, even with these problems and despite the substantially greater risks, most babies born to epileptic mothers (whether they are taking medication or not) are completely normal.

INFECTIONS

A woman may be exposed to a variety of infections during pregnancy. The most frequent of these is the common cold. A cold is a viral infection, and the usual routine of adequate rest and fluids is also appropriate for a pregnant woman. Some nonprescription cold remedies contain drugs that may not be safe during pregnancy. You should check with your physician before you take *any* medication. Most physicians feel that Tylenol is safe to use during pregnancy.

If you have a bad cough or a fever, you should notify your doctor promptly. What begins as a cold may progress to a more serious infection such as tonsillitis, sinusitis, or pneumonia. These infections are often bacterial and should be treated with antibiotics. Some antibiotics, such as tetracycline and chloramphenicol, should be avoided during pregnancy, but others, such as penicillin and erythromycin, are commonly used without any known side effects to the baby.

Urinary tract infections, such as bladder and kidney infections, may also occur in pregnant women. The symptoms of a bladder infection are burning urination, frequent urination, or bloody urine. The symptoms of a kidney infection are low back pain and a high fever. If you have any of these symptoms, notify your doctor promptly. Your urine can be examined microscopically and cultured for bacteria to determine whether you have a urinary infection. A mild infection can usually be treated by an oral antibiotic, but a severe infection may require hospitalization and intravenous antibiotics.

Some infections during pregnancy can cause dangerous side effects to the fetus before birth or to the baby as it passes through the birth canal. These include rubella (German measles), syphilis, gonorrhea, genital herpes, and AIDS. The most serious disease that can be transmitted by an infected mother to her newborn infant is AIDS. (See the chapter on "Sexually Transmissible Diseases.")

A simple blood test can confirm if a woman is immune to rubella. If she is not immune, she should have an immunization against the infection before she becomes pregnant. Because the vaccine contains a mild strain of live rubella virus, it should be given at least three months before a woman becomes pregnant; it should not be given to a woman who is already pregnant.

Unfortunately, it is not until they have become pregnant that many women realize that they are not immune to rubella. In this case exposure to anyone with the infection must be avoided. If you are not immune to rubella and think that you may have been exposed, notify your doctor so that the appropriate blood tests can be taken to see if you develop the disease. Postpartum rubella immunization should be given to prevent this problem during subsequent pregnancies.

If a pregnant woman is or becomes infected with syphilis, the bacteria can travel through her bloodstream and across the placenta to infect the baby. If she is treated promptly with antibiotics, the baby has a good chance of being completely normal. For this reason blood tests for syphilis are done routinely during pregnancy.

In the early stages of gonorrhea a woman may notice a foul-smelling yellow vaginal discharge, although there are often no symptoms at all. In early pregnancy the infection may spread into the uterus and the fallopian tubes, causing a generalized pelvic infection that, if not treated promptly, can cause spontaneous abortion. During the second half of pregnancy, gonorrhea is less likely to spread but may remain in the cervix and infect the baby at delivery.

In the past, babies exposed to gonorrhea while passing through the birth canal often developed gonorrheal eye infections that caused blindness. Today the routine administration of antibiotic or silver nitrate eye drops usually prevents blindness.

A third sexually transmitted infection is herpes genitalis. The initial symptoms of this disease may be painful blisters in the genital area, often accompanied by fever and swollen lymph nodes in the groin. Exposure to the virus as the baby passes through the birth canal can lead to severe infection and death. A woman who has herpes genitalis at the time of labor should optimally be delivered by cesarean section before the membranes rupture to prevent exposure of the infant to the infection. A primary herpes attack (that is, occurring in a woman who has never previously had a herpes infection) in the pregnant mother may pose a risk to the fetus even if it occurs prior to the time of delivery.

RH DISEASE

At your first prenatal visit your blood will be typed to determine whether you are Rh-negative (less than 14 percent of people are) or Rh-positive. If you are Rh-negative, another test will be done to see if you have Rh antibodies. In medical terminology, if you have Rh antibodies you are said to be "sensitized." If you are sensitized and your fetus is Rh-positive, it is possible that your Rh antibodies can damage the fetus's blood cells, causing it to have hemolytic anemia, brain damage, and other serious problems. Sensitized Rh-negative women need to be tested periodically during pregnancy to see if there are changes in their Rh antibody titers. This can give some indication of whether the fetus has any degree of Rh disease. But periodic examination of the amniotic fluid, obtained by amniocentesis (see next page), gives more accurate information about the fetus. If the fetus has Rh disease, intrauterine transfusions and/or early delivery may be necessary. Exchange transfusions may be needed after delivery.

The prevalent use of Rh-immune globulin after deliveries, miscarriages, abortions, and other situations where fetal blood may cross into the mother's circulation has dramatically reduced the incidence of Rh disease.

EVALUATING FETAL HEALTH

Among the many advances that have occurred in the field of obstetrics over the past few decades are the techniques for studying the fetus before birth: amniocentesis, ultrasound, fetal monitoring, and the alpha protein test. More recent advances include chorionic villi sampling, detection of additional genetic flaws, and—the latest and most exciting—a technique first used in France in 1983 and now available in most medical centers in the United States that enables doctors to evaluate, treat, and give blood transfusions to a fetus while it is still in the uterus.

ULTRASOUND

Ultrasound, or sonography, is a procedure that produces an image on a screen (sonogram) by bouncing sound waves through the abdomen. It locates the fetus in a manner similar to sonar locating a submarine. Many physicians recommend an ultrasound examination in mid-pregnancy to confirm the approximate due date, localize the placenta, and survey the fetal anatomy.

Ultrasound may be used to study the growth of a baby that seems to be too big or too small, to evaluate the growth of twins, or to monitor a suspected problem.

AMNIOCENTESIS

Various fetal chromosomal abnormalities and certain fetal diseases can be detected by testing amniotic fluid obtained by a procedure called amniocentesis. The procedure is fairly simple. A sonogram is obtained to determine the location of the placenta, and the lower abdomen is cleaned with an antiseptic solution. A local anesthetic is given, and a long, thin needle is inserted through the abdominal and uterine walls into the amniotic sac. Amniotic fluid is then removed with a syringe. This procedure can be done only by a specially trained person.

The risks of amniocentesis include infection, injury to the fetus or the placenta, Rh-sensitization, leakage of amniotic fluid, and bleeding. In expert hands the overall complication rate of amniocentesis is less than 1 percent.

A common reason for doing an amniocentesis is to determine whether the fetus is genetically normal (genetic amniocentesis). This has usually been done at approximately the sixteenth week of pregnancy, but in some cases the test is now being done earlier. Fetal cells that are in the fluid are cultured and then examined for chromosomal abnormalities, such as Down syndrome. New data reveals that Down syndrome (technically called Trisomy 21 after the number assigned to the abnormal chromosome) increases steadily with age rather than rising dramatically at age 35. Because it is now known that the statistical curve is continuous, amniocentesis has become an accepted procedure and should be considered by all pregnant women over 34 years of age, and perhaps younger, who would consider abortion if the fetus had this genetic defect.

The fluid is also routinely tested for alpha-feto protein. An elevated level could indicate an increased risk of open neural tube defects.

CHORIONIC VILLI SAMPLING

One alternative to amniocentesis in detecting chromosomal abnormalities such as Down syndrome can be done as early as the ninth week of pregnancy; it is known as chorionic villi sampling (CVS). Whereas amniocentesis involves withdrawing of the amniotic fluid by way of a hollow needle that penetrates the mother's abdominal wall, this newer method withdraws a sample of the chorion villus (tissue that surrounds the fetus and eventually becomes the placenta) and removes the sample through the cervix or through a needle stuck in the lower abdomen. Questions about the safety of this procedure were laid to rest in 1994, when a study of more than 150,000 women indicated that it did not increase the risk of birth defects. This risk was placed at 1 percent and attributed to the likelihood that the doctors administering it were not yet fully experienced in doing so. The major advantage of CVS is the fact that it can be done early enough in pregnancy so that, if a woman chooses to have an abortion because of a genetic or other identified birth defect, the abortion can be an earlier and safer one.

ALPHA-FETO PROTEIN ASSESSMENT

Alpha-feto protein (AFP) is produced by every fetus and is present in both its amniotic fluid and its mother's blood. If the AFP level in the latter is abnormally high (positive test) around the fourth month of pregnancy, it may mean that the fetus has an open neural tube defect (an incomplete closure of the neural tube around the spinal cord or brain). It may also mean that there are twins or that the fetus is older than it was thought to be. In any event, sonography is then done, and if it does not verify the possibility of an open neural tube defect, an amniocentesis is done, and its AFP measured. If it is positive (high), there is a 90 percent chance that the fetus has an open neural tube defect. In the United States, 1 to 2 out of 1,000 babies have a neural tube defect (NTD). Couples with a family or personal history of NTD are at some increased risk of having an NTD baby and certainly should have the AFP blood test. But because only 5 percent of all NTD babies have a parent with such a history, couples without such a history may also desire the test, which, although not conclusive, requires no more than a blood sample for assessment. Also, a very low AFP measurement may indicate an increased risk of chromosomal abnormality such as Down syndrome and may indicate the need for further testing to rule out such a disorder.

PRENATAL DNA STUDIES

Through prenatal DNA studies, it is now possible to detect hundreds of genetic, chromosomal, and other birth defects in the fetus. In order to make such discoveries, however, investigators must know in advance which disease is being looked for. Only a few laboratories nationwide are equipped to perform prenatal DNA tests, but those parents-to-be who have genetic diseases in the family or have already had an affected child should know that this option exists. Additional information can be supplied by a genetic counselor or by the March of Dimes Birth Defect Program. (See "Directory of Health Information.")

OTHER PROCEDURES FOR PRENATAL DIAGNOSIS

Fetoscopy is still an experimental procedure, usually performed in the second trimester, to make prenatal diagnoses of hemoglobinopathies and coagulation defects. It involves passing a small-caliber fetoscope through the abdominal wall into the uterus.

One of the most promising developments in prenatal assessment enables doctors to thread a needle into the tiny blood vessels of the umbilical cord and use the needle to withdraw fetal blood samples as well as to inject drugs into the fetus or to supply blood transfusions. This procedure has already revolutionized the treatment of fetuses with Rh disease. It may also be useful in checking to see if the fetus has an infection that the mother may have transmitted to it.

FETAL MONITORS

Many hospitals now have fetal monitors that record the fetal heartbeat and contractions of the uterus during labor. In some hospitals monitors are used for all patients in labor; others have monitors only for patients who have a higher than normal risk of developing complications.

Fetal monitors can be attached either externally or internally. In external monitoring the monitor is placed on the mother's abdomen by means of adjustable bands. In internal monitoring a wire is inserted through the vagina and attached to the fetal head. A catheter may also be inserted through the vagina into the amniotic sac adjacent to the fetus.

The use of a fetal monitor should not prevent the mother-to-be from finding a comfortable position in labor, whether that be sitting or lying on her back or side. There are telemetric monitors that allow the mother to be completely mobile while the fetus is monitored. Although some women do not like the idea of being attached to a machine, it is important to realize that the valuable information obtained in this way may protect the life of the baby, and many women are reassured to be able to "see" the baby's heartbeat on the monitor during labor.

Monitors are used to test for, among other things, abnormalities in the fetal heart rate. For example, a drop in the fetal heart rate may signal that the fetus is not receiving adequate levels of oxygen because of an abnormal decrease in

AMNIOCENTESIS IN EIGHTEENTH WEEK

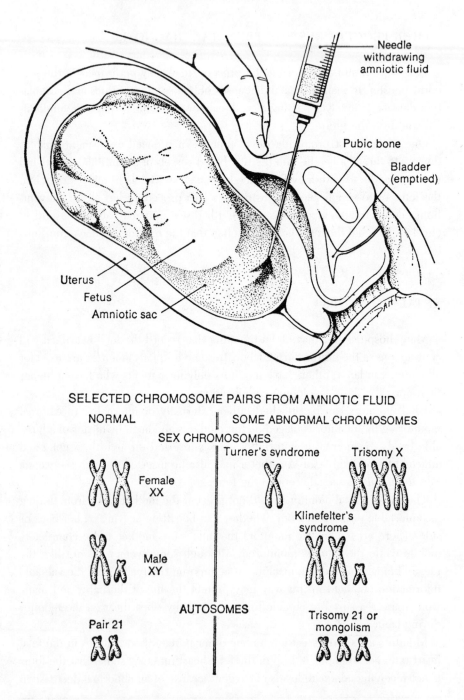

Needle withdrawing amniotic fluid

Pubic bone

Bladder (emptied)

Uterus

Fetus

Amniotic sac

SELECTED CHROMOSOME PAIRS FROM AMNIOTIC FLUID

NORMAL

SOME ABNORMAL CHROMOSOMES

SEX CHROMOSOMES

Turner's syndrome

Trisomy X

Female XX

Male XY

Klinefelter's syndrome

AUTOSOMES

Pair 21

Trisomy 21 or mongolism

blood flowing to the baby during contractions. The decrease might be caused by a twisted or knotted umbilical cord. This problem can sometimes be improved by changing the position of the mother, by giving her oxygen, or by placing additional fluid in the amniotic sac. Many changes in the baby's heart rate on the monitor do not indicate any serious abnormality in the baby.

Monitoring may also be used for patients who are not in labor if the pregnancy is complicated, if the baby is overdue, or if the mother has a medical problem. For example, a fetal monitor can be used to perform the nonstress test (NST), which determines whether the baby's heartbeat accelerates after the baby kicks or moves. A temporary increase in the fetal heart rate after movement is an indication that the baby is in satisfactory condition.

If this test is also nonreactive, a contraction stress test (CST) is done, again using a fetal monitor. Mild contractions are started by stimulation of the mother's nipples or by injection of a dilute intravenous solution of oxytocin, the hormone that is released by the body during labor. A healthy fetus will exhibit a stable heart rate during and after the contractions. On the other hand, a decrease in the fetal heart rate following the contractions may indicate that the fetus is not receiving sufficient oxygen.

Another test now performed in many medical centers finds out if a baby is receiving sufficient oxygen by actually taking a sample of the baby's blood. This test, called a scalp pH, is done only during labor and only if the membranes are ruptured. It may be performed if fetal heartbeat abnormalities are noted or if there are other reasons to believe that the baby may not be receiving adequate oxygen. In a manner similar to the way a blood sample is obtained by sticking a finger with a lance, a small puncture is made in the baby's scalp and a few drops of blood are drawn into a capillary tube. The pH of the blood is an indirect measure of the amount of oxygen being received.

If these tests indicate that the baby is in jeopardy and delivery is not imminent, it will be necessary to induce labor or to deliver the baby by cesarean section. These tests have undoubtedly prevented the deaths of some babies who would not have lived if prompt action had not been taken.

LABOR AND DELIVERY

Normally labor and subsequent delivery occur 38 to 40 weeks (gestational age) after the start of the last normal menstrual period (a term birth). (This is 36 to 38 weeks after conception, but this time reference is rarely used.) Labor that occurs before 37 completed weeks of gestation is considered to be premature or pre-term labor. The mechanisms responsible for the onset of labor at any time are not well identified. Premature labor is more likely to occur when a woman has more than one fetus; has a serious obstetrical condition (pre-eclampsia, placental bleeding); has chronic liver, heart, or kidney disease; or has experienced a serious trauma, either physical or emotional. In most instances, however, there is no well-understood explanation. Premature delivery may also be caused by an incompetent or "weak" cervix, a relatively rare condition.

The problem about premature labor is that it may lead to the premature birth of an underdeveloped premature infant whose chance of survival or of being normal is reduced. The earlier the birth and the more underdeveloped the infant, the smaller the chance. These babies should be cared for in a hospital's intensive care nursery and, if possible, be born in that hospital rather than transported there after birth.

There is a great need to learn more about what causes premature labor so that efforts can be made to prevent it. Sometimes it is possible, particularly if the membranes have not ruptured, to arrest it with various pharmacologic agents and to postpone the birth by days or weeks so that the fetus can develop further prior to birth. However, premature birth frequently follows premature labor.

Labor that occurs after 42 or more completed weeks of gestation is postmature (post-term) labor. After this time, if the dates are certain, the fetus is usually better off in a nursery than in the uterus, and consideration may be given to inducing labor.

NATURAL CHILDBIRTH

Natural childbirth has become quite popular in the United States. Its popularity began after Grantly Dick-Read wrote *Childbirth Without Fear* in 1944. He wrote that labor pain could be eliminated by education in the process of labor and delivery. Despite the substantial contribution of this new theory, it soon became apparent that Dick-Read was not entirely correct, because even with extensive knowledge about labor and delivery, many women still felt pain.

The next step in the popularity of natural childbirth was the Lamaze or psychoprophylactic technique. Psychoprophylaxis is the psychological and physical preparation for childbirth. This technique originated in Russia and was brought to France by Dr. Ferdinand Lamaze in the early 1950s. Its popularity in the United States followed the publication in 1959 of *Thank You Dr.*

Lamaze by Marjorie Karmel, an American woman who became familiar with the Lamaze technique during her pregnancy in France.

The Lamaze technique combines education about labor and delivery with breathing and relaxation exercises. The exercises must be practiced in the months and weeks prior to labor. The partner has an important role as coach. Using the Lamaze breathing techniques, many women are able to go through labor needing little or no medication. Though a purist may insist that a true Lamaze birth means no medication at all, many people believe that the concept is broad enough to include the use of a small amount of medication to relieve pain.

With my observations as an obstetrician and as a woman who has experienced labor, I feel that the Lamaze technique has something to offer to every pregnant woman. I believe that the knowledge of what is happening to your body in labor and delivery can reduce your apprehension and fear and, therefore, reduce the pain of your labor. I also feel that the Lamaze breathing and relaxation techniques reduce, though not necessarily eliminate, the need for medication in labor.

ANESTHESIA

A difficult and painful labor may require some anesthesia or analgesia. Anesthesia may also be required for medical reasons or for a forceps delivery.

The most commonly used medications for labor are pain-killing drugs such as Demerol. With small doses many women are less uncomfortable but still wide awake and able to participate in and enjoy the delivery of their child. However, some women find that even small doses of these medications make them drowsy or nauseated.

Epidural anesthesia involves the insertion of a needle in the mother's back and the injection of a novocaine-type drug into the space next to the spinal canal. An epidural will normally eliminate pain from approximately your waist to your toes and will make it difficult to move your legs. This technique allows you to be completely awake but free from pain. Caudal anesthesia is similar to an epidural, but the needle is inserted at a point much lower on your back.

Epidural or caudal anesthesia requires a specially trained anesthesiologist and is not available at all hospitals. These anesthetics do not always work perfectly, and they may have undesirable side effects. Some women are numbed on only one side of their body or not at all. Sometimes this type of anesthesia can cause the contractions to become less frequent, and in some women it may interfere with the urge to push during the second stage of labor. By lowering the mother's blood pressure, epidural or caudal anesthesia can even cause a temporary slowing of the baby's heartbeat.

Unlike epidural or caudal anesthesia, which can be used to provide pain relief during labor, spinal anesthesia is used to provide relief only for delivery. Saddle block is a type of spinal anesthesia. A needle is inserted into the mother's back and the medication is injected into the space that contains the spinal fluid. Under spinal anesthesia most women are completely numbed from their waist to their toes. When spinal anesthesia is given for a cesarean section, the numbness usually extends to the lower part of the mother's rib cage. The numbness may last for several hours after delivery depending on the type of anesthetic used and the individual's sensitivity to it. A small percentage of women may have a severe headache for several days after spinal anesthesia.

If a woman has not received any medication or pain relief for labor, local anesthesia may be used at the time of delivery to numb the area where an episiotomy is to be cut or a tear is to be repaired.

FIRST STAGE OF LABOR: DILATATION OF THE CERVIX

No two labors are alike. Labor may be long and difficult or it may be short and uncomplicated. Unfortunately, there is no way to predict what your labor will be like or how you will respond to it. When labor begins, you may feel the contractions as mild cramps or they may be very uncomfortable. As labor progresses, the contractions become stronger and more frequent. In active labor the contractions usually occur about every 2 to 3 minutes and last from 45 to 90 seconds. Usually the membranes rupture spontaneously either before or during labor, but if they do not, they are ruptured artificially before the delivery.

The cervix, the lowermost portion of the uterus, must open so that the baby can be born. During most of pregnancy the cervix is firm, thick, and long, with only a very small opening in the center. Late in pregnancy the cervix becomes softer, thinner, and may begin to open before the onset of labor. When labor begins, the changes in the cervix take place much more rapidly. The contractions of the uterus push the baby's head against the cervix and cause it to open. In order for the baby to be born, the cervix must be fully dilated to 10 centimeters (about 4 inches).

The first stage of labor is the time from the onset of labor to the time when the cervix is fully dilated. The length of this stage of labor varies greatly from

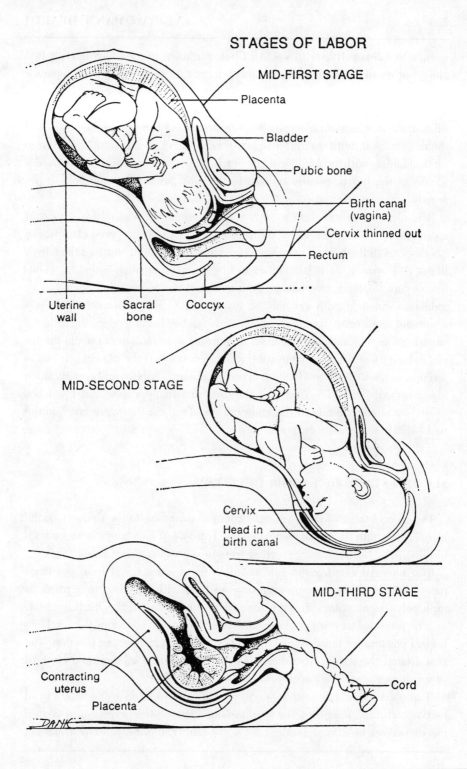

STAGES OF LABOR

MID-FIRST STAGE

- Placenta
- Bladder
- Pubic bone
- Birth canal (vagina)
- Cervix thinned out
- Rectum

Uterine wall   Sacral bone   Coccyx

MID-SECOND STAGE

Cervix
Head in birth canal

MID-THIRD STAGE

Contracting uterus
Placenta

Cord

DANK

woman to woman. It averages 8 to 12 hours in most women having their first child, but it can be much shorter or much longer. In subsequent pregnancies it is usually shorter.

Near the end of the first stage of labor, when the cervix is almost fully dilated, the contractions are usually quite strong and the woman begins to feel the urge to push with them. This part of labor is called transition. After complete dilation, with pushing and the force of the contractions, the baby descends in the pelvis, usually turning to the most favorable position as it descends.

It is sometimes necessary to induce labor instead of waiting for it to start spontaneously. For example, if the mother develops severe pre-eclampsia or has diabetes, if the baby is overdue, if fetal monitoring indicates that the baby's life is in jeopardy, or if labor does not begin spontaneously after the membranes rupture, labor may have to be induced. If the cervix is not favorable for induction, prostaglandin gel may be given in the vagina to make the cervix softer and more ready for labor. In some cases labor is induced by the artificial rupture of membranes. In most cases an infusion of a solution of pitocin (oxytocin), which causes the uterus to contract, is necessary. If the pitocin solution is given intravenously in gradually increasing amounts, labor can be very much like a normal labor. The "horror" stories of unusually strong and fast labor caused by pitocin pertain to the higher doses of pitocin that were given in the past—not to the dosage currently in use.

SECOND STAGE OF LABOR: DELIVERY

The second stage of labor extends from full dilatation to the delivery of the baby. The length of this stage also varies. It may last two hours or more with the first baby but is usually much shorter in subsequent pregnancies.

In a typical United States hospital delivery you are taken from the labor room to the delivery room and put on your back with your legs in stirrups, as for a pelvic examination. In a birthing room the bottom of the "birthing bed" may be removed as you get closer to delivery. In other countries the mother's normal position for delivery may be on her side or in a squatting position. The area around the vagina is washed off with an antiseptic solution and cloth or paper drapes are placed over your abdomen and legs.

If an episiotomy is necessary, it will be done after the top of the baby's head becomes visible. An episiotomy is an incision made in the perineum to expand the vaginal opening to allow the baby to be born without extensive stretching or tearing of the muscles and tissues in this area. Episiotomy was done fairly routinely in the past because it was thought to prevent problems that might arise later in life such as the prolapse of the bladder, rectum, or uterus. Because newer studies have questioned this preventive effect, episiotomy is done less routinely today.

The first part of the baby to emerge is usually its head. Then the shoulders are delivered and the rest of the body slips out easily. After emerging, the baby will take a first breath and cry a first cry. When the baby begins breathing, oxygen is received through the lungs rather than through the placenta and the umbilical cord. At this time the cord is clamped and cut.

In what is known as a "breech" birth, the baby is positioned so that its feet or buttocks lie nearest the birth canal. In such cases, delivery is usually done by cesarean section.

There is no need to become alarmed if forceps are used to assist in the delivery of your baby. Forceps are metal instruments, shaped somewhat like a pair of large spoons, which fit against the sides of the baby's head and are used to guide it through the birth canal. Marks commonly caused by the forceps may remain on the baby's cheeks for several days and are not indicative of any problem. Forceps are often used if an emergency delivery is necessary, as in the case of "fetal distress" or bleeding. However, if these problems occur early in labor, before the cervix is fully dilated, a cesarean section may be necessary. Sometimes forceps are used because the mother is too exhausted to push the baby out or because the baby's head is tilted in a position that makes spontaneous delivery very difficult.

A device sometimes used as a substitute for forceps is a vacuum extractor, a plastic or metal suction cup that is placed over the baby's head to guide it through the vagina. While a vacuum extractor does not leave marks on the baby's cheeks, it may leave a temporary swelling or bruising of the top of the head.

In recent years, many hospitals have modified the environment provided for labor and delivery. In some places routine deliveries may be done in a bed rather than on a delivery table. In other places the delivery room is darkened and soft music played. In still others an attempt is made to give the delivery room a more homelike atmosphere by the installation of curtains, carpeting, and pictures. Such rooms are called birthing rooms. One or two support persons (visitors) are encouraged to be with the woman through labor, delivery, and recovery. In many places, in fact, a support person is permitted to be present in a regular delivery room, even during a cesarean section. In a delivery technique called a Leboyer delivery, lights and noise are kept to a minimum, the child is placed on the mother's abdomen for several minutes before the umbilical cord is clamped, and the baby is promptly given a bath in warm water. This technique was devised to try to ease the trauma of the newborn's entry into the world. However, there is no scientific evidence that this approach has any beneficial effect.

THIRD STAGE OF LABOR: AFTERBIRTH

The third stage of labor involves the delivery of the placenta. Usually within a few minutes after the delivery of the baby the placenta separates itself from the wall of the uterus and is expelled. After this point the episiotomy or any tears are repaired. Dissolving sutures are usually used; there are no stitches to be removed later.

CESAREAN SECTION

Cesarean section is the delivery of a baby through an incision in the abdominal and uterine walls. General anesthesia may be used or the mother may remain awake with either spinal or epidural anesthesia.

In recent years there has been a strong and outspoken reaction against the increase in cesarean deliveries. Many experts are convinced that at least half of these were unnecessary. (The United States stands first in the rate of cesarean deliveries.) Taking note of the fact that this rate has quadrupled since 1970, Dr. Warren Pearce, executive director of the American College of Obstetrics and Gynecology, agreed that the rate should be no higher than 12 to 16 births out of every 100. He also noted that it was by no means always necessary to repeat the cesarean procedure if it was used once before. These repeat performances are among the main cause of the swelling in the statistics. Other contributing factors include an overdiagnosis of abnormal labor and fetal distress (an overdiagnosis partly caused by the ever-present possibility of a malpractice suit) and the fact that the procedure in some cases is more convenient and more profitable to the doctor and hospital.

In 1995 both the American College of Obstetricians and Gynecologists and the Public Citizen's Health Research Group set a national goal to reduce the cesarean rate from the level of nearly 23 percent of all births to less than 15 percent by the year 2000. A major motivation is the additional cost. A cesarean costs on average 20 to 40 percent more in doctor's fees and roughly double in hospital fees. This economic factor is of considerable concern to insurance providers.

Informed critics point out that the substitution of cesarean sectioning for normal labor can increase the risk of illness or death for the mother, in addition to leaving her with an incalculable psychological burden.

A woman who is told during pregnancy that a prenatal diagnosis indicates the need for cesarean delivery would be wise to seek a second opinion, and women who have had one such delivery (estimated at nearly 600,000 each year) should not assume or be led to believe that a second one is inevitable. In the considered opinion of the most informed members of the profession, this point of view is completely outdated. An option selected by an increasing number of women in this category is vaginal delivery. In a survey conducted in 1990 for the American College of Obstetricians and Gynecologists, it was reported that 6 out of 10 women who tried vaginal delivery after a cesarean section were successful; most of the others had to have another cesarean delivery because of such preexisting conditions as diabetes, high blood pressure, or a complicated pregnancy indicating the advisability of surgical delivery. It was also reported that patients of younger doctors who encouraged the newer procedure were more likely to succeed than those whose older doctors were less enthusiastic about it. However, many women still want to have cesareans, according to Dr. Bruce Flamm, an expert in vaginal birth after cesareans and research chairman at Kaiser Permanente, a health maintenance organization, in Riverside, California. In a recent *New York Times* (8/3/95) interview, Dr. Flamm said, "There's a new image, a VBAC [vaginal birth after cesarean] resister, who is a professional woman who schedules a Caesarian between business commitments. After speaking with half a dozen women about their decision, I found that control was indeed the issue."

There are two types of skin incisions used for cesarean deliveries: a vertical incision from the navel to the pubic hairline or a horizontal ("bikini") incision near the top of the pubic hairline. A vertical incision may be necessary if the cesarean delivery is an emergency, if the baby is very large or in an abnormal position, or if the patient is obese. In other cases either type may be used, although many physicians have been trained to use predominantly one type of skin incision or the other. The various layers of the abdominal wall are carefully opened until the uterus is exposed. In most cases a horizontal incision is then made in the lower part of the uterus and the baby is delivered. The uterus is then carefully repaired and the abdominal wall is closed.

Cesarean section may be necessary if the baby is in a position that makes vaginal delivery difficult or potentially dangerous. For example, 4 percent of all babies are in the breech position at the end of pregnancy. The baby's head is

POSITIONS OF THE FETUS

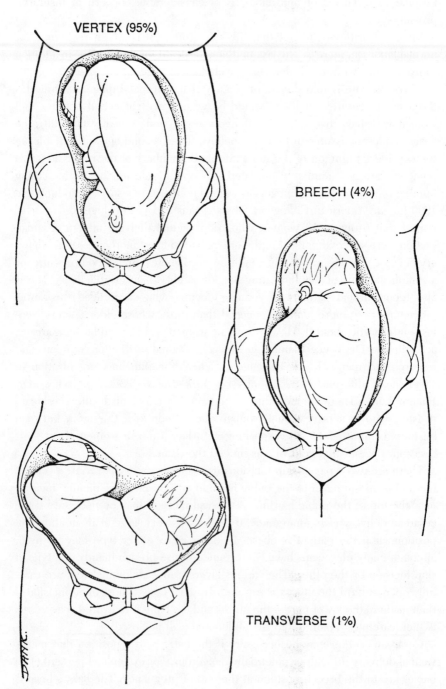

VERTEX (95%)

BREECH (4%)

TRANSVERSE (1%)

the largest part of the baby that must pass through the mother's pelvic bones. When a baby is born head first, the head has a chance to elongate and thus decrease in diameter in order to pass through the pelvic bones. When the baby is breech, the head does not have a chance to accommodate itself to the mother's pelvic bones, and some babies born breech suffer permanent damage. For this reason many doctors now advise a cesarean section in all cases of breech babies unless there is specific evidence that the mother's pelvic bones are large enough to accommodate the baby's head.

A position that makes vaginal delivery impossible is a transverse lie (across the pelvic opening, neither the head nor buttocks down). Unless the baby can be turned into a normal position, it cannot be born vaginally and must be delivered by cesarean section.

Sometimes a cesarean section must be done for the safety of the mother. If the mother has severe pre-eclampsia, severe high blood pressure may be life-threatening to her. If labor cannot be quickly induced, a cesarean section may have to be done. Similarly, any danger to your baby, as evidenced by a drop in the baby's heart rate, may cause your doctor to recommend a cesarean section.

After a cesarean section, you will probably be in the hospital for at least three or four days. As with most abdominal operations, you will receive intravenous fluids for a few days. Moving around will be difficult, but forcing yourself to get up and walk will probably speed your recovery. You will need more rest than if you had a vaginal delivery. Not only is your body going through the adjustment of getting back to a nonpregnant state, but it must also recover from a major abdominal operation.

AFTER THE DELIVERY

Your baby has been born and you are probably elated. You hold your baby in amazement at this new life. But labor has been aptly named and you have been working very hard and are exhausted. You very likely have missed a night's sleep and you will probably sleep soundly for a few hours after the baby is born. Meanwhile your baby will be in a nursery being evaluated and cared for by a pediatrician and nurses. New babies should have a full physical examination to check for congenital or genetic problems and possible infections. A hearing test is recommended when the baby is one day old. A few days later babies should have a blood test to evaluate their thyroid function and to see if they have phenylketonuria (PKU). If either test is positive, proper treatment can prevent major future problems. Babies born to mothers who have diseases such as diabetes or hepatitis B or who are taking certain medications need to be evaluated for any related problems. Although the National Institutes of Health recommended in 1988 that all states establish a universal screening program for sickle cell disease, some states continue to target only the babies born to higher risk groups.

ROOMING-IN

Many hospitals have made "rooming-in" available to mothers. Perhaps you have just had a baby girl. Rooming-in allows you to be with her, care for her, feed her, bathe her, and change her under the supervision of the hospital's nursing staff. Some hospitals offer a modified rooming-in where you can take your baby during the day but have her cared for in the nursery at night. Others allow you to rest for the first day before you take the baby both day and night. The baby is usually taken out of the room when you have visitors.

If you are at all apprehensive about caring for your new baby, rooming-in provides excellent practice with trained people to answer your questions and to give you assistance. Recent experimental evidence, mostly from animal studies, seems to show that prolonged early contact between mother and child (called bonding) may be beneficial to the health and well-being of both mother and child. Rooming-in allows more contact between mother and child during these important early days.

However, you should consider your feelings and physical condition after the delivery. When you leave the hospital, you will be returning to your care of the household with the additional attention and energy the baby requires. If you're very tired and want to take advantage of your days in the hospital to recover your strength, rooming-in is not essential.

HOSPITAL VISITORS

Well-meaning friends and relatives want to visit mother and baby as soon as possible, and if it weren't for hospital rules, the lying-in room would be mobbed from morning to night. A new mother should make sure there's a phone at her bedside not only so that she can keep in touch with the world but also so that she has a tactful way of discouraging unwanted visits and postponing them until after homecoming.

If you're pregnant with your second child, it's a good idea to find out in advance of delivery what policy the hospital imposes on visits by children who want to see the new family member. Many hospitals now allow young children to enter the maternity floor, but most don't permit them to get any closer than the glass partition outside the nursery.

THE "BABY BLUES"

After the first day or two of excitement, new mothers are likely to experience some form of postpartum depression, the "baby blues." While nearly two-thirds have the blues for only a brief period, for about 10 percent the depressive symptoms are prolonged and severe. Recent studies support the theory that the trigger is biological, pointing to the fact that postpartum depression is just as common in rural Africa as it is in the industrialized West. Many things contribute to it—the letdown after nine months of anticipating the birth, hormonal changes accompanying the start of the flow of milk, fatigue from labor, anxiety about the realities of having a baby who needs taking care of.

This depression may recur periodically in the first few months after birth as your body continues to make major adjustments in returning to the non-pregnant state, as you deal with your new role and activities, especially if it is a first child, and as you simply go through the physical stress of not having an uninterrupted night's sleep. Again the depression usually passes quickly. But if the depression persists or if you're increasingly upset by the constant crying and your nerves are ragged because of constant loss of sleep, it is extremely important for your well-being and the building of a satisfactory relationship with the baby *not* to deny your feelings of anger and frustration and *not* to keep trying to suppress your feelings of irritation with the baby because the feelings produce so much guilt. Better by far to deal with the negative feelings, air them, and accept the need for help and support. In such circumstances, don't let anyone—and that includes well-meaning friends and family members—make light of your anxieties. Ask your obstetrician or primary care doctor for a recommendation of a therapist or a support group until you can face the day-in, day-out stress of parenting without feeling overwhelmed. Referrals and additional information are available by calling Depression After Delivery (800)-944-4773. You can also help yourself by resuming as many of your outside-the-home activities as soon as you can handle them.

PHYSICAL RECOVERY

After delivery you will have vaginal bleeding. The blood comes from the uterus and is called lochia. Lochia will be heavy and bright red for the first few days after delivery. Thereafter the flow decreases but may persist as a red or brown staining lasting for several weeks. If you are breast feeding, there may be an increase in bleeding at feeding time. You may also feel cramps during feedings. You may feel your uterus as a firm grapefruit-sized or larger mass in your lower abdomen. The uterus will return to almost normal size within a month.

If you do not nurse, your first menstrual period may come in six to eight weeks, although it may be delayed for several months. If you do nurse, your first menstrual period will normally be later. Some women have no menses while they nurse; others resume having menstrual periods after four to six months.

The return of fertility is also unpredictable. Some women ovulate within a month after delivery and before their first menstrual period; in others the return to the normal ovulatory cycle takes much longer. Although breast feeding may reduce your chances of becoming pregnant, you should not count on this alone to prevent pregnancy. Many women ovulate and become pregnant while nursing. Whether you are nursing or not, if you do not wish to have another baby right away, it is important to use some form of contraception as soon as you resume having sexual relations. Most physicians recommend waiting at least two weeks before resuming sexual relations. Some recommend waiting until after the postpartum checkup, four to six weeks after delivery.

If you have had an episiotomy, you may find the stitches uncomfortable for the first day or two, and you may be given a mild pain medication. The pain gradually decreases, although it may last for several days or weeks. Pain with sexual intercourse may last for several months after the episiotomy is healed. Conscious tightening and relaxation of the perineal muscles surrounding the episiotomy will help healing and will also decrease the pain of the episiotomy. This exercise also helps a normal tone to return to these muscles.

In nursing mothers the hormone balance inhibits vaginal lubrication. Nursing mothers frequently have a problem with painful intercourse. Using a lubricant will help, but other things do not return to normal until after nursing has been discontinued.

Hemorrhoids are varicose veins in the rectal area and are very common in pregnant women, even those who have no evidence of varicose veins in any other place. They develop during pregnancy because of the pressure on the veins from the growing uterus and are aggravated by the constipation that is common in pregnancy. Hemorrhoids often worsen at the end of pregnancy and during labor. In the first few days after delivery you may need an anesthetic cream to help reduce the discomfort. Fortunately, in most women hemorrhoids disappear or become asymptomatic within a few months after delivery.

Some women experience difficulty in urination after delivery. The baby's head presses against the bladder while moving through the birth canal, and this pressure can result in a decrease in the normal sensation in this area for a time after delivery. Anesthetics used in labor and delivery can also decrease the sensation of the bladder. The reduced sensation can cause difficulty in control of urination or difficulty in knowing when the bladder is full. Sensation and control gradually return to normal after delivery.

If you weigh yourself on the day after delivery, you will probably find that you have lost only about 12 to 16 pounds. The weight gained in pregnancy is more than just the weight of the baby, the placenta, and the amniotic fluid. For example, the breasts normally increase by about 1 pound, blood volume increase accounts for about $3\frac{1}{2}$ pounds, and the uterus increases by $2\frac{1}{2}$ pounds. The mother's body also retains fluid and a small amount of fat is deposited. Most mothers shed an additional 5 pounds in the first two weeks after delivery. Mothers who nurse use up some of the additional fat that has been deposited during pregnancy; mothers who do not nurse may have to go on a more restrictive diet than nursing mothers in order to return to their normal prepregnancy weight.

The stretch marks (striae) that may have developed on your abdomen or breasts will gradually fade but will not disappear completely. In spite of many available ointments and home remedies, there is no prevention or cure for a stretch mark.

BREAST-FEEDING

During pregnancy the glands in your breasts develop in order to produce milk after the baby is born. During the last few months there may be leakage of a small amount of colostrum, a thin yellow fluid. Shortly after delivery the amount of colostrum increases substantially, and colostrum is the only food that breast-fed babies receive during the first few days of their life. On the third or fourth postpartum day, production of milk begins. The amount of milk that is produced depends on the amount of stimulation and sucking by the baby. The repeated emptying of the breasts increases the milk supply to meet the needs of a growing baby.

Breast milk is the ideal food for a baby. The Committee on Nutrition of the American Academy of Pediatrics recommends that every mother breast-feed her baby unless there is a specific medical reason why she cannot. Among the many benefits are the following:

- The baby's nutritional needs are more closely satisfied by breast milk.
- Antibodies in the milk confer important immunities on the baby.
- Breast-fed babies are less likely to become overweight.
- Allergies are less likely to develop.
- Nursing contributes to better tooth and mouth development.
- The hormones produced in nursing help in the contraction of the uterus.
- Weight is lost more easily after the delivery.
- Bonding between mother and infant is achieved more naturally.

Every woman who thinks she might be interested in breast feeding should give it a try. Almost all women who really want to can do so if given the proper support and encouragement. You can nail down this support in advance if sometime toward the end of pregnancy you arrange to meet the doctor who will be your baby's pediatrician and make sure that an understanding is reached *before* delivery about your intention to breast-feed the baby. If for one reason or another you sense the doctor's disapproval, find a more sympathetic pediatrician. It is also extremely important that you have a similar discussion with your obstetrician. The nursery nurses must be told that you plan to breast-feed your baby so that the baby will be brought to you regularly for this purpose as often as necessary during your hospital stay. In the past, in many hospital nurseries new babies were routinely formula fed, so that when the baby was brought to the mother for "feeding," it was not interested because it was not hungry, thus defeating the mother's original intentions and causing considerable disappointment. This practice is uncommon today as the benefits of breast feeding have become widely known.

The good nutritional habits of pregnancy must be continued during breast feeding. Most women require more calories each day during nursing than they did during pregnancy, as well as an even higher liquid intake, especially of milk. An occasional glass of beer or wine is acceptable, but alcohol consumption should be kept to a minimum. And if you're still smoking, you must decide to do so outside your home to protect your infant from the disastrous effects of secondhand smoke. (There are mothers so addicted to nicotine that they actually smoke while nursing!) Special caution must be exercised about the risks of various medications and the need to abstain from spicy foods whose flavors might come through in the milk, causing it to be unpalatable to the infant (garlic is a known offender).

Another note of caution for nursing mothers who embark on or return to a vigorous exercise routine as soon as they are able. It has been found that the level of lactic acid in the milk immediately after the mother has exercised is so high that the baby rejects the feeding. If you're following both a nursing regimen *and* an exercise regimen, you have three options: nurse the baby *before* you exercise; wait *at least 90 minutes* after you've exercised before you offer the baby a feeding; extrude a necessary amount of milk at a convenient time to be fed to the baby at your convenience.

Breast infections are not uncommon in nursing mothers, but if promptly treated they need not be serious. A breast infection may result from a clogged milk duct or from a small crack in the nipple. The infected breast is hot and tender to touch, and the woman may have a fever or feel weak and generally ill. Notify your physician promptly if you have any evidence of a breast infection. Usually antibiotics can be given and nursing can continue when the infection improves. If the infection is not treated soon enough, an abscess may develop (a localized collection of pus in the breast). An abscess may respond to antibiotics or may require surgical drainage. Even after this complication breast feeding may be continued if desired.

One of the most difficult problems for a breast-feeding mother is not knowing the amount of milk that her baby is receiving. In the early weeks of life babies often cry for unexplained reasons. The bottle-feeding mother knows how much formula the baby took at the last feeding and can feel with confidence that hunger is not the problem. A breast-feeding mother may worry that the baby is hungry and that her milk supply is inadequate. These doubts may lead her to substitute a bottle at the next feeding or give a supplementary bottle. The baby then nurses less, and as a result her milk supply is decreased. If a mother's milk production is insufficient, continued stimulation by frequent nursing will usually increase the supply. It is important to remember that for thousands of years before infant formulas were available, all babies were raised on breast milk alone.

Alternatively, many women prefer and enjoy the many advantages of bottle-feeding their babies. Perhaps they are planning to return to work in a short time or they are afraid that they will be tied down. To some mothers the idea of breast feeding is simply not appealing. If you feel this way, it is better to make your choice and abide with it. A woman who breast-feeds only because her friends or doctor have urged her to is rarely successful.

If you decide not to breast-feed, you will experience a few days of discomfort from about the third to sixth day after delivery. Your breasts may feel full and may leak a small amount of milk. Your breasts should be tightly bound to maintain pressure on them in order to decrease the production of milk and to relieve the discomfort that you may experience. If the breasts are not emptied, the production of milk ceases and the milk already in the breasts is eventually absorbed. Sometimes hormones are given after the birth to inhibit lactation in women who do not intend to breast feed.

This, then, is the story of childbirth. Too often when I was pregnant, I thought of the labor and delivery as an endpoint. So many thoughts during pregnancy are directed toward that long-awaited day. Of course, I knew that I would go home from the hospital with a baby, but when I was pregnant it was difficult to think of the growing, kicking lump in my abdomen as a real person. I soon found that instead of being the end, delivery is only the beginning of much more. I'm continually amazed at how quickly a child grows and develops. To wait for the first smile, to listen for the first words, to look on breathlessly as the first independent steps are taken, these are some of the first rewards of motherhood. Whatever the frustrations and the sacrifices, enjoy every moment whenever you can!

$\mathscr{I}$NFERTILITY

Kathryn Schrotenboer Cox, M.D.
Assistant Attending Physician, Obstetrics and Gynecology,
New York Hospital-Cornell Medical Center; Clinical Instructor,
Cornell University Medical College

Infertility is usually defined as one year of frequent intercourse without contraception that does not result in pregnancy. Various studies have shown that from 65 to 90 percent of all couples who conceive spontaneously will do so within the first year of trying, and 90 to 95 percent will achieve pregnancy within the first two years. However, fertility and infertility are not always absolutes. "Reduced fertility" would be a better term than infertility in those cases where pregnancy is possible but takes longer than two years to achieve. About 40 percent of "infertile" couples conceive in seven years, including those couples who are considered treatment "failures."

It is currently estimated that infertility affects at least 5 million couples, with at least one couple out of ten experiencing some difficulty in becoming pregnant. Although infertility rates have been constant for at least three decades, the impression of an infertility epidemic has been created because more and more women are postponing childbearing until they are well into their thirties. The 1990s have therefore witnessed a considerable increase in the number of couples seeking infertility evaluation. The desire for a biological child is so profound that couples may find themselves willingly impoverished by their efforts. According to the *New England Journal of Medicine* (7/28/95), the cost on average of successful delivery by in vitro fertilization (IVF) increases from $66,667 for the first cycle to $114,286 by the sixth cycle.

From the very outset, a professional evaluation of infertility may add to the humiliation and sense of failure. The reproductive capacity of both partners will be examined and their sexual relations timed to comply with a doctor's suggestions. There is often an emotional toll when a man is told that his sperm count is below normal or a woman learns she does not produce enough of the necessary hormones. It may be particularly difficult for a woman to find herself infertile if she had a previous pregnancy voluntarily terminated because it was unplanned or inconvenient.

Great advances have been made in the study of infertility in the last 20 years. There are improved diagnostic techniques, such as blood hormone tests and laparoscopy. There are improved surgical techniques, potent new drugs, and better treatment for medical problems, chronic illnesses, and infections. Doctors can now diagnose and often successfully treat 85 percent of cases.

By 1995 thousands and thousands of babies had been born nationwide through in vitro fertilization, following the famous first "test tube baby," Louise Brown, who was delivered in 1978. Through the use of new fertility drugs, tens of thousands more have been brought to term within the woman's body. The down side of these scientifically engineered miracles is that infertility treatment and care have become a big business, a $2-billion-a-year business. In 1985 there were 30 fertility clinics in the United States, and by 1995 there were more than 300. In order to recoup their investments and expand financially, those that are privately owned and operated (as compared with those connected to major medical centers) are being accused by some doctors of performing the riskier and more expensive procedures rather than those that are less complicated. It has also been pointed out that, as in other areas of medical practice, some physicians are choosing a procedure based on what the patient's insurance covers rather than the one that will be most cost effective. There have been many complaints from consumer advocates claiming that the infertility business has not been answerable to outside scrutiny about price, safety, and positive accomplishments. These complaints resulted in the enactment of a federal law requiring all fertility clinics to disclose their pregnancy success rates in a way that will enable potential patients to make better comparisons; to establish uniform standards for clinics' laboratories; and, through an annual government report, to make public the names of those that do not meet them.

Because there are many causes of infertility, there are many tests to evaluate an infertile couple. Often there is more than one contributing factor. Most infertility problems in women are handled by obstetrician-gynecologists; the male partner may be referred to a urologist. Infertility was legitimized as a medical specialty as recently as the 1960s. Those in need of information and referral to doctors with special credentials can consult the "Directory of Health Information."

MALE INFERTILITY

Male factors are estimated to cause about 30 percent of all infertility problems and to contribute to them in another 20 percent. Whatever traditional wisdom may have to say about whose "fault" the problem is, statistics indicate that the responsibility is divided about equally between the sexes. Studies initiated by the National Institutes of Health at six universities are exploring the infertility consequences of the increase of sexually transmitted diseases among the young. At greatest risk are those between the ages of 15 and 19 regardless of socioeconomic differences. The 1995 movie *Kids* provides a frightening view of irresponsibility as it relates to the transmission of AIDS.

CAUSES OF MALE INFERTILITY

The production or quality of sperm may be affected by congenital and genetic abnormalities, injuries to the genital tract, heat, age, sperm agglutination, acute and chronic infection (often sexually transmissible infections), malnutrition, previous surgery, allergies, chronic illness, environmental or occupational factors (such as radiation), varicocele, or certain medications. Among these medications are Tagamet, used in ulcer treatment; drugs used for treating cancer; and some antibiotics (especially those used to treat tuberculosis). Also heavy smoking of marijuana and smoking generally, alcoholism, and stress may result in impotence or inability to ejaculate.

Varicocele, a varicose enlargement of the veins of the spermatic cord, is a potentially curable cause of male infertility. While this condition occurs in many men with normal fertility, it has been found to be present in as many as 40 percent of infertile men. Half of all men with varicoceles have decreased sperm count or sperm motility or other changes in the semen analysis. Theories of the cause of these changes include heat, pressure, and toxic substances from the dilated vessels.

Permanent or temporary damage to the male testis can occur as a result of a genital infection or a systemic infection. Gonorrhea may do enough damage to

CAUSES OF MALE INFERTILITY

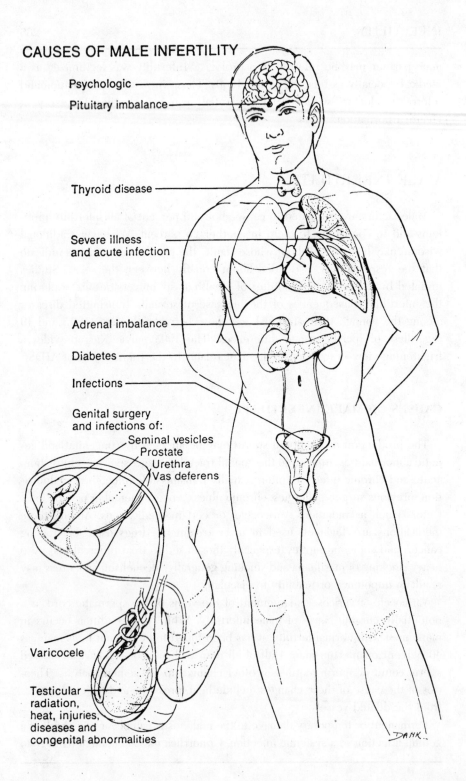

Psychologic

Pituitary imbalance

Thyroid disease

Severe illness
and acute infection

Adrenal imbalance

Diabetes

Infections

Genital surgery
and infections of:
Seminal vesicles
Prostate
Urethra
Vas deferens

Varicocele

Testicular
radiation,
heat, injuries,
diseases and
congenital abnormalities

DANK.

the male genital tract to result temporarily in a marked decrease in the sperm count. Mumps in an adult male may involve one or both testicles and may cause severe testicular damage. Fortunately, usually only one testicle suffers severe impairment, and the sperm count, though possibly reduced, is usually compatible with fertility. Any systemic viral or bacterial infection may cause a temporary depression in the sperm count.

TESTS FOR MALE INFERTILITY

Because many of the infertility tests for women are more complicated and involve more risk than those for men, infertility testing often begins with the male. A semen analysis is a simple test that can provide a great deal of information. The male is asked to submit a recently ejaculated semen specimen to the physician or laboratory. This specimen is then examined microscopically to determine sperm count, their size and shape, and if they are able to move normally. There is no sharp line of demarcation between fertility and sterility in the sperm count. Counts of less than 20 to 40 million per cubic centimeter are often correlated with decreased fertility, although men with counts of 5 to 10 million have fathered children. A high percentage of sperm with abnormal shape, size, or decreased motility is also correlated with decreased fertility. The semen can be analyzed also for antibodies and cultured for various infections. The hormone levels in the man's blood are also measured to make sure his hypothalamus and pituitary glands are functioning normally.

TREATMENT FOR MALE INFERTILITY

Some causes of male infertility are sometimes correctable. A varicocele may be surgically repaired to improve fertility. Treatment with antibiotics of a chronic infection can enable a previously infertile man to become fertile. In some situations where substance abuse is a contributing factor, it may be essential for the male to abstain entirely from alcohol and/or other drugs and to join self-help groups in order to do so. Reevaluation of medications prescribed to treat a chronic illness may produce positive results. A careful study of the man's exposure to occupational hazards such as radiation, lead, or dangerous pesticides may indicate a possible solution through change in employment.

In other cases administration of various hormones can increase a borderline sperm count or suppress sperm antibodies enough to make conception possible. These hormones include testosterone, thyroid hormone, and cortisone. In some situations clomiphene citrate (Clomid) or human menopausal gonado-tropins (Pergonal), medications that are used to induce ovulation in infertile women, may also be given to a man whose pituitary deficiency is the cause of his inability to father an offspring. In vitro fertilization, originally used more for female infertility, is being used increasingly for the treatment of male infertility.

What is being described as a revolution in treating infertile men originated in Belgium in 1993, when researchers produced several successful pregnancies by the direct injection of a single sperm cell into a human egg in a petri dish. The important discovery was that men who had no viable sperm in their semen often had at least a small number in their testes. The problem was that getting the sperm out of the testicles required a very expensive operation and an extended hospital stay. In 1995 American researchers found a much easier and cheaper way to extract the sperm: by aspirating them through a thin needle in a procedure that can be done in the doctor's office. Even though the needle aspiration is not very expensive, it has to be combined with in vitro fertilization and the direct injection of sperm into eggs. The combined procedures, known as intracytoplasmic single sperm injection (ICSI), can cost as much as $15,000, an amount not likely to be covered by insurance.

The extraordinary advantage of this new development is that it has reduced fertilization to getting the sperm's genes into the egg. It doesn't matter whether the sperm can swim vigorously or even if it can penetrate the egg's outer layer. All that matters is that it is alive. Dr. Richard J. Sherins, director of the male infertility program at the Genetics and IVF Institute in Fairfax, Virginia, and the developer of the aspiration technique, believes that it should be of the greatest use to the approximately 10 million American men who have had vasectomies. And according to the *New York Times* (6/19/95), even though the method is expensive, it has resulted in a diminishing market for sperm donors both in this country and Europe.

FEMALE INFERTILITY

It is estimated that there are more than 3 million women in the United States who cannot become pregnant.

CAUSES OF FEMALE INFERTILITY

The problem of infertility appears to be confronting more women than ever before, and according to the Federal Centers for Disease Control, this increase is partially attributable to an increase in sterility-causing diseases. For example, between 1965 and 1976, reported cases of gonorrhea tripled. By the late 1970s, penicillin-resistant gonorrhea had become a major public health problem, and unfortunately not until the 1980s did infectious disease experts realize the full extent of the fertility problems caused by chlamydia. During the same decade, there was a 600 percent increase in the number of women using IUDs, which put them at increased risk for pelvic inflammatory disease, a major cause of infertility. According to a 1985 infertility study, as many as 88,000 women may be unable to conceive because of infections that occurred while they were wearing an IUD. The drop in fertility has also been attributed to the postpone-ment of pregnancy into the thirties because of career demands or because of uncertainty about the long-term stability of the spousal relationship.

Specifically, abnormalities of the fallopian tubes, including scarring from endometriosis or previous infections or surgery, or swelling from a current infection account for about 20 to 30 percent of all infertility problems. Prob-lems with ovulation are thought to be the cause of infertility in about 10 to 15 percent of all cases. Chronic diseases such as thyroid disease, uncontrolled diabetes, or liver disease usually cause infertility by interfering with the com-plex mechanism of ovulation. In approximately 5 percent of the cases there is a problem with the cervix or cervical mucus. Other factors include on-the-job exposure to chemicals and radiation and sustained strenuous exercise, such as marathon running, which can cause temporary (that is, reversible) infertility in some women even though their menstrual cycles may continue to be normal.

Endometriosis is a condition in which tissue that looks like endometrial tissue (the tissue that lines the uterus and is shed each month in menstruation) is located outside the uterus. It is uncertain whether this develops from a backflow of endometrial tissue during menstruation into and beyond the fallo-pian tubes or from an "embryological mistake" whereby endometrial cells de-velop in an incorrect location. Endometriosis is usually located only on the pelvic organs surrounding the uterus, but in rare instances it can be found in other places such as the upper abdomen or lung.

These areas of endometriosis may bleed at the time of the menstrual period just as the uterine endometrium does. This may cause pain, and because there

CAUSES OF FEMALE INFERTILITY

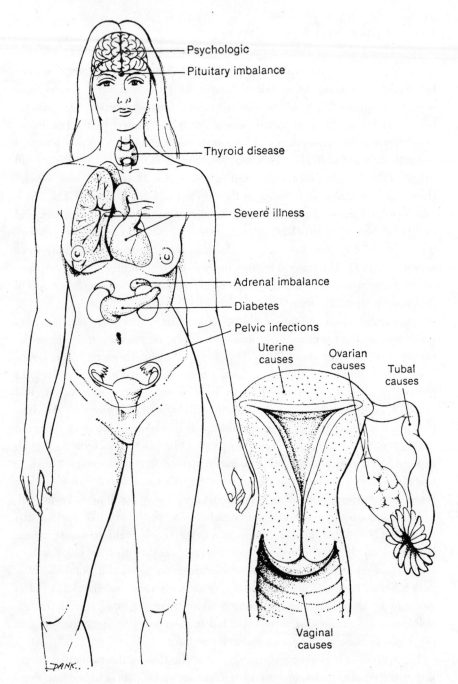

Psychologic

Pituitary imbalance

Thyroid disease

Severe illness

Adrenal imbalance

Diabetes

Pelvic infections

Uterine causes

Ovarian causes

Tubal causes

Vaginal causes

DANK..

is no way for the blood to escape, scarring may develop. This scarring may seal off the ovaries and prevent the egg from reaching the fallopian tube. Even if there are only small areas of endometriosis and the tubes and ovaries are not completely blocked, fertility may be reduced.

Infertility related to tubal blockage and pelvic adhesions is on the rise. An increase in sexually transmissible infections, widespread use of intrauterine contraceptive devices, and the increase in elective abortions are all thought to play a role. The infections include gonorrhea and chlamydia. Women with intrauterine contraceptive devices may have chronic low-grade infections, and some may develop an acute severe infection or a pelvic abscess. Though severe pelvic infection was more common before abortions were legal, a mild infection is not unheard of after an elective abortion today. A ruptured appendix may also cause pelvic infection and scarring of the fallopian tubes. Pelvic adhesions may occur after surgery to remove ovarian cysts, fibroids, and tubal pregnancies or after any other lower abdominal or pelvic surgery.

Irregularities in the shape of the uterus can occasionally cause infertility, although they are more frequently associated with spontaneous abortions than with the inability to conceive. The most common cause of irregularity in the shape of the uterus is fibroids (benign fibrous growths of the uterus). Other causes are congenital or developmental abnormalities. Recently some abnormalities in the shape of the uterus have been found in daughters of women who took the drug diethylstilbestrol (DES) during pregnancy.

Both hypothyroidism and hyperthyroidism and other hormonal abnormalities may cause infertility by unbalancing the delicate and complex regulation of the menstrual cycle. Severe illness of any sort (diabetes, liver disease) can also affect the normal cycle and cause infertility.

A vaginal infection may alter the cervical mucus and the pH of the vagina, creating a hostile environment in which the sperm may be able to live for only a very short time.

The presence of sperm antibodies in cervical mucus or vaginal secretions may cause infertility. There is controversy among physicians about how often this may be a factor because these antibodies may be found in people with normal fertility. In some couples, however, these antibodies appear to kill or inactivate the sperm.

There is a significant number of infertile couples who complete all of the standard testing without any obvious cause of infertility. Many of these couples eventually conceive. Unfortunately, some remain infertile. However, with advances in infertility testing, fewer and fewer cases of infertility remain unexplained.

Timing of intercourse is important. A woman with a 28-day cycle should

UTERINE, CERVICAL, AND VAGINAL CAUSES OF INFERTILITY

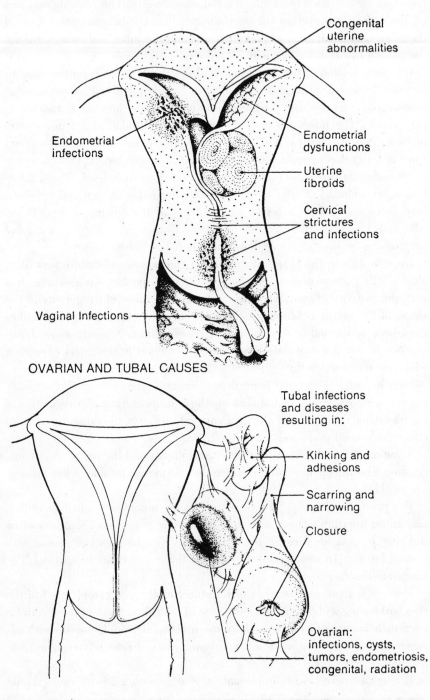

Congenital uterine abnormalities

Endometrial dysfunctions

Uterine fibroids

Cervical strictures and infections

Endometrial infections

Vaginal Infections

OVARIAN AND TUBAL CAUSES

Tubal infections and diseases resulting in:

Kinking and adhesions

Scarring and narrowing

Closure

Ovarian: infections, cysts, tumors, endometriosis, congenital, radiation have intercourse daily from the tenth to the fourteenth day of her menstrual cycle. These are the days of her maximum fertility. A male with a low sperm count should get special intercourse timing instructions, as should the woman with a shorter or longer cycle.

Position during intercourse may also be important. Sperm may reach the cervix more easily when the woman, lying on her back, draws her knees up to encircle her partner's hips. After his orgasm the woman should maintain this position for 10 to 15 minutes or relax with a pillow under her hips.

TESTS FOR FEMALE INFERTILITY

Basal Body Temperatures

Keeping a record of basal body temperatures can be helpful in establishing whether or not a woman ovulates. Every morning, immediately after waking up and before any activity, the woman takes her temperature. Special thermometers that are somewhat easier to read than regular thermometers are available for this purpose. Before ovulation morning oral temperatures usually range from 97.0° to 97.5° F (morning temperatures can be a degree lower than those taken later in the day). After ovulation, because of the effect of increased levels of progesterone, morning temperatures are usually 98.0° F or above until menstruation occurs. Ovulation usually occurs during the day before the temperature rise. Therefore, an accurately recorded temperature chart that shows low temperatures in the early part of the menstrual cycle and higher temperatures for the last 14 days is presumptive evidence that ovulation has occurred.

Ovulation Test Kits

Thanks to ovulation test kits that are easy to use at home, it is now possible to find out when conception is most likely to occur. By measuring the amount of the luteinizing hormone (LH) in her urine each day beginning with the tenth day of her menstrual cycle, the woman will detect a sudden significant increase in the LH hormone by a change in the color of the testing paper. This change occurs about 24 hours before ovulation. Intercourse should take place on the day of the color change and the next day to ensure maximum probability of conception. The ovulation test kits are available over the counter under such

names as Ovukit, OvuQuick, and Q-Test. They are also available through a
doctor.

Endometrial Biopsy

Another test to help determine if ovulation is occurring is an endometrial
biopsy. This test is usually performed on the first day of the period or in the
week before a period is expected. An endometrial biopsy normally can be done
in the physician's office without the use of anesthesia. A speculum is inserted
into the vagina and the cervix is grasped with an instrument called a tenaculum, which may cause a slight pinching sensation. Then a small, thin instrument is inserted into the uterine cavity to take the biopsy. This procedure may
cause a brief cramping sensation. The removed tissue is sent to a laboratory to
be examined microscopically. In addition to confirming whether ovulation has
occurred, this test sometimes can identify other causes of infertility such as
infection and certain rare causes of infertility. Though scarcely ever a problem,
this test has the theoretical risk of interrupting an early pregnancy. Therefore,
if there is any chance that the patient may be pregnant, it should not be done.

Hormone Tests

Measurement of blood and urinary hormone levels can help to give evidence
whether or not a woman is ovulating. For example, because progesterone levels
in the blood rise after ovulation, a blood test taken after ovulation will reflect
this. However, many authorities still consider the endometrial biopsy the most
accurate proof that ovulation has occurred.

Measures of the level of other hormones may also yield information. For
example, certain conditions that are associated with abnormally high male
hormones such as testosterone or cortisonelike hormones can cause infertility.
Also follicle-stimulating hormone (FSH) and luteinizing hormone (LH) are two
messenger hormones that play essential roles in the delicate ovulation mechanism. If these are present in slightly reduced or elevated amounts or do not
fluctuate appropriately during the month, infertility may result. The hormone
prolactin (which plays an important role in breast milk production) may be
abnormally elevated and be the cause of infertility. Treatment of this elevated
hormone level with the drug bromocryptine will in many cases cure the infertility.

Cultures and Serologic Tests

Cervical mucus can be cultured for gonorrhea, chlamydia, and other infectious agents.

Hysterosalpingogram

A hysterosalpingogram is a test used to study the uterus and fallopian tubes. It can be done in a hospital or in the office of a radiologist. A speculum is inserted into the vagina, and the cervix is grasped with a tenaculum. A dye-injection apparatus is then attached to the cervix, the dye is slowly injected into the uterus, and X-rays are taken. Most women feel the injection of the dye to be about as uncomfortable as moderate menstrual cramps. The X-rays show the internal outlines of the uterus and fallopian tubes as the dye fills them. If there is any abnormality in the shape or size of the uterus or a blockage in the fallopian tubes, this may show up on the X-rays. This test also gives valuable information to a DES-exposed woman prior to a pregnancy. The degree of abnormality of the shape of the uterus is predictive of the chances of premature labor during the pregnancy and will help determine how closely such a woman needs to be monitored during pregnancy.

Postcoital Test

A postcoital test (PC test) is a painless, simple test that often can yield important information in the evaluation of an infertile couple. This test is done around the time of ovulation. You must come to the physician's office within a specified number of hours after intercourse. A speculum examination is done, and a small sample of the cervical mucus and vaginal fluid is taken and examined microscopically. This examination will show if the cervical mucus is normal and if the sperm are active and alive. If sperm are alive and active, this is presumptive evidence that sperm antibodies are not a problem.

Laparoscopy

Laparoscopy is often the final step in an infertility workup. This is done in a hospital, usually with general anesthesia, although local anesthesia can be

TESTS FOR INFERTILITY

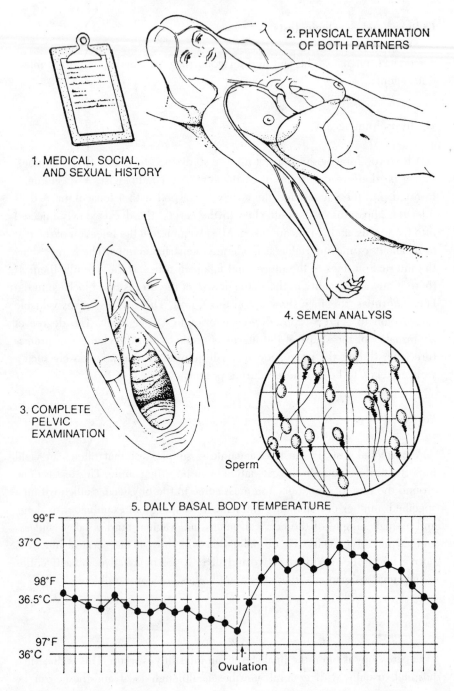

1. MEDICAL, SOCIAL, AND SEXUAL HISTORY

2. PHYSICAL EXAMINATION OF BOTH PARTNERS

3. COMPLETE PELVIC EXAMINATION

4. SEMEN ANALYSIS

Sperm

5. DAILY BASAL BODY TEMPERATURE

Ovulation

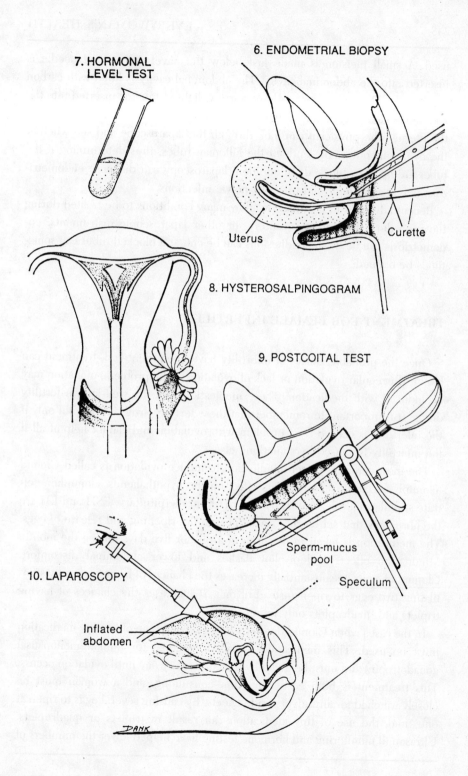

7. HORMONAL LEVEL TEST

6. ENDOMETRIAL BIOPSY

Uterus

Curette

8. HYSTEROSALPINGOGRAM

9. POSTCOITAL TEST

Sperm-mucus pool

Speculum

10. LAPAROSCOPY

Inflated abdomen

DANK

used. A small incision is made just below the navel and a long needle is inserted into the abdominal cavity. The abdominal cavity is filled with carbon dioxide gas. The laparoscope, a long, narrow, lighted tube, is inserted into the abdominal cavity to permit viewing of the pelvic organs. Dye is injected into the uterus. The physician can look through the laparoscope and see whether the dye spills out of the ends of the fallopian tubes, thus determining if the tubes are open or blocked. In addition, laparoscopy can diagnose endometriosis, pelvic adhesions, and previous pelvic infections.

Recent advances in laparoscopy allow many conditions to be treated during the procedure. Using laser, cautery, or other laparoscopic instruments, endometriosis can be treated, adhesions can be cut, and blocked tubes can sometimes be opened.

TREATMENT FOR FEMALE INFERTILITY

Once the probable causes of infertility have been identified, treatment can begin. If irregular ovulation or lack of ovulation is the problem, ovulation may be induced with medication. These medications are the well-known fertility drugs. It is important to remember that these fertility drugs are helpful only if the infertility is caused by a problem with ovulation and cannot help at all if the infertility is caused by something else.

The most commonly used medication to induce ovulation is called Clomid (clomiphene citrate). Through its effect on the hypothalamus, clomiphene citrate stimulates a release of FSH and LH from the pituitary. FSH and LH are the hormones that act on the ovary to cause the ripening and release of eggs. The medication is taken in the form of a pill for five days during the month. Minor side effects include hot flashes and lower abdominal discomfort. Clomiphene citrate substantially increases the chances of having twins by stimulating two eggs to ripen instead of one. It increases the chances of having triplets and quadruplets only minimally.

In the cases when Clomid doesn't work, a second type of fertility medication must be used. This medication is called Pergonal (or human menopausal gonadotropin) and must be given by injection every day until ovulation occurs. This treatment is both costly and time-consuming, and a woman must be closely watched for any adverse side effects. By causing several eggs to ripen at one time, the use of this medication can result in triplets or quadruplets. Ultrasound monitoring and hormone testing have helped lower the numbers of unwanted multiple births. Serious side effects of Pergonal include large ovarian cysts and massive shifts in body fluids.

Problems with the fallopian tubes may be treated surgically. The fallopian tubes may have been blocked as a result of a congenital abnormality, scarring subsequent to a previous pelvic infection or to endometriosis, or previous pelvic surgery. Sometimes the fallopian tubes themselves are normal, but adhesions surrounding them prevent the egg and sperm from meeting.

There is a reasonable chance that the surgical removal of the adhesions will improve fertility. Unfortunately, when repairing the fallopian tube requires major reconstructive surgery (tuboplasty), the success rate is much lower. Even when it is possible to open the fallopian tubes, tubal function does not always return to normal, and the infertility may persist. Frequently operating microscopes, very fine instruments, and lasers are used to improve the success rate of tubal surgery.

An experimental procedure that may eliminate the need for surgery in some cases of blocked fallopian tubes has been adapted from a technique used to unclog coronary arteries. A catheter carrying a small balloon is threaded through the uterus into the blocked tube. When the balloon is inflated, the fallopian tube is stretched, and the obstructive tissue is washed out.

Treatment of endometriosis may improve fertility. In some cases the treatment is surgical: large areas of endometriosis are removed and adhesions that have formed by the scarring are opened. Lasers may be used at the time of laparotomy or through the smaller laparoscopy incision to remove endometriotic implants. In other cases the treatment is medical. Danazol, a drug that can prevent menstrual bleeding for six to seven months can be given to treat endometriosis. Newer drugs to treat endometriosis are the GnRH analogs, given by injection or nasal spray to induce a temporary menopause. After the medications are stopped, normal menstrual cycles begin again and pregnancy may occur. The causes of any hormonal abnormalities should be identified and appropriately treated.

Other treatments are available for other specific causes of infertility. For example, treatment of a genital infection may correct the infertility, especially if the partner is treated simultaneously. Sometimes problems with the cervical mucus may be treated by the administration of low doses of estrogen. Sperm antibodies may disappear if there is no direct contact with sperm for six months, so the use of a condom or sexual abstinence may make future fertility possible. If there is a medical problem, such as thyroid disease, treatment of the medical problem may itself correct the infertility.

ARTIFICIAL METHODS OF FERTILIZATION

ARTIFICIAL INSEMINATION

When both partners are presumed to be fertile, artificial insemination (AI) can be attempted with sperm from the male partner (AIH—husband) if there is an anatomic defect in either partner that prevents the sperm from being deposited near the cervix. These defects include hypospadias (abnormal position of the urethral opening) in the man and an abnormal position of the cervix in the woman. Artificial insemination also may be necessary in certain types of sexual dysfunction. If the male partner is not fertile but the woman is presumed to be, artificial insemination is attempted using sperm from a donor (AID), usually anonymous. The donor, generally matched to the partner in coloring and body build, is found by the woman's physician, either personally or through a sperm bank. The semen from a nonpartner must be screened for a variety of sexually transmissible diseases, including HIV infection, gonorrhea, syphilis, herpes, hepatitis B, and chlamydia. Freezing of sperm decreases the likelihood of infection and allows more time for testing of the donor. This is being used increasingly. At the time of ovulation the sperm is injected into the woman's vagina at the opening of the cervix. In some cases a newer artificial insemination procedure called intrauterine insemination (IUI) is used. The insemination catheter is placed directly into the uterus and bypasses the cervix.

Artificial insemination, which has been practiced for about 200 years, was successfully used in the United States in 1884 for the first time. By 1990 this increasingly popular procedure accounted for the birth of 30,000 babies annually, assisted by 11,000 private doctors, 400 sperm banks, and over 200 fertility centers. It should be noted that there are fewer than 1 percent birth defects when donor sperm are used, compared to 6 percent in the general population.

With few children available for adoption today, artificial insemination is the simplest way that some couples can have a child. However, it is not something to be undertaken lightly because it raises countless psychological, moral, religious, and legal questions. Some men cannot cope with the fact that they are not the biologic father of their child, while other men feel that a child who has their wife's genes and whom they have raised is as much theirs as any child can be.

Couples who choose artificial insemination do not always have the support of others. In fact, because some major religious groups feel that artificial insemination with donor sperm is the equivalent of adultery, many couples who choose this procedure for achieving parenthood do not tell even their families or closest friends.

There are many legal questions about these children that have not yet been answered. Some courts in the United States, England, and Canada have held that they are illegitimate, while other courts have held that a husband who agrees to the artificial insemination of his wife has an obligation to support the child. A few states have passed laws to attempt to clarify the legal position of these children, but further legislation is sorely needed.

In the meantime, in increasing numbers, donor-inseminated offspring and some donors are trying to find their genetic kin. Those who have been successful are complicating our concept of "family," but no more so than egg donors who are enabling postmenopausal women to give birth to babies with whom they have no genetic connection.

IN VITRO FERTILIZATION (IVF)

In the procedure called in vitro fertilization (IVF), a woman's egg is removed surgically from one of her ovaries and fertilized in a glass dish ("test tube"). This fertilized egg is later placed back in her uterus. This method was originally designed for women who have an obstruction of both fallopian tubes but have at least one normally functioning and surgically accessible ovary or in some other situations that cannot be corrected. These conditions exist in about 5 to 10 percent of infertile women.

"SURROGATE MOTHERS"

Overcoming infertility by a commercial transaction with a woman located through an advertisement or a lawyer remains controversial as a result of the notoriety of the "Baby M" case. The procedure, which consists of implanting an in vitro fertilized egg in the uterus of a woman who did not produce the egg (a variant of the original in vitro fertilization approach) has been forbidden in many states as well as in many countries worldwide. Unpaid surrogacy remains a viable option for the woman who can call on the cooperation of a close friend or family member to carry the embryo to term.

FOR FUTURE USE: FROZEN EGGS, SPERM, EMBRYOS

Technically called "cryopreservation," the freezing of eggs, sperm, and early stage embryos fertilized in the lab for future use in IVF cycles has become a routine procedure. For many years frozen sperm banks have been the source for donor insemination, and it is not unusual for men going off to war to leave a supply of frozen sperm to be used in the event of their death in combat. Male cancer patients under 50 who are scheduled to undergo radiation and chemotherapy likely to leave them sterile are advised to have their sperm preserved before beginning treatments. It is anticipated that a woman undergoing chemotherapy, perhaps for breast cancer, will be able to have strips of her own ovary removed, frozen, and put back in place when treatments are concluded, thus preserving her fertility for the future. The first in vitro fertilization birth using a frozen embryo occurred in the United States in 1986, and since that time doctors have been routinely freezing extra human embryos produced by IVF so that they can be stored until the couple asks for them again.

Until definitive decisions are made by the highest courts on who "owns" these embryos in the event of a divorce, litigations abound on the state level. At the same time, medical ethicists and legal specialists admit current laws were formulated at a time when no one anticipated that the essence of life could be frozen and used to create a new offspring even after the father was dead.

GAMETE INTRAFALLOPIAN TRANSFER (GIFT)

Increasingly popular is the technological advance that eliminates any need for third-party collaboration. Known as GIFT (gametic intrafallopian transfer) and developed at the Health Science Center of the University of Texas, it proceeds in the following way: egg cells (usually two to four) that are extracted from the woman by laparoscopy are mixed with about 100,000 sperm from the spouse and again, by using a laparoscope, a catheter is introduced into the open end of one or both of the woman's fallopian tubes and the sperm and eggs injected. Thus the embryo can be fertilized inside the oviduct in its natural environment, where cell division takes place without the need for laboratory culturing. When the procedure works as anticipated, the embryo descends into the uterus and develops into a normal fetus. This procedure takes about one hour and can be performed on an outpatient basis. It is being used when traditional infertility therapies are unsuccessful, especially in cases of endometriosis, low sperm counts, and unexplained infertility. The first pregnancy using the GIFT technique occurred in 1985, and in the year that followed, patients having the procedure increased from 47 to 419. According to the IVF Registry, the overall clinical pregnancy rate in 1987 for IVF was 16 percent, while the rate for GIFT was 25 percent. A recent report by the American Fertility Society puts the success rate at 26.6 percent. A variation of the GIFT technique, known as ZIFT (the Z stands for zygote) transfers the newly fertilized egg, or zygote, into the fallopian tube by laparoscopy, usually within 24 hours after fertilization has taken place in the laboratory.

Although there have been major advances in solving some of the problems of infertility, much more is yet to be learned. There are still couples whose infertility is unexplained, and there are couples with known causes of infertility that cannot be cured. In addition, advances in technology have given rise to problems that concern hospitals and neonatologists who specialize in premature babies. Multiple births resulting from IVF and GIFT are common, and when twins, triplets, and even quadruplets arrive early, the costs for assuring their well-being can be extremely high.

INFERTILITY SOLUTIONS: UNFORESEEN DEVELOPMENTS

Approximately 20 years ago, the birth of the first "test tube" baby was hailed as a miracle. Since that time, in vitro fertilization has become an accepted means of treatment throughout the Western world. In retrospect, it turns out that this procedure ushered in a new era of reproductive technology that has outdistanced the ability of the learned professions and society at large to keep pace with its consequences. The hullabaloo over "surrogate" motherhood triggered by the "Baby M" case continues to resonate in courts of law and legislatures. Fertility clinics are making money by making it possible for couples to make babies not only by providing sperm banks, but since 1990, by providing donor eggs. Donors of both sexes are forcing medical ethicists as well sociologists and jurists to confront the question not only of who is the *biological* parent and what are the rights of that parent, but also of how a "family" and identity itself are to be defined. The normal life cycle of women has become a matter of government involvement following the successful pregnancies of

women in their late fifties. An international furor yet to be resolved was triggered by the announcement of a researcher in Scotland that it would soon be
feasible for infertile women to be implanted with the ovaries taken from
aborted fetuses.

On this latest development, Dr. Robert Levine, an ethicist at Yale University
School of Medicine, has noted (*New York Times* 1/6/94) that a long-standing
principle in ethics forbids the use of a vulnerable population such as prisoners
or retarded children, merely for convenience, if the same studies can be done
with people who freely volunteer, such as women who volunteer to donate
eggs. Are fetuses therefore a vulnerable population? According to Dr. Levine,
that question, which has elicited one of the most divisive debates in society, is
at the heart of the problem.

As for the debates precipitated by the childbearing successes of postmenopausal women, there are those who feel that government restrictions reflect a
paternalistic double standard. "When men have children in their old age, it's
looked on as a crowning achievement—look at the biblical references to Abraham," said Dr. Mark Siegler, director of the Center for Medical Clinical Ethics
at the University of Chicago, in the *New York Times* (1/2/94). "The history of
medicine has been devoted to overcoming the natural lottery, the hand fate has
dealt each one of us. We are already pushing the bounds of attractiveness,
sexuality, human well-being. Why draw the line at reproduction?"

When scientists effect major changes, they are rarely expected to take responsibility for the unforeseen results of their work. Americans have a difficult
time confronting the fact that "progress" always has its price, that everything
has the defects of its virtues. For the infertile couples who achieve parenthood
because of unanticipated advances in the technology of reproduction, these
advances have been a blessing. Whether they have been an *unmixed* blessing
for society at large will be decided in the legislative bodies and law courts,
which reflect the changing attitudes of the general population on how families
are created.

ADOPTION

Until recently adoption, like infertility, rarely received much national attention. Thanks to television, however, millions of people, including many future
adoptive parents, saw the beaming faces of men and women who had become
the legal parents of babies from South America, Romania, China, and other
parts of the world where the children—almost always girls—might otherwise

have been consigned to lives of neglect or outright starvation. In unwelcome contrast, we also saw a screaming child forcibly snatched away by a stranger from the only parents she had ever known. That "stranger" was her biological father, who had been granted the legal right to claim her after she had been given up for adoption by her mother.

It is estimated that in the United States, approximately 50,000 children are adopted every year. At least five times that many people are trying to become adoptive parents. Adoption has always been a hazardous enterprise, but no more so than parenthood itself. During a time when definitions of the family are yielding to social change, practically all the established pronouncements of family law are in a state of contention. The laws affecting adoption vary from year to year, from state to state, and from city to city within the same state. One cheerful note: in response to widespread outcry against judges whose decisions ignored the well-being of the child, the interests of the *child* are now represented by social workers, psychiatrists, and lawyers with at least as much passion and determination as the interests of the embattled adult litigants. (The interests of the child have almost always been represented in divorce and custody cases.) Potential adoptive parents needn't be discouraged by these battles. They should, however, try to keep informed of how legal decisions might affect them.

Having made the decision to investigate the option of adoption, you may scarcely know how and where to begin. If you don't want to be at the mercy of experts, try to collect as much information as possible on your own, and make a habit of jotting down useful names, addresses, and phone numbers in a purse-size notebook. You might begin at your local public library, where you're likely to find several useful books covering all aspects of the subject. You can find out how to contact state and national nonprofit referral organizations, as well as how to get started on the adventure of adopting a child from a foreign country. The librarian can also tell you how to get in touch with adoptive parent support groups in your community. Contact the office responsible for social services in your city or county for additional information.

Lesbians can get some useful leads from comprehensive books on adoption. They can tap into the gay and lesbian grapevine for how to start networking, and they can depend on the Lambda Legal Defense and Education Fund in their community for current rulings that affect them. As of 1995, the national office says that only two states—Florida and New Hampshire—officially prohibit a gay person from adopting. The National Center for Lesbian Rights in San Francisco points out that other states have informal policies on this question depending on the attitudes of social workers, judges, and whether the local citizenry is especially homophobic. Most states make it difficult for a gay couple to adopt *as a couple*. In any case, the guidance of a knowledgeable lawyer is recommended.

All prospective adoptive parents are advised to postpone their efforts to locate a child to adopt until they have consulted a lawyer. Find a lawyer who knows everything there is to know about your state's current adoption laws and who might eventually become the intermediary for the adoption itself. To locate such a practitioner, family members and close friends or the state or county bar association can be helpful. If you trust your judgment about character and decency, you can also look in the local Yellow Pages for an attorney who is a specialist in adoption law and arrange a consultation.

As you begin to get in touch with the many agencies, both public and private, and the many professional individuals, both religious and secular, who may eventually help you find the child you're looking for, *be patient.* Be prepared to spend lots of time and in many cases lots of money (perhaps more than $30,000) along the way. But above all, remember that persistence pays off in pursuing the worthwhile goal of providing a child with a loving family and rewarding yourself with the gift of parenthood.

$\mathscr{G}$YNECOLOGIC PROBLEMS AND TREATMENT

Mary Jane Gray, M.D.

Professor Emeritus of Obstetrics and Gynecology, University of North Carolina Medical School, Chapel Hill, North Carolina

Gynecologists are physicians who specialize in the care of women, with emphasis on matters relating to the reproductive system. Gynecological problems may have arisen for a few of us with the onset of menstruation. More complex problems concern most of us with the beginning of sexual activity, and for all women, regular examinations and cancer tests are a vital necessity.

FINDING CAUSES OF COMMON PROBLEMS

Most women would like to know more about their reproductive system and what may go wrong with it. Because of dissatisfaction with the care they have received, some women have left the mainstream of medical care for self-help groups. These groups are excellent for education in normal function and health maintenance and for emotional support. However, they are sometimes short on medical expertise and may be especially deficient in the use of advanced diagnostic tools and techniques. This chapter is intended to help women understand common gynecologic problems and their treatment (excluding contraception, sexually transmissible diseases, and sexual dysfunction, discussed in other chapters) and to give women the knowledge they need to communicate more effectively with their physicians. A review of the anatomy of the female reproductive system and the physiology of normal menstruation will be helpful to the reader at this point.

DOCTOR/PATIENT RELATIONSHIP

The relationship between a woman and her gynecologist is likely to last a long time and cover many contingencies. Often the gynecologist becomes the woman's primary care physician. It is, therefore, important that the relationship should start out with mutual respect and should proceed in an atmosphere that encourages relaxed communication. Both participants may have an easier time if the first visit occurs when there is no need for crisis intervention but rather because the patient wants to have a complete checkup for preventive purposes. During this first visit, you should be prepared to ask the doctor to answer specific questions after your medical history has been taken. Write the answers down.

More and more, gynecologists are accepting a new patient's request to meet for the first time in the doctor's office, with the patient fully clothed, instead of in the examining room with the patient unclothed and about to assume a submissive posture. Neither the doctor nor the doctor's staff should feel free to address you by your first name. ("Honey" or "dear" is entirely unacceptable.) If the doctor assumes the liberty of using your first name, you should certainly feel entitled to do the same.

The patient should be prepared to describe all problems in detail and be in command of all the facts of her personal and medical history as well as her family history, especially along the matrilineal line. Remember that you can expect your gynecologist to help you with menstrual problems, infertility, contraception and abortion, prepregnancy counseling, prenatal care, childbirth, sexually transmissible diseases, hormone and breast problems, genitourinary infections, and the transitional difficulties of menopause. During the first discussion the gynecologist will ask about the onset of periods, their previous and present character, pregnancies, abortions, and a complete sexual history. In addition, you may be asked about any family history of breast or ovarian cancer. It is essential to be honest in answering all questions.

When the doctor indicates that you can now proceed to an examination room, find out whether you can ask *your* questions before you're examined or after, at the time when you're back in the office for a summary of your present condition. In either case, here are some of the questions you should be prepared to ask:

1. If I have no special problems, how often will I be scheduled for a routine checkup, and will I be notified that the time has come to make an appointment?
2. How often is a Pap smear taken?
3. Is a chlamydia lab report part of every checkup?
4. How often should I schedule a mammogram and where?
5. Do you conduct other cancer screening tests as part of preventive care?
6. What is your hospital affiliation?

If you sense any resentment on the doctor's part about answering these questions (or any others you might want to ask); if you feel that your answers to the doctor's questions have been cut short, or that the doctor has been distracted and interrupted during your time together by several phone calls; if there have been any indications of disapproval of your life-style; if the waiting room is mobbed and there's a backup of appointments that necessitated your waiting for more than an hour for your consultation to begin: find a different doctor.

PELVIC EXAMINATION

The patient should not douche for two or three days before the appointment and should empty her bladder beforehand to make the examination more comfortable for her and more accurate for the physician. (Most gynecologists ask for a urine specimen.) The diagnosis of a gynecological problem is based on a thorough examination, which usually includes taking height, weight, and blood pressure measurements; feeling the thyroid gland; listening to the heart and lungs; and examining the breasts and abdomen before proceeding to the pelvic examination. Laboratory tests will be based on the patient's history and on whether the examiner is assuming primary responsibility for her health (see "Suggested Health Examinations for Women").

The first part of the pelvic examination is an inspection of the external genitals for lumps, sores, inflammation, and general hormonal status. The folds of skin forming the labia are separated in order to expose the urinary and vaginal openings. A woman who has had children may be asked to "bear down" or "strain as if moving your bowels" to demonstrate any weakness of the supporting tissues of the vagina.

Next comes the vaginal examination. After a finger locates the vaginal open-

VAGINAL EXAMINATION

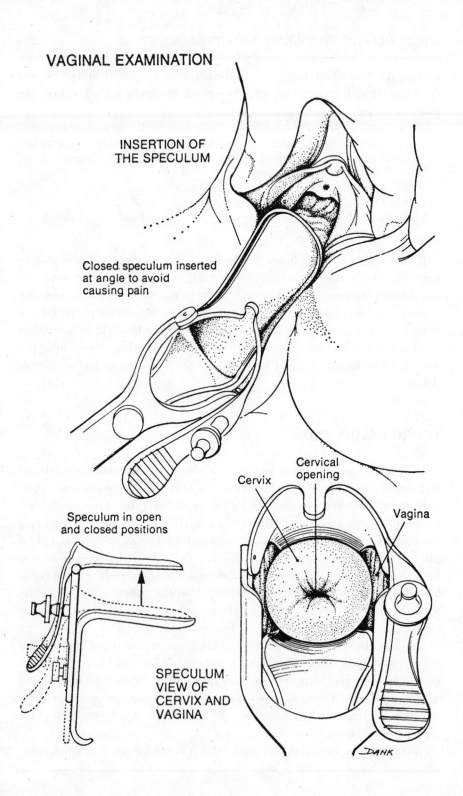

INSERTION OF
THE SPECULUM

Closed speculum inserted
at angle to avoid
causing pain

Speculum in open
and closed positions

Cervix

Cervical
opening

Vagina

SPECULUM
VIEW OF
CERVIX AND
VAGINA

DANK

ing, a speculum is placed inside and opened. The speculum is a metal or plastic instrument that looks a little like two shoehorns hinged together. When opened, it holds the vaginal walls apart and allows the examiner to see the vagina and cervix and check for inflammation or infection, scars or growths, and other abnormalities. A scraping of tissue and samples of discharge are taken for examination under a microscope and for cultures and a Pap test. The woman may request a mirror to follow this part of the procedure.

After the speculum is removed, a bimanual pelvic examination follows. This consists of placing two fingers in the vagina and the other hand on the abdominal wall in such a way that the uterus and ovaries can be located between the two hands and the size, shape, consistency, and tenderness of these structures can be determined. Normal ovaries, like testes, exhibit a characteristic discomfort when examined in this way. Usually the examiner will then put a finger into the rectum to feel both the rectum itself and those structures lying near it in the pelvis.

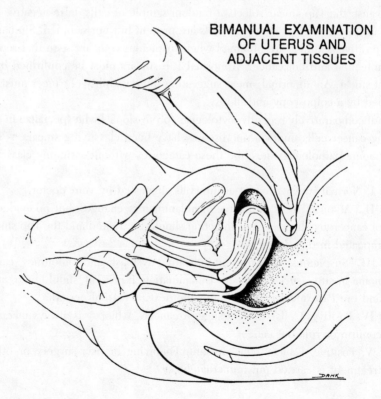

**BIMANUAL EXAMINATION
OF UTERUS AND
ADJACENT TISSUES**

PAP SMEAR

Named for Dr. Papanicolaou, who developed this method for cancer screening, the Pap smear has proved to be an inexpensive and accurate way to diagnose cervical cancer and malignant tumors of nearby organs such as the vagina and endometrium, as well as potentially malignant changes. Cells from the surface of the cervix and vagina are placed on a glass slide and examined under a microscope by a technician trained in recognizing cancer cells and dysplastic cells. Dysplastic cells are cells showing evidence of changes that indicate they might at some time become malignant; dysplasia is the abnormal growth created by the aberrant cells. Recent evidence linking venereal warts and cervical cancer has caused increased attention to be given to cellular changes caused by the wart virus.

Because the Pap smear selects a random sample of cells, false-negative results are possible when abnormal cells are present but not sampled. Similarly, false-positive readings are obtained when suspicious cells are seen that represent infection and not cancer. Abnormal Pap smears must be confirmed by a repeat smear. An abnormal smear suggesting the possibility of cancer must be clarified by a colposcopy and biopsy.

Until comparatively recently, cytologists (professionals who specialize in detecting cancer cells under a microscope) have been classifying smears as follows. Some pathologists describe these categories without assigning classes.

Class I. Normal smear. Repeat at intervals suggested by your doctor.

Class II. "Atypical" cells indicative of inflammatory changes, but no evidence of cancerous changes. Any infection should be treated and the Pap smear repeated in 6 to 12 months.

Class III. "Suspicious" cells present indicating dysplasia and sometimes "carcinoma-in-situ" (surface cancer). Inflammation, if present, should be treated and the Pap smear repeated after the next menstrual period.

Class IV. Positive. Cells strongly suggest cancer. A biopsy is always taken to confirm or rule out cancer.

Class V. Positive. Cancer cells present. Following biopsy, surgery or other treatment is carried out immediately.

In 1988 a new format for classifying Pap smears was developed under the auspices of the National Cancer Institute at a workshop conducted in

Bethesda, Maryland. Known as the Bethesda System, it consists of three elements for reporting Pap results:

1. A statement of whether the specimen is *adequate for diagnosis*. (Under the previous system, "inadequate" samples were referred to as Class O and were repeated.)
2. A *general categorization* of the diagnosis as "normal" or "other." The latter category can include anything from a bacterial or viral infection to cell abnormalities.
3. A *descriptive diagnosis* detailing the findings under "other." (When the older terminology is used, dysplasia and carcinoma-in-situ may be combined as *cervical intraepithelial neoplasia* (CIN), with a subscript indicating degree of severity.) With the newer system, all degrees of dysplasia (and CIN) are separated into two categories:
   a. Low-grade squamous intraepithelial lesions (includes mild dysplasia as well as CIN 1).
   b. High-grade squamous intraepithelial lesions (includes moderate dysplasia, CIN 2, severe dysplasia, carcinoma-in-situ, and CIN 3).

It is anticipated that with the Bethesda System, greater uniformity and accuracy in reporting will result in better patient care.

Frequency of Pap Smears

Guidelines for the frequency of Pap smear screening as presented by the American Cancer Society in 1987 and endorsed by the American College of Physicians and Surgeons, the American Medical Women's Association, and the American Medical Association recommend an annual Pap test and pelvic examination for all women who have reached the age of 18 or who are or have been sexually active. When the results of at least three consecutive tests are negative, the frequency of further tests can be decided jointly by doctor and patient. However, women who are at high risk for any conditions leading to cervical cancer should schedule a Pap smear *at least* once a year. These factors are first intercourse, marriage, or pregnancy at an early age; multiple sex partners or a partner who has had or still has multiple sex partners; many pregnancies; DES daughters; and history of human papilloma virus (HPV) infection (see the chapter on "Sexually Transmissible Diseases").

X-RAY, SONOGRAPHY, LAPAROSCOPY, COLPOSCOPY,

AND HYSTEROSCOPY

If the examination or Pap smear indicates the presence of a problem requiring further information for an accurate diagnosis, several other diagnostic procedures may be followed.

X-rays may be taken to study the structure and location of organs within the pelvic cavity. X-ray is most effective in showing hard tissue, such as bone, or in outlining the urinary and gastrointestinal tracts after the use of contrast material. The uterus and tubes can be outlined by injecting radio-opaque material through the cervix. The resulting X-ray is called a hysterosalpingogram.

Sonography or ultrasound is a technique in which sound waves are sent across the area to be examined and their echoes recorded on a screen. The image on the screen is a sonogram. It provides a picture of soft tissue and can be used to determine the size and placement of organs and to detect any abnormal tissue mass, swelling, or fluid collection. The procedure may be done by a radiologist or in the radiology department of a hospital, but no radiation is involved. More often the procedure is carried out in the gynecologist's office.

Laparoscopy is an increasingly popular surgical procedure in which a lighted viewing tube (a laparoscope) is inserted into the abdomen through a small incision. It allows the visual examination of internal structures. Anesthesia is required, but the procedure can be done without an overnight stay in a hospital.

Colposcopy is the examination of the cervix and vagina with a magnifying device (a colposcope) in order to see details not visible with the naked eye. It is used to identify cervical or vaginal abnormalities, to examine abnormal surface areas, and to locate specific sites for biopsy if a Pap smear indicates the presence of abnormal cells. Because the device enters only the vagina, no anesthesia is required and the procedure can be done in a doctor's office.

Hysteroscopy involves putting a scope through the cervix and looking at the inside of the uterus.

BIOPSY

Biopsy is a surgical procedure that consists of taking a sample of tissue for examination under a microscope to determine whether the tissue is malignant or to identify an unusual growth or infection. In many cases the sample can be taken in the doctor's office with local anesthesia, but biopsies of internal structures or biopsies that involve the removal of a large amount of tissue require hospitalization and surgery. For example, an operating room is necessary for a biopsy of an ovary or for a cone biopsy of the cervix in which a large "cone" of tissue is removed for extensive evaluation. Lasers are often used for such biopsies. Endometrial biopsies and small "punch" biopsies of the cervix are office procedures.

PROBLEMS AND DISEASES

An understanding of the various gynecologic problems and diseases that may occur is important for every woman.

MENSTRUAL PROBLEMS

Too much has been made of the regularity of menstrual periods. No woman starts her first period at 12 and then menstruates every 28 days for 5 days until she reaches the menopause at 49. The numbers 12, 28, 5, and 49 are averages that are not indicative of the wide normal variation. An onset between 9 and 16, an interval from 25 to 35 days, a length from 2 to 7 days, and menopause from 45 to 55 are completely normal. Each woman has a pattern that is normal for her. It is also normal for an individual to skip periods in the early teens and again in the years just before the menopause. Periods will not necessarily be the same at 16 as at 26, 36, or 46. Nonetheless, periods can be too heavy, too light, too frequent, or too infrequent. Some of these deviations from normal will be considered.

Delayed Onset of Periods

Failure to start menstrual periods is termed primary amenorrhea. If a girl has not had a menstrual period by the age of 16, a medical investigation is warranted. A complete history of previous illness is important. The first point to be noted on physical examination is whether breast development shows that the ovaries are secreting estrogen. Then one must discover whether the hymen has an opening and if the vagina and uterus are normal. Other genetic and hormonal tests may follow in an effort to uncover and correct the cause.

Skipped or Delayed Periods

Skipped periods are common in the early teens before the complicated interactions between the hypothalamic area of the brain, the pituitary gland, the ovaries, and the uterus settle into the patterns that they maintain for almost 40 years. Usually nothing need be done unless these irregularities continue beyond the first year or two.

Pregnancy is one of the most common causes of secondary amenorrhea, the absence of periods after the initial onset of menstruation. Whenever a period is delayed a week in a sexually active woman whose periods follow a regular pattern, this possibility should be considered. Other symptoms of early pregnancy may include breast tenderness, nausea, and an increased frequency of urination. At such an early stage a pregnancy test is necessary for confirmation because examination is often inconclusive.

Stress, either physical or emotional, and excessive dieting (leading to a weight loss of 15 to 25 percent of body weight) can also cause skipped or delayed periods. Delayed onset or erratic menstrual patterns are associated with anorexia nervosa and with the excessive physical demands that lead to a low percentage of body fat in relation to total weight experienced by ballet dancers and young athletes, including compulsive runners.

Periods are often delayed one to six months in women discontinuing oral contraceptive pills. Problems with the pituitary, adrenals, thyroid, and ovaries also may delay periods. In the absence of pregnancy, it is usually reasonable to wait at least three months before seeking professional advice about the absence of periods.

Light Periods

The old wives' tale that a heavy period is necessary to rid the body of poisons runs against the facts that wastes are excreted through the kidney and the bowel and that menstrual discharge contains only old endometrium (the lining of the uterus) and a small quantity of blood. Light periods lasting one to three days are normal for many women. Most women on birth control pills have decreased blood loss and a shorter flow, regarded by most as beneficial side effects of the pill. However, a sudden change to a very light period may mean that the period has been skipped and that bleeding from some other cause is mistaken for a period. This sometimes occurs in early pregnancy.

Frequent Periods

Periods that come more often than every three weeks usually take place in the absence of ovulation. If they are regular and not heavy and if pregnancy is not desired, this condition is not serious. Periods without ovulation are most likely to occur during the early teens and premenopausal years.

Heavy Periods (Menorrhagia)

Some women have heavy periods with clots lasting seven or eight days throughout their menstruating life. These heavier than average periods containing clots may be considered normal and not a medical problem. However, the blood lost each month with the menstrual period may lead to anemia in women who do not eat a diet containing sufficient iron. Most women between the onset of menstrual periods and the menopause have less hemoglobin in the blood than men. Heavy periods easily push a woman into iron deficiency anemia, and such women require supplemental iron to be taken as pills.

Bleeding that requires a super tampon or pad that must be changed more than once an hour and continues for more than a few hours is considered unusually heavy and may indicate the presence of a medical problem.

Estrogen from the ovary stimulates growth of the lining of the uterus; progesterone, produced by the ovary after ovulation, matures the endometrium so that breakdown and bleeding are controlled at the time of menstruation. Teenagers and premenopausal women, who often have periods without ovulation and therefore without progesterone, may have very heavy periods with serious blood loss and anemia. Even though women taking the oral contraceptive pill do not ovulate, the progesterone-type compound in the pill produces light, controlled periods. In young women heavy periods may be controlled by giving progesterone. In older women hormones can be used safely after cancer has been ruled out by curettage or biopsy.

Pregnancy may be a cause of heavy bleeding which occurs after a period is delayed. At least one out of every ten pregnancies ends in spontaneous abortion or miscarriage accompanied by heavy bleeding, usually because of abnormal development of the fetus. Removal of the fragments of the pregnancy that are left in the uterus using suction or D&C (dilatation and curettage; see below) stops the bleeding.

In older women heavy periods are often caused by fibroids (benign muscle tumors of the uterus).

Midcycle Bleeding

At the time of ovulation, approximately midway between menstrual periods, there is a transient dip in estrogen levels. In some women this is enough to start the breakdown of the endometrium and consequent bleeding. If, as is usual, estrogen levels rise again, the bleeding stops. Careful attention to the timing of the bleeding usually clarifies this as the cause.

Premenstrual Syndrome (PMS)

For many years it has been recognized that most women experience some changes such as irritability, depression, mood swings, or headache just before the onset of their menstrual periods. Contrary to the belief in some circles that this is strictly limited to American women, an extensive cross-cultural study conducted by researchers at the State University of New York at Buffalo indicates that women in the Third World as well as Western women experience the same cramps, bloating, and emotional disruption that has come to be known as PMS. For some women these symptoms last long enough and are severe enough to interfere with the normal functions of their lives. Distressing symptoms occur 2 to 14 days before the beginning of menstruation and disappear after the period. Almost all medical and psychological conditions become worse premenstrually, making it difficult to delineate true PMS.

Although PMS is clearly related to normal cyclic hormonal changes, the exact mechanism is not consistent. Measures that promote general health are useful. Decreasing caffeine and salt intake diminishes irritability. Depression can sometimes be alleviated by vitamin B_6 in doses of not more than 100 milligrams a day. Higher doses can cause nerve damage. Some women do better on oral contraceptive pills; others don't. Some clinics are using large doses of very expensive progesterone given in vaginal or rectal suppositories, but the effectiveness of the treatment is doubtful. Diuretics can reduce the puffiness, and an increase in exercise can stimulate the flow of endorphins. Relaxation skills, such as deep breathing and guided imagery, are also helpful.

According to Dr. Leslie Hartley Gise, director of the PMS Program at the

Mt. Sinai Medical Center in New York, there are more than 300 treatments for this condition, including vitamins, hormones, tranquilizers, and progesterone. In searching for a solution to their PMS problems, women should avoid being exploited by fly-by-night PMS clinics that offer "sure" cures. Your gynecologist is much likelier to offer dependable treatment, and if you can locate a PMS support group, participation in peer discussions can be very helpful.

Results of a study published in the *New England Journal of Medicine* in June 1995 indicated that women truly disabled by PMS symptoms might benefit from taking Prozac, the world's most popular antidepressant. Some of these women, however, found the side effects of the drug as unpleasant as the PMS symptoms.

Painful Periods

Pain with menstrual periods is termed dysmenorrhea. The most common type of dysmenorrhea starts within a year or two of the first period, is relatively constant, and tends to decrease with age and after pregnancies. This characteristic cramping pain is associated with cycles in which ovulation occurs, and it is considered normal if it is not incapacitating. Recent studies have shown that this primary dysmenorrhea is caused by substances called prostaglandins, which are released when the endometrial tissue breaks down. They cause the uterine muscle to contract and can also stimulate the alimentary canal, causing nausea and diarrhea. Mild menstrual discomfort can be relieved by aspirin, Tylenol, exercise, and a heating pad. More severe pain usually responds to compounds such as ibuprofen (Motrin, Nuprin, Advil), which function as antiprostaglandins. Women who are sexually active can often combine contraception with relief of dysmenorrhea by taking the oral contraceptive pill. Some women who are not having intercourse may also need the oral contraceptive pill for relief if the antiprostaglandins do not give adequate help.

Menstrual pain that begins after years of pain-free periods is usually due to abnormal causes such as endometriosis, polyps, or fibroids. Dysmenorrhea is a frequent accompaniment of the IUD, making this method of contraception a poor choice for women who already have severe cramps. Whenever previously normal periods become painful, the doctor should be alerted.

Pain with Ovulation

Mittelschmerz, literally "middle pain," is pain that occurs when the egg breaks through the tiny cyst on the ovary where it has been growing. In most women this process is painless; in a few it is always painful; in many it is occasionally painful. At times the pain may be severe, mimicking the pain of appendicitis or other abdominal crises. The pain is characterized by an abrupt onset and usually clears within a few hours, although it may last a day or two. It is necessary to know when the last period occurred and what the woman's normal interval is between periods in order to label an episode of abdominal pain as mittelschmerz.

Menopausal Problems

The menopause, the cessation of menstruation, is the objective evidence that the ovaries are aging and secreting less estrogen. Periods become irregular and cease. (Menopause is discussed in detail in the chapter "Aging Healthfully—Your Body, Mind, and Spirit.")

OTHER VAGINAL BLEEDING

Not all vaginal bleeding is related to menstruation but may be triggered by other events.

Bleeding After Intercourse

Bleeding that follows intercourse results either from injuries sustained during intercourse or, more commonly, from tissue made sensitive by inflammation or tumors of the vagina or cervix. Bleeding from tears in the hymen or vagina may occur in children who are sexually abused, in young women who are having intercourse for the first time, or in postmenopausal women who have not recently been sexually active. Sutures may be required to control heavy bleeding. An inflamed cervix or one with polyps or tumors is likely to bleed when touched by the thrusting penis. Such tumors can be either benign or malignant. Careful evaluation is always necessary.

Irregular Bleeding

Bleeding that occurs at random without regard to the menstrual cycle or is unrelated to sexual activity may be a symptom of endometrial cancer (cancer of the lining of the uterus), benign endometrial conditions, or hormonal fluctuations. Bleeding with an IUD in place is usually not serious but requires careful evaluation to distinguish it from other causes. Irregular bleeding in women on oral contraceptive pills is also sometimes hard to evaluate. Occasionally a biopsy or a D&C needs to be done to find the cause.

LOWER ABDOMINAL PAIN

In addition to menstruation and ovulation, other problems can cause acute or chronic pain. Pelvic infection or pelvic inflammatory disease, often abbreviated PID, is a frequent cause of pain. Gonorrhea, chlamydia, and other infectious organisms can cause PID. Such infections are more common in women using IUDs than in others. Whenever there is suspicion of PID, antibiotics should be used to minimize damage to the tubes and later sterility. (For further discussion of PID, see "Sexually Transmissible Diseases.")

Ovarian and uterine tumors, benign and malignant, may cause pain, as may the uterine contractions of an impending miscarriage. Many conditions of the intestinal and urinary tract are painful and must be considered among possible causes. Stress is another factor that may lead to abdominal pain, but organic causes should be eliminated by diagnostic tests before the pain is assumed to be psychological in origin.

VAGINAL DISCHARGE

The increased levels of female hormones that begin to circulate at puberty stimulate the glands of the cervix and increase the thickness and cellular activity of the vaginal wall. Together these changes cause increased vaginal moisture that collects at the vaginal opening as a completely normal "discharge." Observant women notice that this discharge is thickish and profuse about the time of ovulation. A marked increase in vaginal fluid also occurs as the first phase of sexual response and serves as a lubricant to facilitate intercourse. This reaction occurs whenever the woman is sexually aroused, regardless of whether the source of stimulation is dreams, sexual fantasies, or actual touching of the genitals and regardless of whether or not further phases of sexual response are reached.

Leukorrhea is a condition in which the vaginal discharge increases in quantity, changes color, has an unpleasant odor, or produces itching or irritation in the surrounding tissues. Among the circumstances leading to leukorrhea are mechanical irritation by a diaphragm, tampon, or IUD; chemical irritation by excessive douching or the use of vaginal deodorant sprays; vaginal infection by bacteria or fungi, especially candidiasis or trichomoniasis; sexually transmissible diseases such as gonorrhea; benign growths such as polyps or fibroid tumors. Heavy discharge may also be a sign of diabetes or cervical cancer. In most cases it can be cleared up by finding the cause and initiating proper treatment. (See "Sexually Transmissible Diseases.")

INCONTINENCE

Women leak urine; men have trouble voiding. This generalization reflects the problems relating to the short urethra (tube from the bladder to the outside) in the female and the long urethra in the male. It is not unusual for a normal woman with a full bladder to lose a few drops of urine if she coughs or sneezes. The supporting tissue of the bladder is often damaged by childbirth, so that, with stress, incontinence can become a major problem. The problem of incontinence may worsen when estrogen levels drop after the menopause. A variety of solutions should be considered before surgery is recommended. (See "Aging Healthfully—Your Body, Mind, and Spirit.")

The sphincter controlling the rectum and rectal supports can also be damaged by childbirth and may need surgical repair.

PROLAPSE OF THE UTERUS

During childbirth the ligaments that support the uterus may become so stretched and weakened that the uterus falls or drops into the vagina, often causing discomfort. Weakness of the bladder often occurs at the same time, causing difficulty holding urine, especially during the stress of coughing, sneezing, or moving the bowels. Corrective surgery may be necessary. Prolapse should not be confused with a "tipped womb," which is a uterus that tips back toward the rectum. This is now known to be a normal position for the uterus in about one-third of women.

INFECTIONS

Although not all infections of the female genital tract are sexually transmitted, a majority of them are. As with all infections, a search must be made for the organism responsible. Such a search involves cultures, smears that are stained for bacteria, and wet preparations in which a bit of discharge is placed on a slide and examined for organisms. Tests for the presence of antibodies are also common.

Cystitis and Urethritis

Increased frequency of urination coupled with pain on voiding usually means a bacterial infection of the bladder or urethra (cystitis or urethritis). Blood in the urine is a common symptom of infection. Often the bladder is so inflamed that the woman has difficulty holding her urine even briefly. If the infection originates in the kidneys (pyelonephritis), there is likely to be fever and pain in the side.

The diagnosis is made by obtaining the history, by a physical exam, and by a urine culture to find out which bacteria are present and to which antibiotic they are sensitive. If the discomfort is severe, the treatment may be started before the results of the culture are known and changed later if indicated. Treatment may be continued for 10 days, but shorter courses are almost as effective.

Sometimes infection is caused because organisms normally present in feces get into the urethra. To reduce this possibility, the wiping motion with toilet paper after a bowel movement should be from front to back only (away from your urethra).

"Honeymoon cystitis" is a term used for cystitis that occurs after intercourse. It is thought that intercourse and related sexual activity introduce bacteria into the urethra and bladder. Urination prior to beginning sex or, better, soon after coitus helps to "flush out" organisms from your urethra that can cause urethritis or cystitis.

In addition, the use of a diaphragm, especially one that is too large, may obstruct the urethra and predispose to cystitis.

Because antibiotics kill the normal vaginal bacteria as well as those causing infections in the bladder or elsewhere, a yeast or monilia infection often follows treatment. If these infections are a problem, antimonilial drugs can be used during antibiotic treatment.

Interstitial cystitis is an uncommon disease of the bladder wall with symptoms ranging from mild to severe enough to keep the patient housebound. Typical manifestations are acute pain and pressure in the lower abdomen and the need to urinate very frequently. Although the median age of onset is 40, patients as young as 30 may have to consult several doctors before their complaints are taken seriously. Diagnosis is hampered by the fact that no bacteria are revealed in urine cultures, nor does antibiotic treatment eliminate the symptoms. All standard urologic tests show normal results, except cystoscopy and bladder wall biopsy performed under anesthesia. In 90 to 95 percent of patients suffering from interstitial cystitis, tiny hemorrhages in the bladder wall are revealed when a lighted scope is inserted through the urethra. Until the specific cause of these hemorrhages is isolated, treatments vary depending on the symptoms. Effective singly or in combination are dietary changes; elimination of alcohol, caffeine, artificial sweeteners, and smoking; increased exercise; and a wide range of drugs, including antidepressants and antihistamines.

Infected Bartholin's Glands

On either side of the vaginal opening, Bartholin's gland secretions contribute to sexual lubrication. If the opening of the gland is blocked, the gland becomes distended, cystic, and easily infected. An infected Bartholin's gland, called a Bartholin's abscess, is extremely painful. Treatment consists of heat, antibiotics, and cutting into the collection of pus so that it can drain. Often a catheter or drain is left in the gland for a few days so that the infection will not recur. Mere swelling of these glands without infection does not require treatment. Rarely glands of the urethra or other glands in the vulvar area become infected.

Vaginitis

Vaginitis is an inflammation of the vagina that may cause pain and soreness of the vagina and vulva, burning (especially with urination and intercourse), itching, abnormal vaginal discharge, and odor. The discomfort may in some cases be severe enough to warrant emergency treatment.

Because there are so many different organisms and conditions that may result in vaginitis, it is necessary to find the cause by physical examination, cultures, and microscopic examination of the vaginal discharge before attempting treatment. The urethra and bladder are so close to the vulva and vagina that an infection in one area may cause symptoms in the other, making diagnosis difficult.

The most frequent vaginal infection, which is due to a yeastlike fungus commonly called monilia, is technically known as moniliasis or candidiasis. While neither life-threatening nor the cause of permanent damage, this type of infection can be a great nuisance, especially to those who are vulnerable to it. There are some women who can be reinfected monthly, and during the infection sexual intercourse becomes impossible. Even sitting causes great discomfort. Because the fungus flourishes when estrogen and progesterone levels are high, pregnant women and those receiving large doses of these hormones as replacement therapy are at higher risk. The organisms flourish in the warm, moist environment of the vagina and are likely to take hold when antibiotics prescribed for a prior condition have killed the bacteria normally responsible for maintaining the acidity of the vagina. When taking a course of antibiotics, a yeast infection can be prevented by eating eight ounces of plain yogurt a day or by taking acidophilus capsules with all meals. These capsules and yogurt containing live *Lactobacillus acidophilus* cultures, can be bought at health food stores.

Other factors that encourage the fungal growth are tight pants, wet bathing suits, and nylon panty hose and underwear. Scented douches, bath oils, and bubble baths can be responsible for triggering the infection, and for diabetic women the high sugar content of vaginal secretions is an additional factor.

Itching, rash, and inflammation are symptoms of the infection, which is also characterized by a thick white discharge with a yeasty odor. The diagnosis is made by examining a portion of this discharge under the microscope or by growing the organism in a tube. Candidiasis usually responds to treatment with antifungal creams or suppositories. A recent alternative is an oral medication, but because it can have undesirable side effects, its use should be closely monitored by the doctor. The use of this and other drugs by pregnant women or nursing mothers is contraindicated. When the infection has been cleared up, recurrences can sometimes be prevented by wearing loose cotton underpants and avoiding all pants that fit tightly in the crotch. It is also advisable to find out whether the fungus is being harbored by one's sexual partner.

The term "nonspecific vaginitis" or, more recently, "bacterial vaginosis" is used to designate vaginal inflammation caused by miscellaneous abnormal bacteria. A foul-smelling discharge is often caused by the bacteria *Gardnerella vaginalis* together with organisms from the intestinal tract, but frequently the bacteria cannot be identified. Thinness of the lining of the vagina in a child or postmenopausal woman makes the vagina more susceptible to infection. The discharge with nonspecific vaginitis is usually white or yellow and may be streaked with blood. An unpleasant odor and swollen glands in the groin may be present. Nonspecific vaginitis is usually treated with oral antibiotics such as metronidazole. Creams or suppositories are sometimes used. Consideration must be given to treatment of sexual partners.

The vagina depends on a balance of normal hormone effects and normal bacteria to maintain its acidity and health. Strong douches can interfere with this balance. Some women are allergic to soaps, deodorants, and other preparations used around the vagina.

Not all organisms capable of producing vaginal irritations have been identified and, therefore, one should be careful about attributing symptoms to psychosomatic interactions. However, it has been found that for a number of reasons, including inadequate sexual lubrication, women with sexual and relationship problems have an increased incidence of vaginitis. Conversely, most women with vaginitis have dyspareunia.

Certain precautions can be taken to prevent vaginitis.

1. If the area is sore, don't attempt intercourse.
2. A condom can help prevent the spread of sexually transmissible diseases. Lubricate with a spermicidal cream or jelly and not with Vaseline, which can weaken the latex of the condom.
3. Keep the genital area as dry as possible because organisms that cause vaginitis grow well in a moist environment. Cotton crotch underwear allows for more absorption and helps keep the genital area dry. Avoiding tight jeans or panty hose may also help. Sitting for long periods of time in a wet bathing suit is conducive to yeast infections.
4. Practice good general hygiene. Washing the external genitalia thoroughly with soap and water is sufficient. Be sure to rinse thoroughly after bathing. Avoid bubble baths and perfumed soaps that may be irritating.
5. Avoid perfumed tampons, vaginal sprays, and frequent douching, especially with over-the-counter products, because they can be harsh and may kill normal bacteria and alter vaginal acidity.
6. An occasional douche (not more than twice a week) with mild vinegar solution (2 tablespoons to 1 quart water) can be used prophylactically if recurrent vaginitis is a problem or if a woman chooses. Douching is never necessary!
7. Do not douche during menstruation or pregnancy.
8. Do not use other people's towels.

Pelvic Inflammatory Disease (PID)

Pelvic inflammatory disease (PID) is increasing in incidence, in some cases because early symptoms are ignored, and in others because the symptoms are inadequately treated. While overall health risks associated with the use of an IUD are low compared to other birth control methods, its main disadvantage is that it can be associated with serious pelvic infection. The condition itself, which is bacterial in origin, is often secondary to gonorrhea or chlamydia. (PID is discussed in detail in "Sexually Transmissible Diseases.")

Toxic Shock Syndrome (TSS)

Some years ago it was noted that healthy young women occasionally died of an illness that began during a menstrual period and was characterized by fever, severe diarrhea, aching, and rash. Eighty percent of these women used tampons. A toxic substance made by the bacterium *Staph. aureus,* occasionally found in the vagina, has been found to be responsible for the illness. "Super" tampons seem to be more dangerous, perhaps because they are retained for a longer time. The worst tampon has been taken off the market. A few cases have been associated with contraceptive diaphragms and sponges when these have been left in the vagina for more than 24 hours (see the chapter on "Contraception and Abortion").

As women and their doctors have become aware of TSS, the number of cases and the mortality rates have fallen. A factor that has contributed to the decline in infections is the redesign of sanitary napkins so that they are less cumbersome and easier to wear, no longer requiring belts, pins, and other paraphernalia. If you use tampons, do not leave them in place for more than four hours, do not use them to control vaginal discharges, and do not use them for more than five days during the month. If you use napkins, change them frequently. If you use a diaphragm or a contraceptive sponge, remove it promptly, but no sooner than eight hours following intercourse.

TUMORS

The word "tumor," which means "growth" or "swelling," is used both for a malignant growth—cancer that can spread into surrounding tissues and from which pieces can break off and travel to other parts of the body—and for a benign or nonmalignant growth that may cause problems because of size or pressure but does not spread.

Vulvar Tumors

Most lumps that women find on the external genitals or vulva are benign and may be warts, infections, or cysts. Of all the cancers of the female reproductive system, vulvar cancers account for fewer than 5 percent. The first signs are white patches of skin, or lumps that do not heal, accompanied by pain, itching, and a burning sensation during urination. Vulvar cancers are often traced to genital warts. Detection usually occurs during a pelvic examination, and diagnosis is confirmed by biopsy. Early treatment, which may involve surgery and radiation, can lead to a successful outcome.

Vaginal Tumors

Until the advent of a generation of women exposed before birth to high doses of estrogens such as DES, vaginal tumors were very rare. Now they are somewhat less rare. Most vaginal tumors consist of benign changes in the lining of the vagina, but cancer can occur. The colposcope is used to localize areas for biopsy.

Cervical Polyps

Small benign growths called polyps are the most common cervical tumors. These start in the cervical canal and appear at the cervical opening. Polyps are small, red, mushroomlike growths that bleed easily and irregularly. They are removed by a minor operation called a polypectomy, which usually can be done in the doctor's office. Cervical warts are also seen frequently.

Dysplasia

Early changes in the cells of the surface of the cervix that might become malignant are called dysplasia, or cervical intraepithelial neoplasia (CIN). These changes can be mild or severe and sometimes disappear spontaneously. They are usually discovered by a Pap smear and can best be evaluated by a combination of colposcopy and biopsy. Treatment consists of destroying the abnormal cells by means of hot cautery, freezing by cryosurgery, or lasers.

Carcinoma-in-situ

More advanced changes in the cells covering the cervix are called carcinoma-in-situ (cancer in place). Carcinoma-in-situ may be treated by cryosurgery, cautery, or excision biopsy. A new technique, the loop electrosurgical excision procedure (LEEP), permits diagnosis and treatment at the same office visit. Follow-up with frequent Pap smears is necessary to be sure all the abnormal areas have been removed.

Cancer of the Cervix

Invasive cancer of the cervix is one of the most common female malignancies. Risk increases with a history of sexually transmitted infections, especially of viral genital warts (condyloma). Recent studies indicate that smoking and also constant exposure to secondhand smoke are additional risk factors. There has been a significant drop in the number of cases with the advent of Pap smears, which permit early detection and treatment of premalignant lesions. Cone biopsy, also called conization, is the surgical removal of a cone-shaped piece of tissue from the cervix and cervical canal. This procedure is used for diagnosis, but since it may remove precancerous cells altogether, it may eliminate the need for further treatment in early premalignant lesions. Invasive cancer of the cervix can be treated by a radical hysterectomy or by radiation. A radical hysterectomy is one in which the tissue adjoining the uterus—the pelvic lymph nodes, tubes, and ovaries—is removed as well as the uterus. The operation is generally performed by specially trained gynecologic cancer surgeons. Because there is rarely a connection between cervical and ovarian cancer, consideration can be given to leaving the ovaries in place.

Benign Uterine Conditions

Polyps may appear on the endometrium or lining of the uterus and are removed by D&C. Another type of irregular growth of the endometrium is called hyperplasia.

Endometrial Hyperplasia

Endometrial hyperplasia is a condition of the lining of the uterus that occurs when estrogen stimulates the endometrium continuously without the modifying effects of progesterone. Endometrial hyperplasia is reversible. However, if stimulation of the endometrium by estrogen (unopposed by progesterone), whether produced by the body (endogenous) or taken as medication (exogenous), continues uninterrupted for several years, cancer of the endometrium may result. The diagnosis is usually made by endometrial biopsy or D&C. Treatment is by the use of synthetic progesterones or, if severe, by hysterectomy.

Fibroids or Fibromyomata Uteri

Fibroids are very common benign tumors of the muscle of the uterus. Studies indicate that one woman in four aged 30 to 50 has fibroids. In most cases, they produce no symptoms. They are likely to increase in size when stimulated by estrogen, as happens during pregnancy. Following menopause, when hormone stimulation is reduced, the fibroids shrink. Fibroids can be felt during a manual examination of the pelvis. Even when they produce no symptoms, they should be checked twice a year to find out whether they have suddenly grown much larger.

Unless fibroids cause severe pain or pressure or grow to be larger than 4 inches in diameter, they need not be treated. However, even though they do not cause bleeding between periods, they can cause periods heavy or prolonged enough to result in anemia. Enlarged fibroids may press on the bladder, prompting a need for frequent urination. They may also cause back pain, and in some cases they can interfere with conception by blocking the implantation of the fertilized egg.

Size, location, and complications produced by fibroids, as well as the desire for continuing childbearing capability, are all taken into consideration in deciding on treatment. With the use of a laparoscope, for example, surgeons can now remove troublesome fibroids from the outside of the uterus. Women approaching menopause can wait to see whether the fibroids will shrink when deprived of estrogen. If not, a hysterectomy may be recommended. Antiestrogens can be used to temporarily reduce fibroid size. For women who wish to preserve their fertility, the recommended procedure may be a myomectomy, a more difficult operation, in which the fibroids are removed, leaving a scarred uterus. In deciding on treatment, women should be aware that in fewer than 3 cases per 1,000 do fibroids become cancerous.

Cancer of the Uterus

Cancer of the lining of the uterus rarely develops before the menopause, a circumstance indicating the involvement of hormonal changes. Studies show that women who have never had children and women whose menopause began early are likely to be at higher risk. For purposes of diagnosis, a Pap smear is not an effective indicator of uterine cancer. When unusual bleeding, pelvic pain, or abdominal swelling occur, ultrasound and a tissue biopsy can provide a reliable diagnosis of uterine cancer. Standard treatment is a hysterectomy as well as removal of the fallopian tubes and ovaries, often followed by radiation. Early treatment may insure a favorable outcome.

Endometriosis

Endometriosis is a condition in which normal, benign cells of endometrial tissue break away from the uterus and start to grow in other locations in the pelvic cavity—the tubes, ovaries, and surface of the bladder and rectum. This condition is the third leading cause of infertility, affecting almost one-third of all infertile women. Recent research indicates that the disease often affects other tissues as well as the genitourinary tissues and that the symptoms are caused by immune system hormones. During menstruation women shed endometrial cells, but instead of leaving the body as part of menstrual waste, some of the cells move out of the fallopian tubes into the pelvis and abdomen. Researchers believe that the reflux of the endometrial cells causes the body's white blood cells to secrete the immune system hormone interleuken 1. In women who have endometriosis, this hormone circulates in the bloodstream and suppresses bone growth. Thus women with endometriosis are also at high risk for osteoporosis.

Endometriosis can produce many types of pelvic discomfort or none at all but most typically causes pain that begins two or three days before the start of a menstrual period, possibly caused by changes in the endometrial tissue similar to those occurring in the uterus. Abnormally heavy menstrual flow can be another sign of endometriosis. The diagnosis can be made accurately by laparoscopy. Mild endometriosis, which produces no symptoms or effects, may not require treatment. Laser therapy has been used at the time of laparoscopy to destroy early implants. Treatment with progestational agents and synthetic steroids such as danazol is based on the observed fact that endometriosis decreases when ovulation is prevented for three to six months.

A recently developed procedure is known as endometrial ablation. Since it puts an end to monthly periods and makes the uterus inhospitable to newly fertilized eggs, it is becoming increasingly popular not only in treating endometriosis and as an alternative to a hysterectomy but also as a nonsurgical form of permanent birth control. Endometrial ablation uses electric current transmitted through a probe known as a hysteroscope, which is inserted through the cervix to create scar tissue on the wall of the uterus. Although the procedure requires general anesthesia and is usually done in a hospital, there are no incisions and no external scars. The patient can go home the same day. Another positive aspect of this procedure as compared to a hysterectomy is that, because the pelvic organs remain intact, they remain capable of producing hormones.

Cancer of the Tube

Cancer of the fallopian tubes is very uncommon, hard to diagnose, and difficult to cure. The treatment is surgery.

Benign Ovarian Cysts and Tumors

Because the ovary is a complex structure containing many types of cells, including ova (which have the potential of making every type of cell), many different types of tumors can form in the ovary. The most common benign ovarian tumor is the simple cyst that occurs when the small cyst containing the ovum does not rupture at the proper time in the cycle to expel the ovum but continues to grow. Such cysts usually disappear in one or two months, but if they rupture, they may cause pain or internal bleeding and sometimes require surgery. Dermoid cysts, containing hair, fatty material, and often teeth, are common in young women and are thought to be embryonic remnants present before birth. Although benign, they require removal. Other benign ovarian tumors, both cystic and solid, may cause symptoms and require surgery. If an ovarian tumor persists, it must be removed to find out whether or not it is malignant.

Ovarian Cancer

Ovarian cancer is the fourth leading cause of cancer death in women, exceeded only by lung, breast, and colon cancer, and it is the leading cause of death from gynecologic malignancies in the United States. There are many types of cancer of the ovary. The long-term outlook depends on the type, but all are difficult to diagnose early because symptoms do not occur early. However, monitoring on a regular basis is extremely important for women with a personal history of breast, colon, or gynecological cancers and a family history of ovarian cancer. For women in this category the incidence of ovarian cancer may rise to 6 percent, as against 1.4 percent in the rest of the female population. Three screening tests are currently used for women at high risk: bimanual rectovaginal examination (which in itself is not adequately sensitive), transvaginal ultrasonography, and a blood test called CA 125, which measures the level of particular antibodies associated with cell changes in the ovaries. Final diagnosis depends on removal of the tumor at the time of exploratory surgery for microscopic examination. Treatment consists of surgical removal of as much tumor as possible followed by chemotherapy. Women who have taken the oral contraceptive pill have a decreased incidence of ovarian cancer. Other protective factors include breast feeding, tubal ligation, and for women from families with hereditary ovarian cancer, serious consideration should be given to removal of the ovaries (prophylactic oophorectomy) when childbearing is completed.

ENDOCRINE PROBLEMS

The gynecologic problems considered up to this point have been those for which a specific abnormal tissue has been responsible. Because of the complex interrelationship between the ovary, the hypothalamus, the pituitary gland, the thyroid, and the adrenal glands, many abnormalities of the menstrual cycle are caused by dysfunctions or malfunctions of these endocrine glands. These abnormalities include heavy, irregular menstrual periods, called dysfunctional uterine bleeding. Lack of periods and lack of ovulation may also be endocrine problems.

Unraveling the complexities of endocrine malfunction requires many expensive and complex hormone tests to discover the level of hormones in the body and to find out how one endocrine gland responds when hormones from another gland are administered.

Some pituitary malfunctions are caused by severe dieting or physical and emotional stress on the hypothalamus of the brain. Other problems are genetically determined. Treatment depends on the particular abnormality.

TYPES OF GYNECOLOGIC TREATMENT

Because of the number of treatment options available, it is important for women to become as knowledgeable as possible in order to make intelligent decisions.

TREATMENT OF INFECTION

Gynecologic infections may be caused by viruses, bacteria, fungi, spirochetes, and protozoans. Infection caused by each of these types of organisms requires a different type of treatment. Viruses, causing herpes and warts, are impossible to destroy effectively with current drugs. However, symptoms can be relieved and some effects of their presence can be treated. Warts, which are virally induced, can be removed by cautery, cryosurgery, or laser.

Different types of bacteria can be treated effectively with antibiotics. Treatment becomes more difficult when bacteria become resistant to particular antibiotics. Specific agents are available to treat monilia and trichomonads, common causes of vaginal infections. Because effective treatment requires knowledge of the specific nature of the infectious agent, the telephone management of vaginitis and urinary tract infections is not dependable.

HORMONE THERAPY

The vast publicity given to problems associated with the use of the oral contraceptive pill has clouded the fact that the discovery of orally effective estrogen and progesterone compounds has revolutionized the treatment of bleeding problems in women, reduced the number of D&Cs required, and often permitted an alternative to hysterectomy for control of hemorrhage. Surgery is no longer the first therapy for heavy bleeding. The use of progesterones to bring on a period in women with infrequent periods reduces the likelihood of cancer of the endometrium. New synthetic hormones, including gonado-tropin-releasing hormone antagonists, are widely used to treat endometriosis.

Estrogen Replacement Therapy

Estrogens have been used successfully in menopausal women for many years to relieve hot flashes and painful intercourse due to the thinning of the vagina. No other treatment works so well. In addition, estrogen slows osteo-porosis, the thinning of the bones that occurs with aging. Studies indicate that postmenopausal women who are on estrogen replacement therapy for six years or more reduce their lifetime probability of a fracture by at least 40 percent. The recent linking of the use of estrogen during and after menopause with an increased rate of cancer of the endometrium has reminded us that relative risks are always difficult to assess, but this risk is eliminated by the addition of synthetic progesterones.

Recent studies show that women given estrogen have a decreased risk of heart disease. It is only within the past few years that the medical profession has begun to pay sufficient attention to the fact that heart disease is now the leading cause of death of American women aged 50 and over. The most com-pelling evidence to date of the benefits of estrogen in this regard comes from a 10-year study of more than 48,000 nurses conducted by the Harvard Univer-sity Nurses' Health project. The results, published in 1991 in the *New England Journal of Medicine,* indicated that the nurses who were taking estrogen were half as likely to be at risk for heart disease as those who were not. However, the federal Centers for Disease Control issued a report in the same year that, although it found no increased risk of breast cancer for women who used estrogen for less than five years, there was a 30 percent increase in risk for breast cancer among women who had been on estrogen replacement therapy for 15 years or more as compared to women who had not. In trying to make an informed decision, patients and their doctors should explore the benefits and the risks in terms of individual medical history, general health, age, and other circumstances. (See also "Aging Healthfully—Your Body, Mind, and Spirit.")

CAUTERY

Cautery refers to the limited destruction of diseased tissue by the use of chemicals, heat, or cold. The use of heat is termed electrocautery; the use of cold, cryosurgery. It is used to treat venereal warts and to destroy the abnormal cells of dysplasia and carcinoma-in-situ of the cervix. Lasers are a new form of cautery, as is the loop electrosurgical procedure, or LEEP.

SURGERY

Despite the availability of drugs to treat many problems, surgery may be required for certain disorders.

Excision Biopsy

Cone biopsy or conization, described as a diagnostic technique, may also have therapeutic application. The removal of abnormal tissue for diagnosis may be treatment as well. LEEP is frequently used for this. Drawbacks include the need for hospitalization and anesthesia and the possibility of heavy bleeding and infection.

Incision and Drainage (I&D)

Antibiotics cannot get into the center of a cyst or cavity where blood vessels do not penetrate. Whenever there is a collection of pus that does not drain on its own, it is necessary to cut into the cavity to allow it to do so. This minor operation is called incision and drainage. If the abscess re-forms, the incision must sometimes be sewed open to ensure long-term drainage. This procedure is frequently used to treat Bartholin's abscesses. Drainage of a major infection of the tubes and ovaries that does not respond to antibiotics requires abdominal surgery.

Vaginal Surgery

Vaginal surgery is involved in the repair operations carried out in those women whose vaginas and surrounding connective tissue have been stretched and damaged by childbirth. The supporting structures are reached through incisions in the lining of the vagina, excess tissue is removed, the supports strengthened, and the incisions closed. A vaginal hysterectomy can also be carried out in this way.

Polypectomy

The removal of a cervical or uterine polyp is called polypectomy. Cervical polyps can usually be removed in a doctor's office. Because the removal of endometrial polyps involves dilatation of the cervix, anesthesia may be required, either in an office or outpatient operating room or in the hospital.

Endometrial Biopsy

A narrow instrument can usually be fitted through the cervical opening into the cavity of the uterus in order to obtain endometrial tissue for study. Suction may be used to pull the tissue into a container. Although the biopsy is uncomfortable, anesthesia is usually not necessary and the procedure can be carried out in an outpatient clinic or office.

Dilatation and Curettage (D&C) and Dilatation and Evacuation (D&E)

The cervix can stretch wide enough to permit a 10-pound baby's head to pass through it, but at other times it is closed so that only a narrow tube ⅛ inch in diameter can be passed into the uterus. If larger instruments are required for an operation inside the uterus, the cervix is opened by passing metal tubes of increasing diameter through the opening until the cervix will allow the passage of the required instrument. This is called dilatation of the cervix. Alternate methods using dilators that gradually absorb fluid (laminarias) are available.

In order to remove tissue from the uterus, an instrument called a curette, a loop with a sharp edge, is used to scrape the endometrium off the muscular part of the uterus. This procedure is called curettage. The tissue may be removed for examination and diagnosis or it may be removed as part of treatment for heavy or irregular uterine bleeding.

Dilatation and curettage (D&C) may also be performed to terminate pregnancy, as may a similar procedure called dilatation and evacuation (D&E), which uses a suction curette, a hollow tube connected to a vacuum pump, to remove tissue by suction (see "Contraception and Abortion"). Usually local anesthesia suffices for these procedures.

Myomectomy

The removal of a smooth muscle tumor (fibromyoma or fibroid) of the uterus is called a myomectomy. Because fibroids are usually multiple and small ones may continue to grow even though the largest ones are removed and because a myomectomy is technically more difficult to perform and associated with more blood loss than a hysterectomy, these tumors are generally removed by a hysterectomy. Myomectomy is usually reserved for women who want future pregnancies.

Hysterectomy

The second most frequently performed major operation in the United States is hysterectomy, outnumbered only by cesarean section. Both are the subject of ongoing controversy. A radical hysterectomy is a procedure performed for cancer in which the uterus, cervix, two ovaries, and lymph nodes are removed. In a total hysterectomy, the uterus and cervix are removed; in a partial hysterectomy, the cervix is left in place. In any case, this operation puts an end to a woman's childbearing capability. According to consumer advocates, health care economists, and feminists, of the approximately 650,000 hysterectomies performed each year, 25 percent to 50 percent are unnecessary, undertaken before other less costly and less hazardous procedures are considered. Arguments against what are perceived as indiscriminately performed hysterectomies are buttressed by the striking disparity in rates of the procedure nationwide: in the South, for example, 83 hysterectomies are performed annually for every 10,000 women; in the Northeast, 43 for every 10,000, or half as many.

There are several explanations for this disparity. Greed may be the answer in some cases; lack of empathy of male surgeons with female patients is another. Lack of information on the patient's part and her unwarranted confidence in the doctor yet another. A recent survey has found another factor: the *age of the gynecologist* regardless of sex. It appears that younger practitioners are more likely to believe that the uterus performs functions other than a reproductive one and therefore should not be surgically removed if alternative treatments might be effective. Other studies indicate that if women do not immediately accept the need for a hysterectomy, but press the doctor for less drastic alternatives, this can definitely affect the doctor's recommendations.

In an article in the *New England Journal of Medicine,* three gynecologists at

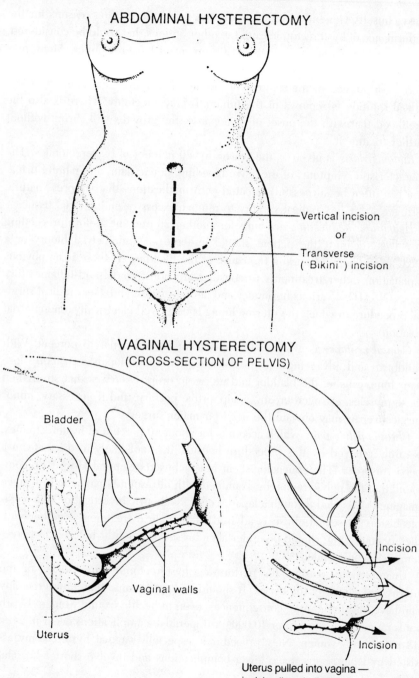

ABDOMINAL HYSTERECTOMY

Vertical incision

or

Transverse ("Bikini") incision

VAGINAL HYSTERECTOMY
(CROSS-SECTION OF PELVIS)

Bladder

Vaginal walls

Uterus

Incision

Incision

Uterus pulled into vagina —
incision lines indicated

Massachusetts General Hospital in Boston listed the leading reasons for the performance of hysterectomies and the other options that could be considered.

Uterine fibroids are the cause of 30 percent of hysterectomies. Many premenopausal women who experience bleeding and pain and who don't want any more children accept the removal of the uterus as a practical solution. A less radical solution is removal of the tumors by myomectomy. There is also the likelihood that with the onset of menopause, the growths will shrink without further treatment.

Endometriosis is given as the reason for 20 percent of hysterectomies. The characteristic symptoms of excessive bleeding, pelvic pain, and painful urination can often be successfully treated with medications that suppress natural estrogen or by less radical surgery to remove excessive endometrial tissue.

Heavy uterine bleeding accounts for another 20 percent. Before proceeding to a hysterectomy, the patient should undergo an endometrial biopsy or a D&C in the hope of finding the cause of the bleeding. If there is no obvious explanation, other treatments to consider are nonsteroidal anti-inflammatory drugs (NSAIDs), various hormones and antihormones, and a less radical surgical procedure in which the uterine lining is destroyed electrically (endometrial oblation).

Genital prolapse is given as the reason for an additional 15 percent. With childbirth and advancing age the muscles that support pelvic structure lose their tone, causing the bladder and uterus to drop. Exercises that strengthen these muscles, estrogen cream, a supportive pessary, and if necessary, minor surgical repair may obviate the need for major surgery.

Chronic pelvic pain, which accounts for about 10 percent of hysterectomies, is rarely relieved by this procedure because it is not likely to originate in a pelvic disorder. The gynecologists at Massachusetts General Hospital recommend that the pelvic region be examined with ultrasound, magnetic resonance imaging (MRI), and through a laparoscope. Psychiatric investigation of a possible history of sexual abuse is advised, and medical treatment together with dietary counseling should be undertaken for several months before a hysterectomy is recommended.

Unambiguous reasons for performing hysterectomies are cancer of the uterus and cancer of the cervix. It should be kept in mind that a hysterectomy can have life-threatening consequences, even in healthy young women. Death rates range from 6 to 11 per 10,000; postoperative complications occur in 24 to 48 percent of women. New procedures, especially vaginal hysterectomy assisted by laparoscopy, have fewer complications and involve shorter hospital stays.

Dr. Sidney Wolfe, director of the patient advocacy group Public Citizen, offers the following advice in a *New York Times* interview (10/25/94): "If a doctor immediately says, 'Have a hysterectomy,' shop for another physician. You need tests to write off all the alternatives."

The unresolved question is whether or not the operation should be performed on women near or past the menopause who have heavy bleeding with no indication of uterine abnormality. Debate continues about the removal of the otherwise normal uterus either as a means of contraception or as a way of preventing future problems, including the possibility of cancer.

Note that the term "hysterectomy" says nothing about the removal of the ovaries and tubes. Decisions regarding the removal of these organs must be made separately. Many gynecologists prefer to remove the ovaries whenever they are performing a pelvic operation on a woman at or near the menopause because the ovaries produce relatively little estrogen thereafter and ovarian cancer, which develops in 1 out of every 100 women, is hard to detect and hard to cure. Sometimes the ovaries must be removed before the menopause because of disease. In this circumstance estrogens should be given at least until the age of normal menopause.

The uterus can be removed through an abdominal incision, either vertical or crosswise, or through a vaginal incision around the cervix at the top of the vagina (see illustration). The operations are called abdominal and vaginal hysterectomies, respectively. Many factors influence the route chosen. The vaginal route is chosen if repair work is required for injuries to the bladder and rectum sustained in childbirth, and occasionally for other reasons. Frequently, with the patient's permission, the surgeon will take out the appendix at the time of an abdominal hysterectomy (it takes only five minutes longer) to prevent future appendicitis. Surgery for cancer is more extensive than other types and is always modified by the extent of the tumor found at the time of the surgery. Ovarian surgery and general exploration of the abdominal organs is easier with the abdominal incision.

A typical hysterectomy usually involves a three- to five-day hospital stay followed by three to five weeks of recovery time at home before resuming normal activities. For the woman previously engaged in a strenuous schedule, some curtailment of demands on energy should be made for at least three months. It is by no means unusual for some women to tire easily one year following surgery, especially if nutritional needs have been neglected or if there is daily exposure to secondhand smoke. In general, speed of recovery is affected by attitude, general health, and emotional support from family members, friends, and colleagues.

The loss of the uterus ends both childbearing and menstruation. The capac-

CROSS-SECTION OF PELVIS AFTER HYSTERECTOMY

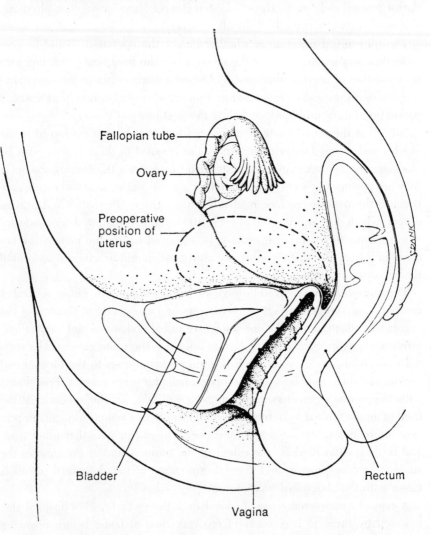

Fallopian tube

Ovary

Preoperative
position of
uterus

Bladder

Rectum

Vagina

ity to bear children has always been very important to women, and the loss of
this potential may be threatening. Among the myths that have emerged regarding a hysterectomy is that sexual response is decreased. Actually, sexual response is usually unaffected. Some women anticipate the onset of obesity. The
fact that physical activity is curtailed for a few weeks may confirm their fear
and start them on an inactive, weight-gaining course. If the ovaries remain,
estrogen production continues to the age of the expected menopause, so that

hot flashes and other menopausal symptoms do not occur until later, even though periods are absent.

The psychological aftermath of a hysterectomy depends on the degree to which the woman regards her uterus as her feminine identity. If she feels that her femininity resides in her womb, she may find the postoperative adjustment hard. If she understands and accepts the operation, she may welcome the relief of symptoms that the operation affords. The adjustment is hardest for the young childless woman; often counseling will be required to help her come to terms with this crisis in her life.

Tubal Surgery

The most common operation performed on the fallopian tubes is the tubal ligation for sterilization (discussed in "Contraception and Abortion"). Less common is the surgery (salpingectomy) necessitated by a tubal or ectopic pregnancy. If the other tube is normal, the surgeon may remove both the tube and the pregnancy because a scarred tube, if left behind, may become the site of a second tubal pregnancy. However, the pregnancy often can be removed and the tube carefully repaired. This surgery is now usually performed using a laparoscope. Many early ectopic pregnancies can be treated with the anti-cancer agent methotrexate without the need for surgery.

Occasionally women who have had tubal ligations for sterilization request reversal of the procedure. The tubes can be put back together using operating microscopes and microsurgical techniques, but such operations are difficult, expensive, and only about 50 percent effective.

Ovarian Surgery

Ovarian surgery involves removing part or all of an ovary because of cysts or tumors. Removal of an ovary is termed oophorectomy. In the case of benign cysts and tumors, as much normal ovary is saved as possible. Pregnancies can occur in women with only half of one ovary. If an ovarian or uterine tumor is malignant, all of the reproductive organs are removed together because the cancer tends to spread to the nearby uterus and the opposite tube and ovary. Severe pelvic infections and abscesses involving the tubes and ovaries that do not respond adequately to antibiotics often require extensive surgery for cure.

Preparation for Surgery

Here are some ways to relieve the anxiety experienced before undergoing surgery:

1. Be sure you understand *why* the surgery is necessary.
2. Find out whether the person who will perform the surgery is a board-certified gynecological surgeon.
3. If you can choose the hospital, select the one associated with a large medical center rather than one that is privately owned.
4. Don't hesitate to ask any questions that occur to you at the last minute.
5. Check your health insurance coverage so that you'll know what to expect in terms of hospital bills, bills from the surgeon, the anesthetist, and other costs. Some insurance policies require a second opinion before surgery.
6. Organize your family life and your job responsibilities so that you don't have to worry about details when you're in the hospital.
7. If you have the time to do so, you can set up an emergency blood supply by donating your own blood and asking a friend or family member with the same blood type to make a donation on your behalf in case of need.
8. If you have prepared a Living Will, bring a copy to the hospital and be sure it is attached to your chart.

In addition, for any but minor office procedures, oral contraceptive pills should be discontinued one month in advance to help prevent postoperative blood clots. (But be sure to use some alternate method of contraception because an unplanned pregnancy can only complicate matters!) Aspirin increases bleeding time and blood loss and should not be used for two weeks before surgery.

· A well-balanced diet with a minimum of caffeine and alcohol helps bring a woman to surgery in optimum condition. Each surgeon is likely to have other specific requests for the period immediately before the operation.

Surgical Complications

Fifty years ago surgery was so dangerous that no one needed to be told that there were risks involved. Now risks may be overlooked. This is a mistake. All anesthesia, whether general or local, involves a small risk of death. Hemorrhage and infection are potential hazards in almost all surgery, although blood banks and antibiotics have greatly reduced these risks. Adhesions, the attachment of one bit of injured tissue to another, occur after most abdominal surgery as part of the healing process and may cause pain or obstruct the bowel. This contingency is reduced by early ambulation.

Pain Control

Postsurgical patients are no longer expected to experience unnecessary pain, nor is there a need to plead for painkillers. Before undergoing surgery, speak to the surgeon and tell him or her that you would like to be in charge of the device that delivers your opiate together with your IV until the acute pain begins to subside.

RADIATION THERAPY

Radiotherapy involving X-rays or radioactive isotopes is reserved either for the treatment of malignancies in which the tumor has spread to areas that cannot be safely removed or for cases where experience has shown that the tumor responds better to radiation or to a combination of radiation and surgery than to surgery alone. Cells that are dividing rapidly are destroyed by irradiation more easily than are normal resting cells, so that growing tumors can usually be treated with minimal damage to the surrounding tissue. Complications involving skin, bowel, bladder, and rectum do occur but have decreased with more powerful sources of radiation that can be more precisely directed to the involved area.

Cancer of the cervix, the endometrium, and the ovary all respond well to radiation, often with a high "cure" rate or five-year survival rate.

CHEMOTHERAPY

The term applied to the use of a variety of drugs for cancer treatment is "chemotherapy." Most of these drugs depend for their effectiveness on the susceptibility of rapidly growing tumor cells to toxic substances. The choice and use of these agents is a very complex, specialized field. Cancer of the ovary and widespread cancer of the endometrium can occasionally be cured by chemotherapy. Trophoblastic disease, or malignant moles, respond exceptionally well to chemotherapy, often replacing hysterectomy. Many more tumors respond well to chemotherapy for months or years before recurring.

PHYSICAL THERAPY, DIETARY ADVICE, HOME CARE

Exercises that can be done in bed even before walking about can be recommended by the staff physical therapist who may make home visits during your convalescence. Be sure to find out from the hospital's social services department whether you can expect regular checkups from a visiting nurse, and ask for a consultation with the staff nutritionist before you go home.

COUNSELING

Many problems presented to the gynecologist involve sexual functioning, interpersonal relationships, and questions concerning contraception and abortion. While a detailed discussion of the issues involved can take place during a regular visit, sometimes a more leisurely appointment needs to be scheduled. The physician may also feel that referral to another source of information or treatment would be in the patient's best interest. Such a referral, whether it be to a psychotherapist, an endocrinologist, a sex therapy clinic, or to one of the many support groups for cancer patients, should be seen not as a rejection but rather as evidence that the referring doctor is trying to find the person who can be most helpful in dealing with your personal area of concern.

A reliable source of information about new procedures and expert practitioners in your community is the American Cancer Institute's hotline: 1-800-4-CANCER. (See also "Directory of Health Information.")

*S*EXUALLY TRANSMISSIBLE DISEASES

Louise Tyrer, M.D.

Medical Director for the Association of Reproductive Health Professionals, Washington, D.C.; Past Vice-President for Medical Affairs, Planned Parenthood Federation of America, Inc.

The specter of venereal disease, long kept in the closet, has emerged in epidemic proportions. In 1994 the Centers for Disease Control (CDC) of the U.S. Department of Health and Human Services reported that more than 12 million Americans are infected with a sexually transmitted disease each year and as many as 55 million Americans already have sexually transmissible diseases. Realistic estimates are very much higher because several sexually transmitted infections do not always cause noticeable symptoms. For example, more than half of chlamydial infections in women show no symptoms. And a person can give no indication for years of having been infected with the virus (HIV) that eventually results in full-blown AIDS. The CDC figures are also inaccurately low because, as we learn more about diseases that can be transmitted from one sex partner to another, it has become apparent that the term *VD* (for venereal disease) is outmoded. VD used to be the "Big Five" diseases reported to most state health departments in the United States—gonorrhea, syphilis, chancroid, lymphogranuloma venereum, and granuloma inguinale. However, chlamydia, which affects 3 to 10 million Americans and is the fastest-spreading sexually transmissible disease nationwide, is far more widespread than gonorrhea. As many as 50 million Americans are believed to be infected with genital herpes, with an estimated 500,000 new cases annually. Each year there are 1 million new cases of genital warts, some of which are likely to be the forerunners of certain types of cancer. And the latest arrival in this somber litany, as we all know, is acquired immune deficiency syndrome, referred to as AIDS.

There are not only many diseases that are sexually transmitted; there are also diseases that may be contracted as a result of low systemic resistance, altered body metabolism, or other causes and then transmitted to a sexual partner. Therefore, the term *sexually transmissible diseases* (STDs) has been adopted to cover this broad spectrum of conditions.

As long as people communicate through touching—and let's hope that this is forever—STD will be a potential problem. So, rather than deny ourselves sexual expression, we should learn about STDs, how to prevent them, and how to recognize their symptoms so that early treatment can be obtained. While we have antibiotics and other drugs that can cure or arrest many STDs, those that are caused by viruses, especially AIDS, continue to present a challenge to the scientific community and a major threat to the world at large.

There are at least 20 diseases that may be transmitted by sexual contact. Many people ask why, with more knowledge about STDs and readily available treatment, haven't STDs been eliminated or at least contained? As with other complex problems, there is no single simple answer. The following are some of the factors responsible:

Increased sexual expression among the young. While teenagers experience higher rates of STDs than any other age group because of their risk-taking attitudes, they are the age group least likely to seek medical care. Since infection in this age group is often untreated and therefore unreported, estimates are unreliable. Some specialists believe they represent one-third of the cases of STDs nationwide.

Contraceptive practices. Today the most effective methods of contraception are the pill, the IUD, and sterilization. However, none of these offer any protection against STD.

Social disgrace. Many people, including health professionals, still attach strong negative judgments to anyone with an STD. This person then reacts with shame and fear and delays diagnosis and treatment. Also, he or she may be unwilling to disclose his or her sexual contact(s), making it impossible to break the chain.

Asymptomatic carriers. Seven of the STDs, including chlamydia, syphilis, gonorrhea, and HIV infection, may occur without any symptoms. People may be highly infectious and be completely unaware of their condition.

Resistant strains. Certain bacteria, particularly the one causing gonorrhea, may become resistant to the usual antibiotics. Because most people believe that one magic shot will cure them, they may not return for "tests of cure" and may still harbor the infection.

World travel. The mobility of our population today accounts for an increased rate of spread of STDs. Also, rare diseases, once indigenous to specific areas of the world, are now spreading globally.

Complacency. Public health agencies have not been spending enough time and money on identifying cases and contacts. This is coupled with an attitude held by many people that reporting of cases and tracing contacts are unimportant because treatment, except for AIDS, is so readily available.

Underreporting of cases. By law, syphilis and gonorrhea (in most states) and recently AIDs and herpes type II (in some states) must be reported to health departments. However, only about one in nine cases of these STDs in the United States is reported. This is frequently related to physician negligence, often because the professional is overly concerned about "protecting" the patient.

Education. Although some communities are mandating curriculum changes that provide essential information and realistic discussion in the classroom, and a few educators have fought for and achieved the distribution of condoms on request, there is insufficient education at all levels regarding STDs' frequency, prevention, recognition, diagnosis, and treatment. Also, educators need to dispel the stigma associated with STD so that it is considered with the same nonjudgmental attitude as other diseases requiring urgent treatment, such as tuberculosis.

WHAT WOMEN NEED TO KNOW ABOUT STD

A woman has a built-in awareness of her bodily functions. Education about symptoms of the STDs can increase that level of sensitivity so that she can notice subtle changes that may indicate the onset of an STD. But what can she do to protect herself against infection and what should she know if she suspects she may have been infected?

There is no way to know in advance that a sexual partner is free of STD. Abstinence is the only guarantee against exposure. Of course, if it is apparent that the partner has a genital lesion or a discharge or admits exposure to an STD, avoidance of sex is the only safe course. A woman must not be bashful about querying her partner or even inspecting his genitals for lesions or urethral discharge, nor should she be offended if he wishes to do the same.

For the woman who is sexually active, the greatest protection against contracting an STD is to develop a monogamous relationship with a partner who is also monogamous. The general rule is, the more partners, the greater the risk of exposure and of contracting disease.

If either partner is not monogamous, insisting that the male use a latex condom affords a woman the best possible protection against her getting or giving STD. She would do well to carry condoms with her in case her partner does not have one available, and should hold firm to the premise "no condom, no sex." Since there is a 7 percent failure rate of condoms because of slippage, tears, or improper use, a woman can supplement this protection if she uses a vaginal barrier (for example, the female condom, the diaphragm with jelly or cream, vaginal foam, or suppositories). The woman who takes the pill or has an IUD can, by the use of a barrier method, not only slightly increase the protection her contraception affords but at the same time have some protection against STD.

If you are concerned that your partner may have a sexually transmissible disease, there are some things you should do to help prevent becoming infected. It is important that your genital area be cleaned prior to and after sex. Also, urinating prior to beginning sex or, better, soon after coitus helps to "flush out" organisms from your urethra that can cause urethritis or cystitis. This approach, however, will not reduce the occurrence of infection in the vagina or the cervix. Immediately wash the vulva with soap and water. Avoid strong medicated or highly perfumed soaps and deodorant sprays because they may be irritating. Insert an applicator or two of contraceptive foam, cream, or jelly high into the vagina and rub it on the external genitals as well. Although the protective effect of after-the-fact use of a vaginal contraceptive has not been documented, its prior use is known to be somewhat effective, so it couldn't hurt.

Douching is not effective and may even encourage bacteria to enter the cervical canal. Also, if you have a chemical vaginal contraceptive in place, douching will remove this effective barrier.

If there is a good possibility you have been exposed—say, your partner tells you of his prior exposure to someone with STD or you were raped—call a clinician (physician, hospital clinic, public health facility) and make an appointment to be seen right away. There are antibiotics that may be given that can provide effective prophylaxis against gonorrhea, syphilis, and chlamydia when taken shortly after such sexual contact. (Antibiotics should be taken only after a known or possible exposure. They should never be taken before expected contact.) The clinician can recommend a plan of follow-up examinations to assure you of proper diagnosis and, if indicated, treatment.

Anxiety about having STD is common. Many people think they have STD when they do not. The only way to be sure is to have an examination and diagnostic tests. If the proper testing procedure is followed and the tests are negative, you can put the matter from your mind while vowing to be more careful in the future. Some women, however, become so obsessed that they imagine all sorts of symptoms, such as itching and abnormal discharge. This is an unhealthy attitude, and if examination, testing, and reassurance do not solve the problem, psychological help may be necessary.

Certain important considerations are applicable to all STDs. The specific diseases are discussed in the next section.

1. A woman should ask her clinician to examine and test her for STDs at the time of her annual health checkup through whatever means are indicated (for example, blood tests, Pap smear, cultures, or examination of a "wet mount" of her discharge under the microscope).

2. A woman may have more than one STD. Therefore, it is important that tests to determine whether several diseases are present should also be considered and done if indicated.

3. In most instances, the sexual partner(s) requires examination and treatment in conjunction with the woman to ensure a cure. The antibiotic used is usually the same for both (presuming no allergy): however, dosages may vary based upon such variables as body weight, site of infection, or stage of disease. With some infections, such as hemophilus vaginalis, use of a condom for about six weeks from the time the woman initiates treatment may be sufficient.

4. If a woman has recurring bouts of vaginal infection, with irritation of the surrounding skin, the local reaction can be reduced and sometimes virtually eliminated by not wearing restrictive and nonabsorptive clothing, such as tight pants or nylon panty hose. Dryness is a very important part of the healing process. During this phase it is best to wear skirts and cotton underpants, which should be changed daily, washed with a mild soap (avoid detergents), and thoroughly rinsed. Deodorant sprays should never be used on the sensitive vulvar skin. They can only cause problems.

5. If a woman masters the technique of internal vaginal and cervical examination, using a speculum, a good light source, and a mirror, and practices it routinely at least once a month (usually best done shortly after the menstrual period when the hormonal influences are at a low level), she may observe changes suggestive of the onset of STD. This will enable her to seek earlier diagnosis and treatment. For example, she may notice a change in the character of the vaginal discharge or an inflammation of the cervix.

6. Certain STDs or their treatment create a special risk for a fetus or a

newborn. Therefore, a pregnant woman should familiarize herself with those STDs that may place her and her offspring at risk; she should talk with her obstetrician about the need for special tests and discuss appropriate options if certain tests are positive. The type of therapy and the dosage of many medications must be made consistent with protection of the fetus. For example, pregnant women should not take tetracyclines, which can affect dental development in the fetus.

7. A woman must inform the clinician, prior to therapy, whether she has any drug allergies, particularly to penicillin or sulfa.

8. Follow-up examinations and tests to assure cure are mandatory after treatment of any STD. The return visit needs to be scheduled at the time of the initial visit.

DESCRIPTION OF SPECIFIC TYPES OF STD

Each STD is discussed below alphabetically (not by frequency of occurrence) with symptoms, diagnosis, and treatment explained.

AIDS (ACQUIRED IMMUNE DEFICIENCY SYNDROME)

See "Human Immunodeficiency Virus Infection (HIV/AIDS)."

BACTERIAL VAGINOSIS

Heavy and unusual vaginal discharge, with or without irritation, is the most common symptom of bacterial vaginosis (BV). Often the discharge has an unpleasant fishy odor, is grayish, and may be frothy. On a wet mount of vaginal secretions examined under the microscope, the causative organism will be seen, identified as "clue cells." It may also be identified in a Pap smear or a stained smear examined under the microscope. Unless combined with such other organisms as streptococcus or *E. coli*, BV does not produce disease. Oral antibiotics such as metronidazole should be curative.

CHANCROID

The first symptom is a group of soft painful ulcers containing pus that bleed easily when touched; they are most commonly found on the external genitalia. The lymph nodes in the groin are likely to become enlarged and sensitive. Chancroid is fairly common in the tropics and becoming more common in the United States. It is transmitted sexually or by skin-to-skin contact and can be transmitted from someone who has no symptoms. Its chief danger is that it may make HIV transmission easier. A diagnosis of chancroid usually is made after ruling out syphilis and genital herpes through laboratory tests. Recommended treatments include a single intramuscular injection of azithromycin or erythromycin taken orally four times a day for a week.

CHLAMYDIAL INFECTIONS

Chlamydia are organisms that cause a variety of infections, some of which are sexually transmitted. The infections are difficult to diagnose. Chlamydia are neither viruses nor bacteria but are called elementary bodies. These bodies are incorporated in cells where they dwell and can be identified by microscopic examination of stained smears of the infected tissue.

Chlamydial infections are the most prevalent form of STD, far more widespread than genital herpes and gonorrhea. They can attack any part of the urogenital tract as well as the anus of both sexes. Infection is spread during vaginal, anal, or oral sexual contact. Babies can get chlamydia during birth if the mother is infected. In newborns, chlamydia can lead to pneumonia and conjunctivitis. Chlamydia can cause sterility when it affects the fallopian tubes, and in young women it is the major cause of pelvic inflammatory disease, which, if untreated, can lead to infertility. In males it is a leading cause of nongonococcal urethritis (NGU), which can result in male sterility. A woman who has had sexual intercourse with a man who has NGU often is treated as if she had chlamydial vaginitis.

Seventy-five percent of females and 25 percent of males show no serious symptoms until infection is quite advanced. Burning and frequency of urination occur most commonly in the male but can occur in females as well.

Chlamydial infections may be diagnosed by a recent test that takes only 30 minutes and is as good as or even better than the previous one, which took four to six days. It is called MicroTrack and consists of taking a cell sample from the sexual organs and adding monoclonal antibodies to the sample. If chlamydial microorganisms are present, they combine with the antibodies, producing a radioactive signal that is visible in an ultraviolet microscope. However, there is still a considerable degree of inaccuracy with this test. Treatment is a long-term antibiotic regimen. If one's sexual partner is infected, treatment should be simultaneous and all sexual contact should be discontinued until cure is accomplished.

Because chlamydial infection is so widespread and often without symptoms, many gynecologists include a test for chlamydia as part of a regular checkup.

CYSTITIS

See discussion under "Infections" in the chapter on "Gynecologic Problems and Treatment."

GONORRHEA

Gonorrhea is the oldest known STD. Commonly referred to as "the clap," "the drip," or "the dose," cases reported to the Centers for Disease Control have been dropping steadily since 1990 except among the 15 to 19 age group, which has twice the number of infections as the 20 to 24 age group. By the end of 1993, the total number of *reported* cases was 336,169, down from the 433,949 cases reported the previous year. Because a large number of cases are unreported, experts put the figure at two million cases a year.

This common STD is caused by gonococcal bacteria *(Neisseria gonorrhoeae)*. A symptom of uncomplicated gonorrhea is a green or yellow-green vaginal discharge, often with a distinctive mushroom-like odor not previously present. The infection may also occur primarily in the throat, producing pharyngitis, or in the rectum, causing proctitis. It has an average incubation period of three to five days. There is an 80 percent chance that a woman infected with gonorrhea will have no symptoms because the infection is located in the cervix, high up in the woman's vagina. In males the infection is in the urethra and causes a pus-like discharge. However, 10 to 20 percent of infected men have no discharge and no other symptoms. The fact that there are many asymptomatic carriers explains why this disease is almost impossible to eradicate. Complications of gonorrhea result from spread of the infection to other organs, causing infection, inflammation, and any combination of the following conditions:

1. Lower abdominal pains.
2. Continuous low back pains.
3. Burning and frequency of urination, sometimes associated with a drop of pus or blood.
4. Swelling and tenderness (abscess) of the Bartholin's gland located near the opening of the vagina.
5. Pleurisy-type pains in the right upper abdomen (perihepatitis) or in the shoulder area.
6. Severe pain in the pelvic area as gonorrhea moves up into the fallopian tubes (pelvic inflammatory disease).
7. Severe generalized abdominal pain as the infection spreads from the tubes to the abdominal cavity (pelvic peritonitis).
8. Pelvic pain as abscesses develop in the pelvis.
9. Sterility, resulting from blocked tubes or surgery necessary to remove abscesses.
10. Other serious complications, such as gonorrheal arthritis and gonorrheal pericarditis.

The eyes of the newborn are particularly susceptible to gonorrheal infection. If prophylactic measures, such as instillation of silver nitrate solution or penicillin injection, are not taken at birth and the infection develops, blindness may result.

In women gonorrhea is diagnosed by a culture taken from the cervix. Other sites of possible infection such as the throat, urethra, or rectum need to be cultured as well if history and examination should indicate possible exposure at these sites. A positive culture provides a firm diagnosis of gonorrhea. However, a negative culture does not necessarily rule out the possibility, particularly if the infection has spread into the tubes or is at a site other than the one that was cultured.

Older strains of gonorrhea can be treated with penicillin or tetracycline. The Centers for Disease Control encourage combining tetracycline therapy with penicillin to treat chlamydia, a commonly associated infection, along with gonorrhea. All individuals undergoing treatment for gonorrhea must return at the appointed time for repeat cultures as a test of cure.

The presence of a strain of gonorrhea that is resistant to penicillin and tetracycline can be revealed by antibiotic sensitivity tests done on the cultured gonococci bacteria. In such cases, two new types of drugs, the cephalosporins and the quinolones, are highly effective. For women allergic to these drugs, a single intramuscular injection of spectinomycin is recommended. This drug although expensive, also cures gonorrhea infections of the throat.

The incidence of infertility (sterility) is higher following each tubal infection. If abscesses form in the tubes and ovaries, surgery may be required, frequently leaving a woman sterile. Early diagnosis and treatment can practically eliminate the need for surgical management.

HEPATITIS B

One of the most contagious and most insidious of all the STDs, the hepatitis B virus can cause a debilitating liver disease that has no known cure or effective treatment. It is spread like the virus that causes AIDS—through blood contact with body fluids that contain it—but is considered to be about 100 times as contagious because it more likely to be spread by contaminated acupuncture needles, dental equipment, and manicuring tools, as well as by saliva exchanged in kissing. It is difficult to estimate the number of people who carry the infection because half of them may develop no symptoms. Of these, many remain contagious for a lifetime, spreading liver disease that makes those contracting it 200 times more likely to develop liver cancer than their noninfected counterparts. While there has been a decline in cases among homosexual men because of a change in their sexual habits, there has been a considerable increase among sexually active heterosexuals with many partners. It is estimated that 200,000 Americans are infected every year and that more than 10 million heterosexuals fall into the high-risk category, according to Dr. Hie-Won L. Hann, director of the Liver Disease Prevention Center at Thomas Jefferson University Hospital.

When an effective vaccine against the hepatitis B virus was licensed in 1980, the Centers for Disease Control guidelines recommended that it be used only by people facing a particularly high risk of infection: health care and emergency workers likely to come in contact with other people's body fluids; people on kidney dialysis because they are frequently exposed to intravenous procedures; intravenous drug users; staff members of institutions whose inmates might bite their caregivers; and anyone with multiple sex partners or whose partners have multiple partners. In 1991, alarmed by the spread of the infection, the CDC recommended that all babies be vaccinated against hepatitis B in the same way they are routinely vaccinated against diphtheria, whooping cough, tetanus, polio, measles, mumps, and rubella. High-risk adolescents have also been added to the list as well as people who live with the 1.2 million Americans chronically infected with the disease.

For women who think they are at risk for hepatitis B infection, three doses of the vaccine provide better than 95 percent protection. The same level of protection is also achieved if the vaccine is given promptly after known exposure to the virus.

HERPES SIMPLEX VIRUS INFECTION (GENITAL HERPES)

Herpes simplex is a virus. Its two variants are herpes labialis, also known as herpes simplex virus type I (HSV-1), and herpes genitalis, or herpes simplex virus type II (HSV-2). Herpes labialis (type I) infection affects primarily the area of the head and neck, where it causes what are commonly called cold sores or fever blisters. However, type I causes about 25 percent of herpes genital infections. Herpes genitalis (type II) is a distinctly different virus that affects primarily the genital area, often causing intensely painful lesions. However, of the 50 million Americans believed to be infected with genital herpes, only one quarter experience any symptoms even though they are capable of transmitting the infection to their sexual partners.

A woman infected in the genital area for the first time with herpes is usually asymptomatic (75 to 90 percent). The symptomatic woman generally will notice one or more small, painful, fluid-filled blisters on the external genitalia within 3 to 20 days after exposure. They may occur also or only in the vagina or on the cervix and may not be noticed, but they can be seen on examination or occasionally be identified by a Pap smear. These soon rupture and, when located externally, form soft, extremely painful, open sores. Secondary infection with bacteria can further aggravate the situation. The lymph glands in the groin may become enlarged and tender.

The herpes viruses have a tendency to remain in the body without evidence of their presence and may reactivate (particularly type II), especially when stimulated by stress or illness. The initial infection usually heals in about 10 to 12 days. Recurrences heal faster and are less painful. The frequency and severity of recurrences vary from individual to individual.

An acute herpes infection of the genital area (both types) during pregnancy may have adverse effects such as abortion, stillbirth, or infection of the newborn as it passes through the birth canal. It is estimated that neonatal herpes kills one-third of the newborns to whom it is transmitted and another one-third suffer from mental retardation. Therefore, when active infection is present at term, delivery by cesarean section may reduce the chance of infecting the baby. The additional concern that remains to be proven is the possible relationship between herpes type II infection and development, years later, of cancer of the cervix.

Herpes simplex infection is usually diagnosed clinically by inspection of the lesions or by a Pap smear, where a typical giant cell is identified. In addition, viral cultures may be taken from the sores for positive identification or a fluorescein-conjugated monoclomal antibody test can be done to differentiate the type.

There is no specific treatment that cures herpes, and no vaccine against it is currently available. However, Zovirax (acyclovir), when taken orally for about five days at the time of an initial infection, is effective in reducing the symptoms of herpes and in shortening its duration. It also is effective, when taken for longer periods—perhaps four months or more—in reducing or preventing recurrences. Further, any recurrence usually is reduced in severity. While side effects from the acyclovir are infrequent, they may include nausea, vomiting, diarrhea, dizziness, and headache. A pregnant or breast-feeding woman should not take this medication unless her physician specifically approves of her doing so.

Additional therapy is directed toward further relief of discomfort and prevention of secondary bacterial infection of open genital lesions, usually with compresses and sitz baths; sometimes prescription pain medication is required. Acyclovir cream applied to the lesions of an initial herpes infection also may diminish its duration and discomfort. Avoidance of sexual intercourse when initial and recurrent lesions are present is best.

Although it is not known whether the use of a condom will with certainty prevent transmission of the virus from an infected male, its use is recommended. However, the virus may be transmitted from genital areas not covered by the condom.

HUMAN IMMUNODEFICIENCY VIRUS INFECTION (HIV/AIDS)

Not until 1992 did it become apparent that the symptoms of HIV infection in women often differed from those in men and that the symptoms specific to women had not been recognized by the medical profession or by the government agencies responsible for tracking AIDS cases. Since that time, the Centers for Disease Control have recognized that certain persistent gynecological dysfunctions and diseases, such as pelvic inflammatory disease, cervical dysplasia, chronic vaginal candidiasis, continuing problems with menstruation, and recurrent STDs unresponsive to treatment, are often HIV-related conditions. This recognition is no small matter, since it extends eligibility for funded treatment and hospitalization to women who were previously excluded from these programs because their illness did not meet the definition of HIV/AIDS, which was specifically based on a male model.

In 1993 the federal government initiated the Women's Interagency HIV study, officially acknowledging for the first time—and after considerable pressure—that HIV/AIDS was by no means the same for both sexes. The purpose of this four-year project is to find out more precisely how HIV/AIDS can affect women, the female reproductive system, and the transmission from mother to fetus.

In 1994 women constituted about 18 percent of AIDS cases in the United States, and their number is increasing every year. Nationwide, HIV infection is the fourth leading cause of death among women aged 25 to 44, and according to the Centers for Disease Control, heterosexual contact with an HIV-infected man has become the most rapidly growing transmission category among women. This category has now surpassed the numbers for transmission between homosexual men.

Through December 1994, the Centers for Disease Control received reports of 58,428 cases of AIDS among adult and adolescent women in the United States. Cases had increased steadily, from 7 percent in 1985 to 18 percent in 1994. The 14,081 women reported with AIDS in 1994 alone represented nearly *one-fourth of the total number of AIDS cases ever reported among women.*

There is still a considerable amount of confusion about the varying conditions between a man or a woman infected with HIV, the virus that eventually results in AIDS, and the health problems of a person described as having AIDS. A person who is HIV-infected may be unaware of the infection unless test results are HIV-positive. It is estimated that in the United States, 75 percent of those who are HIV-infected may have no symptoms at all or only minor ones for as long as 10 years. But once the person carries HIV, whether aware or not, infection of others becomes a lethal potential.

The transition from HIV infection to full-blown AIDS takes place in the following way.

The human immunodeficiency virus (HIV) is the infectious agent that causes AIDS by progressively destroying the immune system, making it incapable of fighting off "opportunistic infections" as they occur. Since it was first recognized in 1981, AIDS (acquired immune deficiency syndrome) has therefore been defined not as a single disease, but as *a progressive vulnerability to many diseases.*

HIV is transmitted (acquired) from one human being to another through direct contact with bodily fluids: semen, vaginal secretions, blood, and breast milk. It enters the body through the vagina, penis, rectum, or mouth, or through a needle puncture of the skin. There is no evidence that the virus is found or transmitted in saliva. HIV infection is not transmitted by coughing, sneezing, embracing; nor by using public swimming pools or water fountains; nor by sharing office equipment, telephones, or eating utensils, or standing very close to people in a crowded train or bus. Modes of transmission are male homosexual or heterosexual intercourse, hypodermic needles shared by infected drug users, mother to unborn child either in the womb or during birth, and blood transfusions, including the transfer of blood from an infected patient to a health professional by accident.

As soon as the virus enters the body, attacker cells known as T-cell lymphocytes, antibody-carrying white blood cells, are produced by the healthy immune system. The invading HIV (technically known as a retrovirus) enters the T cells, multiplies within them, and destroys them. Over the years the destruction of a significant quantity of the T cells causes the qualitative change in the immune system that results in the autoimmune deficiency syndrome, or AIDS.

Recent studies indicate that women are more than twice as likely as men to become HIV-infected during heterosexual intercourse. The presumed biological reasons for this disparity are that the genital surface of women potentially exposed to the virus is much larger than that of men; vaginal secretions from an HIV-infected woman are much weaker than semen from a similarly infected male; and the man's exposure to the virus is limited to the duration of sexual intercourse, whereas the infected semen remains in the woman's body for an indefinite length of time. Another, underlying reason for the disparity is the fact that there are far more men than women in the United States who are HIV-infected, so it is more likely that a woman will have an infected sex partner in heterosexual intercourse than the other way around.

Women who are HIV-infected die more quickly than their male counterparts, according to a study published in the *Journal of the American Medical Association* (10/28/94). The explanation may be that women wait until they are much sicker before they seek treatment, and that doctors need to be more aware of symptoms of infection in women.

To protect herself against HIV when even the slightest likelihood of infection is present, a woman often must overcome cultural and social barriers in order to insist that her partner wear a condom. On this issue, she *must* put herself in the position of power and decision-making. Some women with multiple sex partners choose to use a female condom; others are joining chastity clubs as the surest guarantee against all STDs.

The presence of HIV infection cannot be detected by a direct test. Current tests can indicate only the presence of the antibodies that have formed to fight the virus. It takes about six weeks after infection for the antibodies to be detected. In a few cases, it can take as long as a year following infection for the antibodies to develop. A negative HIV test result does not therefore always mean the absence of infection.

The usual test for HIV infection is performed on blood samples. Technically described as enzyme-linked immunosorbent assay, it is referred to as an ELISA test. This test is not definitive because a positive result may occur in the presence of antibodies responding to some other disease. Only the Western blot test, which is HIV-specific, can provide an unambiguous diagnosis of HIV infection. This test is performed whenever the ELISA is positive.

A woman who tests HIV-positive may show no immediate signs of infection. When early symptoms occur—typically general malaise, swollen lymph nodes, slight fever, diarrhea, night sweats—they may be of short duration and are rarely severe enough to interfere with normal activities. Another early symptom in women is thrush, a fungus-like infection caused by the candida organism, which can occur in the mouth, throat, and/or vagina (candidiasis). Gynecological examination is likely to produce an abnormal Pap smear. Abnormal cells begin to show up in the cervix and vagina. Even though the T-cell count is approximately normal—around 1,000 per cubic millimeter of blood, *it is at this point that HIV infection should be suspected, tested for, and when positive, the latest approved drug treatment for strengthening and protecting the immune system begun, before the onset of more obvious or severe symptoms.* If a woman's primary health care provider does not seem to be well informed about the potential significance of these symptoms, a referral to a more suitable doctor should be sought through community-based support groups. A pregnant woman who suspects she is HIV-infected needs to be tested without delay so that if results are positive, prophylactic treatment for the fetus can begin during pregnancy.

When the immune system becomes more vulnerable, the most common AIDS-defining symptom in both sexes is pneumocystis carinii pneumonia (PCP). Only men experience Kaposi's sarcoma (a skin cancer); women may develop unresponsive pelvic inflammatory disease (PID), cervical cancer, chronic vaginal candidiasis, and latent secondary syphilis; opportunistic infections common to both men and women are tuberculosis and neurological disorders, as well as rapid loss of weight, which cannot be regained. The T-cell count continues to move downward with the development of full-blown AIDS.

At present there is no cure or vaccine for HIV/AIDS. Several drugs are available for slowing the progress of HIV infection: some interfere with the virus's attempts to multiply inside the immune cells; others try to increase the number of fighter cells; all must be closely monitored because of toxic side effects that may develop. Three drugs are currently used to fight PCP. They can be taken by mouth, by injection, or by aerosol spray. Antifungal drugs can control the spread of vaginal candidiasis or thrush. Several experimental vaccines are available that may slow the progress of HIV/AIDS, but none of them can prevent it. A well-informed, experienced doctor can protect patients from exploitation by "healers" hawking "miracle cures" and can also suggest various nonmedical therapies to help counteract the negative effects of stress on the immune system. These include exercise, relaxation techniques, meditation, massage, and yoga. A program of properly balanced meals reinforced by vitamin and mineral supplements can be initiated in consultation with a qualified nutritionist. One of the most effective ways of coping with inevitable depression is participation in a support group.

Through their AIDS hotlines, the Centers for Disease Control provide information about the latest approved medications for treating HIV/AIDS, including how to participate in medical trials for women. Literature on all aspects of the disease and referrals to community support groups are available by calling 1-800-342-AIDS (2347); in Spanish, 1-800-334-SIDA (7432); or by contacting the CDC National AIDS Clearinghouse, PO Box 6003, Rockville, MD 20849-6003 (1-800-458-5231).

HUMAN PAPILLOMA VIRUS INFECTION (GENITAL WARTS)

The group of more than 60 viruses that come under the heading of human papilloma virus (HPV) can cause warts anywhere on the body, but only genital or venereal warts are sexually transmissible. There are various treatments for all warts, but there is no permanent cure for any of them. Genital warts, technically known as *condyloma acuminata,* are usually classified as those that can be seen on the surface of the skin (about 30 percent) and those in which the virus lives in the deeper layers of dermal tissue and produces no visible manifestations. HPV may be detected by a Pap smear. A few types have been linked to cervical cancer and may be among the so-called subclinical infections. Although the exact number of individuals living with HPV infection is not available because it is not a reportable STD, experts put the figure at 50 million, with 1 million new cases every year. Women at higher risk than average are those in their early twenties with multiple sexual partners (or with one sexual partner who has other sexual encounters); women who already have some other STD, such as genital herpes or chlamydia; and women who smoke.

The virus is presumed to enter the body through tiny breaks in the mucous membrane during vaginal, anal, or oral intercourse. It proceeds to deeper layers of dermal tissue, where it may remain invisible and undetected for months or even years. If and when warts appear in women, they are likely to be found on the vulva, on the cervix, in or around the vagina or anus, or in the mouth. The warts may be large or small, raised or flat, single or clumped like a cauliflower. They may be gray or pale pink, and they almost never itch, bleed, or cause pain. When the warts are visible, diagnosis is simple, and a variety of treatments are available. As for the HPV infections that are invisible, diagnosis is difficult since they are not identifiable through a blood test, nor can they be grown in a laboratory. They may become visible when the doctor looks at the suspected mucous membrane areas of the cervix or vagina through a magnifying device called a colposcope. Another helpful procedure consists of swabbing the surface of the cervix and vagina with acetic acid. The swabbed area turns white if HPV infection or other inflamed areas are present below the surface.

While there is no cure for HPV infection, there are many different kinds of treatment: application of medication to the lesions, freezing with liquid nitrogen, burning with an electric current, injecting with the antiviral drug interferon, destruction with a laser, swabbing at home with inexpensive prescription drugs. Over-the-counter remedies are not recommended. Some effective treatments are much more expensive than others; some produce considerable discomfort; others are painless. No matter which treatment is used, one person in four is said to experience a return of the infection within three months. It should also be noted that up to 30 percent of noncervical warts are likely to vanish within about three months of their appearance without any treatment at all. Women undergoing treatment should abstain from sex during healing and should find out whether their sexual partner needs to be undergoing treatment at the same time.

HPV infection is so widespread because it is difficult to prevent. Spermicides may not be effective; neither the scrotum nor the vulva is protected by the male condom. Use of the female condom does reduce risk of infection, and since the delicate surface of the vagina is much more likely to crack when not well lubricated, thereby enabling HPV entry, intercourse should always be preceded by lubrication, either naturally from arousal or by use of a vaginal preparation.

PELVIC INFLAMMATORY DISEASE (PID)

Pelvic inflammatory disease is an infection of the tubes and ovaries and has multiple causes, some of which are STDs. The commonest pathogens that cause PID are chlamydia, *N. gonorrhea*, tuberculosis, streptococcus, and *E. coli*. Among IUD users the most common cause of PID is STD, whether or not the woman is aware of such an infection. If the infection does not respond promptly to treatment, it is best to remove the IUD.

Infectious organisms travel up through the cervix and uterus and cause inflammation and even abscesses of the fallopian tubes, the ovaries, and the pelvis. Typically, a woman who has PID is acutely ill with fever and lower abdominal pain. About 13 percent of women are infertile after their first attack of PID. After three attacks, the proportion is as high as 75 percent. Ensuring that one's sexual partner is not an asymptomatic carrier of an STD can reduce one's risk of reinfection.

The diagnosis of PID is made by history, abdominal and pelvic examination, and laboratory testing. At times the interior of the abdomen is viewed with the laparoscope to differentiate between PID and appendicitis, ectopic pregnancy, or other intra-abdominal emergencies, these conditions being surgical emergencies while PID usually is not.

The treatment is a combination of antibiotics, orally or intravenously. If abscesses have formed that cannot be eliminated with antibiotics, surgery may be required. If so, sterility is a likely consequence, as often the uterus, both tubes, and the ovaries must be removed to effect a cure. However, laser surgery may preserve fertility in some instances. (See the chapter on "Contraception and Abortion.")

PUBIC LICE ("CRABS")

An infestation with pubic lice (crab lice) is almost always sexually transmitted. However, lice or their eggs may be transmitted through infected clothing, bedding, and towels. The adult organisms infest immediately, while their eggs hatch after 3 to 14 days. The most common symptom is intense itching in the pubic hair as a reaction to the bites of the lice.

The pubic louse is yellowish-gray in color, but after it is swollen with blood it becomes dark. It can be found attached to pubic hairs. The eggs are white and give the appearance of a "growth" near the base of the hair shaft.

An infestation of pubic lice can be cured readily with the application of gamma benezene hexachloride, commonly known as Kwell, and other similar preparations, all of which require a prescription. These preparations are available as a cream, lotion, or shampoo. In order to prevent recurrence, the sexual partner(s) must also take treatment, and clothes and bed linen must be washed or dry-cleaned.

Pregnant or breast-feeding women should not use products containing lindane or pyrethrin with piperonylbutoxide.

SCABIES

Scabies is considered an STD because it is usually transmitted by intimate contact; it is also spread through contaminated clothing and bedding. It is caused by a mite $1/60$ inch long called *Sarcoptes scabies*. Because scabies is not a reportable disease in the United States, the exact number of cases is not known. The characteristic lesion is the burrow of the mite under the skin. It appears initially as a small, wavy line, usually located between the fingers, on the wrists, armpits, breasts, buttocks, thighs, and rarely on the genitalia. The face is not usually involved. Itching is present wherever the burrowing parasite is found and is worse at night. Scratching can cause secondary infection of the lesions.

Scabies can be diagnosed by clinical history and the presence of characteristic lesions. Additionally, the burrow can be scraped to obtain the mite, eggs, and larvae, which can be identified under the microscope. Undiagnosed scabies, which may be chronic, is often referred to as "the seven-year itch."

The usual treatment for scabies is lindane, which was known as gamma benzene hexachloride when used as an agricultural chemical. It is applied as a lotion and shampoo, left in place for 24 hours, then washed off. A newer treatment, considered safer for use with children and the elderly, is called permethrin or Elimite, a synthetic based on chemicals found in chrysanthemums. Continued itching after the treatment is related to secondary infection and should be treated symptomatically. Bedding and all clothing, especially underclothing, must be washed or dry-cleaned.

SYPHILIS

Syphilis and AIDS are the most serious of the STDs because both diseases are life-threatening, not only to the woman herself, but to her future children. Syphilis is caused by a spirochete organism known as *Treponema pallidum.* It dies very quickly outside the human body and is killed by soap and water if present on the skin—a good reason for thorough washing after sex. The organism passes from the chancre or skin of an infected individual who is in the primary or secondary stage to an uninfected person through the latter's mucous membranes or a break in the skin. Because symptoms can simulate many other disease conditions or the disease may be asymptomatic for many years, the discussion of symptoms will be divided into the stages of the disease— primary, secondary, latent, and late—and other special situations. The stages describe the *untreated* course of this disease.

The primary sore of syphilis is the chancre. It appears where the organism entered the body, usually on the genitals, and may appear as early as 10 days or as long as 3 months after infection. The chancre is usually a solitary, painless ulceration that feels firm and has a slightly elevated border. In the woman it is commonly located on the cervix or in the vagina hidden from view. The chancre exudes the spirochete and is highly infectious. Often the associated lymph glands are swollen. Even without treatment the chancre heals within 1 to 5 weeks, concluding the primary stage.

The onset of the secondary stage occurs anywhere from 6 to 24 weeks after the untreated primary phase. It is often heralded by a general feeling of ill health. This may include any combination of the following symptoms: headache, muscle or joint aches, pain in the long bones, loss of appetite, nausea, constipation, and a low-grade, persistent fever. Swelling and tenderness of the lymph glands are often present, and the hair may fall out in patches.

The most classical visible symptom of a secondary infection is a nonirritating, highly infectious rash. It may appear anywhere on the body. If the extremities are involved, it is symmetrically distributed. It may also affect the mucous membranes of the body and in women is commonly found around the labia. On the mucous membranes it appears initially as a grayish-white surface that breaks down into sores with a dull red base that ooze a clear fluid loaded with the infectious spirochete. Syphilitic warts may also develop on the genitals. Unless secondary infection occurs, these lesions are not usually painful. Without treatment the secondary phase usually passes in 4 to 12 weeks.

Latent syphilis is asymptomatic, beginning at the conclusion of the secondary phase. It is not infectious to a sexual contact, but the spirochete can spread within a pregnant woman to her fetus. Early latent syphilis has a duration of less than four years, while late latent syphilis extends from four years to the development, if it occurs, of late syphilis.

Approximately one-third of individuals develop manifestations of late syphilis. The other two-thirds do not, but we do not yet know what determines into which group they will fall. The most common manifestations of late syphilis are gumma (syphilitic tumors) in any affected organ, cardiovascular syphilis, and neurosyphilis. Late syphilis can cause insanity and death.

The spirochete of the mother's untreated syphilis at whatever stage invades the placenta and eventually the fetus between the tenth and eighteenth week of pregnancy. If untreated, the risk of stillbirth or of congenital syphilis affecting the newborn is high. It is important for every pregnant woman to be tested for syphilis early in pregnancy so that the disease may be treated before it can damage the fetus.

Most children born to women who have untreated syphilis during their pregnancies will have congenital syphilis. Its effects include blindness, deafness, crippling bone disease, and facial abnormalities. Special blood tests combined with other diagnostic measures are essential when congenital syphilis is suspected.

There are several tests used to diagnose syphilis; their performance and accuracy are related to the phase of the disease. Part of the diagnostic process is a complete physical examination, not limited to the genitals. Diagnostic laboratory tests include the following:

1. Darkfield Microscopic Examination. Fluid obtained from a chancre or other open sores is examined under a microscope to identify the spirochete.

2. Serologic Tests for Syphilis (STS). A number of different tests are done on blood serum to see whether an individual has a pathologic level of antibodies to the spirochete *T. pallidum*. It takes about three weeks following the appearance of the chancre for STS to become positive. Certain tests measure antibodies that show a declining titre concentration in blood serum with treatment and are indicators of successful therapy. Other tests measure antibodies that, when they remain permanently elevated, indicate whether a person has ever had the disease.

3. Spinal Fluid Examination. With latent or late syphilis it is necessary to have a serologic test done on the cerebrospinal fluid to determine whether the infection has invaded the central nervous system because neurosyphilis requires special treatment.

The treatment of choice is long-acting penicillin, which is 98 percent effective at all stages of the disease. The dosage and duration of treatment vary with the stage and manifestations of the disease. In the event of penicillin allergy, alternative therapy is tetracycline or doxycycline. To ensure arrest of the infection or cure, follow-up blood tests need to be done after three months and after six months. Relapses of syphilis following treatment are rare and usually are the result of reinfection.

TRICHOMONIASIS

One of the most common vaginal conditions, trichomoniasis is caused by a simple, one-celled, motile organism called *Trichomonas vaginalis*. The condition may be asymptomatic, and a woman may not know that she is infected until the organism is identified as part of the Pap smear procedure. Usually, however, within 4 to 28 days after exposure, infected women will notice a greenish-yellow, often frothy, vaginal discharge associated with itching and an unpleasant musty odor. The discharge frequently causes irritation and redness of the vulva, and a spotting of blood may be mixed with the discharge. Inspection of the vaginal mucous membranes and cervix may reveal small red dots, commonly referred to as "strawberry marks." The lymph glands in the groin may become enlarged. The infection can spread to the urinary tract, where it may be asymptomatic or may cause symptoms of urinary frequency and urgency. Trichomoniasis is frequently associated with other STDs and may mask their symptoms.

Clinical diagnosis can be made by identifying the strawberry marks on the vaginal wall and cervix. Microscopic examination of the vaginal discharge mixed with saline will reveal the presence of the organism.

Metronidazole is a specific cure for *T. vaginalis*. Alcoholic beverages must be avoided during therapy. Metronidazole must not be taken during the first four months of pregnancy. The sexual partner(s) also needs to be treated simultaneously. Although vaginal creams, suppositories, and douches may relieve symptoms, they are seldom curative.

URETHRITIS

See discussion under "Infections" in the chapter on "Gynecologic Problems and Treatment."

VAGINITIS (NONSPECIFIC)

See discussion under "Infections" in the chapter on "Gynecologic Problems and Treatment."

OTHER DISEASES LINKED TO SEXUAL PRACTICES

Because sexual practices other than vaginal intercourse are not uncommon, certain diseases not generally considered as STDs may be acquired through sexual contact. A woman who practices oral or anal sex as well as genital sex should let the clinician know this so that appropriate tests can be taken to evaluate the possibility of disease of the pharynx or gastrointestinal tract. Gastrointestinally transmitted STDs are much more common among homosexual and bisexual males and, through this route, their female partner(s) may contract the diseases discussed below.

AMEBIASIS

This infection is caused by a single-cell amoeba known as *Endamoeba histolytica*. Symptoms consist of diarrhea, often containing blood and mucus, associated with abdominal distress, low-grade fever, and a general feeling of illness. Infection can occur in the liver and other organs. Carriers of the disease, although asymptomatic, may have cysts in their stool or around their rectum that are highly infectious with oral contact. Microscopic examination of the stool reveals the organism or the cysts. Treatment is individually determined by a physician.

GIARDIASIS

An infection of the small intestine, giardiasis is caused by the protozoa *Giardia lamblia* and is spread between sexual partners by the anal-oral route through fecal contamination with the organism. Symptoms include stomach cramps, bloating, and foul-smelling stools. Diagnosis is made through examination of a fresh stool specimen. The drug of choice for treatment is metronidazole, which must be taken by both sexual partners.

CONCLUSION

Confronting this alarming array of diseases that may be sexually transmitted, one might be inclined to exclaim, "No more sex ever again!" However, the sex drive is a powerful part of human nature and so is a short memory for the unpleasant things described in this chapter. But to be forewarned is to be forearmed. Remember to take precautions to protect yourself against STD, have regular checkups annually that include examinations to detect the presence of such diseases, be alert for unusual symptoms that may suggest the onset of a disease, and seek early diagnosis.

ℬREAST CARE

Margaret Nelsen Harker, M.D.

Adult General Medicine, Morehead City, North Carolina;
Electronics Data Systems (1979–1982), Raleigh, North Carolina;
Assistant Professor of Surgery (1975–1979), University of North
Carolina Medical School, Chapel Hill, North Carolina

A woman's breasts are not only a graceful complement to her womanhood; they are also symbols of her individualism and sexuality. It has been some time since the human breast was thought of as a mere milk gland, primarily useful for nourishing the species. The average woman, however, has little understanding of normal breast structure and function. Two facts are generally known: (1) breast cancer is a leading cause of death in women and (2) therapy often involves removal of the breast. Therefore it is not surprising that the perception of any abnormality of the breast leads to anxiety and fear. Some women respond to this anxiety by seeking immediate attention for what often are normal physiologic changes. Other women respond by ignoring a significant abnormality that should be seen promptly for effective treatment.

It is the purpose of this chapter to alleviate unnecessary anxiety and fear and to encourage all women to participate in their own breast care. By becoming aware of the normal structure and function of your breasts, you can deal more confidently with any needed treatment. The attitudes of women patients and the capabilities of physicians are changing. No longer is the woman willing to be the ignorant recipient of treatment, and no longer are physicians limited to a single form of treatment.

GROWTH AND DEVELOPMENT OF THE BREAST

Throughout your life your breasts reflect changes in your endocrine system as well as changes related to age. Your breasts are formed during gestation and by the time of birth consist of a branching system of ducts that empty into the nipples. In the newborn, due to the influence of the hormones of pregnancy, there is often evidence of a clear milky secretion from the nipple. After a few days this secretion ceases. The breasts then remain dormant throughout the remainder of childhood, consisting chiefly of the nipples and rudimentary duct systems. Occasionally, a mass is noted during infancy or childhood that most often disappears. There is no cause for concern, although there is no satisfactory explanation for such masses.

At the time of puberty, as your ovaries begin to manufacture estrogen, several changes begin to take place. The first changes are noticeable between the ages of 9 and 15. At first the areola, the pigmented skin surrounding the nipple, begins to enlarge and darken. Beneath the nipple and the areola the previously quiescent duct system enlarges and grows. Branches also begin to form. Usually by the time of your first menstrual period, the normal, protuberant, and firm adolescent breast is well developed. As the ovaries produce progesterone and the breast continues to develop, ducts begin to bud at the end of their branches, producing groups of glands. The essential components of the adult breast are now present.

Let us take a more detailed look at the normal adult breast. The breast normally extends from the second to the sixth or seventh rib and from the sternum (breast bone) to the side of the chest wall and into the axilla (arm pit). The average breast extends 1 to 2 inches out from the chest wall, is 4 to 5 inches in diameter and weighs about ½ pound. The weight may almost double during lactation. It is very common to have one breast larger than the other, and most often it is the left breast that is larger. There is no explanation for this sometimes striking difference. The overall size of the breast is greatly influenced by the fat content.

Under the upper portion of the breasts are the muscles of the chest wall and some of the shoulder muscles that are attached to the chest wall. These muscles are the pectoral muscles. The breast itself normally glides smoothly over

DEVELOPMENT OF THE BREAST

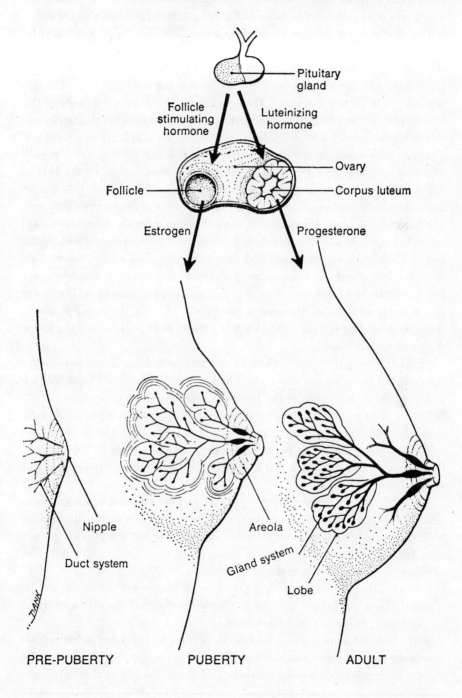

Pituitary gland

Follicle stimulating hormone

Luteinizing hormone

Follicle

Ovary

Corpus luteum

Estrogen

Progesterone

Nipple

Areola

Duct system

Gland system

Lobe

PRE-PUBERTY

PUBERTY

ADULT

all of these muscles and is supported by ligaments called Cooper's ligaments, which rise from the deep portions of the breast to the skin, like guy wires.

The nipple and areola are covered by a modified membrane lubricated by special glands, which appear as little rough areas in the areola. These glands are called the glands of Montgomery and are similar to your other oil-producing glands. Situated in the center of the areola is the conically shaped nipple that has 15 to 25 tiny openings. These openings come from the ducts of the breasts and are very hard to see without magnification. Beneath the areola and nipple are tiny muscles responsible for erection of the nipple when stimulated. They are quite similar to the muscles that cause fine skin hairs to stand on end. The tiny openings on the nipple connect to the duct system of the breast, which radiates away from the nipple like the spokes of a wheel. Just underneath the nipple and areola, these ducts enlarge somewhat to serve as a reservoir for milk. As each duct extends toward the chest wall, it separates into multiple branches. At the end of these branches are the secretory glands of the breast. Each grouping of glands and duct tissue is called a lobe; the smaller branches and glands themselves are called lobules. Between the lobes and lobules are fat and connective tissue, including Cooper's ligaments. The lining of the ducts and glands consists of two layers of cells. Around the glands themselves are tiny cells like muscles that help to move milk toward the major duct system and nipple.

Blood is supplied to the breasts by arteries branching from beneath the sternum and between the ribs as well as by branches from the large axillary artery. Blood is drained from the breast by veins that follow the same routes. Often the veins in and just under the skin of the breast are very visible. Lymph drains from the breast to five major lymph node areas. These areas are in the axilla, just above the collar bone, under the sternum, across to the opposite breast, and through passages that lead to the lymph nodes in the upper abdomen.

The nerve supply to the skin of the breast and the nipple-areola complex is generous and specialized. The nerves are thought to play a role in stimulating milk production. They also explain the increased sensitivity of your breast, skin, and nipple to stimulation of all sorts. These nerves originate low in the neck and from the nerve supply to the ribs.

During early pregnancy the first noted breast changes occur in the areola, which darkens and begins to enlarge. (For more detailed discussion of these changes, see "Pregnancy and Childbirth.")

With the onset of menopause the breasts become less firm due to the regression of the glandular structures. Frequently, too, the supporting ligaments relax and the breasts become more pendulous. It is not unusual to be able to feel the

CROSS-SECTION OF THE BREAST

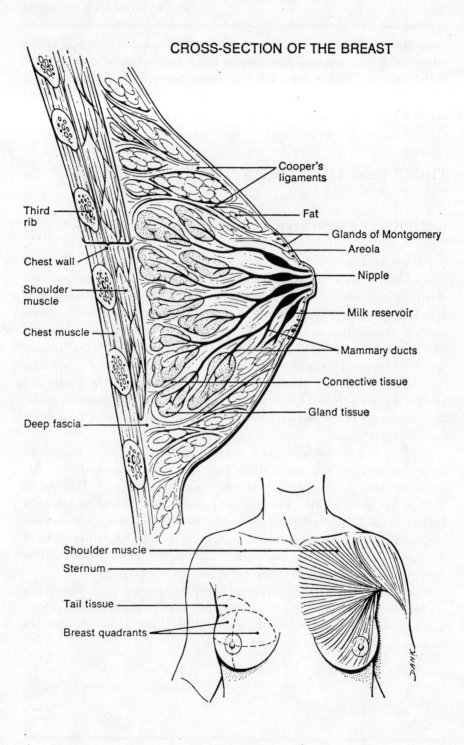

Cooper's ligaments

Third rib

Fat

Glands of Montgomery

Areola

Chest wall

Nipple

Shoulder muscle

Milk reservoir

Chest muscle

Mammary ducts

Connective tissue

Gland tissue

Deep fascia

Shoulder muscle

Sternum

Tail tissue

Breast quadrants

breast ducts themselves in an elderly woman. If, however, a woman is taking estrogens after menopause, there may be less regression of the glandular and ductal structure. Such women will have breast tissue more like the younger adult, although there is still some relaxation and sagging due to lax ligaments and skin.

THREE ESSENTIAL BREAST EXAMINATIONS

BREAST SELF-EXAMINATION (BSE)

Perhaps there is no better way you can safeguard your health than by carefully examining your breasts once a month. You will come to know the subtle details of your breasts better than the most astute physician. With a good knowledge of your normal breasts, you can detect any significant changes yourself. The illustrations on the pages that follow show the proper technique. The National Cancer Institute of the U.S. Department of Health and Human Services recommends that the best time to do BSE is two or three days after the end of your period, when your breasts are least likely to be tender and swollen. A woman who no longer has her periods is advised to pick a particular day, such as the first or last day of every month, in order to make a routine of her self-examination.

Any local unit of the American Cancer Society can put you in touch with further material, such as an excellent five-minute movie demonstrating this technique. Your doctor or your local cancer society may have to help you to learn to find abnormalities, and you can practice on models of breasts with built-in lumps. These models are available at local units of the American Cancer Society and teaching hospitals. As outlined in the illustration, the timing of the examination is important, due to the variations that normally occur during each menstrual cycle. These variations will be discussed shortly.

What should you do if you find something? First, *be sensible!* Most problems are *not* cancer. Seek prompt attention from a competent physician. If you have found an early cancer, you have done yourself the biggest possible favor because early breast cancers are highly curable.

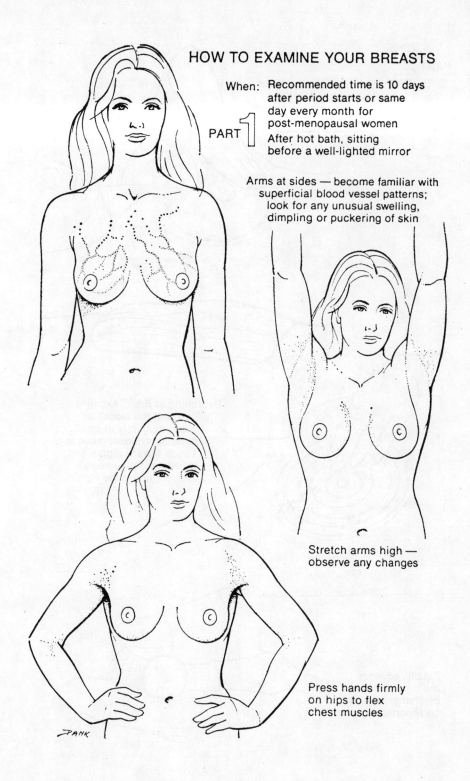

HOW TO EXAMINE YOUR BREASTS

When: Recommended time is 10 days after period starts or same day every month for post-menopausal women

After hot bath, sitting before a well-lighted mirror

PART 1

Arms at sides — become familiar with superficial blood vessel patterns; look for any unusual swelling, dimpling or puckering of skin

Stretch arms high — observe any changes

Press hands firmly on hips to flex chest muscles

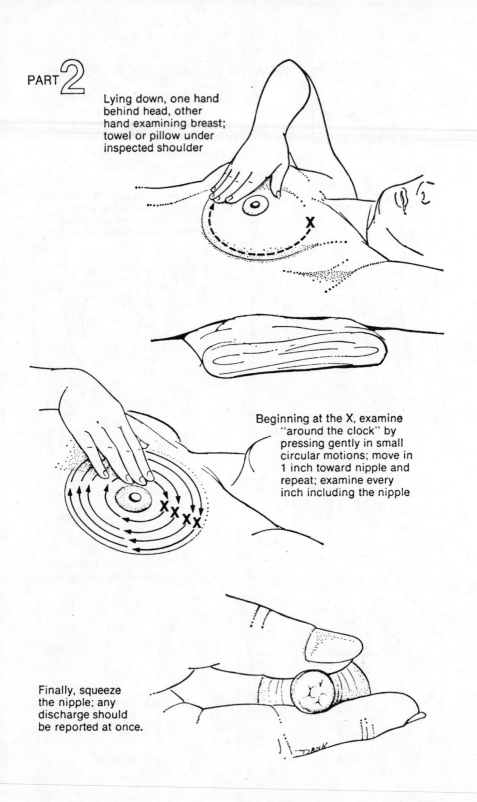

PART 2

Lying down, one hand behind head, other hand examining breast; towel or pillow under inspected shoulder

Beginning at the X, examine "around the clock" by pressing gently in small circular motions; move in 1 inch toward nipple and repeat; examine every inch including the nipple

Finally, squeeze the nipple; any discharge should be reported at once.

PHYSICAL EXAMINATION BY A HEALTH PROFESSIONAL

The second essential step in increasing the chances of detecting breast cancer in its earliest stages is a regularly scheduled breast examination during your routine physical checkups. If this procedure has previously been omitted by your primary care physician or nurse practitioner, ask that it be included. This is the time to call attention to any changes you have become aware of during self-examination. During the exam the health professional feels the breasts and underarm areas with the fingers in a procedure called palpation. The external condition of the breasts is also examined for changes such as dimpling, scaling, or puckering, as well as any discharge from the nipples.

MAMMOGRAPHY

Mammography is the special X-ray procedure considered to be an effective method for detecting breast cancer in its earliest, most treatable stage. High-quality mammography can discover a tumor up to two years before any lump can be felt. A mammogram is an office procedure that takes only a few minutes. Usually two X-rays are taken of each breast—one from the top and one from the side. The effectiveness of mammography as a diagnostic tool depends to a large extent on the clarity of the image achieved by the technician and the interpretation of the image by the discriminating eye of the radiologist who evaluates it.

Several years ago Congress passed the Mammography Quality Standards Act to ensure that mammography as performed in the approximately 11,000 facilities in the United States is safe and reliable. Under this law, government certification is conferred only on those facilities that have met the agency's standards for the training of the technician who takes the X-ray pictures and for the ongoing experience of the radiologist who interprets the pictures. (In a certified facility, the radiologist is expected to interpret a minimum of 40 mammograms a month.) All mammography equipment is monitored on a regular basis by government inspectors to make sure that it generates no more than the necessary amount of radiation and that the images it produces are clear and sharp.

In addition to providing guidelines for facilities that perform mammograms, doctors and patients are given advice that ensures the best possible results. Here are some suggestions for women to follow:

- Call 1-800-4-CANCER for the names and addresses of FDA-certified mammography facilities in your area. This government service is provided free of charge Mondays through Fridays from 9 A.M. to 4:30 P.M.
- If you have been referred to a mammography facility by your doctor, or if the service is provided by a technician in your doctor's office, ask to see the FDA certification. Don't be shy about this, and if the certificate isn't produced or your request is given the brush-off, leave the premises and use the above source for an alternative address.
- If this is not your first mammogram, bring the film from the previous one for comparison.
- Make your appointment at a time during your menstrual cycle when your breasts aren't tender so that the technician can compress the breast as tightly as possible between the two plates without causing undue discomfort.
- Don't apply deodorants, lotions, or powders before your appointment because they can cause a blurry image.
- Give the facility the name, address, and telephone number of both you and your doctor so that both of you can be informed of the results. Find out whom to call if you don't get results within two weeks.

If you are continuing to experience breast changes or discomfort even though your mammogram results are "normal" or "benign," talk to your doctor about the advisability of additional diagnostic procedures and physical examinations or get a second opinion from another physician. Be sure to make all your available mammograms available to this physician for a reading by another radiologist.

SCREENING MAMMOGRAMS

In women above the age of 50, screening mammograms are recommended yearly. They have been shown to be very helpful in identifying previously undetected breast cancer. (Additional discussion can be found in "Aging Healthfully—Your Body, Mind, and Spirit.")

There is continued debate about screening mammography in other age ranges. If you are age 40 to 49, concerned organizations have various recommendations ranging from no routine screening to a screening every one to two years. Taking into consideration available statistics, costs, and general risk factors, I would recommend a screening mammogram some time in your later thirties and thereafter every several years. Individual advice should be sought from your doctor. Call your insurance company to find out about coverage, do not fail to get a recommended mammogram because of insurance problems. There are often programs that your physician will know about to help you.

OTHER METHODS

In addition to the three basic and essential procedures described above—self-examination, physical examination, and mammography—several other methods are also used. *Ultrasound,* also called sonography, sends high-frequency sound waves into the breast to detect changes in tissue. Echoes from these sound waves are converted into an image on a screen, providing information about the breast's interior. While sonography can help the specialist distinguish between solid masses and fluid-filled sacs or cysts, it does not identify small tumors. *Thermography* measures heat patterns given off by the skin. The development of a problem is indicated by changes in the patterns and the presence of "hot spots." While thermography presents no known radiation risk, it is not a substitute for mammography because it does not have the same level of reliability. CAT scanning can be helpful in locating breast lesions difficult to pinpoint in other ways because they are so close to the chest wall. Magnetic Resonance Imaging (MRI) is one of the newer techniques for achieving even more refined images of breast tissue, and laboratory tests are being developed that could be used to detect cancer in blood samples by the use of substances known as tumor markers.

EVERYDAY BREAST CARE

There are no mysteries regarding the care of your breasts. Good hygiene is important here as everywhere. The skin of the nipple and breast can be susceptible to dryness, particularly during the winter, and to allergic reactions to clothing. A cream or ointment that does not contain alcohol can relieve such dryness. Some women prefer to remove the few dark hairs around the areola by plucking them. Care should be taken not to cause infection by doing so. You should not "dig" them out; pluck gently as you would in shaping your eyebrows. Electrolysis may be helpful in some instances. However, it is suggested that you first consult your physician. It is not unusual to have occasional scaling of the nipple, but crusting or bleeding is another matter and must be checked by your doctor.

Women with large breasts can be plagued with rashes and dryness under the breast fold, especially in the summer. Often such simple remedies as baby powder or cornstarch are effective in relieving the condition.

Most women, particularly those with large breasts, wear a brassiere for both support and comfort. The most important thing about a brassiere is fit. Any good department store can help with fitting. Women whose breasts change a great deal with their menstrual cycles may require more than one size brassiere. Many women find that their brassiere size changes after pregnancy and after menopause. It is not necessary to spend a lot of money for a brassiere that fits properly. A widely advertised brand name or features of decorations and luxury fabrics may enhance the cost but not the support.

A well-fitted brassiere is especially important for most athletic activities. This topic is discussed in "Fitness," the chapter on exercise. In general little breast injury has been noted in women athletes.

When should a young girl obtain her first brassiere? Often this is a matter of local social custom, and these customs have changed considerably since the days of the exaltation of the female as pinup girl wearing a tight sweater. If a young girl doesn't need a brassiere for breast support or to protect her nipples against abrasion during running or active sports, there's no reason for her to wear one. If on the other hand, an adolescent has heavy breasts and is self-conscious about them, a brassiere that provides support without binding in any way is a sensible investment. (Mothers should refrain from making *any* derogatory remarks about their daughters' breasts no matter what size they are.)

Once your breasts have developed, hormones have little to do with size, except during pregnancy and nursing. No amount of creams, ointments, or salves will affect your breast size. Exercises can only change the size of your pectoral muscles and rarely make a significant difference in your figure. Plastic surgery can increase or reduce your breast size and in some circumstances such surgery is indicated (see "Cosmetic Surgery").

It is usual for the nipples to become erect during sexual activity, but the absence of this response is not uncommon. It is not a sign of absence of arousal if sexual stimulation and foreplay produce only little change in the nipple. Other breast changes during sexual activity include venous engorgement, an increase in size of the breasts and later of the areolas (primarily in women who have not nursed), and a pink mottling. Injuries can be caused by overenthusiastic sex play. Vigorous sucking and chewing of the nipple can result in cracked nipples that may lead to infection or painful, superficial ulcerations.

While these conditions are not serious, it is sensible to consult your physician if they occur.

BREAST DISORDERS

The common disorders of the breast can be classified according to genetic or congenital abnormalities of anatomy, endocrine dysfunction, normal physiologic changes, benign cysts and tumors, infections, and malignant disease.

ANATOMICAL ABNORMALITIES AND

ENDOCRINE DYSFUNCTION

There are several relatively common congenital anatomical disorders that do not become apparent until puberty. Failure to develop *any* breast tissue due to anatomical abnormality is exceedingly rare. However, "extra" breasts or parts of a breast occur in 1 to 2 percent of Caucasians and more frequently in Orientals. In all mammals, the breasts develop from an embryonic milk-line that extends on both sides of the body from the axilla to the groin. Breast tissue, nipples, or areolas in any combination may be present along this line and may be unilateral or bilateral. This is rudimentary tissue with no physiologic function. Even if enlarged during pregnancy, these incompletely formed breasts will usually regress. A fully formed additional breast, however, may function normally and even provide satisfactory nursing. These more complete breasts are subject to the diseases affecting normal breasts.

Another common problem that appears at puberty is a difference in the size of one breast compared with the other. This is not considered abnormal in most instances. However, because of the adolescent girl's intimate and excessively critical involvement with her body and its development, even a minor difference in breast sizes may give rise to anxiety. Parental reassurance can be helpful, but where the emotional disturbance is severe or the difference in breast size is conspicuous and is not satisfactorily adjusted by a custom-made brassiere, cosmetic surgery might be considered.

Like navels, some nipples are always "inners" rather than "outers." An inverted nipple that a woman has had all of her life is no cause for concern. But when a change occurs, an examination should be scheduled.

Abnormalities in the breasts that are associated with abnormal endocrine gland development or dysfunction are usually not noted until adolescence. Failure of the breasts to develop at all due to endocrine dysfunction is rare. However, this failure may be associated with the absence of ovaries or adrenal glands. Delayed or minimal breast development may be associated with ovaries that are functioning abnormally. Complex relationships between the pituitary, thyroid, and adrenal glands can produce numerous variations of delayed or minimal development. Failure of development of breasts by age 15, with or without associated onset of menstruation, should be investigated. Modern methods of evaluating gland function can usually pinpoint the precise problem. Replacement hormone therapy can often help to stimulate development of the nonadult breast. It should be noted that very small breasts may be completely normal. It is the function of the endocrine glands, not size of the breast, that determines the need for hormonal stimulation in adolescents. It should also be pointed out that hormonal medication will not increase the size of the normal adult breast and should never be considered for that purpose.

In some cases breast development begins early. If it begins before age 8, it is called precocious puberty. It is common for the other secondary sex characteristics, especially pubic hair, growth of the labia, and menstruation, to develop somewhat later than the onset of breast development. In the past it was thought that most of the problems of precocious puberty were related to a tumor of the ovary that caused increasing production of hormones. Because bone maturation and precocious growth often coexist, it now appears that precocious puberty is related to other or more general endocrine problems. A careful and complete endocrine evaluation is necessary to find the source of the disorder.

Children who develop breasts between 8 and 12 are considered to have early puberty, not precocious puberty. Development may be unilateral and may be noted first as a soft, flat, 1- to 2-inch circular mass beneath the nipple. Because the opposite breast will begin to develop in several months, excision of this "mass" is not wise, as the entire normal breast may be removed. It is not until about age 13 or later that some other common disorders such as cysts or fibroadenomas begin to occur.

NORMAL PHYSIOLOGIC CHANGES

During late adolescence and adult life, normal physiologic changes in the breasts occur with each menstrual cycle. These changes do not represent disorders, and understanding them can relieve much unnecessary anxiety and concern. For three or four days before menstruation, the breasts may become engorged, fuller, and more sensitive. In some women there is quite a marked change. There may also be some increase in the nodularity or lumpiness of your breast. Less commonly, you may notice a more distinct lump or cystlike mass, which may be uncomfortable but which disappears with menstruation. The breast may become very tender. Other more general symptoms related to menstruation are fluid retention, mood changes, and pelvic cramps, together known as premenstrual syndrome (PMS).

Variability in symptoms is great. Such changes and complaints may not always occur with every cycle because there are times when, although the menstrual cycle is quite regular, you do not ovulate. The woman whose ovaries are intact after a hysterectomy should remember that menstrual symptoms, including breast changes, may be present, even though vaginal bleeding is absent. Awareness of your own pattern of symptoms and careful self-appraisal in these circumstances can be quite helpful.

Premenstrual breast complaints frequently require no therapy other than a good supporting brassiere and aspirin. Because caffeine has been implicated in the exacerbation of some of these symptoms (but not as their cause), it might be helpful to abstain from all beverages containing it. Physiologic changes in the breast associated with menstruation are sometimes described as cystic disease. To label such normal physiologic changes a "disease" is inaccurate. Other premenstrual symptoms and their treatment are discussed in "Gynecologic Problems and Treatment."

BENIGN CYSTS AND TUMORS

It is during young adulthood that problems of an enlarging mass or masses may begin to occur. Most often these masses are cysts or fibroadenomas (see illustration). Fibrocystic breasts are so common a condition, appearing in from 60 to 90 percent of all women to some degree, that most doctors no longer consider the condition a "disease" and no longer describe it as such. The fibrocystic syndrome rarely makes its initial appearance after menopause, and indeed, menopause frequently "cures" the problem.

Fibrocystic conditions have not been shown to be closely related to increased breast cancer. Women with "lumpy breasts" and their physicians have a little more trouble sorting out the various nodules. It is even more important that such women perform regular self-examination so that if any change is noted, further investigation is done.

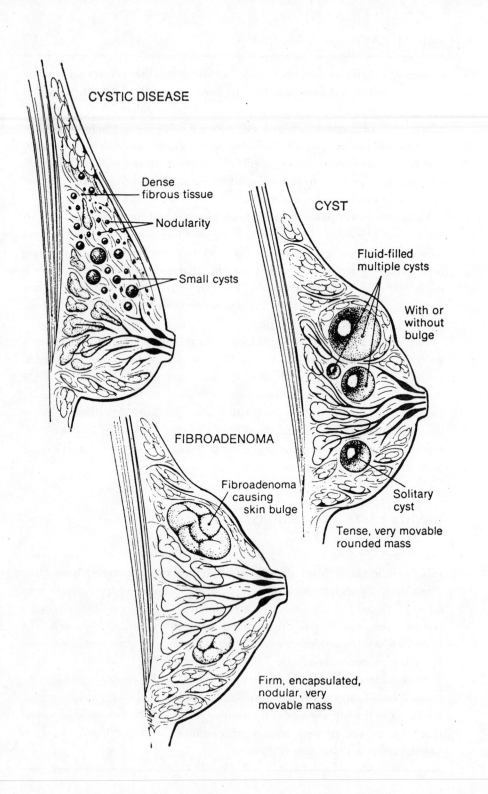

CYSTIC DISEASE

Dense fibrous tissue

Nodularity

Small cysts

CYST

Fluid-filled multiple cysts

With or without bulge

Solitary cyst

Tense, very movable rounded mass

FIBROADENOMA

Fibroadenoma causing skin bulge

Firm, encapsulated, nodular, very movable mass

There is much confusion regarding this group of benign conditions. It is helpful to think of cysts as larger and less numerous in occurrence than the smaller multiple nodularities that characterize the cystic syndrome. Other terms frequently used to describe the syndrome include chronic cystic mastitis and fibroadenosis.

A cyst is a fluid-filled sac like a small balloon. The cause and significance of cysts are poorly understood and a source of controversy among medical experts. At the present time no specific hormone imbalance has been identified, and the entire problem may be a normal result of the cyclic hormonal changes to which the breasts respond. The first general form of the problem is the presence of larger cysts containing fluid that can be withdrawn through a hollow needle. The second form is associated more often with nodularity and often the nodules are shown to be cysts only under microscopic magnification. There are other highly variable cellular changes noted under the microscope in both types of the disorder. Sometimes cysts follow the menstrual cycle. Occasionally a cyst may completely disappear as the menstrual cycle proceeds. In addition, it is common to have chronic and continuing difficulty with cysts or the fibrocystic condition. Whether or not there is an increased risk of cancer in a breast that has had cysts or cystic disease is not proven.

Continued monitoring by both you and your physician is advisable. No specific therapy is indicated. The influence of exogenous hormones, such as birth control pills, is not totally clear.

The most common form of benign tumor is known as a fibroadenoma and is most likely to appear in women under age 40. Initial appearance after menopause is rare. Fibroadenomas are twice as likely to occur in African American women as in other American women. This tumor, like a cyst, may produce a skin bulge. It is also movable and difficult to distinguish from a cyst. Unlike cysts, which are fluid-filled, fibroadenomas are solid, freely movable masses. In general, there is little influence on these tumors by the menstrual cycle and they are seldom painful. Usually they grow very slowly, although in rare cases they grow rapidly during pregnancy. In some few cases they spontaneously disappear or get smaller, particularly with the onset of menopause. There is no nipple discharge and usually no pain. In younger women the diagnosis is often based on personal history and physical examination. Women over 25 should have the diagnosis confirmed microscopically, which means either excisional biopsy (removal of the whole mass) or needle biopsy (withdrawal of tissue sample). If the mass is not producing symptoms and is not enlarging, there is no compelling reason to remove it. However, if there is any doubt in the physician's mind or in yours regarding the diagnosis, surgical removal can be readily done. There is no known relationship between fibroadenoma and the development of subsequent cancer. The role of birth control pills in the natural history of fibroadenomas is not clear.

Less common in the young adult is another benign tumor, an intraductal papilloma. This is a growth of the cells lining the breast ducts, similar in some respects to a kind of wart. These growths can produce nipple discharge, which is often dark and contains traces of blood. The discharge may come from a single duct opening or from several duct openings in the nipple. You may become aware of the discharge because of a stain on your brassiere. Such symptoms, even without a palpable mass, require investigation by a physician. Intraductal papilloma has no known relationship to cancer but can mimic the symptoms of some cancers. There is no known specific relation to the menstrual cycle.

Another benign lesion that can produce nipple discharge is breast duct ectasia. Duct ectasia is the dilatation of the ducts just beneath the nipple with changes in the tissue surrounding the ducts. These changes are variable but can cause new nipple inversion. The lining cells of the ducts are thinned, rather than proliferating as in papillomas. Nipple discharge or discharge along with a slight suggestion of ropiness under the nipple may be the only symptom. Duct ectasia seems to be more common among women who have nursed for long periods of time. Duct ectasia is not malignant, nor is there a known association with cancer. However, bloody nipple discharge and *new* nipple inversion are also signs associated with cancer. Usually excision of the involved area is indicated for diagnostic purposes.

Copious nipple discharge that is clear or milky is called galactorrhea. Detailed endocrine studies can pinpoint the cause of this problem. Galactorrhea may be caused by antidepressant and antihypertensive drugs as well as oral contraceptives. Rarely the cause is a tumor in the pituitary gland.

Sometimes there is a mild, clear nipple discharge for which there is no satisfactory explanation. As age increases and menopause ensues, this problem seems to decline.

Another relatively common breast disorder that makes its appearance in the adult woman and has signs similar to cancer is fat necrosis. Injury to the breast, such as a significant bruise, can cause scarring and damage to the fatty tissue. It can distort the skin, and the damaged area may feel like a hard knot (a sign often associated with cancer). Such symptoms, which may occur long after any recalled injury, require prompt evaluation and usually biopsy to determine the specific diagnosis.

INFECTIONS

The breast and its overlying skin are subject to inflammation, infection, and possible abscess formation. Most infections are related to nursing. Infection of the mammary glands is called mastitis, which may begin with oversecretion or retention of milk. A fissure in the nipple may cause infection, usually with staphylococci bacteria. Symptoms of infection include diffuse redness, swelling of the skin or nipple, a tender painful mass appearing like a boil, fever, and general weakness. Breast infections require appropriate antibiotics. If the infection is not controlled soon enough, an abscess may develop that usually requires surgical drainage in addition to antibiotics.

ESTROGEN REPLACEMENT THERAPY (ERT)

Because the need for post-menopausal estrogen varies, the individual's need must be carefully considered. Disability from symptoms such as "hot flashes," vaginal dryness, and bone changes should be weighed against the possible risk of endometrial cancer. This risk is not yet clearly identified but seems related to the dose given and duration of exposure. There are indications, however, that the risk is reduced when estrogen is combined with the hormone progestin. And on the positive side, recent studies indicate that ERT diminishes the likelihood of a heart attack. Although there is no general agreement among researchers on the possible relationship between ERT and breast cancer, it is recommended that women at high risk for breast cancer because of family history should discuss this matter with their physician. As matters now stand, it appears that most women benefit from estrogen therapy for a limited number of years with careful monitoring of negative side effects by a physician.

BREAST CANCER

An estimated 182,000 new invasive breast cancer cases will occur among women in the United States during 1995, according to the American Cancer Society. Of these, an estimated 46,000 will result in death, making breast cancer the second cause of cancer death among women. (Lung cancer, with an estimated 62,000 female fatalities in 1995, now heads the list.) In recent years there has been a significant decline in the breast cancer death rate among white women (but a small increase among black women). The most important factor in the decline of deaths, especially among younger women, according to Dr. Larry Kessler, director of applied research at the National Cancer Institute, has been the increased use of "adjuvant therapy"—cancer drugs and radiation in addition to surgery. Next in importance is the rise in the rate of women who have routine screening mammograms, which went from practically nothing in the early 1980s to 17 percent in 1987 and to 33 percent in 1990 and is still climbing.

BREAST CANCER AS A POLITICAL ISSUE

Several years ago, when the American Cancer Society announced that "one in nine women are at risk for breast cancer," many researchers took exception to these figures, claiming that they were meant to confuse and frighten women rather than to enlighten them. What should have been pointed out at the time this announcement was made (and widely publicized) is *not* that in any random group of nine women—at the supermarket or at a PTA meeting—one was destined to get breast cancer. The estimate was based on the assumption that, given a life expectancy of 85 years, if all women lived to be 85 years old, one in nine could expect to have a diagnosis of breast cancer at some time within that life span. In point of fact, among women aged 50, one in 50 will get breast cancer. The bottom line risks are being female and getting older.

The "1 in 9" concept developed a life of its own, however, when it became the name of the activist organization on Long Island, New York, where breast cancer cases far outnumbered the national averages. By 1991 the grass roots "1 in 9" groups were among the more than 180 advocacy groups united under the National Breast Cancer Coalition, a voluntary organization that has successfully fought for substantial increases in government funding for basic research into the *causes* of breast cancer. This "women's health issue" went public when the government designated October as Breast Cancer Awareness Month. Nationwide, in the fall of every year, women of all ages and from all walks of life—sufferers, survivors, bereft kin—march together for the benefit of all women, demonstrating by their public presence that breast cancer is no longer only a private concern.

RISK FACTORS

It should be understood that factors known to increase the *risk* of developing breast cancer are not the *cause* of the cancer. Here are some of the known risks:

- **Getting older** Women 65 or older are twice as likely to develop or die from breast cancer as women ages 40 to 64.
- **Family history**–About 10 percent of all breast cancers are thought to be familially linked. In 1994, when scientists identified the mutant gene (BRCA1) responsible for hereditary breast cancer, they estimated that it may account for half the familially linked cases. In 1995 a special mutation of this gene was found to be present in an estimated one percent of American Jewish women of eastern and central European origin. Risks are not necessarily increased for those who have the mutation but do not have a family history of breast cancer. Accurate genetic testing for these mutations is not expected to be available for many years.
- **Reproductive history** Risk is increased for women who began to menstruate before age 12 compared to those who began at age 15; who never had a child or had their first child after age 30 compared to before age 20; who reached complete menopause as late as age 55 compared to women whose menopause at the age of 45 was the result of surgical removal of their ovaries. The impact of early and ongoing use of oral contraceptive pills and of long-term estrogen replacement therapy is still being investigated.
- **Life-style** International variability rates in the incidence of breast cancer correlate with diet, especially fat intake; smoking and alcohol use are under investigation, but caffeine is not considered a problem.
- **Exposure to environmental and occupational factors** The impact of industrial wastes, pesticides, and electromagnetic radiation requires additional investigation.

"The majority of women who develop breast cancer do not have a family history of breast cancer and do not fall into any other high risk category."—National Cancer Institute

"Most risks are at such a low level that they only partly explain the high frequency of the disease in the population. . . . Since adult women may

not be able to alter their personal risk factors in any practical sense, the best current opportunity for reducing mortality is through early detection."—The American Cancer Society

DETECTION OF BREAST CANCER

All studies stress the fact that early detection of breast cancer is of the greatest importance for ultimate cure. In order to be most effective in detecting breast cancer at an early and curable stage, breast self-examination should be practiced faithfully each month. Important signs that require investigation include:

- *Nipple discharge.*
- *Any change* such as the nipple drawing inward or pointing in a different direction.
- Any chronic *scaling* or *bloody secretion of the nipple.*
- Any *change in the contour or the symmetry* of the breast.
- Any breast *lump* or *thickening* that persists through a menstrual cycle.
- Any breast *skin dimpling.*
- Any *new* breast *lumps.*

Generally, there is a lead-time during which a cancer may be quite small and localized. The enlargement and spread may take many months or years. Cancers of the breast usually arise in the cells lining the ducts and glands and then progress outside the ducts (see illustrations). There are rare forms of cancer arising from other tissues of the breasts and even more rare cancers that arise from other parts of the body and spread to the breast. Thus, any suspicious abnormality noted by a woman or her physician requires diagnosis by examination of the area. A palpation of your breasts and examination of the nipples will be performed, first while you are sitting and then while you are lying down. You will be asked to put your hands on your hips and squeeze to tighten your pectoral muscles and to raise your arms above your head perhaps several times. These movements allow the doctor to examine the contour and symmetry of your breasts as well as their movement as you exercise your pectoral muscles. Sometimes very subtle but important changes can be seen in the skin with these techniques. The axillae and the areas above your collar bone will be examined.

Do not be embarrassed or concerned if the physician has some difficulty finding the abnormality you have found. After all, you have been checking

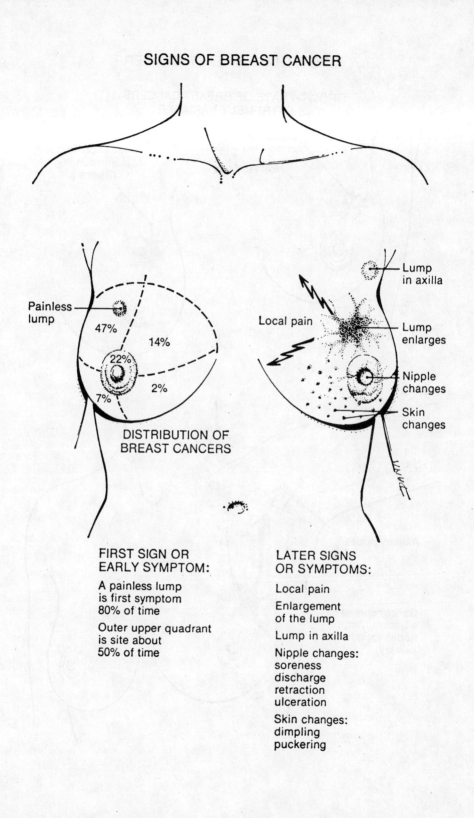

SIGNS OF BREAST CANCER

DISTRIBUTION OF BREAST CANCERS

Painless lump

47% 14% 22% 2% 7%

Lump in axilla

Local pain

Lump enlarges

Nipple changes

Skin changes

FIRST SIGN OR EARLY SYMPTOM:

A painless lump is first symptom 80% of time

Outer upper quadrant is site about 50% of time

LATER SIGNS OR SYMPTOMS:

Local pain

Enlargement of the lump

Lump in axilla

Nipple changes:
soreness
discharge
retraction
ulceration

Skin changes:
dimpling
puckering

GROWTH OF BREAST CANCER

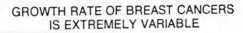

GROWTH RATE OF BREAST CANCERS IS EXTREMELY VARIABLE

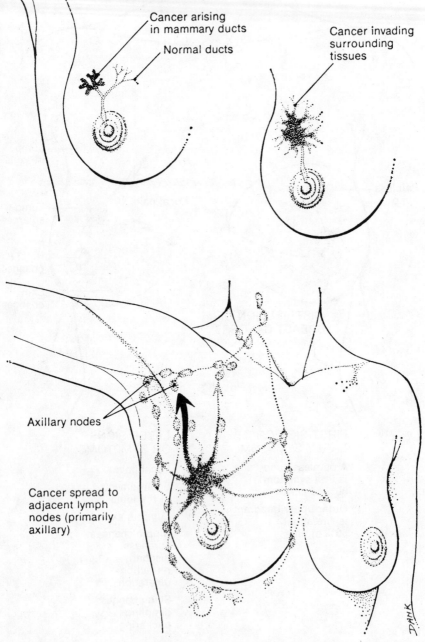

Cancer arising in mammary ducts

Normal ducts

Cancer invading surrounding tissues

Axillary nodes

Cancer spread to adjacent lymph nodes (primarily axillary)

yourself regularly and this may be your first visit to the doctor. You may have to help the physician when such a problem arises. Sometimes, however, a cyst or nodularity that may have been related to your menstrual cycle will have disappeared.

Your doctor may examine your nipple with a magnifying glass and you might be asked to help obtain a sample of the discharge. This may involve some discomfort, but it is necessary. The discharge may be tested for blood or smeared on a glass slide for microscopic study. The remainder of the examination varies greatly. If you have never had a mammogram, you will be asked to have one.

During mammography, each breast is placed on a small examination plate, and up to three different pictures made. Sometimes the radiologist may ask for other views or ask to examine your breasts. For nipple discharge complaints a tiny plastic tube may be inserted into the duct from which the discharge comes, and a small amount of special radiologic dye injected and additional mammograms taken.

In addition to these techniques, the evaluation of a lump or mass in the breast quite often includes a needle aspiration. This aspiration is done using a small amount of local anesthetic in the skin so that a needle can be inserted into the mass. Sometimes several attempts may be needed to set the needle into a very movable mass. If fluid is present, it is removed through the needle. Those masses that are true cysts will collapse when the fluid is removed and usually do not recur. Normal breast cyst fluid varies in color from clear yellow to various shades of green or green-brown. As yet there is no known reason for these color differences. It is not always necessary to have normal-appearing breast fluid examined because cell abnormalities are rarely noted. Abnormal fluid may be cloudy and/or contain blood or tiny tissue fragments. This fluid requires microscopic examination. Even if no fluid is obtained, there may be enough cells in the needle for a pathologist to examine.

If the mass does not completely disappear with aspiration of the fluid, if a solid tumor is noted, or if a diagnosis cannot be made from the fluid or cells in the needle, a biopsy is indicated. The biopsy may be performed either with a much larger needle or through an incision, depending on individual circumstances. Such biopsies can frequently be performed in the office or clinic under a local anesthetic and have several advantages. They avoid the risk involved in general anesthesia. They do not require hospitalization, which is expensive, interrupts activities, and may be more anxiety-producing than outpatient treatment. There is no rush with pathological analysis as there is when the patient is under general anesthesia and the surgeon is waiting to proceed with treatment. If the results do indicate treatment is necessary, you and your physician have time to discuss all the therapeutic alternatives. There is no evidence that in the case of breast cancer (as in some other forms of cancer) proceeding in this manner will "spread the cancer."

After a needle aspiration, needle biopsy, or incisional biopsy there is some bruising. Sometimes after an incisional biopsy a small, thin, rubber drain may be left in place for one or two days. Generally, there is some discomfort that can be controlled by aspirin or other mild analgesics. It is very important to follow your doctor's instructions regarding activity and changing surgical dressings after such biopsies.

Hospitalization and a general anesthetic are indicated for the removal of intraductal papillomas, plastic surgery, extensive biopsy, and other major breast surgery. Fibroadenomas can usually be removed on an outpatient basis.

Any examination of fluid, tissues, or cells that have been removed may take several days. A "frozen section" is faster but not considered as final as a more detailed study requiring three to four days. The pathologist may have difficulty with some cases and require longer than several days for a specific diagnosis. The time it takes to do a careful examination of the tissue is time very well spent.

Most frequently now, a specific diagnosis is first established and the full extent of disease evaluated before definitive therapy is undertaken. Tissue studies, including hormone receptor tissue, can then be completed before treatment plans are finalized. Definitive treatment and various potential alternative treatments (including breast reconstruction) can then be discussed and clarified. The psychological benefit to the patient is obvious. No longer is it necessary to "go to sleep not knowing what will happen."

TREATMENT OF BREAST CANCER

Rapidly accumulating data from national and international studies make it imperative that any woman who has a diagnosis of breast cancer discuss her treatment plan with her physician on an individual basis. It is also advisable to seek a second opinion if there is reason for a well-informed patient to disagree with the first one.

Patients in many parts of the country now have an additional way of exploring their treatment options. Recently developed interactive video programs enable women to feed their personal characteristics into a computer that contains a very large amount of backup data on a broad range of breast cancer circumstances. When the patient provides information about her age, the stage of her cancer, and other relevant facts, the computer describes her available treatment choices plus simple explanations of the risks and benefits of each choice. The video begins with interviews with three attractive women of different ages who are breast cancer survivors. Each one tells the viewer what facts led her to make her particular treatment choice and her postsurgical therapy. Two videos of special interest to breast cancer patients are among a series developed at Dartmouth Medical School and available at approximately 175 breast cancer treatment centers in the United States and Canada: *Treating Your Breast Cancer: The Surgery Decision* and *Treating Your Breast Cancer: Adjuvant Therapy*. For information about the availability of these interactive videos in your area, consult the Foundation for Informed Decision Making, P.O. Box 5457, Hanover, NH 03755; phone: (603) 650-1180.

Local Treatment

Surgery (mastectomy) is, and for many years has been, the cornerstone treatment of breast cancer that has not spread at all or at least has not spread beyond the axillary lymph nodes. If the cancer is found to have spread beyond the axillary nodes at the time of initial diagnosis, surgery will be of no or only limited benefit. The amount of tissue removed (type of mastectomy) depends on certain characteristics of the cancer such as its size and location, on the general health and age of the woman, and on her and her physician's personal preferences. There are eight surgical procedures used in the United States at the present time.

1. Subcutaneous mastectomy. Breast tissue is removed but overlying skin is not. The axillary nodes may or may not be removed. The nipple may be removed or left in place depending on the individual situation. The nipple may be temporarily grafted, usually in the groin. This procedure is not often used to treat carcinoma.
2. Lumpectomy (also called tylectomy or local excision). The breast lump is removed along with a small amount of surrounding tissue. The breast is not removed and may or may not be smaller. (Of the 500,000 women undergoing breast surgery in 1986, approximately 100,000 had lumpectomies, and by 1990, 40 to 50 percent had been treated the same way.
3. Partial mastectomy, segmental resection, or wedge resection. The tumor and a fairly large amount of surrounding breast tissue are removed. The breast is not removed but will be smaller. If the axillary nodes are also removed, the procedure is called a partial radical mastectomy.
4. Simple or total mastectomy. This is like the extended simple mastectomy (below) except that no, or only one, lymph node is removed.
5. Extended simple or extended total mastectomy. The breast is removed and a few

The Types of Mastectomies

Shaded areas indicate what is removed in each procedure.
Cancer is designated by black spot.

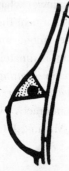 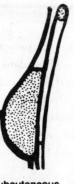 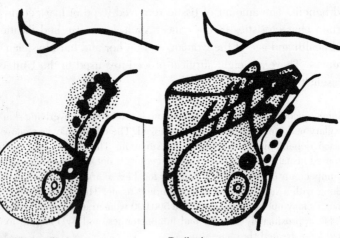

Lumpectomy
Removal of
cancer and
nearby tissue.

Subcutaneous
Removal of
interior breast
tissue. Since
procedure is
usually done as
a preventive
measure, no
tumor is shown.

Simple
Removal of
breast, nipple
and skin only.

Modified radical
Removal of breast,
lymph nodes and
nearby tissue. Option
chosen by Nancy
Reagan, if she has
cancer.

Radical
Removal of breast,
lymph nodes and
underlying muscle.

SOURCE: American Cancer Society

axillary lymph nodes are removed for microscopic analysis to see if the cancer has spread to them. The pectoral muscles are not removed.

6. Modified radical mastectomy. This is like the classical procedure (below) except that the pectoral muscles are not removed.

7. Classical or standard mastectomy (also called a radical mastectomy or the Halsted procedure). The breast, all the axillary nodes, and the pectoral muscles are removed.

8. Supraradical or extended radical mastectomy. The breast, the pectoral muscles, which cover the chest, and the axillary and substernal lymph nodes are removed. To remove the latter, some sections of the rib must also be removed. Some surgeons also remove the supraclavicular lymph nodes (where the neck joins the shoulders). This procedure is rarely done now.

It must be stressed that the specific type of surgery is tailored to the individual circumstances. Surgery is *local treatment,* and the type of surgery performed is greatly influenced by the specifics of location, size, and microscopic type of the cancer as well as other medical conditions. Also it is now common to consult with other oncologists (cancer specialists) regarding the complete treatment plans of which surgery may be one part. Should you require surgery for breast cancer, you should be certain you understand the proposed treatment.

Depending again on your individual circumstances, treatment may include surgery followed by endocrine (hormone) treatments, radiation therapy, and/or chemotherapy. The presence of microscopic involvement of lymph nodes often indicates that such postoperative treatments are advisable.

Tumor tissue is now also analyzed for hormone (estrogen and progesterone) receptors. The presence or absence of these receptors indicates a great deal about the "behavior" of the particular tumor, including the potential response to chemotherapy and hormone therapy. Other studies on the behavior of breast cancer relate to cell turnover, susceptibility to such treatments as radiation, chemotherapy, and immune therapy. These studies may soon have clinical application outside of experimental programs and are likely to add to treatment options. There is also some correlation with predicted survival (also, of course, taking into account the stage or extent of spread and other factors mentioned earlier).

Radiation. While radiation treatments can sometimes destroy a tumor that cannot be reached surgically, it is most frequently used after a lumpectomy as insurance against recurrence. Treatments are usually administered every day over a period of several weeks. Advances in technology now make it possible, when using radiation to shrink a tumor, to focus more precisely on the tumor itself, thus keeping destruction of adjacent healthy tissue at a minimum. The side effect most frequently noted is a feeling of fatigue toward the end of the series of treatments.

Radiation treatments are local treatments and are effective in the area irradiated, just as surgical treatments are effective in the area operated upon.

If you have surgery, of whatever specific type, and radiation treatment, you may also be advised to have other treatments such as hormonal manipulation, some form of chemotherapy or, perhaps eventually, some form of immunotherapy. These other forms of therapy are systemic and reach beyond the local area to the rest of your body and can be very important in providing the best chance of a complete cure.

Systemic Treatment

Hormone therapy can be most helpful. These include adding hormones or blocking them. Female hormones (estrogens), male hormones (androgens), or blocking medications (antiestrogens) can be utilized. At times surgical removal or radiation destruction of the ovaries is indicated. Other hormones (for example, prednisone) are also sometimes used. About two-thirds of women with breast cancer have estrogen-receptive positive tumors and can benefit from hormonal therapy. According to the National Cancer Institute, when a biopsy indicates that a tumor has both estrogen and progesterone receptors, there is an 80 percent chance that the cancer will respond to hormone treatment.

Chemotherapy is the most commonly used treatment following surgery. It consists of using various drugs in combination with the purpose of "poisoning" the cancer cells. Because of the toxicity of the drugs, they can cause unpleasant side effects, especially nausea and vomiting. Queasiness and more serious stomach discomfort are now effectively controlled by various antinauseants that do not produce such undesirable side effects as either drowsiness or agitation. Even baldness is no longer an inevitable consequence of chemotherapy. While some drug combinations cause hair loss after therapy begins, healthy hair will often regrow after therapy. Progress has also been made in reducing the number of leukemia cases caused by chemotherapy because of less harmful drug combinations.

Other Therapies

Immune treatment (immunotherapy) is also being studied. This treatment can stimulate your body's own defense mechanisms against cancer—much as a vaccine stimulates your defenses against polio and tetanus. Dietary "chemoprevention tests" are being conducted in Italy, where women already treated for breast cancer are given 4-HPR, a synthetic form of vitamin A, in hopes of preventing cancer in the other breast. The potential therapeutic value of other vitamins is also being tested.

One further point must be made regarding breast cancer treatment. If, at any time of diagnosis, the cancer has spread to body parts beyond the lymph nodes, no form of mastectomy may be indicated. To determine this, you may be asked to undergo multiple tests. Some of these are blood tests, bone scans, X-rays, and possibly biopsies of areas other than the breast.

Recent drug treatments. Tamoxifen is an estrogen-blocking nontoxic agent in use since the 1970s. At first it was found to be very effective in the treatment of advanced breast cancer, especially in older women who have completed the menopause. The study of the presence of hormone receptors in the original tumor specimen has greatly advanced the effective use and helpfulness of this drug. There has been some indication that there are other positive benefits to other organ systems.

In 1992 the National Cancer Institute launched a five-year trial of 16,000 women to find out whether this medication can be used to *prevent* breast cancer in high-risk women. The identification of these women presents many difficulties, and because the preventive value of tamoxifen is still uncertain, it may have serious adverse consequences. It should not be used by healthy women outside the study because its long-term effects are unknown. Many cancer centers nationwide are taking part in this investigation. More information can be obtained from your local cancer center or the National Cancer Institute's information service: 1-800-4-CANCER.

Taxol is a compound derived from the bark of Pacific yew trees. This drug has been used with some success in treating ovarian cancer as well as breast cancer in its late stages. A more recent drug, Taxotere, became a competitor of Taxol in 1995. Both drugs are administered intravenously and must be carefully monitored for powerfully adverse side effects. These two drugs are treatments of last resort when other options have been unsuccessful.

AFTER SURGERY

Breast reconstruction following surgery is most often done by plastic surgeons. Reconstruction options should not be the major deciding factor in selecting the exact type of surgical procedure, as this selection depends on many

individual factors and as the first purpose is to save your life. (Excellent book-
lets dealing with all aspects of breast surgery are available from the American
Cancer Society. See also "Cosmetic Surgery.")

There are many myths regarding the psychosexual aftermath of breast surgery. It is clear that the most important goal is building and maintaining a
positive self-image. There are no physiologic or sexual capabilities lost when a
breast is lost, except the capacity to nurse. You are as fully capable of joyful sex
and sexuality as you were prior to surgery. There are certainly severe stresses
related to returning home, going back to work, and coping with the problems
presented by a spouse's or a lover's reactions.

Support groups such as the Reach for Recovery Program of the American
Cancer Society can help. The women volunteers in this organization have had
mastectomies and will visit you in the hospital and help you when you return
home. They have been trained to help other patients and understand the
anxieties, fears, and problems accompanying breast surgery. Your doctor or
nurse can readily contact them. The volunteer will usually bring you a temporary breast prosthesis to wear home and can accompany you when it is time to
obtain a permanent one.

Relationships with your family, husband, lover, and friends will be affected
as they would by any other serious and difficult problem in life. Seldom are
sturdy relationships seriously harmed. Weak or difficult relationships are sometimes strengthened but can deteriorate. Unmarried or divorced women patients have told me that the true worth of a developing relationship is strongly
tested following breast surgery. Most physicians caring for cancer patients are
now more aware and trained to discuss patients' psychosexual problems. Self-
help groups can be a life-line during periods of depression and morale is
inevitably boosted by active participation in educational and lobbying programs with other survivors. If professional help is necessary, cognitive therapists can be especially effective in guiding you toward healthy new perceptions of your worth as a woman no matter what scars your body has sustained.
The reassuring fact seems to be that consideration and communication—not
breasts—are central to loving relationships.

Whether your risk of breast cancer is high or low, here are some practical
preventive measures within your control:

- **Detection** Perform self-examination on a regular basis and consult your
  doctor promptly about any changes. Schedule a mammogram at the intervals recommended for your age group and individual history. Ask for a
  copy of the results to keep in your own files.
- **Diet** Although some studies indicate that a diet high in animal fats in-

crease breast cancer risk, a far more important dietary factor for reducing the risk appears to be the consumption of lots of fruits and vegetables. Soybeans and products derived from them (like tofu and sprouts) and green tea have been singled out because they are rich in phytoestrogens, substances thought to block the tumor-promoting effects of natural estrogens. Losing excess weight is more easily accomplished with these nutrients too.

- **Exercise** Several studies indicate that for premenopausal women, moderate exercise pursued on a regular basis significantly reduces cancer risk.
- **Alcohol** While there are no definitive statistics about the role of alcohol in relation to breast cancer, it is known that even two drinks a day will raise estrogen levels, which presumably increase breast cancer risks.
- **Smoking** A 1995 study conducted at the University of Buffalo indicated for the first time that smoking can be carcinogenic to the breast. The risk was shown to be highest among women who began to smoke as teenagers and those who smoke more than one pack daily.
- **Prevention trials:** Women at high risk can consult their doctor or call the Cancer Information Service at 1–800–CANCER about participating in one of the many trials of medicines and procedures being conducted throughout the United States.

The purpose of this chapter has been to provide you with a better understanding of the structure and function of your breasts so that you can be a knowledgeable participant in their care. Try to keep informed about new developments and discuss them with your doctor so that you can find out how they apply to your particular situation.

COSMETIC SURGERY

Maxine Schurter, M.D.
Late, Clinical Professor of Surgery, George Washington University School of Medicine, Washington, D.C.

Gordon Letterman, M.D.
Professor Emeritus of Surgery, George Washington University School of Medicine, Washington, D.C.

Kathryn Lyle Stephenson, M.D.
Late, Santa Barbara Cottage Hospital, Santa Barbara, California

Cosmetic surgery is a specialty within the larger field of plastic surgery. Plastic surgery includes the repair of congenital defects (such as a cleft lip) and the restructuring of parts of the body damaged by disease (as in the case of breast cancer) or by injury (such as might be sustained in a fire, in war, or in an automobile accident). Cosmetic surgery is usually elective. Its purpose is to improve an individual's appearance by changing the shape of the nose (rhinoplasty), removing wrinkles from the face (rhytidoplasty), correcting the wrinkles or bulge of the eyelids (blephaorplasty), altering the relation of the ear to the head (otoplasty), reducing or augmenting the size of the breast (mammoplasty), or removing excess fat by excision (lipectomy) or suction (lipoplasty).

Cosmetic surgery is not a sharply defined area. An operation of any kind should achieve a good cosmetic result, even an appendectomy or a back operation for ruptured disc. Also, many cosmetic operations have a functional as well as cosmetic aspect, such as upper eyelid surgery to improve the field of vision, or breast size reduction to alleviate neck, back, or breast pain.

By virtue of common usage, cosmetic surgery has become an acceptable term. There are some plastic surgeons, however, who prefer the term aesthetic surgery. *Cosmetic* is derived from the Greek word *kosmos,* meaning order, beauty, or improving on beauty. *Aesthetic* is derived from the Greek word *aisthētikos,* meaning to perceive by the senses, or pertaining to the senses of the beautiful.

There is nothing new about the desire to look younger or more attractive. Improving self-image is an acceptable concept in today's health regime. Most American women discuss restorative surgery with their friends and family, and they do not feel guilty about having such surgery performed. Of course, they do not usually advertise their operation and sometimes ask how they can camouflage the postoperative look so that they can return to work as soon as possible.

Many factors account for the increasing popularity of cosmetic surgery. Contemporary culture in the United States is preoccupied with youthful appearance. Women who are threatened with the loss of a job because they look too old may have cosmetic surgery for monetary reasons. Unfortunately, many employers value the look of blooming good health associated with youth rather than years of experience and a mature sense of responsibility. The "baby boomers" in the workplace are well aware of this. Now entering their fifties, this generation was the first to enjoy the many advantages of modern medicine. They enjoyed the protection of the polio vaccine and the life-saving advantages of antibiotics. Fitness programs and better eating habits have contributed to their good health, but do they have to face the consequences of growing older? Not if they can afford to schedule regular visits for surgical nips, tucks, and smoothing away of wrinkles. The computer screens in the surgeon's office can help them make up their minds when they see how much better they look with the lines removed. And for young women contemplating a "nose job," the computer screen removes the uncertainty about which nose shape to choose by superimposing the possible changes on an image of the young woman's face.

Another factor that accounts for the recent increase in cosmetic surgery is the publicity it has received in newspapers, women's magazines, and the media. Prior to 1979 ethical plastic surgeons did not advertise. Then the Federal Trade Commission declared that this restriction created a monopoly, which was illegal. Now physicians, even those not trained in plastic surgery, can advertise, and they do. As a result, the number of people, particularly women, seeking cosmetic surgery has increased. So, too, has the number of the qualified and unqualified practitioners.

Only diplomates of the American Board of Plastic Surgery are recognized by the American Board of Medical Specialists as specialists in plastic surgery. They have been trained in general surgery and subsequently in plastic surgery and therefore are qualified to operate on the entire body. Other groups of physicians operate above the clavicle (collar bone) on the head and neck. Dermatologic surgeons perform chemical peels, a popular way to defeat the skin's aging process.

Improvements in instruments and refinements in technique, particularly in microsurgery and craniofacial surgery, are constantly being made. With the ongoing advances in medicine and anesthesia, operations can be undertaken with greater safety and more assurance of a successful result. The most recent development in achieving physical enhancement is endoscopic plastic surgery, used mainly for removing facial wrinkles. The procedure and its advantages and disadvantages are discussed later in this chapter.

Who pays for cosmetic surgery? Being elective, it is usually paid for by the patient. (Surgery to correct congenital deformities such as cleft lip and palate, deformities resulting from accidental injury, and cancer ablation deformities such as mastectomy may be covered by insurance.) Some women forgo vacations, and others spend practically no money on clothes for years so that they can save up for cosmetic surgery. Some borrow money; others sell a valuable piece of jewelry. Girls in their teens are sometimes given money to spend on a "nose job" for their sixteenth birthday.

DECIDING TO UNDERGO COSMETIC SURGERY

Cosmetic surgery cannot perform miraculous changes in physical appearance or reconstruct basic personality defects such as self-rejection, incurable envy, the "if-only" syndrome, or hopelessly childish notions about beauty and romance. A woman with unrealistic expectations about results is almost certain to be disappointed. A woman with a specific and limited problem—whose livelihood is at stake because of premature wrinkles or bags under the eyes or who feels socially inadequate because she is flat chested or has localized areas of obesity that limit the type of clothes she desires to wear or who loathes her nose—is likely to be pleased with the solution cosmetic surgery can provide. When her impaired physical appearance, whether apparent to others or only to herself, is corrected, her improved self-image results in greater self-confidence, which carries over into her relationships with others.

While a face lift won't save a marriage that's on the rocks or guarantee a better job or a bigger salary, it can be helpful in building the self-esteem and assertiveness that often play a crucial role in competitive situations. However, women who are obsessed with looking young and are terrified of aging might benefit more from sustained soul-searching or psychotherapy than from sur-

gery. Any woman who wants to get the best return for a considerable investment of money and time should therefore be as honest with herself as possible
about the motives that bring her to the surgeon's office.

Past or present psychotherapy for unresolved emotional problems need not
rule out the use of cosmetic surgery as one way, but never the only way, of
dealing with psychological stress. The surgeon should be informed of the therapeutic situation and perhaps consult with the psychotherapist to evaluate the
patient's suitability for the desired operation. Cosmetic surgery performed on a
schizophrenic person is fraught with hazards. Women who for many years have
focused on some aspect of their appearance that is unsatisfactory to them as the
reason for sexual or professional inadequacies should be sympathetically
guided toward what may be painful introspection about major flaws in their
behavior and away from obsessive concentration on the minor flaws they see in
the mirror.

Surgery should not be undertaken when the patient's emotional stability has
been threatened by a shocking experience. There is no doubt that some
women who have experienced an unusually stressful crisis such as a divorce, a
sudden death in the family, the unanticipated loss of a job, or the unexpected
responsibility of taking care of an invalid child or parent can benefit from the
positive effects of a long-postponed improvement in appearance, but psychic
stress has an adverse effect on the physiology of the body and in many cases
can slow down the healing process.

Ideally, a person about to undergo elective surgery should be in the best
possible physical and mental condition, always taking into account the fact that
if the surgery is to be extensive, it will inevitably produce some feelings of
anxiety in the patient about the outcome. A reputable surgeon will take a
detailed medical history, including past illnesses, present chronic conditions,
whether the patient is addicted to alcohol, smoking, or any drugs such as
tranquilizers or sleeping pills, and if she is a chronic user of any medication
such as aspirin and antihistamines. Surgery may have to be delayed until she
has ceased smoking or using alcohol or drugs for sufficient time so that they no
longer affect the body. Some medications such as aspirin and antihistamines
reduce the body's blood clotting efficiency, thereby increasing the potential
hazard of intraoperative or postoperative bleeding. A patient addicted to certain types of drugs may require dangerously high doses of sedatives for adequate relief from pain. Estrogen medications may affect pigmentation or enhance bleeding tendencies following certain procedures. A patient who has
been taking cortisone presents special problems and needs more than the usual
amount of monitoring by an internist and an anesthesiologist before, during,
and after the operation.

Before any woman goes to a cosmetic surgeon, she should attempt an honest assessment of her appearance and know precisely how she wishes it to be changed. Where exactly is the problem? Does the chin need strengthening? The nose need altering? Are the ears too outstanding? Does a body contour need to be changed? Take a good look in the nude. Perfect symmetry of either the face or the figure is usually out of the question. In fact, it is the slight asymmetry of the facial bones that gives most faces interest and individuality. Over time the concept of beauty has changed and is not unassociated with the position of women in society and their activities. Today most females desire to be thin and full breasted. With the development of prostheses and the relative simplicity of the operation, breast augmentation has been requested frequently. Probably the concept of the type of nose that is most desirable has changed most in the last fifty years; again that is a highly individual matter. Computerized imaging can be helpful in reaching the most desirable—and achievable—results.

Advice from friends and family about cosmetic surgery should generally be avoided. Conflicting opinions of friends who do not understand the problems involved can be extremely confusing. Close relatives may be offended at the idea that a physical trait shared by the family is offensive to one member. While they may be as tactful as possible, their feelings or ethnic pride may be severely wounded. One or the other parent may refuse to permit a daughter to have her nose changed. In other cases a teenager may not have strong feelings one way or the other—in fact, may feel that her nose is exactly like a classic portrait—but her mother may want her to have her nose trimmed or straightened. With young people in particular, if those close to the patient take a negative view of prospective surgery, this attitude is likely to persist after the operation, causing the patient to be unhappy about the result. When the decision for surgery is finally taken, it should be based on a realistic assessment of options and information and should be arrived at as independently as circumstances permit.

CONSULTATION WITH THE COSMETIC SURGEON

Once the decision is made, the individual should seek a properly accredited surgeon. At a minimum, the physician's credentials should read American Board of Plastic Surgery Accredited. For the names of properly accredited surgeons in your area, write to Directory of Medical Specialists, 121 Chanlon Road, New Providence, NJ 07974, or call 1-800-521-8110. This directory can also be found in most libraries. Professional societies for plastic surgery or cosmetic surgery can also be consulted. Among these are the American Society of Plastic and Reconstructive Surgeons, Inc., 444 East Algonquin Road, Arlington Heights, IL 60005 (phone: 708-228-9900), and the American Society for Aesthetic Plastic Surgery, Inc., 3922 Atlantic Avenue, Long Beach, CA 90807 (phone: 213-595-4275). The two societies also will provide educational materials on request.

More and more cosmetic surgeons are creating mini-hospitals in their own offices to lower the costs of hospitalization. Therefore it is important to check with the local hospital association to learn if the doctor is permitted to do a particular surgery in that hospital. It is also important to check the facility. Is it accredited by the American Association for Accreditation of Ambulatory Surgery? Does it have cardiorespiratory equipment, monitoring for blood pressure, EKG, arterial oxygen tension, and pulse? Is there a certified nurse or anesthesiologist to monitor the patient throughout the procedure?

When making an appointment with a surgeon for a first visit, the prospective patient should ask how much the consultation fee will be. All other questions relating to fees should be discussed in great detail at the time of the first visit in order to avoid future misunderstandings. The patient would be well advised at that time to ask about the cost of the surgery, additional fees for possible X-rays, other laboratory fees, anesthesia fees if there are any, hospital or operating room fees, and any other costs. It may come as a shock, but most cosmetic surgeons expect to be paid in full in advance of the operation. Unless the commitment to have the operation is made final by prepayment, cancellations and postponements can accumulate to the point where the surgeon cannot maintain any kind of schedule.

During the consultation, the surgeon will question the patient about her medical history and her physical condition. The woman who is not entirely honest or is evasive in her answers is asking for trouble and being unfair to herself and to the doctor. Special problems associated with previous surgery should be described in detail. Any bleeding tendencies should be mentioned. Drug dependencies and the use of any medication must be discussed. A history of hypertension, diabetes, asthma, kidney or heart disease, allergy, or mental illness must be mentioned. The patient should expect the surgeon to supply detailed answers to questions about the problems ordinarily connected with the particular type of surgery requested, the patient's suitability or unsuitability for it, realistic limitations of the procedure and expectations of the results, potential complications, preparations essential before the surgery is performed, the actual technique by which the surgery is performed, and the nature and length of postoperative recovery. It is advisable to come to the consultation with the questions *written down,* and noting the answers is helpful for future reference, especially if more than one surgeon is to be consulted.

If, after this discussion, the patient wishes to proceed with the surgery and the surgeon feels she is a suitable candidate for it, photographs will be taken either during the first visit or during a subsequent preoperative visit. Some surgeons think computerized imaging is helpful, but this is debatable. It is one thing to see an image altered on the screen, but it is better to know that the surgeon can produce it in the living patient. The surgeon evaluates the photographs with the patient at a subsequent visit prior to surgery. It is during this visit that the patient should feel free to ask any and all questions that still remain unanswered.

It must be especially emphasized that the patient should make a determined effort to hear what the surgeon says to her. Controlled studies of patients undergoing plastic surgery have shown that few patients remember postoperatively the statements made to them by the surgeon before the operation. The reason for this memory lapse appears to be the fact that in most instances patients have so firmly decided in advance to have the surgery that they are incapable of absorbing the information communicated to them by the surgeon. There are also those patients whose anxiety about the procedure or the presence of a physician prevents them from hearing anything that is said to them. This has been called the "white coat syndrome." They simply do not listen to the surgeon's recounting of the limitations of the procedure, the possibility of having to undergo secondary surgery, the immediate and delayed anticipated results, the time necessary for recuperation, or the potential complications. Hence the recommendation that the patient take notes during the consultation.

While complications are not common, they do occur. There is no operation that is risk-free. Hemorrhage may occur at the time of surgery or immediately following it; adverse response to anesthesia may occur despite all precautions and impeccable techniques; postoperative infection may complicate and delay healing and recovery. Incisions, although designed and sutured by the surgeon to be as inconspicuous as possible, do result in scars and these scars are permanent. Some individuals form elevated red scars termed hypertrophic or keloidal. Some scars stretch regardless of the physician's technique. How conspicuous the scars will be varies with the area of the body involved and with the patient's type of scar formation. One of the most compelling reasons for the increasing interest in endoscopic face lifts is the substantial reduction in scarring.

SURGICAL PROCEDURES

Cosmetic surgery procedures are performed on practically all parts of the body—facial features are changed, breasts are enlarged, thighs are diminished. Techniques for accomplishing these changes are constantly being refined in order to achieve maximum results with a minimum of discomfort to the patient.

The procedures described in this section are standard practice with individual modifications; however, a growing number of practitioners have been using endoscopy for facial cosmetic surgery as well as for performing breast implants through the armpit or belly button. Other applications are also being explored.

Endoscopy is a surgical technique used for many years to perform knee operations and gall bladder operations. It has only recently been applied to cosmetic surgery, especially for the removal of facial wrinkles. Other applications include eyelid surgery and liposuction to remove fatty neck deposits. In this innovative procedure, tiny incisions are made in the skin through which are inserted small straw-sized tubes containing a viewing scope and microsurgical instruments. The viewing scope, which functions like a camera, is connected to a video monitor onto which it projects a greatly magnified image, enabling the surgeon to operate by viewing the surgical site on the screen.

Women who would like to find out more about this new option can discuss it with their surgeon. Information is also available from the previously mentioned professional societies.

RHINOPLASTY (NOSE ALTERATION)

Rhinoplasty, or alteration of the contour of the nose, is one of the most frequently requested cosmetic operations. It is usually not done before the age of 16, when facial bone development is complete. It is best, however, not to postpone the surgery indefinitely. The overlying soft tissue on the bridge of the nose is not sufficient to conceal even the slightest irregularity. With aging, the skin loses elasticity and may not adapt to the new shape. Development of scar tissue beneath the skin may alter the result desired by both patient and surgeon.

Rhinoplasty requires great attention to detail. The concept of an attractive nose is very individual—what one person likes, another does not. A nose may protrude too much or not enough. It may be hooked or depressed. The tip may be bulbous or pinched; it may turn up or turn down. The septum may deviate, or it may be markedly crooked. The nose is rarely symmetrical; even the beauty queens of Hollywood constantly request that the cameraman take their "best" side.

It is necessary for the surgeon to understand exactly what the patient is looking for. The patient's desires and the surgeon's abilities can be clarified by the study of black-and-white photographs. The desired changes can be drawn on the photos until both surgeon and patient are satisfied.

Rhinoplasty can be done under local or general anesthesia. Young people often prefer to be asleep during the operation. If general anesthesia is used, endotracheal intubation is performed: a breathing tube is inserted through the mouth into the trachea (windpipe) to prevent blood from getting into the lungs while the patient is unconscious. When general anesthesia is used, most surgeons also inject local anesthesia containing epinephrine into the tissues to limit bleeding that may obscure the operative field. The anesthesiologist must be able to prevent excessive bleeding, which is not only dangerous for the patient but difficult for the surgeon.

The surgery itself is performed through incisions within the nostrils unless the nostrils themselves are to be decreased in size or otherwise shaped. Through these incisions, the soft tissues are separated from the underlying bone and cartilage. The cartilage of the tip is modified, and the undesirable bony hump is removed by saw or chisel and filed for smoothness. The lateral nasal bones are fractured inward to recreate the pyramidal form of the upper part of the nose.

If, on the other hand, the dorsum (ridge) of the nose needs to be augmented, cartilage or bone can be inserted into the pocket between the bone and skin. Nasal septal cartilage is often used. Larger defects can be filled with some type of synthetic material.

When crookedness of the nose is caused by deviation of the septum (the cartilage on the inside of the nose that separates the two nostrils), a modification or resection of the septum is indicated.

There is increasing popularity in the use of external incisions (open rhinoplasty). The soft tissues of the nose are elevated so that the surgeon has a direct view of the underlying bone and cartilage, which can then be altered.

Following completion of the surgery, most surgeons insert packing into each nostril. Many also apply an external splint to maintain the new position of the bones, limit postoperative swelling, and protect the operated sites. The packs are removed within a few days. The splint, if used, may remain for as long as two weeks while being changed every few days. Postoperative pain is negligi-

COSMETIC SURGERY OF THE NOSE

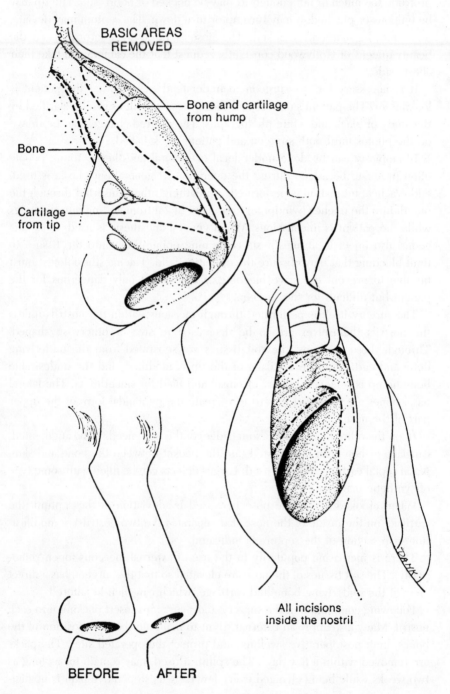

BASIC AREAS REMOVED

Bone and cartilage from hump

Bone

Cartilage from tip

All incisions inside the nostril

BEFORE

AFTER

ble, but the eyelids usually become swollen and discolored. While the nose is packed, mouth breathing causes dryness of the mouth and throat. The nose may feel stiff and numb, but the numbness disappears gradually. Although the greatest amount of swelling is gone in about two weeks, it takes about six months for the nose to assume its final shape. Exercise should be eliminated for about three weeks, and contact sports should not be engaged in for about six months.

It is important to be aware of some of the most common complications that may follow this procedure. The formation of excessive scar tissue may result in distortion and a less delicate contour than anticipated. Asymmetry or deviation may occur. A flat arch and pinched nostrils or even partially occluded nostrils may present a postoperative problem. Profuse bleeding may occur with septal surgery; there may be a perforation of the septum or a collapse of the bridge of the nose. While most of these complications rarely occur, the patient embarking on a septo-rhinoplasty should take these possible failures into account.

Sometimes the nose appears too large because the chin is too small. This is determined by measuring the angles of the face on the black-and-white photographs. At the time of the rhinoplasty, some septal cartilage may be inserted over the chin bone through an intraoral incision. A more severe retrusion may be treated by sliding a section of the chin forward and fixing it there.

RHYTIDECTOMY (FACE LIFT)

The patient's face should be evaluated to determine which areas are most wrinkled, sagging, and unattractive. The procedure may then include a forehead lift, cheek lift, or neck lift. Any excess fat in the neck can be removed at the same time, either by suction or scissors.

While the surgery can be accomplished under local anesthesia with adequate preoperative sedation, some surgeons prefer to use supplemental intravenous or inhalation anesthesia as well. If that is the case, there should be an anesthesiologist or certified nurse anesthetist in charge of the patient.

A face lift consists of separating the skin and subcutaneous fat from the underlying muscles, pulling it back and up, and cutting away the excess tissue. Today the trend is to be more and more aggressive. The level of dissection may be as deep as the facial bones. The surgeon must have a complete knowledge of the branches of the facial nerve because inadvertent section would result in paralysis of the part supplied by this nerve.

If a forehead lift is to be included, the incision extends across the top of the

COSMETIC SURGERY OF THE FACE

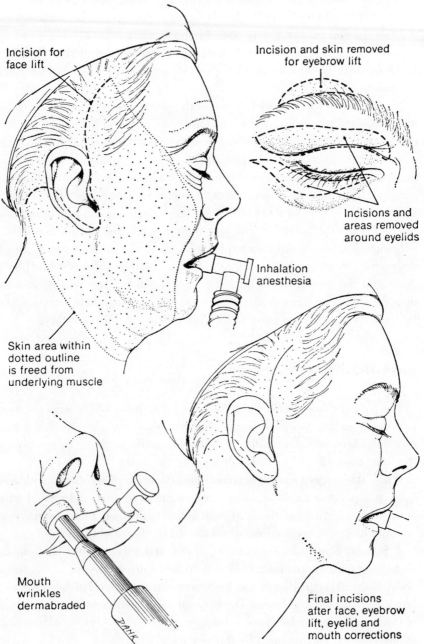

Incision for face lift

Incision and skin removed for eyebrow lift

Incisions and areas removed around eyelids

Inhalation anesthesia

Skin area within dotted outline is freed from underlying muscle

Mouth wrinkles dermabraded

Final incisions after face, eyebrow lift, eyelid and mouth corrections

DANK

head from ear to ear in the shape of a crown; hence the procedure's other name, coronal lift. Some surgeons prefer to make the incision just below the hairline, especially in a very high forehead, because this part of the forehead is raised during the operation. Many people have deep frown lines between the eyebrows. For this reason, the muscles between the eyebrows are cut and a portion removed. The coronal lift is designed to accomplish four things: elevation of the eyebrows, removal of deep wrinkle lines across the forehead, improvement of crow's feet, and removal of deep creases between the eyebrows.

The incisions vary according to each surgeon's preference. Some think that they get a better or longer lasting correction of the sag if the tissue overlying the parotid (mumps gland) and adjacent muscles is elevated and firmly sutured there, the excess being cut away or sutured behind the ear.

On completion of the surgery, some surgeons insert drains under the skin which are attached to a gentle suction reservoir. Blood and serum are removed, leaving less bruising and less postoperative swelling. Some surgeons do not apply any dressings, while others use an around-the-head occlusive dressing.

Postoperatively there is some pain, especially in the muscles at the sides of the neck. It should be treated with some form of light narcotic. Each surgeon has a particular timetable for suture and bandage removal. The patient should plan on three weeks for recovery to the point of no bruising or swelling.

Of all the possible postoperative complications, the most common one is the formation of a hematoma (a swelling containing blood). This is most likely to occur in individuals who have untreated hypertension or uncorrected blood clotting factors and those who are taking aspirin or who smoke. A large hematoma may lead to loss of tissue and infection. Smaller hematomas result in the development of heavier scar tissue, which may appear as a dimple or a lump that can take up to six months to soften.

Other complications involve injury to nerves and changes in pigmentation. Loss of skin sensitivity may occur but gradually diminishes. As the nerves regenerate, the patient may experience a tickling sensation similar to that which is produced by an insect crawling on the skin surface. The transection of a motor nerve may lead to permanent paralysis, but more often the immediate appearance of limited muscular activity is due to the swelling or compression of the nerve, and when healing is complete, normal action returns spontaneously. When there is a change in skin pigmentation, it is most apt to occur in the neck. It is to be expected that the hairline will change, as the skin elevation also causes hairline elevation.

Six months after surgery, recovery is usually complete and the maximum effect on appearance is attained. Of course there are individual variations due to heredity, age, quality of the skin, and general health. At that time additional minor surgical correction may be indicated in order to achieve optimum results. In the 40 to 50 age group, the time at which this surgery is most commonly undertaken, both the skin and the underlying adipose (fatty) tissue have already begun to lose their elasticity. The facial and cranial bones have begun to decrease in size. For these reasons, among others, not all wrinkles can be removed, and a face lift should not be undertaken with that expectation.

The length of time the improvement will last varies with the individual factors mentioned with regard to immediate recovery and also the amount of stress experienced; general health; maintenance of a constant weight; avoidance of excess exposure to the sun and overindulgence in alcohol, smoking, and drugs. There may be some relaxation at the end of six months that may be improved by minor surgery.

Six to eight years after surgery is an average time at which the patient who recalls the original improvement is likely to wish to repeat the procedure. If they are not undertaken too frequently, repeat procedures will produce equally satisfactory results. And whether or not a patient does have repeat face lifts, she will continue to look younger than if she had not had the surgery in the first place.

No other procedure produces such a high degree of euphoria in such a large number of patients. Some of this sense of well-being may be due to the character of the women who seek the improvement: usually they are energetic, determined to cope with life's more unpleasant realities, and eager to participate in the activities of the world around them.

DERMABRASION AND CHEMOSURGERY

Dermabrasion is the removal of the outer layers of the skin. Scars caused by acne can be improved by beveling the edges if they are not the deep-pitted "ice pick" type, although the abrasion may have to be repeated several times to achieve a skin surface that approaches normal in appearance. It is not always possible to estimate the depth of the scars, and therefore the results are not usually predictable. Dermabrasion can also be done to smooth fine wrinkles, especially of the upper lip. Because elevated levels of estrogen affect the pigmentation of the skin, the procedure should not be done on a woman who takes estrogen as replacement therapy or as a contraceptive.

The procedure can be done under local anesthesia or by topical refrigeration (spraying on a solution that freezes the skin surface), but because dermabrasion takes a long time, many patients elect to have general or supplementary intravenous anesthesia. Most surgeons prefer to work on the entire face in order to blend the margins at the hairline and beneath the jawline. If spotty areas are done, blotches of depigmented skin may result. Sandpaper or a rotary diamond fraise or a rotary wire brush may be used.

If the skin is properly dressed with Vaseline gauze topped by dry gauze, there is no pain and no crusting. After the dressings are removed, redness may be present for six or more weeks. It is absolutely essential that for six weeks the patient totally avoid exposure to the sun by wearing a large-brimmed hat and using a sun block. If the face is exposed too early, spotty pigmentation may occur. In general, treated skin is lighter than it was before surgery. If for some reason the skin has brown pigmentation, a local medication can be used. Sometimes there is a formation of milia (white papules caused by the retention of sebum). This can largely be prevented by cleansing with fine soap granules.

Chemosurgery consists of the application of an acid to the skin. The acids that are used today are a 50 percent solution of phenol, one of the chloracetic acids for a lesser exfoliation (the phenol peel), or one of the fruit acids, such as glycolic acid, which can be used by the patient at home.

The phenol peel is probably the treatment of choice for wrinkles around the mouth. Anatomical segments may be peeled, or the entire face may be treated. At one time there were reports of some cardiac irregularity during the procedure. Since then the EKG monitor has been used, and no further reports have been made. The face is carefully cleansed, and the patient is heavily sedated. As the surgeon applies the phenol solution with an applicator, the patient experiences a stinging sensation. A waterproof adhesive tape mask is applied in overlying strips and left in place for 24 to 48 hours. The patient has marked pain during the first 16 hours. Following removal of the tape, thymol iodide powder is applied to dry the weeping surface. Today many physicians prefer to use Vaseline in place of adhesive tape, and Neosporin powder in place of thymol iodide. After removal of the mask, there is intense redness, which may take as long as six months to subside.

Complications following this procedure are similar to those following dermabrasion and are more apt to occur. The patient must protect her face from the sun as long as the redness persists. Keloids (thick red raised scars) may result, which have to be treated with prolonged injections of cortisone. Perhaps these complications can best be avoided by following the advice of dermatologic surgeon Harold J. Brody, chairman of the American Academy of Dermatology's Task Force for Chemical Peeling Guidelines. In a January 1995 Vogue interview, Dr. Brody advises those interested in a chemical peel to be sure to seek out an ethical, board-certified physician through the American

Academy of Dermatologists because "dermatologists and dermatologic surgeons are the only ones specifically trained during their residency for this
procedure."

SCARPLASTY

Scars are basically permanent in nature, but in some instances they can be
made less conspicuous by redesign of tissue. Procedures such as Z-plasty or
W-plasty are used to change the direction of the scar and also lengthen the
scar so that there is no contracture. Keloids may be improved by the injection
of cortisone or the application of pressure by paper taping or elastic pressure.
These techniques may be used singly or in combination.

MAXILLOPLASTY, MANDIBULOPLASTY, MENTOPLASTY, AND

MALARPLASTY

The premaxillary portion of the facial bones (the upper jaw) just below the
nose may protrude or recede too much for an attractive appearance. While
some correction can be obtained from orthodontia, if the malocclusion is severe, maxilloplasty, the surgical recession or advancement of the bone itself,
may be advisable. This is major surgery that demands careful preoperative
study, hospitalization, and longer postoperative care than most cosmetic surgery procedures. While it does in fact improve the patient's appearance, maxilloplasty does not generally come under the heading of cosmetic surgery.
Rather, it is considered reconstructive surgery because function, namely,
proper occlusion of the teeth, is nearly always involved.

Severe malocclusion may also be corrected by mandibuloplasty, the re-
secting or advancing of the mandibular (lower jaw) bone. Frequently, the addition of bone, cartilage, or some type of silicone implant is used to bring the
chin forward to achieve better facial balance. This surgery is often performed
in conjunction with a rhinoplasty, making possible the use of the bone and
cartilage removed from the nose for the reconstruction of the chin. As an
additional procedure accompanying a face lift, it is especially valuable to the
individual whose chin has receded excessively because of the premature loss of
the lower teeth.

Chin surgery (mentoplasty) is undertaken under local anesthesia unless it is
necessary to obtain bone from some other part of the body. The incision is

made either inside the mouth or just beneath the chin, where the scar will be inconspicuous. The incision beneath the chin is used for the removal of excess bone to reduce an excessively long or prominent chin. After the operation the patient is limited to a soft diet for about 10 days. While complications are rare, a nerve may be damaged, producing numbness and lack of mobility of the lower lip either temporarily or in rare instances permanently. Another postoperative complication may be the deviation (separation or slippage) of the material inserted. This is corrected by a secondary adjustment.

The appearance of some women is enhanced by malarplasty, the augmentation of the malar eminence of the cheekbone. Bone or block silicone is inserted to achieve greater prominence of the cheekbone. The incision may be made in the mouth, through the lower eyelid, or behind the hairline in the area above the ear. A pocket for the insertion of the implant is created by separating the overlying tissue from the bone beneath. If the inserted material drifts, it may create a grotesque effect. In thin individuals it may be apparent on close inspection.

BLEPHAROPLASTY (EYELID LIFT)

Blepharoplasty is the correction of puffy or wrinkled eyelids. Fullness or puffiness of the eyelids may occur even in young women, and it is often a familial characteristic. In this condition the orbital fat that cushions the globe of the eye weakens the orbital muscle and a pseudohernia develops. The resulting puffiness of the lower eyelids becomes conspicuously wrinkled. In older women the wrinkling may occur without the puffiness. In some cases the overhang of the upper lid interferes with peripheral vision. The surgery can be and usually is performed under local anesthesia, but because most patients are nervous about surgery close to the eye, supplemental intravenous or inhalation anesthesia may be advisable. The additional anesthesia relaxes the patient who may suffer some pain when the fat is being removed. Vision is checked before the operation. Some surgeons insert plastic lenses for the protection of the eye, and others do not. The surgeon also makes an estimate of the amount of tissue to be removed and usually draws an outline on the eyelid with a colored solution.

The incision on the upper eyelid is ordinarily made in the fold of the lid. The scar is thus concealed when the patient's eye is open. The incision on the lower lid is usually made just beneath the lashes, where it will be hidden. Some surgeons prefer a conjunctival (inside the lid) incision for the lower lid, which eliminates an external scar. The excess skin is removed and the muscles separated so that the fat is exposed and can be gently extracted. Following suturing of the skin, ice compresses may be applied in order to give comfort and limit swelling and discoloration. The sutures are removed in several days. By the tenth day after surgery, the patient generally is presentable without dark glasses. The use of subcuticular (under the skin) sutures eliminates suture marks.

In most instances the eyelid tissue heals with practically no visible evidence of surgery, although the patient should not anticipate the removal of all wrinkles. In some cases excessive swelling may turn the lower eyelid out. This postoperative condition almost always disappears with time, but if too much skin has been removed or if there is abnormal scar formation, the drooping eyelid may be permanent and must be corrected with a skin graft. Another possible postoperative condition is interference with the drainage of tears through the tear ducts, but it is usually temporary. A few cases of loss of vision in one or both eyes have been recorded. The patient must be informed of this possibility. Should symptoms arise, she should immediately be treated.

Some surgeons today like to anchor the under surface of the upper eyelid skin to fascia or cartilage (anchor blepharoplasty). They feel that it gives a better definition to the upper eyelid fold.

EYEBROW LIFT

There are some women whose eyebrows have sagged so low that it is better to remove skin from above the brows rather than from the upper eyelids. The brows may be elevated from various locations: in the scalp (the coronal lift), just below the hairline on the forehead (the forehead lift), in a wrinkle line across the forehead, or above the eyebrows.

OTOPLASTY

Cosmetic surgery for the alteration of ear contour may involve reducing the size or form of the entire ear, the lobe, or the rim, but the most common operation is the correction of protruding ears. The protrusion results when the midportion of the ear (the concha) is too deep or the upper portion of the ear (the auricle) does not have as well-developed or acutely angulated folds as the normal ear. Making ears lie closer to the head can be accomplished only by surgery.

The surgery can be undertaken any time after the age of 6 when the ear has reached almost full development in most children. It should be done before the child has suffered psychological damage from taunts by thoughtless class-mates and equally thoughtless relatives, but it can be done on adults.

The surgery is usually done on an outpatient basis in a hospital or an accred-ited free-standing ambulatory clinic. With proper medication and a quiet reas-suring environment, the operation can be performed on most children and adults under local anesthesia, although a restless or apprehensive child may require a general anesthetic. Most frequently the incision is made near the crease that separates the ear from the head. If the surgeon prefers to perform the operation from the front side, the incision is made just inside the rim. The soft tissue is elevated, and then the ear cartilage is revised by cutting the cartilage, excising an ellipse, or thinning it by abrasion or cross-hatching, and then suturing the tissue into the desired position. After the muscles and the skin are sutured, a bandage is applied around the head to splint the ear in the new position and to protect it.

The first dressing is often left in place for one week unless there is bleeding or the patient complains of pain. Pain may be caused by a bandage that is too tight or for some other reason that should be investigated. In most cases after the first day little medication is required. A head band may be substituted later and worn for four to six weeks while the fractured cartilage is healing. The postoperative numbness or insensitivity of the ears usually disappears within a few months.

The scars are well hidden and complications minimal. The cartilage of the revised ear may not become reunited. If the cartilage does not reunite sponta-neously, it may be necessary to resuture it. The gentle anterior curve may be too angular and necessitate a minor corrective procedure. While possible bleeding and infection can never be ruled out entirely, they occur infre-quently.

MAMMOPLASTY

Mammoplasty may be performed either to augment or decrease the size of the breasts.

Augmentation Mammoplasty: Silicone Implants

When augmentation mammoplasty is mentioned, some people dismiss it because they believe it is a frivolous operation and that the woman wanting it should learn to live with what nature gave her. What they fail to realize is that many small-breasted women feel inferior, unattractive, unfeminine, and incomplete. For them, breast size is a very serious psychological problem.

The use of implants of the patient's own body tissues for breast augmentation was a good idea, but it was never particularly satisfactory. When silicone-filled breast implants were introduced in 1964 by Dow Corning (a joint venture of the Dow Chemical Company and Corning Inc.), they were accepted with enthusiasm. Within about 10 years, however, complaints began to accumulate about leakage and other complications, and by 1992, following hearings, headlines, and complaints about the health problems they were causing, the FDA called for a moratorium on the use of silicone breast implants. By 1995 approximately half a million women who had filed complaints were expecting to collect damages amounting to billions of dollars.

The complaints included pains in the joints, chronic fatigue, scleroderma, impairment of the immune system, and a combination of symptoms that some rheumatologists consider to be a new and as yet unidentified disease. The FDA continues to categorize breast implants as an "investigational product"—which means that this agency sees the need for additional tests and research to guarantee their safety. The American College of Rheumatology has taken quite a different position, claiming that there has been no evidence that silicone breast implants caused the diseases attributed to them. In a formal statement quoted in the *New York Times* (10/25/95), the board of directors of the college said that recently completed studies "provide compelling evidence that silicone implants expose patients to no demonstrable additional risk for connective tissue or rheumatic disease," and the group added that it was time for the courts and the FDA to stop giving credence to the anecdotal evidence that implants cause these diseases. As an indication that the last word has by no means been spoken, a letter by a member of the professional organization appeared in the same newspaper one week later saying that "there were certainly members that strongly disagreed with the statement," pointing to a study indicating that women with implants have up to 59 percent increased risk of rheumatoid arthritis.

In the meantime, cosmetic augmentation of the breasts continues in large numbers using a silicone sac containing saline (a salt solution) that is an inflatable prosthesis. The silicone sac may be obtained with a textured surface, which many surgeons believe decreases the incidence of capsular contracture.

Before the operation, the size and shape of the prosthesis is determined by considering the patient's body measurements and the amount of tissue available to cover it. The surgical incision may be below the breast (submammary), at the armpit (axilla), or at the junction of the areola with breast skin. This latter approach has become more common now that the inflatable prosthesis is used, since a smaller incision is adequate.

Reduction Mammoplasty

Not only do large breasts interfere with a woman's ability to wear strapless clothes or other fashionable garments, but they may actually interfere with normal activities. Because of their excessive weight, the breasts become increasingly pendulous, alter posture, and may produce neck pain extending into the arms. Deep grooves are produced on the shoulders by the pressure of brassiere straps, and persistent dermatitis under the breasts is a common hot-weather complaint. After reduction mammoplasty, there is relief from daily discomfort and pain, increased facility of body movement, and improvement in the body's appearance both with and without clothing.

Reduction mammoplasty is a major surgical procedure that is usually performed in a hospital. Endotracheal anesthesia is preferred for many reasons, one of them being that some surgeons like to have the patient in a sitting position. If blood loss is well controlled at the time of the operation, transfusion is rarely required. Should an unusual situation be present, the patient may donate her own blood in advance, which can be given to her during surgery if required. This minimizes the possibility of an adverse reaction to the transfusion of someone else's blood and the transmission of the HIV virus or hepatitis.

There are a great many different ways of performing breast reduction. The majority of the scars are in the form of an inverted T, although at present there is a tendency to reduce the length of that part of the T which is in the fold under the breast. There are several designs that place the scar in an oblique or lateral position rather than in the shape of the inverted T.

Basically, the difference in methods reflects the way in which the nipple and areola are carried upward. In some cases the nipple is oriented on an up and down piece of breast tissue, sometimes on a transverse piece of breast tissue, and sometimes on a triangular piece of breast tissue or dermis (deep skin). Not infrequently the nipple and areola are removed and then, after the reduction

COSMETIC SURGERY OF THE BREAST
REDUCTION MAMMOPLASTY

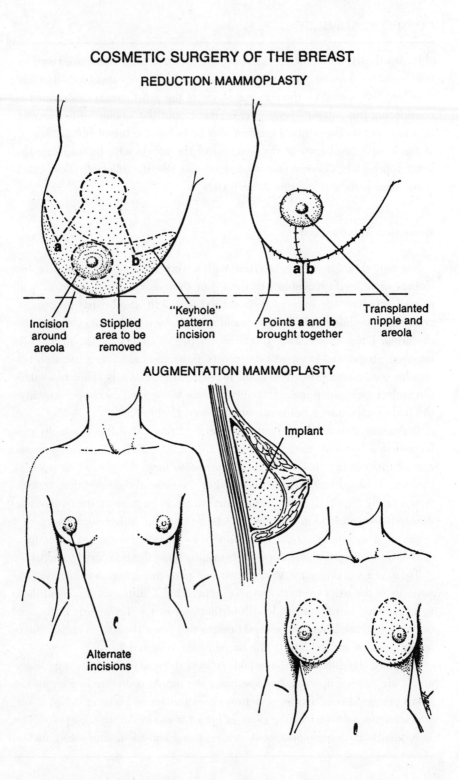

Incision around areola

Stippled area to be removed

"Keyhole" pattern incision

Points **a** and **b** brought together

Transplanted nipple and areola

AUGMENTATION MAMMOPLASTY

Implant

Alternate incisions

and formation of a new breast cone, are placed at the apex of the breast as a free graft.

Before the surgery is performed, the patient may be questioned about the importance of nipple sensitivity, her desire to nurse a new baby, what size she wants to be, and her understanding of resulting scars. Measurements are helpful in determining which of the above methods is most appropriate.

Many surgeons insert drains attached to suction for the removal of blood, serum, or liquefied fat that might accumulate postoperatively and jeopardize the final results. Some patients are discharged later on the same day as surgery, usually because of insurance limitations. Most patients stay overnight in the hospital, since they have had a three- to four-hour operation with general anesthesia. The healing period is about two to three weeks. Athletic activities may usually be resumed in four weeks.

The nipple may be hypersensitive for a while, and there may be some permanent decrease in sensitivity and erectility. With time, the breasts will gradually become more pendulous than they were in the immediate postoperative period. Following a procedure in which the nipple is secured into a higher position, a woman can usually breast-feed a baby. Breast-feeding is impossible when the operation involves free-grafting the nipple because the ducts from the breast tissue to the nipple have been cut.

Mastopexy

Breasts naturally sag with the passage of time, even when they are not abnormally large. The elevation of the sagging breast is much less complicated for the patient than a reduction. The designs of the incisions and the surgical procedure for lifting the sagging breast are similar to those for reduction mammoplasty, but because the procedure takes less time, there are fewer complications. The results, however, are less permanent because the skin over the breast will once again lose its elasticity. Some plastic surgeons therefore advocate augmentation at the same time to increase the permanency of the operation.

PLASTIC SURGERY FOLLOWING MASTECTOMY

After a radical mastectomy, if spread or recurrence of the cancer appears to be unlikely, consideration can be given to breast reconstruction. If the surgery necessitated a skin graft for coverage of the chest wall defect or if radiation was necessary, it is occasionally possible in a small-breasted individual to recreate a breast from an adjacent flap of skin and fat. If this is not possible, it is necessary to bring fat and skin from another part of the body. Many surgeons use a flap from the back or the abdomen. In centers where microvascular surgery is performed, the tissue may be obtained from the groin, buttocks, or thighs. Sometimes these procedures require two or more operations.

During the past decade or two there have been many trends in breast reconstruction after mastectomy for cancer. At first, a silicone gel prosthesis was inserted under the skin to give breast prominency. This was thought to be sufficient for appearance in clothing. Later, techniques became more sophisticated. In the absence of sufficient skin and soft tissues, local tissues from the back and lower abdomen were transferred to reshape the breast. Sometimes this could be done without implants, especially if the tissue was from the lower abdomen. Sometimes implants and tissue transfer were combined.

Then it was realized that the skin and muscle could be expanded by the use of an inflatable prosthesis that could progressively increase in size by the injection of saline into the prosthesis from a direct or adjacent port. When the desired size was obtained, the inflatable prosthesis was removed and a permanent prosthesis was inserted.

All of these operations are costly, time-consuming, and may result in complications of tissue loss due to lack of adequate blood supply or drainage. Most of them are performed under general anesthesia in a hospital and require a longer period of hospitalization than other types of breast surgery.

The nipple and areola reconstruction may be formed from grafts from the inner thigh or arm, and there are numerous patterns for nipple projection. Today many or most surgeons rely on tattooing of these areas with a red or pink pigment.

In addition to the possible complications outlined relative to other breast procedures, other considerations involved in this surgery include prolonged hospitalization, the inevitable scarring at the site from which the tissue was taken for reconstruction, the timing of the procedure, and finances. The timing of the procedure depends on the decision of the surgeon with regard to general suitability for the surgery and especially the degree to which the patient equates her breasts with her femininity. She must realize that although the goal is to recreate a normal breast, it cannot be totally achieved. In some instances a good simulation will be the result, and at the very least the patient will look better in her clothes.

With increasing frequency the surgeon performing the mastectomy recommends that the patient consult a plastic surgeon prior to the surgery. Some surgeons in consultation with a plastic surgeon are of the opinion that there is no reason not to undertake the reconstruction at the time of the mastectomy. Others prefer to wait for six months, after which time the scar tissue will be more pliable than if done a few weeks after the initial surgery. Delay does permit a period of observation for evidence of recurrence.

Another consideration with regard to this surgery is financial. This surgery has been recognized by most insurance companies as rehabilitative rather than strictly cosmetic and is covered by insurance. Nevertheless, each individual should check her policy because it is very costly and often there are several periods of hospitalization.

LIPECTOMY*

Although the most desirable way to reduce the body fat is through diet and exercise, there are some body areas that cannot easily be reduced in this manner—especially the lateral thighs, where what has been called the riding britches deformity occurs. Pendulous skin with dependent fat, as in the abdominal apron, is also difficult to reduce in this manner.

There are two ways to remove fat from the body by surgery. One is to cut the fat out with a sharp instrument (lipectomy). If the overlying skin is also cut away, it is a dermolipectomy. The second method is lipolysis or liposuction, in which a cannula is inserted into the deposit and the fat cells are removed by suction.

Abdominal Lipectomy

Abdominal lipectomy was originally undertaken to correct extreme cases of obesity by removing some of the skin and fat of the grotesquely pendulous lower abdomen. Today this surgery is also performed for the correction of the excessive flaccidity of the skin that may result from pregnancy or weight loss and for the improvement of the striae (stretch marks) caused by pregnancy. Often a lax, obese abdomen is associated with weakened or separated central abdominal muscles, and to obtain a good result in such cases it is necessary that the fascia surrounding these muscles be placated (folded over and sutured) across the midline to pull the muscles together.

The patient should be in excellent health before the surgery is scheduled because this is a major procedure performed under general anesthesia. If the patient smokes, she should give up this habit before contemplating surgery.

* The pronunciation of the letters *lip* in this group of terms is *lype,* not *lip.*

Nicotine in the blood causes constriction of the blood vessels and may result in death of some of the tissues. The patient is usually requested to bathe with antiseptic soap for several days before entering the hospital. Preceding surgery, the pubic hair is shaved. The incision is usually made just above the pubic area and extends laterally across the area that would be covered by the lower part of a bikini. If there is an old midline scar, if improvement of the waistline is to be accomplished, or if the surgeon decides it would be more advantageous, a midline incision may be made instead of a horizontal incision. In some cases both incisions are made. The skin and subcutaneous tissue are separated from the underlying fascia as far up as the rib margin and sternum. The patient is placed in a flexed position, with knees and upper torso elevated so that the maximum amount of tissue can be removed. The excess is cut away, and the navel is relocated in a new opening made for this purpose. Drains attached to suction may be inserted because there may be some postoperative ooze and liquefaction of fat as in a reduction mammoplasty. The flexed position is maintained as the wound is dressed. Various types of dressings are used, but most of them are designed to exert pressure and are similar to a panty girdle. The wearing of a supportive girdle for six weeks after the surgery is recommended to compress the scars and help prevent keloid formation. Ambulation usually begins on the third day and gradually increases as healing proceeds and the patient gradually becomes more upright in position.

Postoperative bleeding may occur and drainage may be excessive. Because the area is one of fatty tissue with a relatively small blood supply, infection may occur, but this is rare. Loss of tissue can occur because of a hematoma, excessive tension, or inadequate blood supply. When tissue loss does occur, a second procedure may be required for correction. Scars may be conspicuous. Rarely are all stretch marks removed. Those that were located in the excised skin are, of course, gone, but those in other areas remain. However, because the skin is more taut, the remaining striae are less conspicuous.

Thigh, Hip, and Arm Lipectomy

Excessive flabbiness of skin or excessive fat or both can also be removed from hips, thighs, and arms. The preoperative preparation and procedure are fundamentally similar to those required by the abdominal lipectomy, and potential complications are the same in all. The excision of arm tissue is the simplest but leaves an unattractive scar.

The incision for the removal of excess tissue from the hip is usually made in the gluteal fold where the buttocks join the upper thigh. If the problem exists over the lateral portion of the upper thigh (trochanteric) area, the incision may extend around three-quarters of the thigh or at a slightly higher level where the scar will sometimes be hidden by a bikini.

For removal of excess skin from the inner thigh, a modified T incision is made extending vertically at the midline of the inner thigh and extending forward and backward for a limited distance at the groin.

To remove the excess skin and subcutaneous tissue of the upper arm, a modified T incision is made, with the vertical portion of the cut placed along the least visible portion of the arm and the horizontal cut extending into the armpit. The scar will be visible when the arm is raised. In deciding whether to have this surgery, the patient must choose between flabby arms and a visible scar.

For all these procedures, three weeks of disuse should be anticipated. After three weeks scars may increase in width but they also become paler and less conspicuous.

LIPOSUCTION

Liposuction is used for the removal of localized fat and to facilitate other cosmetic procedures. Since its introduction into the United States in 1982, it has become this country's most popular cosmetic procedure, not only among models and performers, but also among healthy women with resilient skin and limited areas of fat. The procedure is *not* intended for significant weight reduction but rather for reshaping specific parts of the body, most often hips and thighs. The development of several types of cannulae in the past few years has permitted the surgery to be performed with deceptive ease and has resulted in many unqualified practitioners attempting the surgery. It is not without danger and has in some instances resulted in death for the patient. Therefore special care should be exerted in the selection of a surgeon before the decision is made to undertake this procedure. The credentials to look for are "Board-certified plastic surgeon," and inquiries should be made about hospital connections.

Liposuction is major surgery, and the patient should be in good health and not suffering from any major disease. The same preoperative prohibitions as for other major plastic surgery procedures pertain. Preferably the patient is under 40 because the overlying skin is more elastic and will adapt better to the new contour. It can be used for older persons who are not concerned with the

appearance of the overlying skin after the surgery and are in better than average health for their age.

Preoperatively, the patient is prepared as for a lipectomy. Some doctors
insist on an electrocardiogram a few days before the surgery as well as a course
of antibiotics. The procedure is done under general anesthesia or intravenous
sedation supplemented by local anesthesia. A small incision in the skin is made
in an inconspicuous area. In the abdomen it is usually above the pubis or
adjacent to the umbilicus (navel); for the hips or thighs, in the bikini area. The
cannula (a blunt metal tube with perforations) is inserted approximately one
inch below the skin and suction applied. It is reinserted at a different angle in
a more or less radial fanlike pattern until the fat is removed from the previously designated area. Fat cells and fluid of disrupted fat cells as well as plasma
and blood are removed with the suction. The amount to be removed at any one
time should not exceed 2 liters. (One liter equals about $2\frac{1}{2}$ pounds on the
scale.) The risk of the operation increases with attempts to remove excessive
amounts of fat at one time, and it is *not* intended for significant weight reduction. Since the number of fat cells is fixed, the weight loss in the selected area
is likely to be permanent. The fat cells that remain may expand somewhat with
weight gain, but subsequent gain, if it occurs, usually accumulates in areas not
liposuctioned.

Postoperatively, the involved area is strapped, or an elastic pressure dressing
is applied such as an elastic panty girdle on the abdomen or thighs. If there has
been excessive bleeding, some surgeons may decide to insert drains, although
this usually is not necessary unless a large vessel has been damaged. Overnight
observation, preferably in a hospital, is essential. The patient is required to
wear an elastic dressing or garment for three weeks, and activity is sometimes
limited for a longer period depending on the area involved. Because this "cor-
seting" cannot "breathe," it is advisable to schedule the procedure for times
other than July and August.

Liposuction is useful not only for limited amounts of fat localized in the
abdomen or thigh and hip areas but also for fat at the inner knee, medial thigh,
ankle, arm, breast, and beneath the chin. It is often used to facilitate lipectomy.

Essentially it is a blind procedure, and complications such as blood and fluid
loss can less easily and promptly be detected. Embolism (a clot) may enter a
vessel and be carried to the lung, head, or heart and may be lethal. Venous
stasis may lead to occlusion of a major vessel (thrombosis). In most cases.
however, liposuction is accomplished satisfactorily, without any serious long-
term consequences. Under current investigation are new techniques using
ultrasonics, which have the advantage of reducing blood loss and promoting
faster healing. As matters now stand, the operation may take from 30 minutes

to 2 hours, depending on how extensive the area involved. Bruising, swelling, soreness, and numbness are normal aftereffects. Some women require heavy painkillers for several days, but the aches become tolerable soon after, diminishing gradually until they vanish completely. If the site of the liposuction is the hips or thighs, normal activities can usually be resumed according to the following schedule: walking—1 week; swimming—2 to 3 weeks; aerobic classes or dancing—4 to 5 weeks; running—8 to 10 weeks.

SUMMARY

More than in any other type of surgery, cosmetic procedures involve the entire person. Women who are to have these operations are encouraged to be in good mental health and to give up any habituating drugs, especially cigarette smoking. They should be as close to their ideal weight as possible. This will involve an exercise routine, together with a knowledge of fat, carbohydrate, and protein metabolism. When the mind and body are in good condition, improvement in appearance can bring much happiness to the patient.

ƒUBSTANCE ABUSE

Anne Geller, M.D.

Chief, Smithers Alcoholism Treatment and Training Center,
St. Luke's–Roosevelt Hospital Center, New York City;
Associate Professor of Medicine, College of Physicians and
Surgeons, Columbia University

Helene MacLean

Medical Writer and Editor; Author, *Caring for Your Parents,
Relief from Chronic Arthritis Pain;* Coauthor, *Recovering
from a Hysterectomy, Migraine: Beating the Odds*

Substances that alter mood and change perceptions and feelings have been used by humans since history was first recorded. They have been used in religious rituals to produce states of ecstasy or frenzy. They have been used to increase endurance and overcome fatigue. They have been used to lessen pain and suffering. They have been used in social gatherings. Recognizing the powerful effects of these substances, societies have developed rules and customs regulating their use.

In the United States attitudes and customs surrounding the use of mood-altering substances are extremely variable. They vary among ethnic and religious groups, they vary from region to region in the country, they vary according to age and to socioeconomic standing, and they vary from time to time depending on circumstances.

Today there are many points of view about how to define a mood-altering substance and about what standards to apply to "substance abuse." Is sugar a mood-altering substance? Is compulsive overeating "substance abuse"? Are smokers really drug addicts? Are you a drug addict if you can't get going in the morning unless you have a strong cup of coffee? Which drugs can legitimately be used by athletes?

On questions of substance abuse, there is not only a great deal of ambiguity; there is also considerable ambivalence. Take alcohol, for example. The so-called Prohibition Amendment to the United States Constitution is the only amendment that was ever repealed. Although progress is being made in apprehending drunk drivers and keeping them off the road, images of convivial gatherings almost always include beer, wine, or a bottle of hard liquor. Nor does the war on drugs or the war on crime ever spell out the role of alcohol in these plagues of society, especially their role in the physical abuse of women and children within the home.

Consider the ambivalence about smoking. The addiction to nicotine is responsible for higher costs to the nation and more deaths than any other addiction. Although cigarette vending machines are no longer accessible to children, and advertising campaigns with special appeal to youngsters are being more carefully scrutinized, smoking as a women's issue has never been addressed by the women's movement. The tobacco industry continues to capitalize on the lure of the liberated and sophisticated image or the subtext of Virginia Slims, a brand name that encodes one of the most successful advertising campaigns of all times: "Reach for a Lucky instead of a Sweet." We need to hear it said more often: *Smoking is a women's issue because women,* not men, *continue to smoke so that they won't gain weight.*

A recent development in medical circles is the specialty known as addiction medicine. Specialists in this field debate whether people can be "addicted" to gambling, exercise, or sex in the same way that they are addicted to nicotine or cocaine. (There are now dozens of addictions being addressed by 12-step groups modeled on Alcoholics Anonymous.) In calling this chapter "Substance Abuse," the authors have limited their concerns to conform to the protocol of the official diagnostic manual of the American Psychiatric Association. Physicians now make the formal diagnosis of "psychoactive substance dependence" when at least *three* of the following statements are true:

- The substance is taken in larger amounts or over a longer period than the person intended.
- There is a persistent desire or unsuccessful efforts to stop.
- The person spends a great deal of time trying to get the substance, taking it, or recovering from its effects.
- Using the substance disrupts important social obligations or work activities.

- The person continues to use the substance despite knowing that it is causing problems (such as drinking even though it makes an ulcer worse).
- There is marked tolerance: the person needs markedly increased amounts of the substance to become intoxicated or has a marked reduction of the desired effect if using the same amount.
- There are withdrawal symptoms.
- The substance is taken to avoid the withdrawal symptoms.

In this country the most widely used addictive substances are alcohol, nicotine, cocaine, crack-cocaine, amphetamines, and heroin. But in terms of sheer numbers, caffeine addiction leads all the rest in the form of coffee, tea, and cola drinks. Other inappropriately used psychoactive substances include sleeping pills and tranquilizers.

Perhaps taking the substance dependence test above will shed new light on your life-style choices. Each woman, except for those whose religious beliefs determine every aspect of their daily lives, must determine her own attitudes and her own patterns of behavior. There is a tremendous mythology surrounding alcohol and drug use: for example, that you can't become an alcoholic if you drink only beer or that cocaine is not addicting. And distressing as it may be, there has been considerable publicity about the high rate of substance abuse among physicians themselves. This professional problem has many consequences, not the least of which is a denial of the patient's addictions as a way of avoiding a confrontation with one's own.

Thus, a woman who wishes to make personal choices in terms of her physical and psychological well-being must inform herself and act in her own self-interest, free of social pressure and trendiness as well as of dependence on any single source as the final authority for what's good for her. As an autonomous adult, she can decide when to say "No," when to ask questions to get more information, when to contradict authority by presenting a body of facts, and, especially, when to seek help at the first sign of trouble.

It is hoped that the information that follows will enable you to meet the challenges of substance abuse. Also, if you are concerned about your own or someone else's alcohol or drug use, the sections on problem use and dependency should give you some guidelines. The section on obtaining help and information will enable you to take some action if necessary.

ALCOHOL

It is not known when the special properties of fermented fruit and grain were discovered, but from mute testimony of archaeological evidence it would seem that alcoholic beverages have been part of the human experience since before recorded history. Each society has had customs and rituals surrounding the use of alcohol. In some social and religious groups it is prohibited entirely; in others ritual use is permitted but intoxication proscribed. In our own pluralistic world, it is very difficult, perhaps impossible, to chart a course through the morass of conflicting views and to determine what is acceptable social drinking for a woman today. The problem has worsened as more and more women climb the corporate ladder or move into jobs where having a few drinks "with the guys" takes on the aura of a professional obligation. At the same time that this problem has intensified, however, many more men and women are joining their colleagues for lunch and dinner and, without any embarrassment or fuss, ordering a nonalcoholic beverage without skipping a beat. Even more important is the fact that business organizations in increasing numbers have established company policies that forbid the use of alcoholic beverages at any and all times when business is being conducted.

For women who do drink moderately and would like some guidelines to help them determine what constitutes a safe drinking pattern over which they have total control, here are some helpful facts. Alcohol is metabolized at a constant rate of ³⁄₄ ounce of absolute alcohol per hour. This is equivalent to one drink that contains 1½ ounces of 100 proof hard liquor, 4 ounces of wine, or 8 ounces of beer. If you drink faster than this, the blood and brain alcohol level will rise and you will experience some mood and behavior changes (see Table 1). Not only do women become drunk more quickly than men because they generally weigh less and also have proportionally more body fat to water, but if a woman matches drink for drink with a man, she will have a higher level of alcohol in her blood than he will because women have less of the stomach enzyme that breaks down alcohol before it goes into the bloodstream. A study published in the *New England Journal of Medicine* (1/90) reported that, because of this difference, women get about 30 percent more alcohol into the blood than men of similar weight who drink the same amount. You will therefore become drunk more quickly. Food in the stomach will delay the absorption of alcohol, but it will not prevent you from becoming intoxicated if you drink enough to do so.

TABLE 1

Weight (lbs.)				Blood Alcohol Level in Milligrams %	Behavior/Mood
100	125	150	175		

NO. DRINKS PER HOUR

100	125	150	175	Blood Alcohol Level in Milligrams %	Behavior/Mood
1–2	1–2	2–3	2–3	50–99	Euphoria, poor judgment
2–4	2–4	3–6	4–7	100–199	Poor coordination and thinking
4–6	5–7	6–9	7–10	200–299	Staggering, slurring, confusion
6–8	7–9	9+	10+	300–399	Anesthesia, memory lapses

For women the effect of a given amount of alcohol, say three drinks in an hour, varies with the stage of the menstrual cycle. This is because the amount of body fluid changes. Just before menstruation, when fluid is retained, there is more water in the body for the alcohol to be distributed in. Therefore the alcohol is present in a lower concentration and its effect on the central nervous system is reduced. Three drinks in one hour for a 130-pound premenstrual woman may make her happy, carefree, a little loquacious, impulsive, perhaps a bit clumsy. Taken in the middle of the menstrual cycle, the same amount is likely to cause stumbling, unfocused attention, uncontrolled giggling, and what can only be called socially inappropriate behavior.

Alcohol has a biphasic action. The initial effect is to stimulate thought, action, and social outgoingness and to induce a pleasant emotional state. If drinking continues, the depressant effects on the brain predominate with increasing disturbances in thinking and coordination. The pleasant mood evaporates, replaced by unpredictable mood swings, irritability, and depression. Because the initial effect is so pleasant, it is natural to try to recapture it or intensify it by drinking more. Alas, this cannot be done. Sensible social drinkers learn to bask in the evanescent glow provided by a drink or two, to sustain it by maintaining a low blood alcohol level, and then without regret to let it go.

The risks of drinking increase with the number of drinks you have. These include injuries from falls; inappropriate behavior; bumping into things; driving accidents; pedestrian accidents; being the victim of robbery, physical abuse, or date rape. And for women who have to go to work or have to meet the demands of small children at home, a hangover can cause serious problems.

WOMEN AND DRINKING PROBLEMS

Most people who drink do not consider themselves "problem drinkers." However, it is only since the 1970s that any research has been focused on women and alcohol. Here are some of the facts that have emerged.

According to the Fact Sheet issued by the National Council on Alcoholism and Drug Dependence in 1995:

- 4.1 million American women ages 18 and older can be classified as alcoholic or problem drinkers. Of these, 3.7 million are white and 0.3 million are nonwhite.
- A national survey of women's drinking found sexual dysfunction to be the most consistent predictor of chronic problem drinking.
- Alcohol is present in more than one-half of all incidents of domestic violence, with women most likely to be battered when *both* partners have been drinking.
- Moderate consumption of alcohol for women is defined by the federal government as no more than one drink per day.
- Women metabolize alcohol less efficiently than men, leading to higher blood concentrations over a shorter period of time and higher vulnerability to liver damage.
- Some studies suggest that alcohol consumption may be associated with a 10 percent increase in a woman's risk of developing breast cancer.
- Among college women there is a strong link between dieting and eating disorders and problem drinking.
- Women make up nearly a quarter of the individuals in treatment for alcoholism.
- Lack of child care is one of the most frequently reported barriers to treatment for alcoholic women.
- Alcohol problems that are more pronounced for women than for men include serious reproductive and sexual dysfunctions; rapid development of dependence; victimization by others, particularly spouses; and sexual victimization.

According to a recent study conducted by the Center on Addiction and Substance Abuse at Columbia University, the number of college women who drink excessively has tripled in the last 20 years, to the point where as many women as men engage in drinking in order to get drunk. The study said that the increased rate of drinking by women led to rape, violence, and accidents; 90 percent of all campus rapes occurred when alcohol had been used by either the assailant, the victim, or both. In addition, 60 percent of college women with sexually transmitted diseases like herpes or AIDS were drunk at the time of infection.

According to a study published in the *Journal of the American Medical Association* (7/12/95), women who are heavy drinkers are more at risk of developing a type of irreversible heart disease than men who drink even more. The condition, known as cardiomyopathy, is an overall weakening of the heart muscle.

For women who deny they have any "problems" with drinking but often find themselves drinking more than they "intended" to, there are many warning signs along the way: having an auto accident after leaving a party in a state of intoxication, missing work, being late to work because of a hangover, not getting the housework done, neglecting to feed and walk the dog, having memory lapses, having intercourse with someone distasteful, fighting with friends or hitting one's children, being preoccupied with drinking, getting sick or throwing up, and spraining an ankle because of stumbling. The list is inexhaustible and covers damage to physical health, psychological well-being, social relationships, employment, and legal standing. Women who have a problem connected with alcohol use may be reluctant to think about it or to seek advice for fear of being labeled alcoholic. What is important is not the label "alcoholic" but what is happening to you when you drink. If you had a problem connected with the use of alcohol in the past year, what did you do about it? Were you able to change your drinking pattern so that the problem was resolved or have the same or other problems recurred?

The test below, which you can give to yourself, can help you determine your profile with regard to drinking.

(The Michigan Alcoholism Screening Test—"MAST")

Directions: If a statement says something true about you, put a check in the space under YES. If a statement says something not true about you, put a check in the space under NO. Please answer all the questions and add the total number of points scored.

		YES	NO
1.	Do you feel you are a normal drinker?		2
2.	Have you ever awakened the morning after some drinking the night before and found that you could not remember a part of the evening?	2	

QUESTIONNAIRE ABOUT DRINKING PROBLEMS (*Continued*)

		YES	NO
3.	Does your wife/husband (or parents) ever worry or complain about your drinking?	1	
4.	Can you stop drinking without a struggle after one or two drinks?		2
5.	Do you ever feel bad about your drinking?	1	
6.	Do friends or relatives think you are a normal drinker?		2
7.	Do you ever try to limit your drinking to certain times of the day or to certain places?	1	
8.	Are you always able to stop drinking when you want to?		2
9.	Have you ever attended a meeting of Alcoholics Anonymous (AA)?	5	
10.	Have you gotten into fights when drinking?	1	
11.	Has drinking ever created problems with you and your wife/husband?	2	
12.	Has your wife/husband (or other family member) ever gone to anyone for help about your drinking?	2	
13.	Have you ever lost friends (girlfriends or boyfriends) because of your drinking?	2	
14.	Have you ever gotten into trouble at work because of your drinking?	2	
15.	Have you ever lost a job because of your drinking?	2	
16.	Have you ever neglected your obligations, your family, or your work for two or more days in a row because you were drinking?	2	
17.	Do you ever drink before noon?	1	
18.	Have you ever been told you have liver trouble?	2	
19.	Have you ever had delirium tremens (DTs), severe shaking, heard voices, or seen things that weren't there after heavy drinking?	5	
20.	Have you ever gone to anyone for help about your drinking?	5	
21.	Have you ever been in a hospital because of your drinking?	5	
22.	Have you ever been a patient in a psychiatric hospital or on a psychiatric ward of a general hospital where drinking was part of the problem?	2	
23.	Have you ever been seen at a psychiatric or mental health clinic, or gone to a doctor, social worker, or clergyman for help with an emotional problem in which drinking played a part?	2	

QUESTIONNAIRE ABOUT DRINKING PROBLEMS *(Continued)*

		YES	NO
24.	Have you ever been arrested, even for a few hours, because of drunk behavior?	2	
25.	Have you ever been arrested for drunk driving or driving after drinking?	2	

If you score: 0–3 points   You are probably a social drinker
                   4 points   You are borderline alcoholic
                   5 points or over   You are probably an alcoholic

Other good questions to ask:

Have you ever wondered whether you might be an alcoholic?
Have you ever felt you should cut down on your drinking?
Have you ever felt bad or guilty about your drinking?
Have people annoyed you by criticizing your drinking?
Have you ever had a drink first thing in the morning to steady your nerves or get rid of a hangover (eye-opener)?

ALCOHOL DEPENDENCE (ALCOHOLISM)

In the United States, alcohol dependence affects about 18 million adults and 4 million teenagers, and one arrest in three involves intoxication. For those who are alcohol-dependent, there is no consistent ability to control alcohol intake. Drinking takes place in response to intense psychological and physiological demands of which the drinker is often not aware. Although an alcohol-dependent drinker may be able to control intake for a time, sooner or later she drinks outside her intention, either drinking when she intended to abstain or drinking more than the limit she had set for herself. Because women who become alcohol-dependent drink for all the reasons normal drinkers do and often do not know they are at risk, and because the process of becoming addicted may take several years, it is not surprising that women deny to others and also to themselves the extent of their difficulties with alcohol. However, as more and more women enter the job market out of economic necessity, and as the compelling need to be gainfully employed comes into conflict with the compelling need to drink, more women than ever before are seeking treatment for their alcoholism. Thus, one in every three members of Alcoholics Anonymous is female, and many women are attending on-the-premises alcoholism treatment programs initiated by their employers. Also, women are becoming more aware of the need to take responsibility for their own health. Their consciousness has been raised by television programs and radio discussions that stress the negative effects of alcohol.

In addition to the personal misery and social distress suffered by the alcoholic woman, her life span is shorter by about 15 years than that of the average woman because of accidents while drinking and because of damage to organs in the body that can be fatal. Alcohol abuse eventually damages the heart, the liver, the ovaries, the brain, the nerves, the muscles, and the blood cells. It causes damage directly by attacking the delicate membranes surrounding cells and indirectly because of poor nutrition that usually accompanies heavy drinking. In addition to causing death from liver failure, fatal hemorrhage, or severe brain damage, alcohol causes illnesses such as inflammation of the liver (hepatitis), inflammation of the pancreas (pancreatitis), heart failure, damage to the bone marrow causing anemia, and severe memory loss. Alcoholic women may have irregular menstrual cycles, reduced fertility, and recurrent vaginal infections.

Coming from a family where there is alcoholism markedly increases the risk of developing the disease. If there are alcoholics in your family, you should be extra vigilant about your alcohol use. Being in an environment where there is heavy drinking will increase your exposure and, therefore, the risk. As an example of sensible disease prevention, if your father was an alcoholic you would be wise to avoid working in a cocktail lounge or being part of an office clique that makes a ritual of getting drunk after work on Fridays.

You should also be aware of some drinking patterns that are risky and may signify trouble with alcohol. These include being intoxicated more than once or twice a year; drinking more than a glass of wine or an occasional beer when alone; drinking specifically to relieve stress; drinking to allay anxiety before meeting someone or doing something; drinking to relieve symptoms such as insomnia, tension, depression, or pain; drinking after the party is over; and, of course, drinking the next morning to relieve the hangover.

ALCOHOLISM AS A FAMILY PROBLEM

Late-onset alcoholism is a problem only recently researched and publicly discussed. It is estimated that from 10 to 15 percent of the elderly in this country abuse alcohol. Of the approximately 2 million men and women in this category, about two-thirds have a long history of alcoholism, but as many as 700,000 older Americans develop the dependency after the age of 60.

The condition is usually precipitated by an emotional upheaval or a family crisis: the death of a spouse, divorce, retirement, or onset of a serious illness. Very often it is connected with a deepening depression caused by aging and the loss of independence.

If you spend time with your aging parents or relatives, be alert to the following symptoms and don't be quick to dismiss them as the inevitable consequence of growing old: falling asleep in social situations, slurred speech, unsteady walk, deterioration in personal appearance or compulsive neatness, improvised explanations about reclusiveness or memory losses, black and blue marks resulting from falls, general hostility and paranoia. In many instances, it is a concerned family member who calls the condition to the doctor's attention rather than the other way around. It is also important to keep in mind that not only does the susceptibility to the effects of alcohol increase with age but that older women are frequently taking various medications whose interaction with even small amounts of alcohol can produce disastrous effects.

Alcohol treatment programs designed for the elderly are not easy to find, and it takes great tact to get an older person to admit that the problem exists. But help is available through social services for the elderly and through geriatric clinics in some hospitals. And, of course, you may get the support you need and some useful referrals from Al-Anon.

Leaving aside the specific problem discussed above, it is difficult to say whether it is more painful to be an alcoholic, to be a daughter of an alcoholic, to be married to one, or to watch a child in the throes of alcoholism. It is not uncommon for women to have suffered through all four conditions, because alcoholism does run in families and children of alcoholics themselves not infrequently marry alcoholics. In the course of a lifetime, few of us are fortunate enough to be untouched by alcoholism. If not in ourselves or our immediate families, we may encounter it among our friends, our colleagues, our students, our employees. It does not spontaneously cure itself. If ignored it will continue. An alcoholic, like all addicted persons, is powerless to arrest the disease by herself. If it affects someone close to you, you will have to intervene.

First, find out where in your community an alcoholic can get help and also where you can get help if necessary. Next, confront the alcoholic person calmly and directly with your observations and concerns about his or her drinking behavior and with a list of the places where he or she can get help. You will be more effective if you intervene together with other people who are close to the alcoholic, but you can act alone as well. Then you have to set about changing your own behavior around the alcoholic's drinking, recognizing that you cannot control it by nagging or hiding the bottles; that you did not cause it, whatever the alcoholic person may imply; and that you cannot cure it. If, after your intervention, there is no significant change in the drinking, then you must consider what you have to do to improve the quality of your life. If the alcoholic is a spouse or a lover, you may decide that you must leave, but do not threaten to do so unless you intend to carry out your threat. Think of your own interest; paradoxically, this will be best for the alcoholic too. In the case of a friend you may say, with regret, that you cannot continue to see her while she is still drinking. Sometimes the actual loss of a spouse, lover, or friend will be the critical factor for recovery in an alcoholic. Al-Anon, an organization for the family and friends of alcoholics, can be a wonderful support during these crises.

In addition to and as an adjunct of Al-Anon several organizations have been formed as a result of recent investigations into the special problems of children of alcoholics and the psychological warp caused by growing up in a home where family dysfunction is caused by alcoholism. Al-Ateen maintains a schedule of self-help meetings for the younger offspring, and Al-Anon conducts meetings for the adult offspring. The National Association for Children of Alcoholics (founded in 1983) has a growing number of chapters nationwide, publishes literature, holds regional conventions, and supplies community guidance in the form of lectures and educational meetings. The Children of Alcoholics Foundation (founded in 1982) publishes pamphlets and acts as a clearinghouse for meetings of the various groups (including Al-Anon) that conduct self-help sessions attended by the adult children of alcoholics in the greater New York area.

Since its small-scale beginnings in 1935, the pioneering organization known as Alcoholics Anonymous (AA) has led the way in demonstrating to the professional world how uniquely effective the concept of self-help can be. As a result, there are now similar organizations that attempt to duplicate its success in coping with the many problems confronting all of us nowadays.

In a little more than 50 years, it has grown to a worldwide membership of more than 2 million people who attend meetings in over 90,000 groups on the five continents. The United States and Canada account for 51,000 meetings attended by over 1 million members with a common goal—to maintain their sobriety one day at a time.

If you want help with your addiction problems, look in your phone book. Make a call to find where and when a meeting is held, and go. All that will be asked of you will be your first name, a handshake at the door, and your attention when speakers tell their stories. You will soon learn that you are not alone if you have a drinking problem. There are millions of people in AA who share this problem and are helping each other—as they can help you—to deal with it. There is one woman to every two men among new AA members now, compared to one to ten 20 years ago, and the gap is narrowing. Larger cities have groups for women only; some areas have lesbian groups.

For those who feel the need for professional treatment, there are physicians, psychologists, social workers, clinics, alcoholism units in hospitals, and rehabilitation centers where expert care can be found. Use caution, though. Not all health professionals are equally knowledgeable. Many have not had formal training in this area. The National Council on Alcoholism has affiliates in major cities that maintain a list of treatment sources. Finally, local hospitals usually have inpatient alcoholism units for detoxification and/or outpatient clinics that can be contacted for both treatment and information.

A recent development that should be investigated is the drug naltrexone, used for the treatment of heroin addiction and approved in 1995 for the treatment of alcoholism. It is the first drug to be approved for this use in 45 years. Specialists emphasize that to maximize the effectiveness of naltrexone, it should be combined with counseling and other treatment components.

ALCOHOL AND PREGNANCY

Since 1989 the federal government has required that the following message be conveyed on the labels of all containers of alcoholic beverages: "GOVERNMENT WARNING: According to the Surgeon General, women should not drink alcoholic beverages during pregnancy because of the risk of birth defects."

The birth defects that characterize the condition that has come to be known as Fetal Alcohol Syndrome (FAS) include prenatal and postnatal growth deficiency, central nervous system dysfunction, and organ malformation. It is the third leading cause of mental retardation and the only one that is preventable. In milder cases the baby's birth weight is low, physical malformations are less dramatic, and behavioral problems are less easily identified. Making a diagnosis of fetal alcohol syndrome at birth is difficult because facial features that appear distorted may right themselves in a short time, and behavioral problems and deficient cognitive functioning do not become apparent until later. Hospital birth records are therefore not entirely reliable as a source of information about how many babies are born with health problems because their mothers drank too much during pregnancy. In 1995 the Centers for Disease Control's Birth Defects Monitoring Program, which uses the FAS diagnosis made during the neonatal period, reported that the rate had increased from 1 in 10,000 births in 1979 to 6.7 per 10,000 in 1993. The sixfold increase during the 15-year period occurred in spite of aggressive education campaigns and warnings on liquor bottles.

Medical authorities are not prepared to say exactly how much alcohol is harmful to the developing fetus; however, because there is evidence that even small amounts can be damaging, many doctors recommend no drinking at all. For example, a study sponsored by the federal government's Department of Health and Human Services indicates that pregnant women consuming between one and two drinks a day are twice as likely as nondrinkers to deliver a growth-retarded infant weighing less than 5.5 pounds. The same study warns that newborns whose mothers drink heavily (an average of five drinks per day, especially in the last three months of pregnancy) may show signs of alcohol withdrawal, such as tremors, sleeping problems, constant crying, and abnormal reflexes.

For women who want to know the risk of any drinking at all during pregnancy and what is a safe limit, our advice is that it is safest to abstain, although you shouldn't go through agonies of guilt if you have a glass of champagne to celebrate an important event, nor should you be filled with anxiety if you drank moderately before knowing you were pregnant. If you do have trouble abstaining, it would be a good idea to get some help.

SMOKING

Early in 1995 Dr. David A. Kessler, the commissioner of the FDA and a pediatrician by training, said that smoking was fundamentally a pediatric disease because most addiction to tobacco begins among teenagers. He added that a person who hasn't started smoking by age 19 is unlikely ever to become a smoker. This conclusion is borne out by the sales strategy of the tobacco industry, which has been targeting younger and younger children. As one top advertising executive puts it, "If the last ten years have taught us anything, it is that the tobacco industry is dominated by companies who respond most effectively to the needs of the younger smokers."

Dr. Kessler has also concluded that nicotine is a drug that should be regulated. This decision followed the revelation that the world's largest tobacco company had conducted 15 years of research on the effect of nicotine on smokers' bodies, brains, and behavior, and according to a Philip Morris scientist who participated in this research, the most crucial finding was that "the company could reduce the tar but increase the nicotine. . . . After all their work, they realized that nicotine was not just calming or stimulating, but it was having its effect centrally on the brain, and that people were smoking for brain effects."

In a *New York Times* interview (6/8/95) on the significance of publicizing the Philip Morris research, law professor Richard A. Daynard, chairman of the public health advocacy group Tobacco Products Liability Project, made the following comment: "These studies are extremely important. It seems that their own documents prove that they knew about the role of nicotine and the role of physiological need versus habit, and that they deliberately manipulated nicotine. It means that they understood more than they publicly acknowledged, even up to today."

The FDA's attempts at regulating nicotine are supported not only by these studies but also by the federal law stating that a substance must be regulated as a drug if the manufacturer intentionally uses it to "affect the structure or function of the body" of consumers. Although tobacco executives continue to deny the deadly nature of their product, the overwhelming majority of Americans say that cigarettes are addictive and that tobacco companies do not tell the whole truth in acknowledging the health risks of smoking. Considerable progress has been made in state and city laws that control where smoking is permissible, but members of Congress who have a tobacco-growing constituency are not likely to countenance categorizing nicotine as a drug that requires regulation.

A new understanding of exactly how nicotine exerts such a powerful influence on the thinking, alertness, mood, and addiction of smokers has been provided by researchers at Columbia Presbyterian Medical Center in an article in the journal *Science* (5/95). It appears that nicotine speeds up the flow of glutamate, a major neurotransmitter chemical that carries signals within the brain. Increasing the speed with which the signals are carried is likened to turning up the volume of a radio. Even a slight increase in the amount of nicotine in the blood delivered to brain tissue can heighten alertness and sharpen short-term memory. The chief author of the new study, Dr. Lorna Role, clarifies the addictive aspect of nicotine in this way: "Nicotine reaches the limbic part of the brain that includes the so-called reward system in which information is encoded that says 'That was good. Do it again.' As a result, the effect on the brain is to command the repeat of actions that keep up the nicotine levels in the bloodstream, prompting smokers to light up again. Thus people tend to self-administer in order to keep up the nicotine level." Her hope is that this research will help scientists learn how nicotine mimics natural brain substances that encourage rewarding behaviors. "It is important to understand why people are willing to inhale a couple of hundred class A carcinogens in order to get this agent nicotine."

Teenage girls say they smoke because it's "cool and sophisticated"; many women say they're hooked because it's the easiest way to stay thin; others find that smoking helps them deal with stress. Here are some of the hard facts and figures about women's addiction to nicotine:

- The risk of dying of lung cancer is 12 times higher for women smokers than for people who never smoked.
- Lung cancer death rates among women who smoke increased sixfold from the 1960s to the 1980s.
- Pack for pack, cigarettes may pose more of a lung cancer threat to women than to men.
- Early smoking apparently increases the risk of colorectal cancer for life, even if the smoker quits.
- Cigarette smoking increases women's risk of fractures by robbing the bones of their mineral density.
- The more a mother smokes after giving birth, the more behavioral problems her children are likely to have.
- Women who smoke are more susceptible to facial wrinkles than those who don't.
- Women who smoke 10 cigarettes a day are twice as likely to have a stroke as women who have never smoked, and those who smoke two packs a day are six times as likely, according to the American Heart Association.
- The benefits of estrogen replacement therapy in preventing bone fractures is wiped out for women who smoke, according to a 1992 report in the *Annals of Internal Medicine.*
- Women who smoke double their risk of heart disease. In some cases the risk is tripled.

In addition to the damage smoking inflicts on their own bodies, women must also consider the effects of smoking during pregnancy. A recent study published in the *Journal of Family Practice* (4/95) estimates that smoking by pregnant women causes the death of about 5,600 babies and 115,000 miscarriages every year in the United States. According to the American Cancer Society, smoking increases the likelihood of below normal weight of the newborn baby even if the delivery is at full term. Also, according to several studies in the United States and elsewhere, smoking may impair a woman's ability to breast-feed her baby. It has also been observed that women who smoke stop breast-feeding their infants much earlier than nonsmokers because nicotine lowers the levels of prolactin, a pituitary hormone that stimulates the production of milk. A recent study conducted at the University of California and published in the *Journal of the American Medical Association* (3/8/95) concluded that nursing mothers who smoke and caregivers who expose babies to cigarette smoke may double or even triple the infant's risk of dying of sudden infant death syndrome. (Among babies of nonsmokers, breast-feeding is associated with a 60 percent reduction in the risk of crib death.) As for older children whose respiratory problems are increased by exposure to secondary smoke, mothers who smoke are losing court battles for their custody in favor of a nonsmoking father or other family member.

On the other hand, a nonsmoking mother should make every effort to safeguard her health as well as the health of her children by preventing family members who smoke from doing so indoors.

SECONDARY SMOKE:

A MAJOR HEALTH HAZARD FOR CHILDREN

All over the United States nonsmokers are increasingly protected from the hazards of exposure to secondary smoke by laws that prohibit or restrict smoking in public places and require that employers strictly limit the workplace areas in which smoking is permitted. Such protection is not provided for the children of parents who smoke at home in spite of the rapidly accumulating evidence of the damaging consequences to their well-being. Results published in 1991 of an extensive study conducted by the National Study for Health Statistics indicate that children who live in households with smokers are almost twice as likely to be in fair or poor health as children never exposed to cigarette smoke. It is calculated that half of all children in the United States who are 5 years or younger live in households polluted with cigarette smoke. This means that about 10 million children are

- breathing in poisonous carbon monoxide, a substance in cigarette smoke that stays in the air for hours and increases the likelihood of respiratory disabilities;
- experiencing speeded-up heart rates and increased blood pressure levels;
- more likely to have debilitating asthma attacks;
- more likely to miss attending school because of respiratory ailments.

Other studies report similarly alarming facts: Children under 5 whose mothers smoke no more than 10 cigarettes a day in their presence have positive blood tests for nicotine and cancer-causing chemical compounds. A 12-year study publicized by the American Lung Association indicates that children exposed to cigarette smoke early in life have significantly impaired lung function that can last into early adulthood. Scientists have also reported that children of smokers scored lower on tests of reasoning ability and vocabulary than children of nonsmokers. These results have been attributed to the fact that breathing in tobacco smoke may reduce oxygen to the brain, thus impairing thinking ability, and also increases the frequency and seriousness of middle ear infections. Whatever the details of the effect on children, the bottom line has been articulated by Dr. Louis W. Sullivan, former secretary of Health and Human Services: "I can't think of a more compelling reason for parents to quit smoking than insuring their children's chance for a healthy life."

IT'S QUITTING TIME!

"I'd like to quit but I don't want to gain 25 pounds."

Yes, it's true that women who stop smoking do gain some weight even if they don't eat any differently or exercise less. According to a study published in the *New England Journal of Medicine,* it is the nicotine in cigarettes that makes smokers burn more calories. A weight gain of 6 to 8 pounds is therefore inevitable over a 5-year period and should not be a cause for guilt. Even women who gain more weight than that over a longer period enjoy the health benefits of having stopped smoking.

"I've tried several times to quit 'cold turkey' but I seem to need a transitional crutch. What about nicotine gum?"

Nicotine-laced chewing gum was approved by the FDA in 1984 and is available without a prescription under the trade name Nicorette. It is most effective when used according to instructions and when the smoker is involved in an organized support program. Although its use seems to be trading one addiction for another, there is ample evidence that it is much easier to quit the gum than to quit smoking. In addition, the gum is less of a threat to health because it does not carry with it the dangers to the lungs of inhaling smoke and tars. Nor does it provide the powerful impediment to stopping that smoking does, namely, about one-fourth of the nicotine that enters the lungs when inhaling cigarette smoke reaches the receptor cells in the brain in 7 seconds, whereas the nicotine in the gum is absorbed through the cheeks and takes almost one-half hour to reach peak level in the bloodstream. Thus, it provides the drug "fix" without providing the quick "rush" that cigarette smokers count on.

"I hate chewing gum. Are the nicotine patches just as helpful?"

Nicotine transdermal systems, known as "skin patches," are designed to help smokers quit by continually releasing nicotine directly into the bloodstream through a patch worn on the arm. More than 4 million smokers use nicotine patches every year in their efforts to stop smoking. The three products on the market since 1992 have FDA approval and are available only by prescription. Of the three—Habitrol, Nicoderm, and ProStep—ProStep is the only one whose advertising makes it clear that it can be effective only in connection with participation in a stop-smoking program that helps overcome psychological addiction. Specialists say that it is too soon to predict with certainty whether the patches provide a *permanent* solution to giving up smoking. A study in the *Journal of the American Medical Association* (6/22/94) indicates a quarter of smokers using the patches continue to abstain after six months. This study has also found that smokers were as likely to quit if they wore the patch for 6 to 8 weeks as they were if they wore the patch for the recommended 10 to 18 weeks. The 8-week regimen costs approximately $224; the 12-week regimen costs about $350.

While a few women can go through all the withdrawal discomforts on their own, 95 percent of all smokers can kick the addiction when they are cheered on by a support group such as Smokers Anonymous or through attending such programs as those run by the American Cancer Society or the American Lung Association. Programs are also available through hospitals, community organizations, and corporate health efforts. Some hospitals now have inpatient programs that use behavior modification and changes in diet.

Some women have achieved success through treatment by an acupuncturist or a hypnotist. If you're contemplating either of these practitioners, be sure to check on licensing and credentials. Also of benefit are relaxation and breathing exercises and meditation techniques that provide more wholesome ways of dealing with stress than smoking. (See "Alternative Therapies" for details.)

For most women who truly want to stop smoking, it may take several attempts over a period of three or four years. The more serious the intentions, the greater the likelihood of success. It is generally agreed that the most effective techniques are based on behavior modification and self-monitoring of habitual reflexes. Here are some practical suggestions from the American Cancer Society:

- Throw away all your cigarettes at bedtime the night before you stop smoking.
- As soon as you wake up, take a cool shower and drink a glass of orange juice.
- Switch from coffee to tea or low-calorie chocolate milk at breakfast, don't linger over it, and leave the house fast.

- At your workplace, get busy at once, and if you must spend time on the phone, doodle on a scratch pad.
- Because smoking is forbidden in many places of employment but a cigarette break is allowed in restricted areas, use this time to stand up and take deep breaths.
- Drink at least six to eight glasses of water a day.
- When you return home, avoid alcoholic beverages including wine at dinner.
- Keep busy and change the chair in which you customarily watch television.
- Exercise as much as possible.

Remember that 40 million Americans have stopped smoking, and for a considerable number it took more than one try. Some women find that if they take a "one-day-at-a-time" approach, they can breathe a nonsmoker's sigh of relief each night. Others work at developing a new self-image: not "I'm trying to stop smoking," but "I'm a nonsmoker" and "I have too much self-esteem to smoke."

Many women who have been heavy smokers for many years and who have stopped complain that no one prepared them for how long it would take to get over the withdrawal effects. Be prepared for months or even a year of unfocused anger, sleeplessness, headaches, a disrupted gastrointestinal system, and slower mental responses. But in the final accounting, what a relief to be able to say, "I was once a drug addict and I'm not anymore."

CAFFEINE

More people use caffeine worldwide than any other psychoactive substance. It is found in plants everywhere and has been favored throughout history (and probably prehistorically) as a mood elevator that combats fatigue, increases alertness, and promotes clear thinking. It is ingested by drinking tea, coffee, cola beverages, and in many places, by chewing the leaves and beans of the cacao plant. American women consume large amounts of caffeine in over-the-counter painkillers (Anacin, Excedrin, Midol) as well as in such prescription drugs as Cafergot, Fiorinal, and Darvon. Chemically its effect on the brain and central nervous system is similar to but somewhat milder than that of amphetamines. In most women one good cup of coffee can produce a "high" that lasts for several hours. Other effects on the body: caffeine dilates the arteries that feed the heart, thereby increasing blood flow to that organ, and constricts the arteries in the head, making it a helpful treatment for migraine.

While few women suffer ill effects from caffeine and many develop a high tolerance to it, there are those who are especially sensitive to it, complaining of insomnia and digestive problems when they drink only two cups of coffee a day. Although they are likely to switch to decaffeinated coffee or tea, they may not be aware of how much caffeine they are consuming in cola beverages and over-the-counter medications. However, drinking decaf beverages appears to be part of a health-conscious life-style that includes regular exercise, vitamin consumption, and eating more broccoli.

Most women consume an average of 200 milligrams of caffeine a day, the amount contained in three cups of coffee. Consuming fewer than five cups of regular coffee seems to create no additional cardiac risk. Beyond that limit, the risk of heart trouble increases both for smokers and nonsmokers and especially for women who have high blood pressure. Ongoing studies of caffeine consumption and breast cancer do not confirm a positive connection, nor does caffeine consumption cause fibrocystic breast syndrome, although it may increase the symptoms. The debate continues about whether heavy caffeine consumption is the cause of bladder cancer, but the answer is a definite yes in regard to loss of bone density. An ongoing Yale University study has found that older women who consumed over 800 milligrams of caffeine a day were three times as likely to suffer a hip fracture as those who consumed no caffeine. Conflicting conclusions continue to be published about whether immoderate caffeine consumption reduces the ability to conceive or results in low birth weight babies or increases the likelihood of miscarriage. Dr. James L. Mills, a researcher at the National Institute of Child Health and Human Development who studies caffeine's effects on pregnancy, says, "I don't think caffeine is the problem, but during pregnancy, you should be cautious about any substance that has a metabolic effect" (New York Times, 9/13/95).

Caffeine has always been recognized by the FDA as a drug, and scientists accept the fact that of the millions of Americans who consume it, a small number are addicted to it in the same way that others are addicted to alcohol or nicotine even when it represents a serious threat to their well-being. The strength of this dependency is not necessarily related to the amounts consumed. A woman who drinks only two or three cups of coffee a day and decides to go "cold turkey" may suffer the same withdrawal symptoms as one who depends on the effect of two or three times that amount: lethargy, depression, intense headaches, anxiety attacks, and functional impairment.

If you're determined to cut down on "real" coffee or eliminate it altogether eventually, go about it gradually. To minimize withdrawal symptoms, experts recommend cutting down your intake by 20 percent a week over a period of about a month. It may be easier to measure your success by using instant coffee until you reach a goal of half a teaspoon a day in half a cup of water. And remember not to cheat with cola drinks or caffeine-laced headache remedies.

PRESCRIPTION AND NONPRESCRIPTION DRUGS

Because prescription tranquilizers, sleeping pills, and painkillers have a high mood-altering potential, they are easily misused. Misuse unfortunately can become abuse, that is, using them in greater amounts or for purposes other than those for which they were prescribed and thereby developing a psychological and/or physical dependency.

Does this mean that sensible women should avoid these drugs altogether? No. Nothing so extreme is being suggested. However, *all* drugs should be given serious evaluation both by the doctor and the patient. (See the chapter on "Plain Talk About Medications" for details about the most widely used prescription and nonprescription drugs and how to use them responsibly. Special information is included about those medications that are potentially addictive.)

ILLEGAL DRUGS

The harm to health of the legal drugs alcohol, nicotine, and caffeine have been described in detail. And while some women have abused prescription drugs, the vast majority of users of these drugs are not taking them in order to get high, get a kick, get a rush, be sociable, or be in fashion. Street drugs or "recreational" drugs are quite different. No one is using them innocently as medication only to discover by accident that they have attractive and compelling mood-altering effects. They are being used specifically for these effects from the start. There is, however, a good deal of innocence and ignorance about the nature of these mood changes, the side effects, the dangers of addiction, and the hangover effects.

Whether they are willing to admit it or not, women who use illegal drugs are actively contributing to crime on the streets, and street crimes make waves powerful enough to affect *everyone's* safety. When you turn down offers of illegal drugs, you safeguard not only your personal health and well-being but also the well-being of your family and your community.

Knowing about the dangers of street drugs is one of the best ways to be armed against them.

COCAINE

Cocaine is found in the leaves of *Erythroxylon coca*, a shrub growing in the Andes. The natives of Peru have for centuries chewed these leaves for their stimulant effects, their suppression of hunger, and the euphoria that counteracts the demands of unremitting hard work. However, the amount of active drug extracted in this fashion is quite small, sufficient to produce a sense of well-being and increased energy but not enough to cause the devastating dependency resulting from the use of the highly concentrated drug available for the past century in Europe and the United States.

The United States is now in the midst of its second cocaine epidemic. The first occurred in the late nineteenth century when cocaine was hailed as the wonder drug by, among others, Sigmund Freud. It was widely used in patent medicines and, of course, was the prime ingredient in Coca-Cola. It was not long before serious problems with intoxication and dependency began to surface. In 1914 its use was legally restricted by the U.S. government. Interestingly, its use declined when amphetamines became available, only to rise again 50 years later when amphetamines fell out of favor. (It has also been used as a local anesthetic since 1984.)

Cocaine is sold on the street as a fine white powder sometimes called coke or snow. It can be snorted, smoked, or injected intravenously. The effects, which last for about 30 minutes, include a feeling of euphoria, heightened self-confidence, a rush of energy, and intensified sensuality. It is an effective appetite suppressant, and whatever the route by which it is taken, it gets into the bloodstream quickly, producing a more intense effect than amphetamines or other stimulants taken by mouth.

Cocaine is currently the second most widely used illegal drug following marijuana. It is estimated that 30 million men and women in the United States have tried cocaine and more than 5 million use it regularly. Because the high is so rapidly succeeded by the low as the effects wear off, there is a compelling desire to take it again as soon as it is available. When the drug becomes habitual, users suffer from increasingly damaged self-esteem, nervousness, insomnia, inability to concentrate, fatigue, anxiety, and depression. Women can become nonorgasmic and men impotent.

Cocaine carries with it the same risks whether it is snorted or injected into the skin, muscles, or veins. Eventually, in addition to risks of addiction, it can painlessly and permanently injure the heart muscle, leading to dangerously irregular heartbeats that can result in sudden death. Convulsive seizures and hallucinations are not uncommon. Although there is a widespread belief that cocaine is an aphrodisiac, long-term use produces difficulties in maintaining an erection and producing ejaculation in men, and difficulty in reaching orgasm for women. Used during pregnancy, cocaine can cut off the supply of oxygen to the fetus and kill it or it can cause premature delivery of low birth weight babies who have tremors and are unusually irritable.

About one in every three cocaine-dependent people in the United States is a woman. It is estimated that 53 percent of the women referred for treatment are under 30, and of these a significant number are also addicted to alcohol and amphetamines, spending as much as $500 a week on their addictions. They are usually in middle- or upper-income brackets, well educated, in competitive demanding jobs, or dissatisfied with their lives.

An increasing number of women who enter AA are determined to put an end to their dependence on all drugs, both legal and illegal. Help is also available at many special treatment centers, both on an inpatient and outpatient basis.

Emergency information and referral can be obtained by dialing the 24-hour hotline 1-800-COCAINE (262-2463).

In the past few years, cocaine in its smokable form, known as *crack*, has become the street drug most closely associated with inner city crime. (The term crack refers to the crackling sound heard when the cocaine rocks are heated for smoking.) The processing results in a much more powerful form of cocaine than the white powder that is snorted. The small chunks of cocaine rocks are smoked in a pipe, placed in regular cigarettes, or combined with marijuana in a joint. Crack is deadlier than ordinary cocaine because it delivers a concentration of the drug to the brain and bloodstream high enough to lead to respiratory and cardiac failure. Although the intense "high" produced by smoking crack lasts only a few minutes, it produces a craving powerful enough to become a lifetime addiction.

HEROIN

Unlike cocaine, heroin is a narcotic substance that belongs in the category of opiates, a category that derives from the opium poppy and also includes morphine. The term *opiate* has come to be used interchangeably with the term *narcotic*, which is defined (in *Webster's Tenth New Collegiate Dictionary)* first as "a drug (as opium) that in moderate doses dulls the senses, relieves pain, and induces profound sleep, but in excessive doses causes stupor, coma, or convulsions." Thus, strictly speaking, although cocaine is *not* a narcotic but a stimulant, the term *narcotic* has come to be used generically to cover practically all illegal drugs.

During the nineteenth century and into the twentieth, opiates were legal and widely used not only to alleviate pain but also, especially in the form of laudanum, to minimize the discomfort of headaches, menstrual cramps, and gastrointestinal distress. The widely advertised "little pink pills" and "magic elixirs" were innocently used as "nerve medicine" by millions of women who were quite literally drug addicts without anyone's especially noting the nature of their dependence. (Audiences have been made aware of one woman's descent into morphine dependence at the turn of the century in Eugene O'Neill's great play *Long Day's Journey Into Night.)*

Heroin itself was considered a blessing when it first became available because it seemed a viable solution to the morphine addiction that had become so widespread among the wounded soldiers of the Civil War. Thus, heroin once stood in the same relation to morphine that methadone now stands to heroin.

Heroin can be used by skin-popping, snorting, injecting it under the skin, or injecting into a vein. The latter procedure is called "mainlining." Its effects are produced quickly, and they last from three to four hours. Heroin use goes all the way up the social scale, and many middle-class users as well as entertainers and athletes are in methadone maintenance programs.

While only a limited number of susceptible women become alcoholics—and only after at least five years of heavy use—heroin addiction can develop more quickly and with chronic use comes a large number of serious physical disorders: lung abscesses, liver impairment, and brain/mind dysfunction. The result of injecting the drug with a contaminated needle is the AIDS death penalty. Death can also result from an overdose large enough to suppress the actions of the central nervous system to the point where heart and lungs cease functioning.

In 1994 it began to be reported that high-grade heroin that could be smoked rather then injected was replacing cocaine as the drug of choice on both coasts, especially among trend-setting young people in the film, rock, and fashion industries. Hospitals were reporting an alarming surge in heroin-related emergencies; federal law enforcement officials noted that the increase in heroin use was crossing socioeconomic lines, with the most dramatic surge occurring among the rich and educated. Heroin-related celebrity deaths did nothing to counteract the notion that it was "hip to be high." What took heroin out of the ghetto was its new availability in a purer, cheaper form resulting from bumper crops of the drug-yielding poppies in Southeast Asia and Latin America. Declining prices led to the increasing purity of the product sold on the street—skyrocketing from 4 percent to an average purity of 65 percent. This new potency was making it possible to get high by snorting or smoking the drug, eliminating the need to inject it and removing the fear of the needle and the attendant possibility of contracting the AIDS virus. Although more expensive than crack, even high-quality heroin was becoming cheaper than cocaine, with the advantage that a heroin high could last as long as six hours—much longer than the rush produced by cocaine.

On Monday, August 14, 1995, the *New York Times* ran a story with the headline "The Middle Class Rediscovers Heroin: Its Improved Image Suits the 90s and Entices More Professionals." The event that prompted the headline was the death of a female stockbroker and mother of two children, the death resulting from an all-night heroin-snorting binge with her husband. When tested by the police, the heroin recovered from their apartment was reported to be 80 percent pure.

This highly potent heroin, called black magic on the street, is especially lethal to new users, who have a tendency to treat it like cocaine, which requires larger doses to produce a high. It is also more insidious in producing addiction because its hold on body and mind is subtle enough to give the user a false sense of security about being in control of the habit.

Professional women, women on college campuses, creative women in the arts, and health professionals are turning up in ever-larger numbers at treatment centers. They are discovering that breaking the habit is quite different from giving up cocaine or cigarettes. Former addicts describe withdrawal symptoms that are difficult to endure—heavy sweating, tremors, hot and cold flashes, cramps, anxiety, and above all, a profound craving for the drug. None of these symptoms is life-threatening, and, in fact, some addicts who have kicked the habit "cold turkey" have survived to tell the tale with pride.

Treatment with the synthetic opiate methadone substitutes one addiction for another, but it enables those who participate in such programs in a disciplined way to function as productive members of society. Therapeutic residence communities have been attracting women who want to be rid of *all* drug dependencies. Information and referral for methadone programs and other types of treatment as well as support groups can be obtained through hospitals and social service groups in the community.

MARIJUANA

The source of this mildly hallucinogenic drug is the hemp plant *Cannabis sativa,* a common weed that has been used as an intoxicant for about 5,000 years, making its way from Asia to North Africa, and by 1800, to Europe. It has also been known for centuries in the Western hemisphere, but its use in the United States did not become popular until the 1920s, and it was not until the 1960s that marijuana peaked as the illegal drug of choice among the young. At the same time that marijuana smoking declined among high school and college students in 1986, cocaine use as well as the use of alcohol increased.

Like the tobacco leaf, the leaf of the marijuana plant is dried, crushed, and smoked in the form of a cigarette. It is estimated that more than 60 million people in the United States have tried it, including men and women of impeccable social and intellectual credentials, and about 25 million use it regularly because of the pleasurable state of relaxation it induces. It also causes some changes in perception: colors may appear to be brighter and the sense of time is lost. Because memory, logical thinking, and coordination are impaired, driving and smoking marijuana can be a deadly combination.

By 1994 pot began to make a major comeback among teenagers, and because of more efficient methods of harvesting and processing, the marijuana they are using is about 20 times more potent than the pot that used to be sold on the street 20 and 30 years ago. Pointing to new findings about the nature of addiction and the effect of marijuana use on memory, the lungs, and the immune system, Dr. Richard S. Rosenthal, president of New York–based Phoenix House, the country's largest residential drug treatment organization, says that the most recent information suggests that pot was never harmless. Sociologists and law enforcement officials believe that with the increase in teenage violence and the threat of AIDS, any drug use that lowers inhibitions represents a threat to the community.

Many of today's young marijuana users are the offspring of middle-class parents who have fond memories of their participation in the laid-back drug culture of the sixties, and because these parents feel they suffered no permanent ill effects from their use of marijuana, they may feel it won't hurt their children either. But many of their children are beginning to smoke a very much stronger product, and they're beginning to smoke it even before age 14, when their growing bodies are considerably more vulnerable to its negative effects. (In 1993 marijuana use among eighth graders increased twice as fast as in the previous year.) Mothers should know that something needs fixing if schoolwork suffers, too much time is spent alone, and physical activities are ignored altogether. Short-term counseling at this stage by an experienced professional may keep the situation from getting out of control through parental neglect.

The responsible adult woman who uses marijuana as a recreational drug ("responsible" certainly means *not in the presence of her children)*, should be informed of the extent of its effect on her health. There is no evidence that prolonged use causes permanent changes in the nervous system or impairment of brain function, nor is there evidence of permanent damage to the normal cardiovascular system. However, because it does cause changes in heart and circulation performance characteristic of stress, it poses a threat to anyone who suffers from hypertension, cerebrovascular disease, and coronary atherosclerosis. There is no clear connection between marijuana use and cancer.

According to a report issued by the Institute of Medicine of the National Academy of Sciences, there is no evidence of marijuana's harmful effects on male or female fertility. There is evidence, however, that the active ingredient in the drug does pass into breast milk, producing undesirable effects in nursing infants.

Chronic heavy use can result in loss of energy and drive, slow thinking, and apathy. Marijuana can certainly cause psychological dependence, where the user is preoccupied with the drug, experiences a craving for it, and is unable to do without it. Withdrawal symptoms, typically restlessness, irritability, and anxiety, do occur when the drug use is stopped. Dependent users suffer from considerable emotional distress regarding their drug use as well as disorganization in their daily life and often loss of jobs and family. As with alcohol, signs of dependence include preoccupation with obtaining an adequate supply, unsuccessful attempts to cut down, guilt and unwillingness to talk about the drug, personality changes, increasing isolation, and social dysfunction.

LSD (LYSERGIC ACID DIETHYLAMIDE)

This most publicized and widely used of the synthesized hallucinogenic substances was created in 1943 by a Swiss scientist trying to find a remedy for migraine headaches. About 10 years later, the CIA conducted experiments with it hoping to find a "mind-control" drug. Somewhat later still a few psychotherapists used LSD to induce "experimental psychosis," thinking that in this way they might be able to gain greater understanding of the biochemical basis of mental illness.

The use of LSD was eventually democratized at Harvard University by Timothy Leary, who carried his offbeat messages far and wide. Leary was an offbeat psychologist whose behavior throughout his life continued to be that of an antiestablishment adolescent. His early promotion of LSD made it one of the favorite turn-ons of the sixties drug scene. It was promoted as a transcendental experience that expanded perceptions, offering sounds and colors impossible to duplicate in the real world. But an accumulation of adverse publicity about permanent neurological damage, irreversible psychosis, accidental deaths, and suicides resulting from casual use put an end to its widespread popularity—for the time being. In the nineties LSD began to make a comeback on campuses as well as in clubs where the cocaine crowd congregate. LSD is no longer connected with rebellion but rather has been taking its place in the list of street drugs considered to be part of the smart recreational scene. Women tempted to "try" LSD should be aware of the following consequences: even a minimum amount can produce a state resembling acute psychosis and should therefore never be ingested when one is alone. A bad trip, or a "bummer," may cause acute panic and may lead to a suicide attempt. (A euphoric trip may lead the user to believe she can "fly" and attempt to do so by taking off from the nearest open window.) The psychotic effect usually wears off in 12 to 18 hours, but a recurrence may occur without warning at any time in the future. Like other hallucinatory drugs such as mescaline, LSD increases the heart rate and blood pressure and causes sleeplessness. Long-term use is known to cause mental impairment, including irreversible memory loss and abbreviated attention span. An overdose can be fatal.

CONCLUSION

Understanding the hazards of substance abuse can be comparatively simple. The legal drug that can kill you before your time and impair the health of your children is nicotine. The legal drug that can lead to a dependency in which you have lost control over your life is alcohol. Legally prescribed drugs such as tranquilizers and sleeping pills can result in addiction unless they are used only for the period and the purpose for which they have been prescribed. And as for the whole range of illegal drugs, from comparatively harmless marijuana to life-threatening cocaine—saying "No" is the easiest way to ensure your well-being as a law-abiding citizen and as a woman who makes intelligent choices to safeguard her physical and mental health.

DOMESTIC VIOLENCE, SEXUAL ABUSE, AND RAPE

Dorothy J. Hicks, M.D.

Professor of Obstetrics and Gynecology, University of Miami School of Medicine; Consultant, Rape Treatment Center, Jackson Memorial Hospital, Miami, Florida

The increasing violence in our society is reflected in the growing incidence within the family of sexual assault and the battering of children, women, and the elderly. Psychologists, sociologists, and other professionals point out that these crimes usually occur when an accumulation of frustration and rage can no longer be contained. The result in many cases may be an explosive assault so violent as to be life-threatening to the victim, who is always physically weaker than the perpetrator. While alcohol is a common factor in many of these occurrences, even more common is the fact that the perpetrators themselves have been victims of sexual abuse or repeated beatings in their own past.

The definitions of abuse and battering have also been expanded to include prolonged and unremitting psychological abuse and threats short of violence but completely demoralizing to the victims.

In recent years, many of these crimes have come out of the closet and onto the television screen in the form of documentaries about incest, docudramas about battered women who eventually murdered their husbands, and news stories about battered children brought to the hospital dead on arrival. The category known as "date rape" is becoming increasingly familiar, and the term "grannybashing" is heard in family courts to distinguish this particular crime from one in which an elderly person is attacked at home or mugged on the street by an unknown assailant.

Thus, the general public is being enlightened through films, plays, community forums, and newspaper editorials so that as activists, citizens, and potential jurors, they can achieve a better understanding of these crimes and as possible victims, they can know how to seek protection and help.

Equally important are the increasing efforts to broaden the awareness and deepen the sensitivity of lawmakers, police, doctors, social workers, and hospital personnel to the widespread nature of assaultive and sexually aberrant behavior in the home. It is hoped that because of these efforts, problems of rape, incest, and domestic violence will be viewed not only in terms of the "sickness" of individuals or of the pathology of the family but from the point of view of the laxity and inadequacy of the legal and criminal justice system. Among the results of these efforts is the formation of advocacy groups and coalitions to lobby for legislation that takes reality into account rather than denying it.

DOMESTIC VIOLENCE

In 1994, after years of lobbying, Congress passed the Violence Against Women Act and earmarked $1.6 billion for its programs. That same year saw the passage of domestic violence laws in several states, including New York, New Jersey, Connecticut, and California, providing for mandatory arrests in cases of complaints, more stringent penalties for repeat offenders, and training for law enforcement officials on how to respond to domestic violence. In March 1995 the Clinton administration established the Violence Against Women Office within the Department of Justice. This new agency controls a six-year budget of $800 million, of which more than one-quarter will be distributed to the states. While half the state funds are to be earmarked for bolstering law enforcement and prosecution, at least one-quarter must be allocated for local nonprofit victim services and advocacy groups. (These funds are likely to be reduced by $50 million by a Congress bent on cutting government spending.)

Though these projects had been under consideration for many years, some

A Woman's Body

STRUCTURE AND FUNCTIONS IN FULL COLOR

Illustrated by Leonard D. Dank

SKELETAL SYSTEM

VOLUNTARY MUSCULAR SYSTEM

CIRCULATORY SYSTEM

ENDOCRINE SYSTEM

RESPIRATORY SYSTEM

DIGESTIVE SYSTEM

NERVOUS SYSTEM

URINARY SYSTEM

REPRODUCTIVE SYSTEM

THE BREAST

EMOTIONS AND THE BODY

SKELETAL SYSTEM

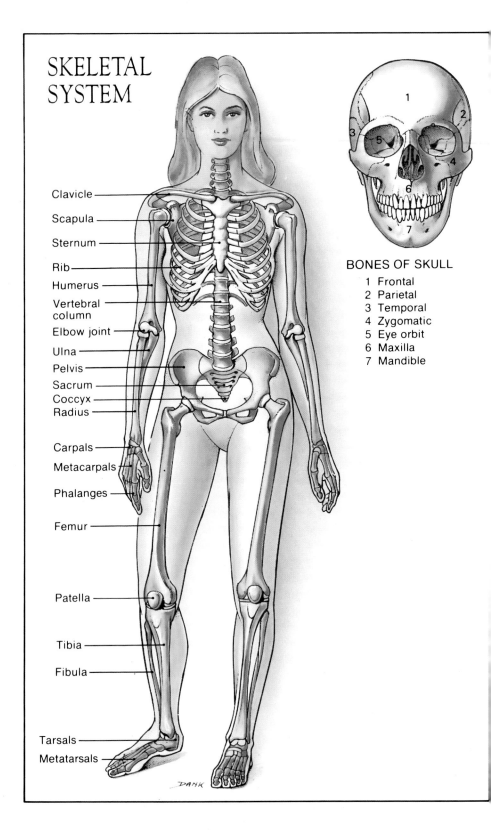

Clavicle

Scapula

Sternum

Rib

Humerus

Vertebral column

Elbow joint

Ulna

Pelvis

Sacrum

Coccyx

Radius

Carpals

Metacarpals

Phalanges

Femur

Patella

Tibia

Fibula

Tarsals

Metatarsals

DANK

BONES OF SKULL

1 Frontal
2 Parietal
3 Temporal
4 Zygomatic
5 Eye orbit
6 Maxilla
7 Mandible

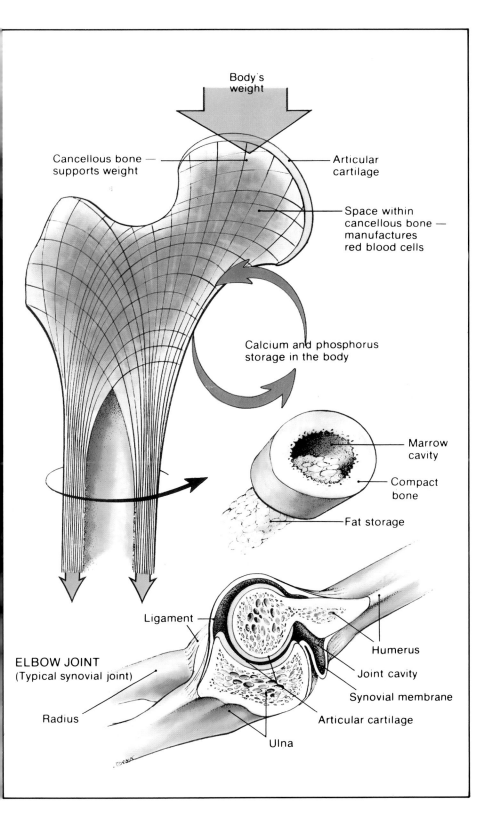

Body's weight

Cancellous bone — supports weight

Articular cartilage

Space within cancellous bone — manufactures red blood cells

Calcium and phosphorus storage in the body

Marrow cavity

Compact bone

Fat storage

ELBOW JOINT
(Typical synovial joint)

Ligament

Radius

Ulna

Humerus

Joint cavity

Synovial membrane

Articular cartilage

ENDOCRINE SYSTEM

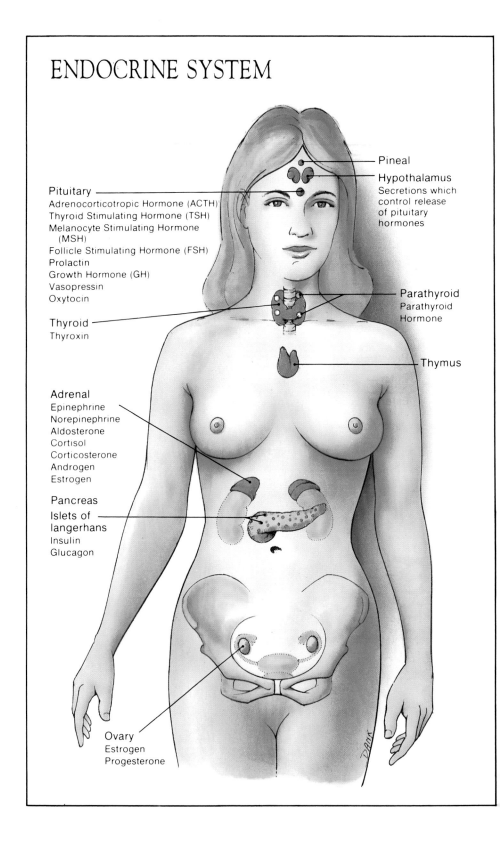

Pineal

Hypothalamus
Secretions which
control release
of pituitary
hormones

Pituitary
Adrenocorticotropic Hormone (ACTH)
Thyroid Stimulating Hormone (TSH)
Melanocyte Stimulating Hormone
(MSH)
Follicle Stimulating Hormone (FSH)
Prolactin
Growth Hormone (GH)
Vasopressin
Oxytocin

Thyroid
Thyroxin

Parathyroid
Parathyroid
Hormone

Thymus

Adrenal
Epinephrine
Norepinephrine
Aldosterone
Cortisol
Corticosterone
Androgen
Estrogen

Pancreas
Islets of
langerhans
Insulin
Glucagon

Ovary
Estrogen
Progesterone

RESPIRATORY SYSTEM

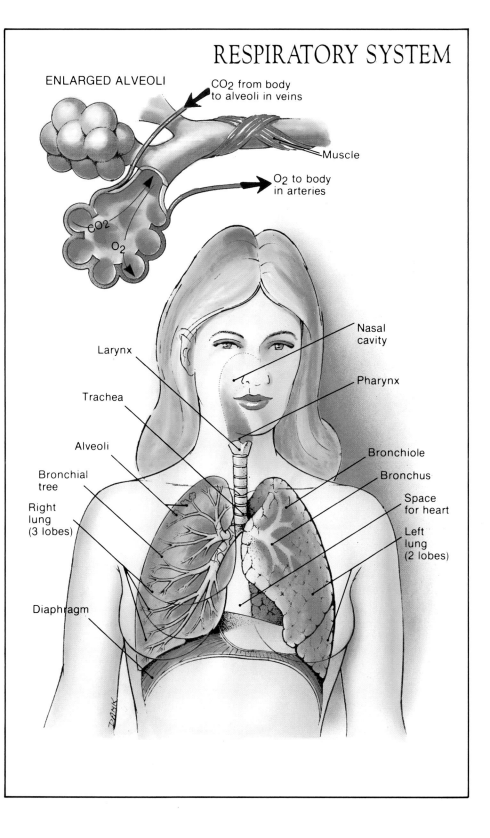

ENLARGED ALVEOLI

CO2 from body to alveoli in veins

Muscle

O2 to body in arteries

CO2

O2

Larynx

Trachea

Alveoli

Bronchial tree

Right lung (3 lobes)

Diaphragm

Nasal cavity

Pharynx

Bronchiole

Bronchus

Space for heart

Left lung (2 lobes)

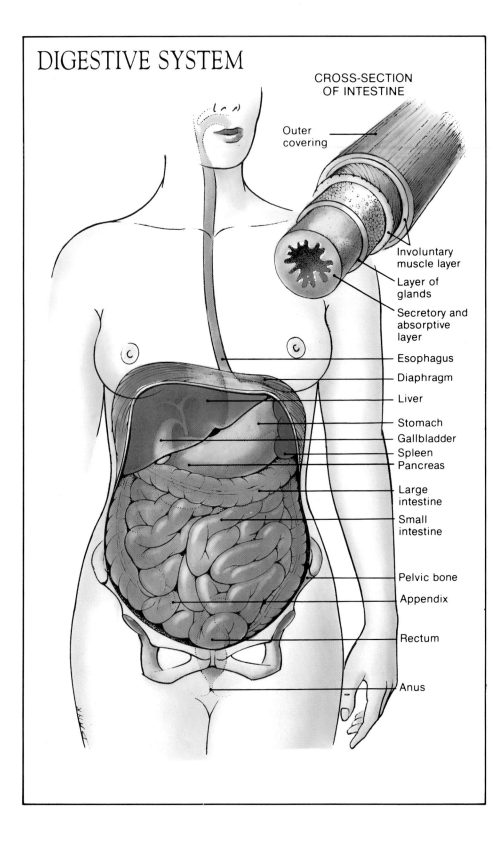

DIGESTIVE SYSTEM

CROSS-SECTION OF INTESTINE

Outer covering

Involuntary muscle layer

Layer of glands

Secretory and absorptive layer

Esophagus

Diaphragm

Liver

Stomach

Gallbladder

Spleen

Pancreas

Large intestine

Small intestine

Pelvic bone

Appendix

Rectum

Anus

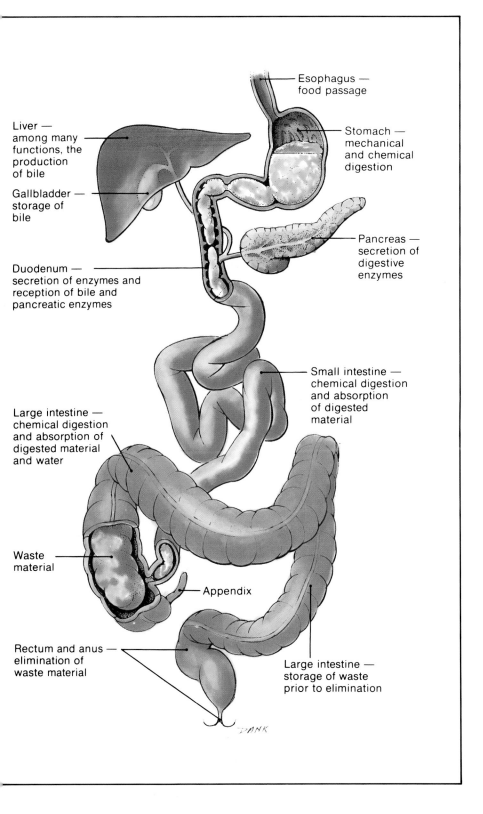

Esophagus —
food passage

Stomach —
mechanical
and chemical
digestion

Liver —
among many
functions, the
production
of bile

Gallbladder —
storage of
bile

Pancreas —
secretion of
digestive
enzymes

Duodenum —
secretion of enzymes and
reception of bile and
pancreatic enzymes

Small intestine —
chemical digestion
and absorption
of digested
material

Large intestine —
chemical digestion
and absorption of
digested material
and water

Waste
material

Appendix

Rectum and anus —
elimination of
waste material

Large intestine —
storage of waste
prior to elimination

DANK

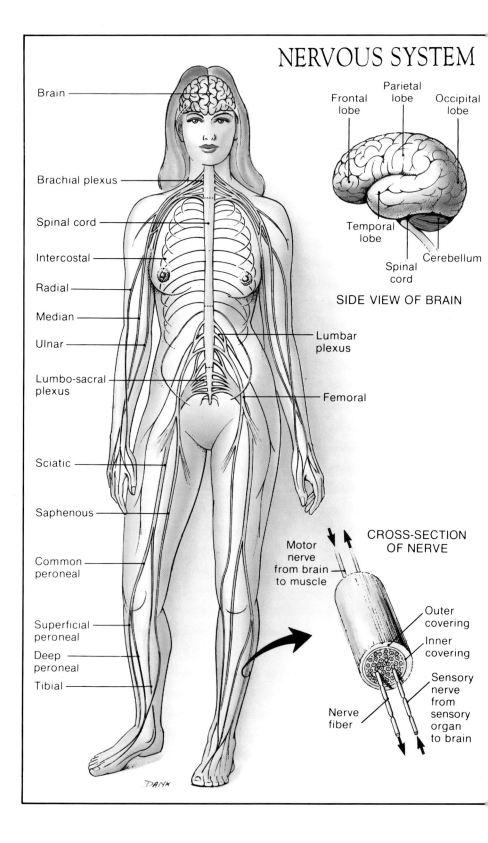

NERVOUS SYSTEM

Brain

Brachial plexus

Spinal cord

Intercostal

Radial

Median

Ulnar

Lumbo-sacral plexus

Sciatic

Saphenous

Common peroneal

Superficial peroneal

Deep peroneal

Tibial

Lumbar plexus

Femoral

Frontal lobe

Parietal lobe

Occipital lobe

Temporal lobe

Cerebellum

Spinal cord

SIDE VIEW OF BRAIN

CROSS-SECTION OF NERVE

Motor nerve from brain to muscle

Outer covering

Inner covering

Sensory nerve from sensory organ to brain

Nerve fiber

DANK

URINARY SYSTEM

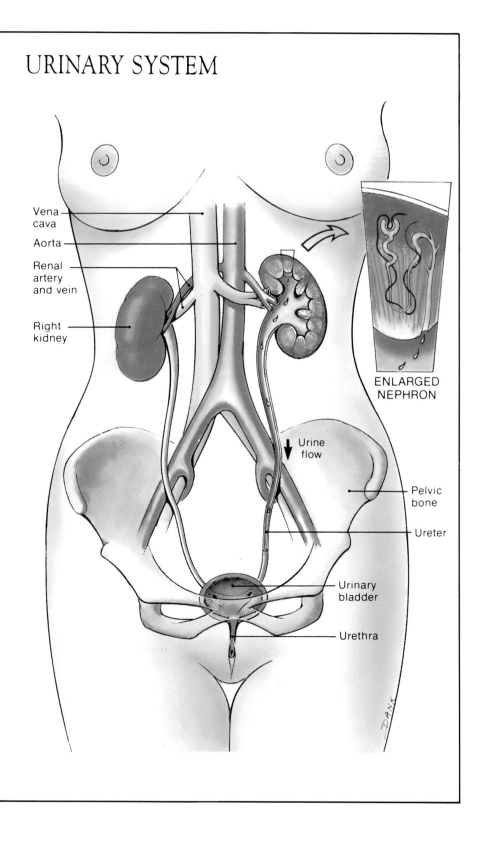

Vena cava

Aorta

Renal artery and vein

Right kidney

ENLARGED NEPHRON

Urine flow

Pelvic bone

Ureter

Urinary bladder

Urethra

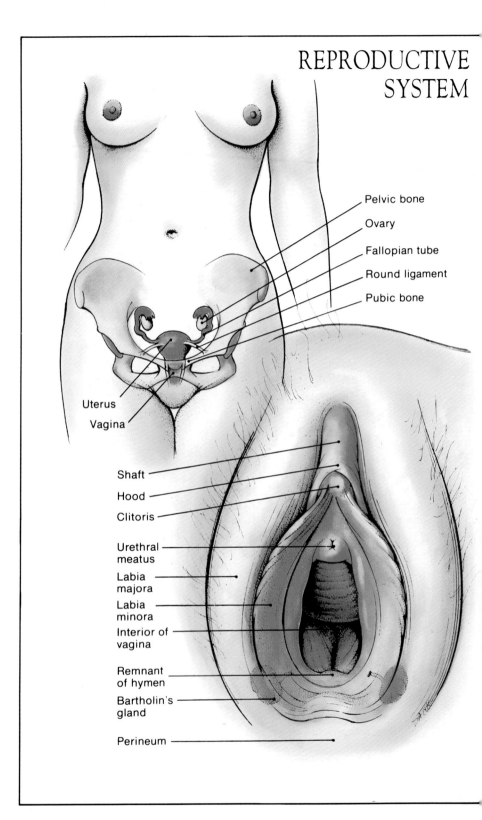

REPRODUCTIVE SYSTEM

Pelvic bone

Ovary

Fallopian tube

Round ligament

Pubic bone

Uterus

Vagina

Shaft

Hood

Clitoris

Urethral meatus

Labia majora

Labia minora

Interior of vagina

Remnant of hymen

Bartholin's gland

Perineum

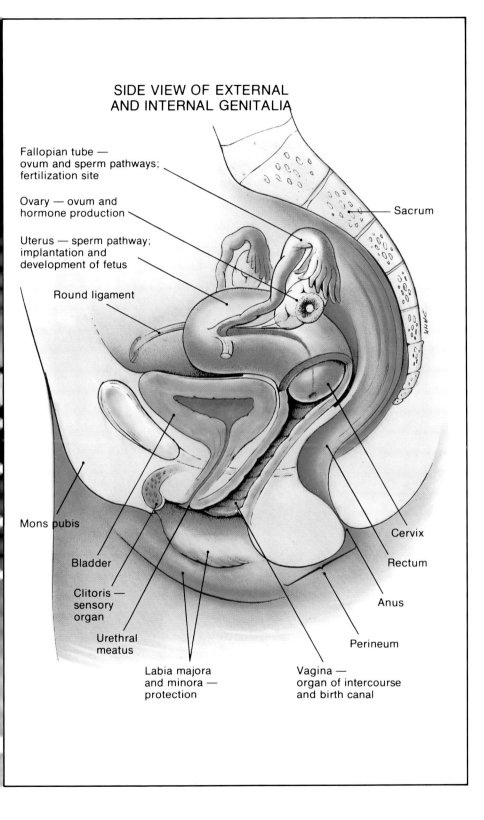

SIDE VIEW OF EXTERNAL AND INTERNAL GENITALIA

Fallopian tube —
ovum and sperm pathways;
fertilization site

Ovary — ovum and
hormone production

Uterus — sperm pathway;
implantation and
development of fetus

Round ligament

Mons pubis

Bladder

Clitoris —
sensory
organ

Urethral
meatus

Labia majora
and minora —
protection

Sacrum

Cervix

Rectum

Anus

Perineum

Vagina —
organ of intercourse
and birth canal

EMOTIONS AND THE BODY

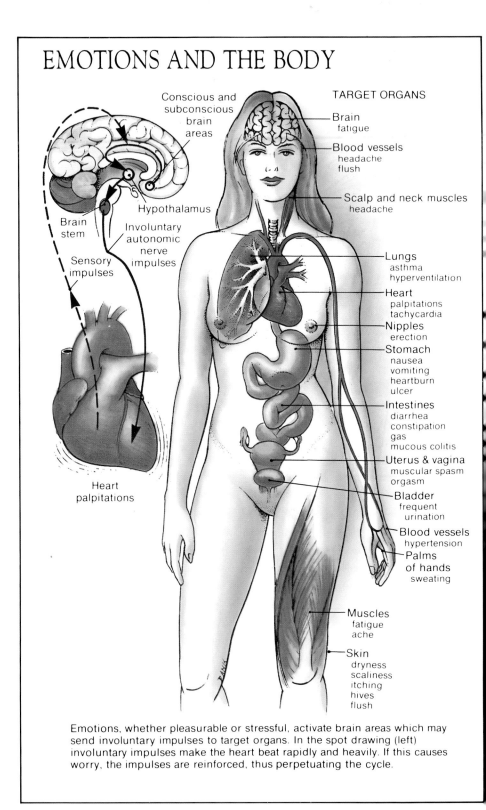

Conscious and subconscious brain areas

TARGET ORGANS

Brain stem

Hypothalamus

Involuntary autonomic nerve impulses

Sensory impulses

Heart palpitations

Brain
fatigue

Blood vessels
headache
flush

Scalp and neck muscles
headache

Lungs
asthma
hyperventilation

Heart
palpitations
tachycardia

Nipples
erection

Stomach
nausea
vomiting
heartburn
ulcer

Intestines
diarrhea
constipation
gas
mucous colitis

Uterus & vagina
muscular spasm
orgasm

Bladder
frequent
urination

Blood vessels
hypertension

Palms
of hands
sweating

Muscles
fatigue
ache

Skin
dryness
scaliness
itching
hives
flush

Emotions, whether pleasurable or stressful, activate brain areas which may send involuntary impulses to target organs. In the spot drawing (left) involuntary impulses make the heart beat rapidly and heavily. If this causes worry, the impulses are reinforced, thus perpetuating the cycle.

specialists believe the O. J. Simpson case was the determining factor in their passage. In a *New York Times* story (10/13/95) headlined "Nicole Simpson, in Death, Lifting Domestic Violence to the Forefront as National Issue," Neil Jacobson, professor of psychology at the University of Washington in Seattle, whose specialty is domestic violence, was quoted as follows: "This case is to domestic violence what the Anita Hill–Clarence Thomas case is to sexual harassment. Sexual harassment has not left the public eye since the Congressional hearings on that case. I think this case will have the same effect on domestic violence." A different view was expressed by the social workers at various shelters for battered women. They quoted the many callers who said that "since Mr. Simpson's acquittal, they are being threatened by boyfriends and husbands emboldened by the verdict." Perhaps the most accurate assessment has been made by another authority who believes that the effect of the case has been only marginal compared to the forces already in motion. Peter B. Edelman, the government specialist who helped coordinate the work of the National Advisory Council on Violence Against Women for the Department of Health and Human Services, said, "This is a long-term effort to change the fundamental culture." A contribution to this effort was made by President Clinton in a radio speech on October 14, 1995, calling on the nation's men to pledge to "never never lift a hand against a woman for as long as we live." Clinton, who as a youngster intervened to stop his stepfather from beating his mother, said he was making the appeal "not just as a president, or a father or a husband, but also as a son who has seen domestic violence first hand."

When politicians talk about "family values," the following facts about the fundamental culture should be taken into account:

- Half of all women will experience some form of violence from their spouses during marriage.
- In the United States about one-quarter of all murders involve family members, and even in Denmark, where homicide has practically been eliminated, the family is the setting in which it is most likely to persist.
- Upwards of 4 million American women are beaten annually by current and former male partners, and between 2,000 and 4,000 are murdered, according to the National Woman Abuse Prevention Center.
- According to former U.S. Surgeon General C. Everett Koop, domestic violence is the number-1 health problem for American women, causing more injuries than automobile accidents, muggings, and rapes combined.
- In some states, a man who strikes a stranger is committing a felony, but a man who attacks his wife is committing only a misdemeanor.
- It was not until 1977 that New York state made wife-beating a crime.

- Nearly 20 out of every 1,000 women with incomes over $40,000 report severe violence.
- There are three times as many animal shelters in the United States as shelters for battered women.
- Violence against women is the most committed and least reported crime in the United States.
- Women at special risk are those whose ethnic and religious origins maintain that obedience to a man is a lifetime obligation: to one's father, then to one's husband, and finally to one's sons.
- It has been well documented that men who physically harm their partners also hit their children.
- Sociologists find that the cultural norm continues to be that parents have the right and the obligation to use physical force to train, protect, and control a child. Eighty-four percent believe that it is sometimes necessary to discipline a child with a hard spanking.
- In the article on family violence in the *Encyclopedia of Sociology*, published in 1992, the author points out that "Just as parenthood gives the right to hit, so a marriage license is also a hitting license. American society has a long way to go before a typical citizen is as safe in his or her own home as on the streets or in the workplace."

There is also little doubt that early exposure to violence is reinforced by the outside world through stereotyped imagery in mass media and social interaction. The stereotyped masculine hero uses physical violence to achieve his objectives and is successful. Therefore, violence is not only acceptable but to be admired.

The data supports the theory that family violence is a learned response. Almost all the husbands came from homes in which there had been physical abuse between their fathers and mothers. Although the connection was not as common in the case of the wives, many of them did come from violent homes. Both husbands and wives in this group came from families in which physical punishment was used regularly to discipline the children. Because parents serve as powerful role models, this behavior teaches their children not only that violence is a useful and effective way to accomplish desired behavior but also that it is morally correct.

Another thing that the child learns from violence within the immediate family is that males are stronger than females and that if a battle is lost verbally, it may be won through the use of physical force. The male child learns from watching his mother's reaction that she is afraid of the father, even if they do not fight physically. He may apply this knowledge in adulthood by using violence or the threat of violence to maintain superiority over family members whose traditional rank is subordinate to his and to control those who challenge his authority.

Although the middle class tends to identify family violence with lower income status and ethnic minorities, family violence is not limited by economic class or social status. Perhaps violence within the family seemed more common among the poor because more of these cases become police matters, but that perception has been permanently altered by the images of the battered rich and beautiful Nicole Brown Simpson.

BATTERING

According to activists who have survived battering, legal specialists and advocates, and the National Coalition Against Domestic Violence, battering is a pattern of behavior that results in establishing power and control over another person through fear and intimidation. It often includes the threat or the use of violence. It occurs when the batterers believe they are entitled to control their partners. Not all battering is physical. It can include a whole spectrum of behavior used to establish and maintain power, including economic abuse, sexual abuse, threats, intimidation, isolation, and exploitation of children. Whether physical or not, battering usually escalates. It may begin with threats and violent actions such as kicking a pet or smashing furniture, and then escalate to punching, sexual assault, beatings, and then proceed to life-threatening actions, such as breaking bones, choking, and brandishing weapons.

In answer to the question, "Who is battered?" the National Coalition Against Domestic Violence replies, "Rural and urban women of all religious, ethnic, racial, economic, and educational backgrounds and of varying ages, physical abilities and life-styles. There is not a typical woman who would be battered."

Consider these facts:

- Although there are cases in which women have assaulted their spouses, men commit 95 percent of all assaults against spouses or ex-spouses, according to a recent National Crime Survey.
- Using data gathered by the FBI, Professor Murray Straus, codirector of the Family Research Laboratory at the University of New Hampshire, found that 43 percent of women who are murdered are killed by another member of the family, most often their husband.

- Each year, more than one million women seek medical help for injuries caused by battering.
- In 1992 the American Medical Association recommended that doctors should routinely screen their female patients for signs of domestic violence because it had become so common. Doctors should be aware that domestic violence may present itself not only in the form of a physical injury, but in chronic pain, gynecological disturbances, or sleep and appetite disorders. (In 1994 a mandatory reporting law went into effect in California requiring doctors and other health professionals to report suspected battering just as they must report suspected child abuse.)
- Studies reported in 1992 by the National Women's Health Network indicate that 40 to 60 percent of battered women were abused during pregnancy, and 25 percent say they were beaten for the first time during pregnancy.
- When the extent of the problem began to emerge in the mid-1970s in the wake of the women's movement, feminists said, "Leave the relationship." But they didn't take into account that more than two million wives are trapped by their economic dependency, their fears, and their confusion about what is best for their children.
- Although the report of the 1990 U.S. Conference of Mayors listed many of the more obvious causes of homelessness in American cities, the physical abuse of women and children was not among them. In fact, domestic violence was the main reason that women with children were homeless in Oregon. According to the Pennsylvania Bar Association, domestic violence is the cause of 42 percent of homeless families in Philadelphia. And according to a report prepared by the Senate Judiciary Committee in 1990, 50 percent of all homeless women and children in the United States are fleeing domestic violence.

Next to acceptance of the learned response of violence, economic survival is perhaps the most important reason that the battered wife does not leave home. Many women have been conditioned since childhood to have no expectation for a career and therefore are not trained for employment. A woman still has fewer job opportunities than a man and often earns less holding a similar job. Because she is usually responsible for an unequal portion of the child care, her time is more limited and therefore her earning further restricted. Upper-class women whose wealth depends entirely on the discretion of their husband are fearful about going public in dealing with abuse because they don't want to disgrace the family and because they cannot depend on the social services available to less "advantaged" women.

Even a court award of child support to the woman with children who does leave is no guarantee of economic stability. Fewer than half the husbands comply even during the first year, and efforts to make the fathers contribute are not only expensive but often futile. She therefore feels bound to stay for the economic good of the children. Wives who are fully dependent on their husbands for financial support often feel they cannot even call for help. They need some kind of job and strong psychological support before they can find the courage to break away.

While many researchers continue to focus on individual and family pathology as the basic causes of the abuse of women, feminist-oriented investigators of battering are asking quite different questions, questions concerned with social policies, community attitudes, and the norms that tolerate battering. The work of these researchers is extremely important because new findings and statistics are influential in the formulation of broad social policies affecting the definition of crime and the meting out of punishment.

For example, it has been the considered judgment of many investigators that the most effective way to end domestic violence is to arrest the perpetrator for a brief period and make arrangements for compulsory therapy and counseling when he is permitted to return home. But as recently as 1984, many members of the Attorney General's Task Force on Family Violence thought the problem was strictly a private family matter. However, when the Task Force concluded that physically abusive husbands should be arrested, police departments nationwide began to respond. (Evidence had already accumulated that domestic violence was twice as likely to recur in households when the police attempted to mediate the dispute rather than arresting the assaulter.)

The most dramatic change in the attitude of law enforcement agencies resulted from a New York City jury's decision in 1984 to award $2 million to a woman who sued the city for failure to protect her after she had begged repeatedly for police protection when her husband attacked her with a butcher knife. As a result of this case, assault arrests for domestic violence jumped 62 percent. In most such cases, when the police arrive, the assaulter says, "You can't arrest me; that's my wife," and is genuinely astonished when he is handcuffed and removed from the premises.

In a landmark decision handed down in July 1984, Chief Justice Robert N. Wilentz of the New Jersey State Supreme Court ruled that expert testimony on the behavior of women who have been subjected to sustained abuse from husbands or lovers is admissible to help establish claims of self-defense in murder cases. One purpose of this ruling was to negate the myths that battered women enjoy being abused, that they provoke their spouse's violent behavior, and that they are free to leave their abusers whenever they wish. When experts testify on the battered woman's circumstances, they emphasize that the syndrome is one of learned helplessness: she is convinced that she has nowhere to go and that if she tried to leave, the beatings would get worse. She is likely to believe that marriage is forever, that her husband is omnipotent, and that if she can figure out the magic formula, her husband will change.

In 1992 what is considered to be the country's model for the most effective domestic violence intervention program celebrated its tenth anniversary. Known as the Domestic Abuse Intervention Project, it gave Duluth, Minnesota, the distinction of becoming the first local jurisdiction in the nation to adopt a mandatory arrest policy for misdemeanor assaults. Its effectiveness is based on more than police action. The message it conveys is that every agent of the justice system—police, prosecuting attorneys, probation officers, judges— must stress that domestic violence is a crime the community will not tolerate. The project estimates that 1 of every 19 men in Duluth has been through the program during the same decade, with the result that not one Duluth woman has been the victim of a domestic homicide.

Here's how the Duluth program works: A first-time offender is incarcerated overnight, and if he pleads guilty, he is sentenced to 30 days in jail and put on probation, during which time he must complete a 26-week batterer's program. If he misses three successive classes, he is likely to be sent to jail. Unfortunately, while intervention is a great step forward, not much progress has been achieved with prevention. The *New York Times* (2/16/92) reported that, five years after going through the Duluth procedures, 40 percent of the men who had been treated ended up by reoffending (or becoming suspects in assaults), either with the same woman or with a new partner.

Experts are inclined to doubt whether any therapies will work with the most violent batterers. Dr. Daniel O'Leary, a psychologist at the State University of New York at Stony Brook, said in a *New York Times* interview (6/22/94), "If a husband repeatedly batters to the point where his wife ends up injured, then the best route for now seems to be arresting the husband and finding safe shelter and supportive counseling for the wife. But the arrest itself does nothing to make the man less violent in the future."

Can domestic violence be predicted? Clues to the possible development of violence can be found in the affirmative answers to these questions:

- Did your partner grow up in a violent family?
- Does your partner have a nasty temper and does he overreact to small problems and the usual frustrations of daily life such as being deprived of a parking space or constantly getting a busy signal when trying to make an important call?

- Does your partner have low self-esteem?
- Are there frequent examples of cruelty to animals?
- Does your partner have rigid old-fashioned ideas about the place of women in the family and his role as undisputed dictator of the family's way of life?
- Are you and all women regarded as second-class citizens who should know their place?
- Does your partner want to know where you are and with whom at all times? Are you given any free time that is entirely your own?
- Does your partner constantly talk about "getting even" with others and play with weapons as a way of showing off?
- Does your partner show signs of rage if you can't figure out what is wanted or expected of you?
- Does your partner alternate between kindness and cruelty in an unpredictable way?
- Did your partner "rough you up" during dating or when you were living together? If he did, don't assume you'll be able to change abusive behavior when you're married.

It has also become increasingly clear that for many battered women, verbal and emotional abuse can be just as destructive as physical abuse. Because it is insidious in its cumulative effects, the victim may end up by doubting her own judgment and even her sanity. Here is a checklist compiled by the National Coalition Against Domestic Violence. How many of these things has your partner done to you?

1. Ignored your feelings.
2. Ridiculed and insulted women as a group.
3. Ridiculed your most cherished beliefs, your religion, your ethnic origins.
4. Withheld approval, affection, or appreciation as punishment.
5. Called you names, criticized you, shouted at you.
6. Humiliated you in front of the children or in public.
7. Refused to socialize with you.
8. Kept you from working or controlled all your money.
9. Taken car keys or money away from you.
10. Regularly threatened to leave or told you to leave.
11. Threatened to hurt you or your family.
12. Punished or deprived the children when angry with you.
13. Threatened to kidnap the children if you left him.
14. Without any foundation in fact, harassed you or accused you of having illicit affairs.
15. Manipulated and confused you with lies and contradictions.
16. Destroyed furniture, punched holes in walls, smashed precious objects.

Rarely is there a close relationship in which none of this behavior is occasionally manifested or in which a spell of irritability doesn't produce actions and words that are later regretted. However, the critical questions for the victim of psychological abuse to ask herself are: Does she think she's going crazy? Is she really afraid of her partner? Is she constantly asking permission to do things and no longer making decisions on her own? Does she feel increasingly powerless?

A consequence of this type of abuse is that no positive messages get through to the battered woman because she is usually isolated by the batterer from family, friends, and neighbors. So what can a battered woman do?

Testimony from battered women in court cases, in interviews, and on TV talk shows emphasizes that the first step is to admit that the abuse exists as a real problem. The next step is to stop hoping and imagining that the problem will go away. Once an abused woman recognizes that she has every right to feel safe in her own home, free of physical harm and psychological impairment, she is on her way to finding a solution. Here are some practical recommendations from "Plain Talk About Wife Abuse," a publication of the National Institute of Mental Health:

A woman can do a number of things to protect herself. She can hide extra money, car keys, and important documents somewhere safe so that she can get to them in a hurry. She should have a place to go, such as an emergency shelter, a social service agency, or the home of a trusted friend or relative.

During an actual attack, the woman should defend herself as best she can. As soon as she is able, she should call the police (the emergency number for calling the police is 911 nationwide). Most important she should leave the house and take her children with her. She may need medical attention too, because she might be hurt more severely than she realizes. Having a record of her injuries, including photographs, can protect her legally should she decide to press charges. In many states, the man who has inflicted visible injuries is arrested on the spot whether or not the victim presses charges.

• • •

A woman needs to talk to people who can help. Good friends can lend support and guidance. Organizations that are devoted to women's concerns and not bound by society's traditions can assist her. They might help her explore her options in new ways. Emergency shelters for women, hotlines, women's organizations, social service agencies, community mental health centers, and hospital emergency rooms are all possible sources of support. Among the emergency listings in the blue pages of local telephone directories is an 800 number for the BATTERED WOMEN DOMESTIC VIOLENCE HOTLINE. Some cities are collaborating with security alarm systems that provide threatened women with an emergency pendant. The victim simply presses the pendant, and unbeknownst to her attacker, an electronic signal is transmitted to the alarm system, which in turn immediately summons the police to the scene. Another innovative program provides battered women not only with alarm systems that secure their homes against invasion by their attackers, but also with cellular phones so that they can call for help if confronted outside the home.

And what about the children who are the silent victims of domestic violence? We know that O. J. Simpson's children were someplace in the house when their mother was being beaten, but we don't know—nor will we ever know—how they were affected by what they heard. Two studies made public in 1994—one by the *Journal of the American Medical Association,* the other by the American Bar Association—concluded that it is worse for children to witness violence in their own homes than to watch shootouts in the street. They are likely to confuse hitting with caring, and when they grow up, the boys are likely to become abusers and the girls victims. Women who endure domestic violence for the sake of "keeping the family intact" should consider that even though the children may be spared physical assault, they are being abused too.

Domestic Violence Resource Network

In October 1993 the U.S. Department of Health and Human Services, Administration for Children and Families, allocated the funds to establish a network of four domestic violence resource centers. These centers work in partnership with domestic violence programs on all levels, ranging from those based in the community to state and federal government agencies. Women with a personal and/or professional interest in the latest developments in these programs regarding research, policy, and practice can contact:

> The Texas Council on Family Violence has established a domestic violence hotline that operates nationwide. The toll-free telephone numbers are 1-800-799-SAFE (7233) and 1-800-787-3224 (TDD).

National Resource Center on Domestic Violence   800-537-2238
Battered Women's Justice Project   800-903-0111
Resource Center on Child Protection/Custody   800-527-3223
Health Resource Center on Domestic Violence   800-313-1310

ABUSE OF CHILDREN: WHAT YOU CAN DO

If you're a single parent suffering from stress, get supportive therapy and join a
    self-help group of parents with similar problems so that your frustrations
    don't lead you to "take it out on the kids."

If your husband expects you to stand by while he beats the children, report his
    behavior to the proper child protection agency so that family therapy can
    prevent an eventual tragedy.

If you're a new mother with signs of postpartum depression and anxieties that
    you'll harm your baby, don't permit family and friends to pooh-pooh your
    feelings. Talk to your pediatrician or to the baby care clinic personnel and
    arrange for supportive therapy or counseling.

If you're a teacher, always be alert to signs of physical abuse and neglect of the
    children in your daily care. Investigate constant absences because of "ill-
    nesses" and insist on meetings with parents of young children who show
    signs of physical or emotional battering.

If you're a friend or neighbor of a troubled family where children are at risk of
    being abused or are actually being mistreated, speak to the adults responsi-
    ble for the well-being of the children and, if they tell you to mind your own
    business, report your suspicions to the local child protection agency.

If you have the time to become a volunteer, seek out a child welfare agency
    and lighten the burden of overworked and underpaid professionals.

If you're a concerned citizen, work for the election of legislators who under-
    stand that spending money on social services for children and needy or
    troubled families is a vital investment for the future health of the whole
    society.

ABUSE OF THE ELDERLY

It is only within recent years that the problem of elder abuse has come to
public attention. The problem is not news to family court judges, social workers, neighbors, and relatives who have been dealing with it day in and day out.

However, now that practically all states have passed laws requiring mandatory reporting of suspected cases of elder abuse as well as laws providing protective services to elderly victims, "grannybashing" is less of a secret than it used to be.

According to reports in the *New York Times* and *Modern Maturity*, the magazine of the American Association of Retired Persons (AARP), about one million older Americans—or one in five—are abused each year. Females are likelier victims than males, and 84 percent of reported physical abuse is perpetrated by sons. In cases of neglect and psychological abuse, daughters are the usual miscreants.

A typical case can be described as follows. The victim is a 75-year-old woman who may be ailing. She may be heavily sedated; her money is taken; essential medication and food are withheld; and she is locked in her room, denied visitors, and forbidden phone calls. Her complaints are met with a barrage of threats followed by beatings. Victims usually live with their abusers, and the problem cuts across racial, religious, social, and economic lines. The abuse is difficult to detect because the victims do not regularly spend time at centers where the bruises are noticed, or they are so vulnerable that they rarely go out at all.

Causes of the victimization are generally the same: a long history of poor interpersonal relationships, an adult child "repaying" an abusive parent, an impatient and greedy wish to gain control over the older person's money. Alcohol and drug dependence may play a significant role, and when women are the abusers of an aged parent, the cause is often unremitting caregiver stress.

There are many reasons for the victims' toleration of the abuse. In some cases, they feel guilty when attacked by their own offspring because, after all, it was they as parents who created these monsters. Or they remember that they themselves used to beat their children as a way of controlling them. Thus, the situation is one of transgenerational violence, with the abuser avenging an earlier history. Also, there are many older people who have been led to believe, or who imagine, that the alternative to their present misery is to be taken out of the family and forced to live among strangers or to be shipped off to a nursing home. With this possibility in mind, many victims have been disinclined to report their situation to any authorities.

With increasing awareness of the problem, however, most communities have established intervention services: elder abuse hotlines that operate around the clock can be contacted by concerned family members or neighbors whose fears about being sued for making false accusations are allayed by counselors. Where physical abuse is charged, the perpetrators are more likely than in the past to be charged with a crime punishable by incarceration followed by counseling. As in the case of the swift removal of the wife batterer from the premises, abusers of the elderly are likely to mend their ways when faced with a jail sentence.

At the request of the AARP, the Department of Family Medicine at Wayne State University undertook a comprehensive study of elder abuse. The study resulted in the following recommendations that could provide solutions to the problem. Raise the awareness of police, home health care workers, nurses, and doctors to signs of this aspect of family violence. Supply support services to relieve the stress of caregivers, especially such services as senior day care centers, chore helpers, and respite arrangements. Create neighborhood watch programs alert to the unexplained "disappearance" of elderly family members.

As a concerned citizen, you should report any instances of family abuse of the elderly to the relevant agencies—elder abuse hotline, protection services for the elderly, legal advocacy, and/or the social services division of the Area Agency on Aging. After you have made your complaint, follow through within a suitable time interval to find out whether any action has been taken.

If you are an elderly woman who is increasingly infirm and financially dependent on an already overburdened family and you have already experienced some abuse and neglect, you should take the necessary steps to protect yourself against further victimization. Here are some suggestions: *Don't isolate yourself.* Stay in touch with your friends and try to participate in community activities for seniors. *Find out about community resources that can help you.* If you want to make every effort to stay in your own home, investigate your entitlement to home health aid, housekeeping services, and other help. Look into *alternative housing plans* if you want to avoid living with hostile, abusive, violent, or alcoholic family members. *When your situation has gone out of control,* ask for help from your doctor, lawyer, or religious pastor. Find out how to connect with a qualified social worker who specializes in helping older women.

If you're a prime caregiver whose nerves are getting frazzled and who has trouble controlling her anger, try to find ways of lightening your load of responsibilities instead of permitting your enfeebled and demanding parent to become the target of your temper. Ask your local Area Agency on Aging about respite services. Look into adult day care centers that offer a broad spectrum of services to the elderly. Some are covered by Medicare, some by Medicaid, and most charge fees based on the ability to pay. Get in touch with the local Self-Help Clearing House and join CAPS (Children of Aging Parents) where you can share your frustrations, air your anger, and enjoy a feeling of solidarity with many others who are dealing with similar problems. For information about a CAPS group in your area, write to CAPS, 1609 Woodbourne Rd., Levittown, PA 19057, or phone (215) 945-6900.

Both generations—adult offspring and aging parents—should be alert to a form of abuse of the elderly that has become increasingly widespread thanks to telemarketing. Telephone scam artists are nothing new, but in recent years, it has become much more difficult for the unwary to distinguish legitimate callers from con artists. Telephone marketers caught in an FBI sting operation admitted that elderly people, especially widows who live alone, are their prime target. Victims are easy to locate through mailing lists of retiree and community organizations. According to the *New York Times* (5/21/95), telemarketing fraud is believed to be a $40 billion business. Unfortunately, many instances of this form of elder abuse remain unreported because "I was too mortified to tell my grown children that I had been exploited." The exploitation may arrive by mail inviting the recipient to participate in a contest; it may begin with a sweet-talking salesman presenting a surefire investment scheme. Within a few months, the mystery man has absconded with thousands of dollars, in some cases, with the savings of a lifetime.

The *Times* adds that "The elderly are also prime targets for cults, many of which flourish in the nursing homes and sunnier climes where senior citizens are clustered." According to psychologist Margaret Singer, a leading authority on the subject and author of *Cults in Our Midst*, "Cults recruit the elderly on the basis of their loneliness. They're going for their assets, not to benefit their lives."

To protect aging parents from the predators whose specialty is inspiring trust in the unwary, adult children are advised to maintain close contact and to issue warnings about smooth talkers who offer easy profits or spiritual salvation in exchange for a regular investment of cash. Perpetrators of fraud should be reported without delay to local authorities.

CHILDHOOD SEXUAL ABUSE

Contrary to Freud's assumption that accounts by his Viennese patients of sexual molestation during childhood by a father or an uncle were wish-fulfillment fantasies, sexual abuse by a family member or family friend is far more common than most people are willing to believe. According to the federal National Child Abuse and Neglect Data System, about 140,000 children under 18 are sexually abused each year by their caregivers. In substantiation of these statistics, most of the women who have publicly spoken of this victimization point out that the offender was not the beguiling stranger we teach our children to avoid; it was someone they had been taught to obey and respect. Oprah Winfrey has spoken publicly about being raped at the age of 10 by a cousin who was 10 years older. Patty Duke recalls being sexually molested by the adult couple who took charge of her life and career from the time she was 7 years old. Marilyn Van Derbur, a former Miss America and one of the founders of the Kempe National Center for Prevention and Treatment of Child Abuse and Neglect, feels that "the greatest achievement of my life was surviving incest." Another woman remembers receiving messages that were not an obvious physical assault, but their incestuous intent was obvious, and she recalls them as being more humiliating than flattering: a father, stepfather, uncle, or older brother who constantly made obscene remarks, smacked his lips, rolled his eyes, and held his crotch at the sight of her when she was a little girl in a party dress, a 12-year-old in a bathing suit, a teenager in shorts.

Many women suppress these memories well into adulthood, until they seek out a therapist to help them cope with sleep disorders or compulsive promiscuity or free-floating anxiety resulting in panic attacks. Dr. Karin C. Meiselman, a clinical psychologist and authority on the trauma of sexual abuse within the family, believes that one of the most detrimental long-term effects is the inability of the victims to trust other people or their own instincts: "As a result, they have difficulty in establishing a committed adult relationship; victims may either totally avoid intimacy or tolerate abusive relationships, seeing themselves as a bad person who doesn't deserve much, therefore picking partners who fulfill that prophecy" (*Ladies Home Journal*, 4/95).

Women who have been avoiding any revelation of their memories of childhood sexual abuse and who believe the psychosexual scars they bear are permanent may achieve a healthy equilibrium by confronting their anger and guilt through one or another type of one-to-one psychotherapy. Participation in a local self-help group can be especially helpful for those women who have been unable or unwilling to verbalize their feelings, especially with those closest to them.

In addition to the resources mentioned earlier in this chapter, the following organizations can supply useful information and referrals:

- Adults Molested as Children United, 615 Fifteenth Street, Modesto, CA 95354; phone: (209) 572-3446
- Survivors of Incest Anonymous, PO Box 21817, Baltimore, MD 21222-6817; phone: (410) 282-3400

As a parent, you can prevent the sexual abuse of your own daughter by being alert to some of the symptoms. In a young child, watch for nightmares, compulsive masturbation, and soreness in the genital area, especially after visits with an estranged husband. In a preadolescent, be aware of withdrawal from friends, secretiveness, and depression. In a daughter who is entering adolescence, notice whether her father or stepfather is beginning to behave like a suitor, is jealous of her boyfriends, and is hostile to her friends of both sexes. Remember that other family members—a grandfather or an uncle—are not above suspicion. You can prevent the full flowering of sexual abuse by being aware of sensual fondling, overheated kissing, and constant invitations to lap sitting. Such behavior should be discouraged in a casual but firm tone of voice. Parents should not make a habit of casual nudity, nor should their young offspring be invited to share their bed, bath, or shower after reaching the age of three. If you are the single parent of a young son (no matter how young) try not to flirt with him, and never tell him he's your favorite boyfriend.

SEXUAL ASSAULT: RAPE

Rape is a violent crime, not an act done for sexual reasons, and it precipitates a crisis situation in the victim. The degree of the stress involved becomes more understandable if rape is viewed as a crime against one's person. This places it in the same category as other aggressive crimes such as robbery, assault, and the ultimate act of aggression, murder. In fact, as far as damage to the innermost self is concerned, rape is the most traumatic act short of murder.

HISTORY

The threat of rape has been a fear of women from prehistoric times to the present. It is interesting to research ancient laws and historical practice to see how they approached the problems posed by rape.

In ancient times, the Babylonian Code of Hammurabi and Mosaic laws allowed capture by force of women from outside the tribe. Such women were considered to be prizes of warfare. Acquisition of women within the tribe required payment of goods or money to the family. Perhaps this was a basis for the concept of criminal rape: to take the virginity of a maiden was equivalent to destroying property or stealing the goods and money she would have brought to the family.

Under the Code of Hammurabi a female had no independent status. She lived as a virgin daughter in the house of her father or as a wife in the house of her husband. A married woman who was raped shared the blame with her attacker and both were bound and thrown into the river, although her husband was permitted to rescue her if he chose to do so. A virgin who was defiled was held innocent and the rapist slain.

Hebrew laws were similar. The "offending" wife and her attacker were stoned to death. A virgin raped within the city walls was considered guilty because she could have screamed for help, but a maiden raped in the fields was considered guiltless: the rapist paid the girl's father a fine, and the two were forced to marry. If the virgin had been betrothed before the incident, the rapist was stoned to death.

Tales of rape and similar stories are found in the Bible and in the folklore of all peoples. Variations on the story of Potiphar's wife, the woman who unjustly accused Joseph of rape, are found in Moslem, Christian, and Hebrew folklore as well as in the myths of the Celts and the Egyptians as far back as 1300 B.C. The moral of the story is that a woman can cause a man a lot of problems by falsely crying rape.

The practice of forcible seizure of women for mates was for centuries considered acceptable. One way to obtain property in the Middle Ages was to abduct an heiress and marry her; it was not until the fifteenth century that this was considered a felony. Arranging marriages was a common method of acquiring property during these times, and in some forms this practice continues today.

In Europe in the eighteenth century an assault was not considered rape if a woman conceived, because it was believed that if she did not consent, she could not have conceived. The law was very vague about the rape of women who were not virgins. There are few records; apparently these victims were not taken seriously and the accusations quashed.

In the United States during the days of slavery it was accepted practice to use slave women as the owner desired, and it was common for them to be raped by the men in charge. There was no attempt to maintain a slave family, but instead the women were considered to be "breeders" and were valued as such.

During wars and occupations of conquered countries, women are always considered a part of the spoils of war and are ravished by invading troops. The primary basis for the assaults is not sexual gratification but rather is part of the psychology of conquest—the right of the conqueror to overwhelm and humiliate his victims. The highly publicized recent rapes in Bosnia are the latest example of twentieth-century brutishness.

Old laws about rape and the attitudes about what was, and in many cultures still is, considered acceptable behavior, reflect the need to preserve social stability and to protect property. The protection of women as individuals against a criminal act is a comparatively recent and by no means universal concept.

MYTHS ABOUT RAPE

Many myths have persisted throughout the ages about the crime of rape, and they must be corrected if we are to make progress in dealing with this problem. Although we cannot deal with them all, here are some of the most prevalent.

1. *The rapist acts to satisfy sexual desires.* From the work that has been done with convicted sex offenders, it is now well known that sexual gratification is not the reason for sexual assault. The need of the attacker is to overpower, degrade, and humiliate. Violence, not sex, is expressed by the attack. The majority of rapists have a sexual partner with whom they identify and have a relationship and many have children.

2. *A woman cannot be raped if she doesn't want to be.* This is absolutely untrue. The primary reaction of a woman to a rapist is fear. Whether her attacker is a stranger or someone she knows, she is fearful of being maimed or killed.

3. *If women did not wear sexy clothes and act in a provocative manner, they would not get raped.* Because violence and not sexual gratification is the motive for the attack, what the woman wears and how she acts have nothing to do with it. Many are assaulted in their own homes; many are asleep in their own beds. Many victims are older women. A significant number are girls between the ages of 12 and 15.

4. *Rape is part of the sexual fantasies of women, or all women want to be raped.* It may be true that some women have sadomasochistic sexual fantasies in which varying degrees of force play a part and that some women at some time and for a variety of reasons want to take a submissive role in sexual relations. However, these thoughts are completely different from and are unrelated to fantasizing rape in the sense of wanting to be the unwilling victim of a violent, nonsexual criminal act.

5. *Most rapes are reported to the police.* Even the most optimistic observers feel that at best one in four attacks is reported to authorities; some think it is only one in ten. Rape situations that usually go unreported because the victims are convinced that no one will believe them include women known to be

sexually promiscuous, women raped by a family friend or neighbor, women in mental hospitals, professors' students, doctors' patients, and lawyers' clients.

6. *You can tell a rapist by looking at him.* Rapists come in all shapes and sizes and from all socioeconomic and educational levels. Most rapists are attractive males and have no problem finding female companions. At least 50 percent have a steady sex partner, married or unmarried, and the partners have no idea that their men are sex offenders.

Shortly after William Kennedy Smith was acquitted of rape charges by a Florida court, TV newsman Peter Jennings hosted a panel discussion on men and rape at Palm Beach Community College. Here are some of the observations made by the participants:

From a male psychologist: Teaching boys how to behave with girls must begin at home with mothers talking to their sons.

From a woman in the audience: How about having the boys taught about civilized behavior by their fathers?

From a detective, after a man in the audience said that women shouldn't put themselves in unsafe situations: There's no way a woman can arrange to be safe from a rapist's attack. She can be dragged off the street, dragged out of her car, followed into an elevator.

From a probation officer: Rapists are constantly being rearrested. It's very difficult to make generalizations about them, but it appears that men who have been sexually abused as children make up a large number.

From the psychologist: Preventing rape depends on reexamining socialization factors. The culture breeds men to be potential rapists. Listen to locker room talk. Men are expected to "score" on dates.

From a woman in the audience: Sexual assault prevention programs should begin in kindergarten and remain as part of the school curriculum on every level.

From a law professor: The law is at fault for letting rapists free to go rape again. Can a rapist be "cured?" You can't punish *rage* out of a rapist, and many come out of prison angrier than when they went in. An outstanding example of recidivism was the man arrested and freed on seven different occasions, with his attacks on women becoming more violent every time until he was finally incarcerated for life under Senator Arlen Spector's Career Criminal Act. Rape must be viewed as a *civil rights violation.* When the law recognizes this, the victim is entitled to her own lawyer rather than having to depend on a prosecutor from the district attorney's office.

UPDATING THE LAW

The word "rape" comes from the Latin *rapere,* "to take by force." Other meanings are to plunder, to destroy, to seize and carry away by force. The traditional legal definition of rape is carnal knowledge (vaginal penetration) of a female through the use of force or the threat of force without her consent.

Although present laws vary from state to state, most states have changed or are in the process of changing their old rape laws so that they now speak of "sexual assault" or "involuntary sexual battery" and have degrees and penalties similar to those found in the laws for murder. Oral, rectal, and vaginal contact, as well as penetration, are grounds for conviction. A witness to the crime is no longer necessary. Because sexual assault is usually a one-on-one crime, requiring a witness is clearly ridiculous. There is a range of penalties for the offender. These newer statutes are far more realistic in terms of the nature of the crime and the effect on the victim. Women and girls can be damaged psychologically as much from an attempted rape as they are from an actual rape. Penetration of the oral or rectal cavities is often more humiliating than vaginal penetration and the effects more serious. The key concept in defining the crime of rape is the *absence of consent.* While the legal definition of rape may differ slightly from state to state, it is generally defined as forced sexual intercourse perpetrated against the will of the victim. It is by this definition that rape is a felony that can be characterized as a felonious assault. (The crime of *statutory* rape belongs in a different category. It is defined as "sexual intercourse with a female who is below the statutory age of consent." The age of consent differs from state to state.)

Women in increasing numbers are filing civil lawsuits against persons, property owners, employers, and institutions that may be considered partially liable for the occurrence of a rape. Landlords and management companies have successfully been sued when a rape victim could prove that unsafe conditions had not been corrected after notice had been given about them; colleges and universities have been named as defendants for not maintaining safe conditions in the first place; hotels, motels, and condominiums have been making out-of-court settlements to avoid the negative publicity of courtroom trials. Many women have come forward after years of silence to speak out against their attackers. In one case of delayed vindication, the Supreme Court of California reinstated a judgment against the City of Los Angeles, which had been ordered by a jury to pay $150,000 to a woman raped 10 years earlier by a city police officer. The officer had detained her under suspicion of drunk driving, then raped her. In addition to receiving the financial award, she had the satisfaction of knowing that the officer was ordered to serve 18 months in jail for the crime.

More and more women are suing rapists even though the perpetrators usually have very little in the way of assets. In a civil court the woman has much more control because she can hire her own lawyer to prove her case, whereas in a criminal trial she simply appears as a state's witness at the discretion of an assistant district attorney. In addition, the evidence needed in a civil case is likely to be less than what is required in a criminal trial to convince a jury that the accused is guilty "beyond a reasonable doubt." It is generally agreed both by rape victims and their counselors that seeking recourse in the civil system can be part of the healing process, empowering the victim and giving her a measure of control over her life. Women's advocates, including an impressive array of law professors, are convinced that laws must be uniformly changed nationwide so that rape is recognized as a civil rights violation.

RECENT STATISTICS

No matter who compiles the figures, rape statistics continue to be ambiguous. When the figures are presented by law enforcement agencies, they are likely to be far too low because of classifications established by these agencies. A rape is classified in one of three ways: forcible rape (this includes attempted rape but not statutory rape or homosexual rape), child molestation, or rape-homicide. On the national average, 15 percent of the rapes reported to the police are dismissed as unfounded, that is, the police establish to their satisfaction that neither forcible rape nor the attempt to rape occurred. Victims also contribute to the inaccuracies because of the perceived stigma attached to being a victim of sexual assault and the perception that the victim is guilty of having provoked the assault. Marital rape has only recently been recognized in many states as a punishable crime. When the rape has been perpetrated by an acquaintance on a date or by an intimate of the family or by the family doctor himself, it may take months or even years for the victim to be able to confront the reality that she has been raped.

A significant finding about rape statistics is that if researchers ask the right questions, they find significantly more sexual violence than has previously been reported. A Justice Department report covering 1992–93 and published after the passage of the Violence Against Women Act found 500,000 incidents of sexual assault a year, twice as many as in previous reports. The explanation for the new results lies in a revision in the types of questions asked in the Justice Department's national crime victimization survey.

In previous surveys only general questions were asked about attacks and threats, leaving it to the interviewee to mention rape. The new survey puts the questions directly: Have you been raped or sexually assaulted in the previous year? Was the assailant a stranger, casual acquaintance, or someone well known to you? In previous studies, responses indicated that more than half the rapists were strangers; the new survey found that 80 percent of rapes were committed by someone known to the victim. The disparity occurs because many rape victims do not define themselves as such, since they persist in the mistaken belief that forced sex can be rape only if the rapist is a stranger. Another misconception that accounts for faulty statistics is that rape victims do not label themselves as such because they assume that rape means only vaginal penetration.

The following statistics reveal some additional facts about rape in the United States:

- Only 12 percent of the time is the perpetrator a *total* stranger to the victim. That means that in 88 percent of all cases, the rapist was an acquaintance, neighbor, friend, family member, lover, or husband. No matter what the relationship, if the woman did not consent to have sex, the act is defined as rape.
- More than 50 percent of all rapes occur in the victim's home.
- More than 90 percent are between people of the same race.
- More than 6 out of 10 sexual assaults occur before the victim reaches the age of 18.
- More than 90 percent of all rape victims say they would be less likely to report the assault to the authorities if their names were to be made public.

MARITAL RAPE

One of the greatest accomplishments of the Fourth World Conference on Women held in Beijing in 1995 was the passage of the declaration asserting a woman's right to make sexual decisions free of coercion or violence. For the first time, the inclusion of this assertion in a United Nations document recognizes that a woman is not just a reproductive machine, but a sexual being with human rights. It is expected that this most recent declaration of human rights will be used as a social and legal tool to provide greater protection for women who live in countries where a husband can legally force a wife to have sex even when he is known to be infected with HIV, the virus that causes AIDS.

Marital rape is recognized as a criminal offense in a growing number of countries worldwide, including Scotland, Canada, Israel, and New Zealand. About one-third of American states recognize nonconsensual sexual intercourse with one's wife as marital rape, usually under the heading of sexual assault. But unfortunately, even in these states, most cases of marital rape go unreported, and in the cases where husbands are charged with the crime, most of them are not convicted because the women decide not to pursue the case. New York's Linda Fairstein, chief of the Manhattan District Attorney's sex crime unit, points out that victims withdraw before going to trial because of fear of reprisals or because of mixed feelings and inbred societal attitudes. Another factor affecting the decision to drop charges is the fear of financial hardship if the wage earner receives a prison sentence. However, there are occasionally cases where the justice system sends a clear message to potential marital rapists. In a recent marital rape conviction following a jury's "guilty" verdict, Justice Franklin R. Weissberg of the state supreme court in New York sentenced the husband to a prison term of 10 to 20 years, declaring: "There are far too many places on this earth where the rape, assault, and battering of a wife by her husband is considered acceptable, or at worst a trivial offense. This state and this courtroom are not such places." Unfortunately, when it comes to defining, prosecuting, and penalizing crimes of marital sexual assault, state laws vary widely, and according to the National Clearinghouse for Marital and Date Rape, a group based in California, there remain six states in which marital rape is not a crime if the couple is living together: Missouri, New Mexico, North Carolina, North Dakota, Oklahoma, and South Carolina. The assumption of the legislative bodies in these states is that when a woman gets married, she has conferred "conjugal rights" on her husband and given up her right to say "no."

Coalitions of human rights activists, women's groups, lawyers, and organizations concerned with reducing violence within the family present their position in more or less the same way: in whatever way the state law defines rape, no exception is to be made for a spouse.

DATE RAPE

Many rapes in this category occur as a spur-of-the-moment event preceded by the male's consumption of a considerable amount of alcohol and growing out of the man's conditioning to believe that when a woman says "no," she really means "yes" and is using resistance as a teasing maneuver. About 20 percent are committed by two or more assailants (this is known as a gang rape, or colloquially, a gang bang) and can occur at a drunken party, in the back room of a bar, or in the back seat of a car. Gang rapes also occur in the military, where sexual harassment has been known to end up as sexual assault.

The problem of date rape has become of increasing concern to corporations. In 1985, following the rape of a female employee by a company customer, DuPont established a rape prevention program, the first of its kind in the country. Primarily for the enlightenment and protection of DuPont's 22,000 female employees, the program also conducts workshops for male managers. The aim of these sessions is to overcome the male stereotyping of the female victims as having "asked for it." Career women, who don't like to think of themselves as vulnerable, are exposed to videotapes alerting them to where rape can occur: in the office after hours, in hotels during conferences, on business dates with colleagues. The videos indicate ways of fending off an attacker, whether it be a boss, an associate, or a business contact. The videos also make a special point of forms of protection when traveling in foreign countries on company business. In this pioneering program, which, it is hoped, is serving as a model for other corporations, employees who are raped can receive paid leave, counseling, legal aid, and if the case becomes public, help in dealing with the media.

Date rape has become so prevalent on college campuses, especially in fraternity houses, that women's Take Back the Night marches have been the dominant form of student protest in recent years, resulting in special seminars to alert possible victims to the problem, to warn possible perpetrators of the unpleasant consequences, and to counsel the victimized. Hobart College in Elmira, New York, has a mandatory course on date rape for all undergraduates. Amherst College in Massachusetts has student-run support groups for rape survivors and men's groups devoted to raising the consciousness of male undergraduates about the various forms of sexual harassment. But it was the "Ask First" policy instituted at Antioch College that occasioned the most widespread publicity and parody. The policy was developed after a series of sexual assaults on campus revealed the absence of any clear disciplinary guidelines for defining date rape. Under this new policy, clear verbal consent is required before proceeding to any new level of intimacy: "Do not take silence as consent; it isn't." Nor does having had a certain level of intimacy with someone in the past constitute tacit consent on another occasion. "You must still ask each and every time," the policy states. Although the details are still being developed, and it is generally agreed that the "Now may I touch your breasts?" approach can get pretty silly, date rape is much less likely to occur if participants are encouraged to talk about sex and to establish ground rules instead of presuming that nice women don't say "yes," and real men don't listen to "no."

Imperfect though the "Ask First" approach may be, it is far superior to what goes on in those schools where attitudes can be said to reflect those of the general public. For example, the following responses resulted from a midwestern campus survey in which men and women were asked, Is it all right if a male holds a female down and forces her to engage in sexual intercourse if "he spends a lot of money on her?" (39 percent men and 12 percent women said "yes"); "she has had intercourse with others?" (39 percent men and 18 percent women answered "yes"); "she says she will have sex and then changes her mind?" (54 percent men and 31 percent women responded "yes").

One of the reasons so many women—whether undergraduates or working women—have been hesitant about going to court to accuse an acquaintance of rape is that they have internalized some of these attitudes too. Instead of seeing themselves as a victim of a punishable crime, they are likely to blame themselves for what happened. They are also aware of how typical jurors are likely to view them. Even though most states now have "rape shield" laws that prohibit questions about the victim's sexual history, lawyers often ask such questions anyway, with the knowledge that they must be stricken from the record.

Unfortunately, jurors take more seriously the rape of a woman who appears chaste and conventional and are more likely to exonerate the man if the woman is known to be sexually active or if she knew her assailant. Thus, a majority of jurors nationwide are likely to make harsh judgments of a woman who keeps late hours, goes to bars, uses birth control pills, or has the same address as her boyfriend.

PROTECTING YOURSELF

What can you do to prevent being raped by a stranger? Most important is to recognize that you are a potential victim. Every female is vulnerable to attack regardless of her age. Sexual assaults occur in broad daylight as well as in darkness; in suburbs as well as in the downtown areas and ghettos; in homes as well as in parking lots, alleys, and automobiles.

Your home should be protected as well as possible. Use initials rather than your first name on the mailbox and in the telephone directory. If you live alone, add a fictitious name on your door so that the fact that you are alone is not apparent. Install good-quality locks and dead-bolts. When you move into a new house or apartment, change or rekey the locks on the exterior doors so that the old keys will no longer work. Never leave an extra key in the mailbox, under the door mat, or over the door: these are the first places an intruder will look. Instead, give a key to a close friend or a trusted neighbor. Lock the door whenever you leave, even if you will be gone for only a moment; all a rapist needs is an opportunity. If you live in a multiple dwelling, arrange to meet with all the tenants to discuss ways to maximize everyone's safety. Insist on the installation of an intercom system if the front door is opened by a buzzer. Never open your door to strangers. It should be fitted with a peephole with a 180° angle so that you may see who is there without being seen yourself. In most states, a peephole is a legal requirement in multiple dwellings and is essential because a chain on the door is not likely to be strong enough to prevent forced entry. If there is any doubt about the identity of the person at the door, do not open it. Ask that utility men, repairmen, and servicemen of all kinds slip their identification under the door before you admit them. If you are not satisfied with the authenticity of the ID, call the company to verify the identification. If a stranger wants to use the telephone because of an emergency, offer to make the call and ask him to wait outside. Fund raisers, poll takers, and the like should be told that their requests will be given your attention if they are submitted by mail. People with long questionnaires for political or product surveys should be told to phone you (but only if you wish to honor their requests).

Be alert to suspicious telephone calls. Never let the caller know you are alone and never give personal information about yourself, your family, or your neighbors. If you receive calls that are obscene or those in which the caller is silent or hangs up, notify the telephone company immediately. The police should be notified if threats are made. If you have a message-recording tape on your phone, the message to the caller should never indicate that "No one is home at this time" but rather that the caller has reached your phone number and can leave a message. Many women who live alone screen their calls via the answering machine before they pick up the phone and respond in person.

Walking alone, especially after dark, can be hazardous. Never stop to give directions to a stranger: just keep walking so that your questioner has to walk with you, and keep far enough away to avoid being grabbed. Walk with a purpose, be aware, and don't wear shoes with very high heels, you may need to run. If you think you are being followed, check by crossing the street and reversing your direction. If there is any doubt, find a populated area and call the police.

Jogging alone in deserted areas day or night is inadvisable. Many women arrange to be accompanied regularly by a "buddy"—not only for safety but for human companionship.

Driving an automobile, especially when alone at night and/or in an isolated or unfamiliar location, can present special problems that necessitate precautions. Keep the car properly maintained so that breakdowns are less likely and keep the gas tank at least half full. Also keep a tire iron under the left front seat and telephone change in the glove compartment along with the number of a 24-hour towing service. Women who frequently travel by car on business or because of family responsibilities should have a portable cellular phone (not a "car phone") in order to avoid the risk of leaving the car to use a pay phone in an emergency. A traction mat, shovel, and bag of sand should be kept in the trunk in case you get stuck in snow or ice. Whenever you are in an unfamiliar area, lock the doors with the windows up. If possible, park your car in a central, well-lighted place and have your key out and ready to use when you return to it. Be sure that no one is crouched in the back seat before you enter the car. If your car becomes disabled, lock yourself in with the windows up, put on the four-way flasher, and wait until a uniformed police officer arrives. If strangers offer help, ask them to call the police for you. If you are in an isolated place and have a flat tire, drive slowly to a service station or public area. Sound your horn if you are in danger. Never pick up a hitchhiker. Never stop for a disabled vehicle or accident: use your cellular phone or go on to the nearest safe telephone and call the police.

These are some of the measures you can take to avoid becoming a victim. Above all, however, is the necessity to realize that you can be assaulted even though you do nothing to encourage the offender.

More and more women are enrolling in women's self-defense courses offered by community groups such as the local "Y" or the extension division of a local college. These courses usually discourage attempts to master the martial arts unless the woman is really serious about becoming a karate or tai chi expert, and if such is the case, she is directed elsewhere. Practical self-defense courses emphasize the inadvisability of carrying a knife or Mace because such devices can be taken away by the attacker and used against the victim. A police whistle worn around the neck is recommended instead. In addition to these practical tips, such courses provide an increase in awareness of possible dangers, an increase in self-confidence, and a strong feeling of identification and fellowship with other women.

WHAT YOU SHOULD DO IF ATTACKED

No one knows how she will react when actually confronted by an attacker. Age, physical condition, previous experience and training, religious convictions, and basic personality traits all come into play in a crisis situation. Of considerable importance is whether the attacker is a total stranger, an acquaintance, or in any way known to the victim. It is also of some consequence if he is not only physically more powerful than she is but more powerful in other ways, that is, if the relationship is that of professor/student, psychiatrist/patient, or husband/wife. Dr. Howard Barbaree, a psychologist who directs a treatment program for sex offenders in Ontario and has conducted in-depth research on the mind of the rapist, had this to say in a report published in the *Journal of Consulting and Clinical Psychology* (10/91): "Rapists often recall being intensely angry, depressed, or feeling worthless for days or even months leading up to the rape. Frequently they say that the trigger for the rape was when a woman made them angry, usually by rebuffing a sexual overture." Dr. Neil Malamuth, a psychologist at the University of Michigan, conducted a study of 2,652 men and found that those who had admitted having forced sex on a woman tended to have a hostile adversarial relationship with women. "These men feel they have to be in control of their relationships with women, even in conversation," he said in his report.

Whether your attacker is a stranger, an acquaintance, or someone you thought you knew very well, what you must keep uppermost in your mind is the fact that rape is a violent crime and that the need to humiliate and overpower, not sexual gratification, is the motivation for the attack. This will help you to prevent panic and to think clearly and make the best decisions possible.

If you are being threatened by attack, some of the following tactics may be used to try to avoid the attack. A loud noise such as that made by a police whistle or a Freon horn may be enough to frighten him off. Sometimes screaming will do the trick. Yell "call the police" or "fire." Do not yell "help": no one wants to help, but almost everyone wants to see a fire. Try to be sure there is someone near enough to hear the noise or your scream. Otherwise, you may infuriate the attacker, and if no one is there to respond, the problem may be intensified.

Stalling is another tactic that may help. Several ploys have proven to be useful. Among these is feigning a fainting attack or a convulsion. Pretending to have severe pains in the abdomen or chest may be effective. Vomiting or urinating on the attacker are other tricks that have aborted an attack.

Running to a safe place may be a successful tactic if the circumstances are favorable. However, you must be able to run fast and have a safe place within a reasonable distance to run to. If you are in an isolated area, any attempt to flee may make the situation worse by angering the rapist.

If it is impossible to avoid the attack, try not to do anything that will threaten the attacker. If you stay calm and do not antagonize him, it is usually possible to defuse his anger and prevent any serious physical injury. If he is a date who is drunk, stalling for time can be helpful because he may eventually pass out. (Also, a man who is drunk enough is not likely to be able to have an erection.)

Talking may be the best way to abort an attack if it is impossible to frighten him away or escape. It is necessary to talk calmly "with" him, not "to" him. Enhance his ego. Never cry, plead, moralize, or make small talk: this may be just what he is looking for and expects to hear. Although he may not have picked out a specific victim, the rapist has carefully planned the scenario for the rape and operates within this fantasy. Therefore, if the victim can talk with him and make him see her as a person, rather than as an object, and himself as a worthwhile individual, instead of some kind of monster, he may come to his senses and stop, ending the attack. Some women have talked about their families, religion, plans for the future: try anything to break his fantasy.

Fighting is the last tactic to use. All rapists are potentially violent and are capable of inflicting serious physical harm. If he has a weapon, he will not hesitate to use it. Many victims have been sprayed with their own Mace or shot with their own guns, and several "fighters" have had broken bones and other severe physical injuries in addition to genital trauma. Fighting is not the method of choice unless you have been well trained. Surprise and speed of reaction are necessary if you are to be successful. You must be able and willing to overpower and disable the attacker because the struggle itself may enrage him and increase his violence. The risk of serious injury is definitely increased when the victim responds with physical force. Remember the emotional stimulus for rape is anger and hostility not sex.

If an attack is inevitable, try to get it over with as easily and as quickly as possible. Submit and try to show no emotion. Although it is not necessary to cooperate, do not resist unless he is going to beat or maim you. Be alert to anything that may help to identify the man: height, weight, skin color, eye color, hair type and color, scars, language, odors, clothing. You can help the police immeasurably if you are alert and do not panic.

Remember rape is a crime and there is no more reason for you to feel embarrassed or ashamed than if you had been the victim of any other crime.

You will need help because the psychological trauma of the attack, even if physical rape was not completed, can be destructive to you and others close to you. Some studies report that 50 percent of the victims are separated from the man in their life within two years after the rape.

The police should be called. (Unfortunately, because of persistent attitudes toward rape, there may be personal reasons for not wanting to call the police. For example, in one case a woman involved in a custody battle felt her husband might use the attack as evidence of her promiscuity.) Remember, rape is a violent crime; you are the victim of a crime. The police understand this and will be supportive and helpful. Rapists are repeaters, and the police may be able to identify the attacker just from your story. The victim can change her mind anytime, but unless the crime is reported, it will never be known how many rapes actually occur. It is not necessary to prosecute just because the crime is reported. The police will usually take the victim to a hospital or rape treatment facility for skilled care and will provide transportation in any case.

It is important to go "as is." No shower, bath, or douche should be taken, and the same clothes should be worn. Bed sheets, towels, and so forth should not be disturbed if the police are to be involved. Semen samples must be available as incriminating evidence and for HIV testing. The "scene" should be preserved, and all physical evidence of the attack saved.

If you do not want to call the police, call a rape crisis counselor (practically all phone books have such a listing), or you can ask the operator if there is a crime victim's hotline. Either source can recommend a physician who will examine you and give any medical treatment that is indicated. Either the counselor or the doctor will give you the psychological support and care you need. Do not underestimate the psychic trauma of sexual assault. Rape victims have special needs. Seek help from people who have been trained to counsel rape victims. This skilled care is necessary if you are to survive the attack successfully and have no permanent emotional damage.

TREATMENT

All victims of sexual attack need care and counseling. If the problem is not dealt with properly at the time, the effects may surface weeks, months, or even years after the attack and may take longer to resolve than if it had been taken care of at the time of the incident.

Comprehensive care, both medical and psychological, should be available to every victim of sexual assault. No one who does not understand the problems of these victims should be involved in their treatment. Trained specialists in this area must have empathy, not sympathy, for the patient. Understanding is essential; sympathy is degrading. Rape is a legal not a medical diagnosis; therefore, no judgments should be made by the medical team.

Today most areas have some kind of treatment facility available to the rape victim. Large cities have crisis centers, and many smaller communities have volunteers who are ready to counsel victims of sexual assault. This is especially true in university towns and those cities in which women's groups are well organized. A properly staffed rape treatment center is organized so that expert treatment is available at all hours. It may be connected with a hospital or be freestanding. Under ideal circumstances, the team should consist of a gynecologist, a nurse, and a social worker, all of whom have been trained in crisis counseling and caring for the specific needs of the victim of sexual assault.

Because the victim has just been through an ordeal during which she felt completely powerless, it is absolutely necessary that the victim regain control of her life as soon as possible after the attack. One way to accomplish this quickly is to encourage her to make all necessary decisions. It is essential to explain to her that even if she does not wish to report the crime, she needs a medical examination and may need medication to prevent venereal disease and pregnancy. She must also face the possibility of having been infected with the AIDS virus. A test for AIDS may not be necessary at this time. Even if the test is negative at the time of initial examination, it should be repeated at 3, 6, and 12 months because it may turn positive later. She and those close to her will need professional counseling if they are to handle this crisis properly and go on with their lives. However, it is the victim who should have the decisive voice in determining what is to be done after all options and their possible consequences have been spelled out for her. In most cases, cooperation is forthcoming when this procedure is followed.

The examination of the patient should be done with only the physician and the nurse in the room unless the patient requests the presence of someone else. The police should never be in the room, even if they are involved.

The medical examination varies depending on the history of the attack. It is not only unnecessary but cruel to do procedures not indicated by the history. All examinations, however, should include careful documentation of injuries; tests for gonorrhea, chlamydia trachomatis, syphilis, and AIDS (if the patient wishes); and tests to see if semen is present in the vaginal canal. If the police have been called into the case, specimens such as vaginal fluid, foreign bodies, pubic hair, venous blood, and saliva are collected as evidence. Photographs of any injuries are essential because most bruises and abrasions are healed by the time the case goes to court; the patient has no visual evidence of the attack.

Severe injuries should, of course, be treated before the routine examinations are done. In several instances in our experience the specimens to be used as evidence were collected in the operating room while the patient was under anesthesia.

Prophylactic medication should be offered for sexually transmissible disease (STD), and the patient should be encouraged to take it. Although the reported incidence of gonorrhea following rape is only 3 percent and of syphilis 0.1 percent, proper medical attention can ensure that neither is contracted because of a rape. If there has been abrasion of the skin, tetanus prevention may be indicated.

The incidence of pregnancy following a rape is reported as 1 percent. Despite this low risk, medication to prevent conception should be offered unless the victim is already pregnant or on a method of family planning or the assault occurred more than 72 hours before the examination. Pregnancy secondary to rape is not a pleasant prospect, and prevention is less traumatic than menstrual extraction or interruption of the pregnancy after conception has occurred. Several contraceptive methods may be offered, but the one most commonly used is Ovral (two tablets at initial exam, two 12 hours later); the classical morning-after pill (diethylstilbestrol, or DES), or other forms of estrogen. If estrogen is used to prevent pregnancy, it must be given within 72 hours after the exposure. Insertion of an intrauterine device has been suggested, but this is questionable. Placing such a device is not always a simple procedure in women who have not been pregnant. In addition, any unnecessary manipulation in the vaginal area only adds to the trauma of the rape victim.

If the patient was treated with prophylactic or contraceptive medication, she should be reexamined and retested six weeks after the initial examination to be sure that she has not contracted a sexually transmissible disease or become pregnant in spite of the medication. If no antibiotics were given, the patient should be reexamined for gonorrhea two weeks after the attack.

The psychological assessment and counseling of the patient should begin as soon as the patient reaches a treatment center, although the formal counseling usually occurs after the physical examination. The doctor, nurse, and counselor evaluate the victim's mental state and her ability to cope with the situation as they talk with her.

The rape experience precipitates a crisis, and the trauma fits within the framework of the general crisis theory. A crisis is an event that produces stress and comes with suddenness: there is no opportunity to prepare for the emergency. The reaction of the rape victim is similar to that of grief. However, in addition to the deep sense of loss that the rape victim experiences, she must also deal with the emotions resulting from the threats to her safety and the invasion of her body. The loss of self-esteem and the threats to her relationships with others close to her only add to her difficulties. An inability to develop or recapture her sense of self-worth and realize that she is a worthwhile person is one of the long-term problems of a rape victim that can jeopardize her future success. It is reassuring when the victim can talk with a counselor and find that the emotions and reactions she is having are the same as those of other women who have been sexually assaulted and that she is not the only victim who has felt that way.

In the rape trauma syndrome the victim goes through three stages of recovery: the acute stage, the outward adjustment stage, and the integration stage. The length of time needed to pass through these stages may vary with the basic personality and previous experiences of the victim, but all rape victims go through these steps. Since 1980, the American Psychiatric Association has recognized the rape trauma syndrome as an authentic disorder. Following that recommendation, state courts around the country have been struggling with the question of whether expert testimony about this effect is admissible. In 1990 New York's highest court approved testimony about the emotional side effects of sexual assault when the intent is to educate jurors about the seemingly cool behavior of the victim, depending on what stage of the trauma she is undergoing at the time of her courtroom appearance.

During the acute stage the woman experiences a gamut of emotions including shock, anger, fear, hostility, disbelief that it could happen to her, and often denial that it did happen. It is essential that she receive practical help as well as medical and psychological support during this time. Some of the practical problems that arise are whether she will tell her family or friends, where she will stay, if she needs money, whether she will report it to the police. All these things must be dealt with almost immediately after the attack.

She may have many physical complaints that will persist for weeks after the attack. Some of these are headaches due to the tension, inability to sleep, nightmares, abdominal pains, loss of appetite, and even nausea. Usually all these somatic complaints are the result of the psychological trauma she has experienced. It is important to make her realize that she is not to blame for the attack and that the offender is a criminal to be caught and punished.

It is during this first phase that it is so important for family and friends to provide adequate support and, if there is a special man in her life, for him to be understanding and realize the sexual fears she may have. If no one is available to understand and support her during this early phase, the victim may become disorganized and thus unable to regain a healthy self-image and unable to function or relate to others as she did before the attack.

The outward adjustment stage is the period during which the patient seems to be doing well, sometimes too well. She resumes her life, returns to work or school, and is apparently adjusting to and coping with the trauma. It is common during this phase for the patient to suppress her feelings, and she may be depressed. She may try to forget that the assault ever happened, and unless she is forced to, she may not face the problem and may stay in limbo for weeks. The longer this phase persists, the more difficult it is for the patient to begin the reorganization process.

Once the patient has faced the problem, she begins the integration stage. This is the period during which resolution of the rape experience takes place, and it may be several months or even years before this phase is completed. It is common for a patient to change her residence and telephone number in an effort to prevent the attacker from finding her and perhaps doing it again. She may seldom go out alone even during the daylight hours. The support of friends and family is again essential. The counselor encourages the victim to seek support, but at the same time expresses confidence that she will again be able to function at least as well as she did before the assault.

During this period the woman is willing to discuss her experience and can talk about it without becoming distraught. She may even be angry and be eager to punish the offender. However she reacts, she is ready to face her anxieties and verbalize her fears; she is ready to recover and return to her world.

If the woman decides to prosecute the offender, she will need ongoing support from her family and from the police and prosecutors. The court procedures are not easy, and it is difficult to win rape cases if the victim is young and pretty and has not had serious physical injuries. The police investigation is often long and tedious. The actual trial does not take place until months after the attack. It is impossible for the victim to resolve the experience and get on with her life until the trial is over. However, many victims, once they realize that the rapist is a criminal and repeats his crime over and over, are quite willing to prosecute and try to send him to jail "so he can't do this to another woman."

A woman raped by her husband or a family member (such as a stepfather or an uncle) or by a neighbor or friend has to deal with special problems. It will be no simple matter to establish and maintain her credibility and face the possibility of becoming a pariah in her family and her community because she is accusing an "innocent man who is a respected citizen." Support not only from legal counsel and a psychotherapist but also from women's groups and self-help groups is indispensable during the period following the assault.

Women who decide to prosecute the rapist should look at themselves as trail blazers. Ten years ago the case would not have gone to court; 20 years ago no one would have listened to them at all.

Women who have been victims of sexual assault—and domestic violence— also have the right to expect their personal doctors to take the time to listen to them. Having decided that many male doctors are often too embarrassed or too uncomfortable to counsel women in need of someone to confide in, the American Medical Association issued new guidelines in 1995 to help their members be more supportive. Describing sexual assault as a "silent violent epidemic" in which the perpetrator is often a lover, friend, acquaintance, or relative, the guidelines point out that although doctors are in a good position to recognize and treat victims, they are not likely to ask routine questions of their female patients about violence in their lives, nor are women likely to initiate discussions about such matters. The new guidelines, which have been distributed among doctors and nurses, urge all health care professionals to be alert to signs of physical as well as emotional abuse. When a female of any age panics and withdraws from a doctor's touch during an examination, the doctor can play a critical role in helping such a patient recover from many of the consequences of sexual assault.

HEALTH SAFEGUARDS FOR WORKING WOMEN

Frances M. Love, M.D.

Late, Specialist in Occupational Medicine; Retired Southwestern
Regional Medical Director, Gulf Oil Corporation

Helene MacLean

Medical Writer and Editor; Author, *Caring for Your Parents, Relief
from Chronic Arthritis Pain*; Coauthor, *Recovering from a
Hysterectomy, Migraine: Beating the Odds*

Here are some facts and figures of particular interest to gainfully employed
women as well as to women who work as homemakers and mothers, many of
whom are likely to enter or reenter the workforce in the future.

What percentage of the total labor force is made up of women? Women
account for 46 percent of the total U.S. labor force. This figure is expected to
rise to 48 percent by 2005.

*What percentage of women aged 16 and over in the United States are in the
civilian labor force?* Of the 102 million in that age group, a record 60 million—
more than 50 percent—are in the civilian workforce or are looking for work.

Where are most women likely to be employed? The largest proportion work
in technical, sales, and clerical jobs.

Which jobs continue to be viewed as "women's" work? One figure that remains unchanged since 1940 is that 74 percent of teachers are women. A figure
that remains largely unchanged since 1950: one in five working women holds a
secretarial or clerical job. Most professional nurses, bookkeepers, bank tellers,
librarians, cashiers, and telephone operators are women.

In what fields have women made the most substantial progress? More jobs have been obtained in managerial and professional occupations as a result of expanding educational gains and equal employment opportunities. The number of women economists, lawyers, pharmacists, doctors, and stockbrokers has grown dramatically, to the point where more than half (52.8 percent) of all professional workers are women; however, because of the larger numbers of women in clerical and low-wage service work, 75 percent of working women still earn less than $25,000 a year.

Have women made significant progress in the areas of business and finance? Only a few at the very top. In 1994, for the first time, more than half of the country's largest corporations had at least one woman on their board of directors.

Are practically all employed women working full time? In 1994, of the 57 million women employed in the United States, 41 million worked full time (35 hours per week or more) and 16 million worked part time (less than 35 hours). Of this number, 3.3 million held more than one job, mainly for economic reasons: to meet regular household expenses, to pay off debts, and to save for the future.

Has the gap between men's and women's median weekly earnings been decreasing? Yes, but the discrepancy still exists. In 1965 the ratio of women's median weekly earnings to men's was 59 percent. It has gone up to 76.4 percent, but even in traditionally female occupations, where women outnumber men, such as registered nurses and elementary school teachers, women continue to earn less than men. In fact, even though there have been breakthroughs in nontraditional areas, as soon as women become the majority in any given field, the pay and the prestige go down.

Of the 68.5 million families in the United States, how many are maintained by women (no husband present)? Eighteen percent, or 12.4 million: 8 million are white, 3.8 are black, and 1.5 are Hispanic.

What is the income differential when a woman maintains the family? When no husband is present, the median income is $17,443; for families maintained by men with no wife present, the figure is $26,467; for married couples, where both husband and wife work, the median income is $43,005.

What is women's occupational outlook for the future? Here are some highlights from the U.S. Department of Labor's 1993 overview, *Women Workers— Trends and Issues:*

- The four fastest-growing occupational groups during the next decade are projected to be (1) executive, administrative, and managerial; (2) professional specialties; (3) technicians and related support; and (4) services. Some 13.3 million workers are expected to be added by 2005. As in the preceding 15-year period (1975–90), the majority of newly created jobs will be nonfarm wage and salary jobs in the service-producing industries, especially retail trade, hotels and lodging services, business and repair services, health services, and public administration.

- Of the 3.2 million government jobs to be created by 2005, almost all (3 million) are expected to originate at the state and local level.
- Women are expected to be granted 42 percent of all first professional degrees by 2001.
- The projections show faster rates of employment growth for occupations that require higher levels of education and training and slower rates of growth for those that require less formal education and training.

HOW WORKING WOMEN SEE THEIR PROBLEMS

A recent survey of working women conducted by the Women's Bureau of the U.S. Department of Labor yielded information not expected by the bureau's director, Karen Nussbaum. In a *New York Times* interview (10/15/94), she observed: "The concern about discrimination and equal pay surprised me. I was also surprised by the consensus that emerged. We tend to think of training as a blue collar issue, child care as a low income issue, the glass ceiling as something professional women care about, and discrimination as a concern for women of color, but each of these issues cuts across all lines." Other information that emerged: Although four out of five women said they liked their jobs, their top priorities for improvement were better pay and health insurance. Most respondents agreed that the number-one conflict requiring the attention of the president was the difficulty of balancing work and family. Stress was identified as a health problem by 60 percent of women, especially by single mothers and women in their forties holding professional or managerial jobs. (Stress is discussed in detail later in this chapter.)

Women whose well-being has been affected by gender discrimination, not only in blue-collar jobs, but on the managerial and professional level, have been speaking out in congressional hearings, in the courts, and in the press. Gender bias has been cited in the highest ranks of the CIA and the FBI, in the top management of the movie and television industries, and in the most prestigious law firms. Women are especially concerned about their underrepresentation in science and engineering and in the ranks of tenured professors at Ivy League universities. Lesbians in the military continue to fight for less restrictive policies about acknowledgment of their sexual identity.

"MOM THE PROVIDER"

Under this headline a *New York Times* editorial (5/14/95) called attention to the fact that wives are sharing equally with their husbands in supporting the family. According to a Louis Harris survey, almost half of the married women questioned said their earnings provided half or more of their family's income. The editorial made explicit what millions of American women know: "Imagine it: in all those suburban streets, half of the houses, half of the computers, half of the new pairs of Nikes and mountain bikes and orthodontists' bills, paid for by mother."

The latest information about mothers employed outside the home emphasizes that these women work to support the family, not because they "want something interesting to do" or "to earn extra money." Thus, a family style dependent on two incomes has become the norm in American society. As for single-mothers, the trends toward later marriages and more divorces indicate a higher likelihood that women will head their own households at some time in their lives. A recent report reveals that while 67.8 percent of married mothers are labor force participants, 73.2 percent of previously married mothers (now divorced, separated, or widowed) are employed.

Contrary to what some people think, most mothers do not feel guilty about working outside the home. What most of them feel is anger about the lack of affordable day care. Of the 22 million preschool children whose mothers work, less than half are in day care centers, including the unregulated ones operated out of someone's home. The majority are looked after by a relative, a neighbor, a baby-sitter, or an older sibling. And when these arrangements unexpectedly fail, the mother or the father—if he's available—must stay home, or one parent may have to take the child to work (a not uncommon solution). Some large companies provide on-site day care facilities, thereby eliminating some of the anxieties for working mothers, but these facilities rarely offer supervised after-school programs for the millions of youngsters in the 6 to 13 age group.

WORKING WOMEN AND ELDER CARE

When the Family and Medical Leave Act was signed by the president in 1993, the responsibility for elder care had already begun to disrupt the lives of many working women. Entitled by this legislation to unpaid leave, those who cope with sporadic crises in the family find themselves trying to make up for lost time by working extra hours and taking more work home. Andrew Scharlach, a University California professor who specializes in the problems of aging, estimates productivity losses from elder care at $2,500 per employed caregiver per year based on time missed from work and the cost of replacing caregivers who leave their jobs altogether. With the scattering of family members, more and more women, as they themselves age, are looking out not only for parents, but also for grandparents, aunts, and uncles. Solutions vary depending on workplace flexibility and career demands. Thirty-seven percent of women in the workforce will be age 40 to 54, the prime time for caring for elderly parents, by 2005. It is to be hoped that between now and then, politicians who talk about family values will have improved the long-term care system for both generations.

WELL-BEING IN THE WORKPLACE

In 1970 Congress passed the Occupational Safety and Health Act (OSHA). One of its provisions is that the employer is responsible for the safety and health of employees in the workplace. Another provision states that employees must be informed of known and suspected occupational health hazards. This "right to know" clause implies that those who have the information are obliged to communicate it to concerned employees.

The National Institute for Occupational Safety and Health (NIOSH) is the research and investigatory arm of OSHA. Any company, union, or committee of three employees may submit a formal request to NIOSH's Health Hazard Evaluation Program.

It is only in recent years that women's on-the-job health has become a matter of interest and concern to special groups. While it is true that many men face life-threatening occupational hazards, women are especially vulnerable, and in ever-increasing numbers, to the pervasive problems of stress-induced illnesses, and, more seriously, to the irreversible damage to childbearing capabilities caused by exposure to radiation and chemicals.

In hearings conducted on June 23, 1982, by the House of Representatives' Subcommittee on Education and Labor, testimony was given by a speaker on behalf of 9 to 5, the National Association of Working Women. Judith Gregory, research director of the Working Woman's Education Fund of the parent organization, pointed out that American management's idea of the office of the future means little more than a recreation of the factory of the past. "Women office workers are on the front line of the new wave of automation," and women must therefore stress the need for more research on the cumulative negative effects of the new technology on their health.

By the end of 1986, a NIOSH report described in compelling detail the substantial health problems resulting from work overload, lack of control over one's job, limited job opportunities, and feelings of dehumanization attributable to technological "advances" in the workplace.

The 1980s also witnessed another development of major importance: the revival of interest in job-related illness. A landmark article published in March 1990 in the *New England Journal of Medicine* begins by noting that until as recently as the past decade, "The clinical discipline of occupational medicine [has been] largely unstudied, untaught, and unpracticed in major medical centers." The article in two successive parts provides the American medical profession with its first overview of occupational diseases and their causes, beginning with lung diseases (going far beyond miner's "lung" and farmer's "lung" and including more than 50 substances causally linked to asthma in the workplace) and continuing with disorders of the kidney and blood caused by exposure to toxic chemicals; irreversible damage to the nervous system, liver, and gastrointestinal system; and damage to male sperm from the same types of exposure. The authors of these two articles—Dr. Mark R. Cullen and Dr. Martin G. Cherniak, staff members of the Yale–New Haven Occupational Medicine Program, and Dr. Linda Rosenstock of the Occupational Medicine Program of the University of Washington School of Medicine in Seattle—have attempted to be as inclusive as possible in alerting their colleagues to health hazards in the workplace, discussing not only cancer and the chemicals known to cause it but also the assorted musculoskeletal disorders that are now disabling an ever-increasing number of "high-tech" employees. An indication of the lag between the problems workers have been experiencing and the medical profession's recognition of the problems is the fact that these researchers include under the heading "New Problems in Occupational Medicine" discussions of video display terminals, the sick building syndrome, and multiple chemical sensitivities. For many years working women have been talking to their doctors about headaches, allergies, breathing problems, and assorted pains that originate in the workplace. It is hoped that when you call your doctor's attention to this two-part article, your complaints will no longer be ascribed to imagination, suppressed anger, or psychostress but will be given the serious consideration they merit.

In the pages that follow, some of the more common health-threatening workplace conditions are discussed together with suggestions for how to deal with them.

ACHES AND PAINS

If you spend most of your working day sitting down, the chair you use should be suitable for the body movements your job requires, and it should be adjustable to your own body dimensions. Unless these requirements are met, the result over a long period will be musculoskeletal aches and pains, especially in the shoulders and lower back. The first requirement of a chair is that it be sturdy and stable. Many accidents could be avoided if all office chairs, no matter what their other features, were designed so that the seat can swivel on a column that is set into a five-pronged base with casters that lock.

Whatever tasks you perform while seated, your hips and knees should be bent at right angles. If you have to operate a buzzer or a foot pedal, the seat height should be adjustable so that these movements can be accomplished comfortably. If you spend most of your time reading and writing at a desk and you don't operate a machine, your chair should have a firm straight back. If you work with your hands in a forward position on a keyboard, your chair should have a small flexible backrest that supports your lower back.

One of the most effective ways of reducing back problems is to develop and maintain good sitting posture. It's also helpful to set up a routine of exercises designed to strengthen the muscles that support your spine. Backaches can be reduced by varying your work posture from time to time, alternately sitting and standing. Try not to stand in one position for too long, and be sure that your shoes are giving you proper support. Neither very high heels nor running shoes nor "barefoot" sandals are the right footwear for a job that requires hours of standing. Leather (not plastic) pumps or walking shoes with medium heels or low-heeled oxfords are the best choice.

If you have to lift heavy objects, be kind to your back by lifting them the right way. Don't bend over in a hairpin curve and hold the object at a distance from your body in order to keep your clothes clean. And don't try to prove your prowess as a weight lifter by attempting to pick up and carry anything that weighs more than about 25 pounds. That's just about the weight of a large plant, five reams of copying paper, or five encyclopedia volumes. Do bend from the knees, and when you raise the object, hold it close to your chest.

In addition to lower back discomfort, pains in the joints of the neck, lower arm, wrist, and fingers are associated with keyboard work, especially those operations during which your back moves very little and your wrist and fingers are constantly flexing and bending. These rapid repeated movements can lead to musculoskeletal disorders now grouped together under the term repetitive strain injuries (RSIs) or repetitive motion injuries (RMIs). Most commonly, such injuries include tendinitis (inflammation of the fibrous tissue that connects the muscles to the bones), tenosynovitis (inflammation of the tendons and the membranes that line and lubricate the joints), "tennis elbow" (inflammation of the lateral muscles of the forearm), and carpal tunnel syndrome, which is caused by nerve damage in the fingers and is characterized by sharp pains as well as tingling sensations in the thumb and fingers. Some pains in the fingers and wrist, especially in the left hand, are attributable to the "q w e r t y" typewriter keyboard, in which the left hand does 60 percent of the work, and only 30 percent of the work is done on the easy-to-reach center keys. Unfortunately, and in spite of more sensibly designed keyboard arrangements, the old "q w e r t y" design was formally adopted as the international standard in 1971 and has since been built into the keyboards of the new technology. However, recent improvements in keyboard design have reduced the elevation between rows and sloped the key surfaces farther forward. Both these innovations have decreased the wear and tear on joints and tendons.

Sharp pains in the forearm (the catchall term is "tennis elbow") may be caused by constant flexing of the wrist or by maintaining an uncomfortable arm position at the desk. The latter problem may be solved by moving the chair closer to or farther from the desk at the same time that your back is correctly supported. Or try raising or lowering the chair seat to see whether the position of your arm on the desk is improved.

If pains interfere with work efficiency and/or with sleep, discuss the problem with your doctor and be sure to describe the nature of your job. If the doctor understands that the problem originates in your job, you may be advised to take anti-inflammatory medication at the same time that you try to alternate jobs with someone whose work doesn't require the same repetitive motions. In some cases of tenosynovitis, surgery can be helpful.

Women who work in the performing arts—especially dancers and instrumentalists—are often subject to musculoskeletal problems that produce immobilizing pain. Through the use of such alternative therapies as acupuncture for pain control and the Alexander Technique for posture correction, many have been able to avoid overmedication and surgery. These treatments, as well as others that are noninvasive, are often recommended in pain control centers by physiatrists, the doctors who specialize in treating pain and rehabilitation by means other than medicines. (See the chapter on "Alternative Therapies.")

BAD AIR

In the interest of energy conservation, most modern office buildings are designed with windows that can't be opened, and they are equipped with central air-conditioning that recirculates filtered air. The result in many workplaces is a combination of complaints known as *sick building syndrome.* This condition is characterized by irritation of the mucous membranes of the eyes, nose, and throat. While these symptoms seem to have much in common with an allergic response, they result not from an allergy but from indoor air pollution and inadequate ventilation. Typical irritants include asbestos and glass fibers from insulating materials; formaldehyde gases from foam and furniture (this slow exudation is known as "outgassing"); hydrocarbons from copying machines, fax machines, laser and bubble-jet printers; dirt and detergent residues in floor coverings; and where legal restrictions have been slow to recognize the health hazards of exposure to secondary smoke—cigarette smoke.

According to a recent *Wall Street Journal* story (10/26/95) at least 30 percent of the nation's 4.5 million buildings other than residential and industrial have indoor air problems severe enough to expose 60 million to 120 million people a year to contaminants that make them sick. Many lawsuits are being filed on behalf of employees who claim to have been permanently disabled because of day-in day-out exposure to toxic indoor air, and some estimates calculate that the sick building syndrome is costing this country as much as $100 billion in medical costs and absenteeism.

No workplace environment is free of bad air risk if standards for flushing out contaminated air and bringing in fresh air are not scrupulously followed. Air-conditioning ducts, humidifiers, and drain pans must be cleaned out regularly to prevent the accumulation of mold, viruses, and bacteria, some of which can be life-threatening. Recently designed central filtering systems combined with individual filters at work sites are reducing absenteeism caused by airborne toxins.

Women who work in art departments or with arts and crafts materials should be especially aware of fumes and vapors from solvents and other necessary supplies that can have a harmful effect on the skin and respiratory system. It is especially important to read all labels carefully because they may contain warnings about contents linked to chronic diseases as well as to fetal damage. Especially toxic are solvents used in silk screening, which are associated with neurological damage, respiratory disease, and miscarriage. Ventilation requirements should be strictly observed in all cases.

Women who develop health problems attributable to faulty ventilation should find out whether women in other offices in the same building are having similar problems. If this is so, it should be possible to initiate an investigation of the entire system. It should be kept in mind that air cannot be cleaned of pollutants by fans, which merely circulate the noxious substances.

While the ailment known as multiple chemical sensitivity has not yet been recognized as an authentic complaint by doctors and scientists, sufferers insist that even the trace amounts of certain chemicals in perfumes or carpets can trigger acute headaches and respiratory problems. In spite of the uncertainties of the medical profession about multiple chemical sensitivity, it has been declared a disability under the Americans with Disabilities Act, and some state workers' compensation boards are recognizing claims based on lost earnings due to this problem.

One of the most widespread developments in this area is the recognition that strong odors of any sort can make people sick. As a consequence, to accommodate those who are scent-sensitive, many businesses have been banning fragrances—perfumes, hair spray, air fresheners—in the workplace. If your office mate uses a fragrance that causes you to wheeze and sneeze or gives you a headache, you are within your rights to ask her or him (politely of course) to stop wearing it to work. When it's the boss's strongly scented perfume or after-shave lotion that's causing the problem, it would probably be advisable to discuss the matter with the director of human resources!

VDTs

The automation of producing, transmitting, manipulating, and storing information is proceeding at a dizzying pace thanks to VDTs (video display terminals). These links between people and computers are also called word processors. Of the 50 million VDT work stations in use in 1992, it was estimated that 80 percent were operated by women.

In the NIOSH study of 130 occupations, in which secretaries ranked second only to day laborers in the incidence of stress-related diseases, it was also found that the secretaries who operate VDTs face higher stress than all other groups, including air traffic controllers. There is not yet sufficient information about the cumulative threat of VDTs to women's health (occupational diseases often are not sudden and acute but slow and insidious). However, a recent

Massachusetts survey indicates that VDT operators suffer from a higher rate of musculoskeletal discomfort, headaches, and fatigue than other clerical workers. In some parts of the country, and in many places of employment where office and professional workers are represented by unions, collective bargaining has resulted in special medical insurance coverage for VDT operators. Also, committees on occupational safety and health that are part of most state legislatures now have subcommittees whose special concern is the consequence of VDT work.

When NIOSH discovered that VDT workers had higher levels of complaints about aching and swollen joints than other office workers, it was found that musculoskeletal stresses could be decreased by adjusting as many parts of the work station as possible, particularly screens, lighting, and chairs, to the woman's needs. Backaches and neck and shoulder stiffness can be prevented in the following ways: stretch regularly (after each hour at the screen, exercise your fingers, shrug your shoulders, tilt your head from side to side); sit with your feet flat on the floor and legs as far apart as clothing and modesty permit; adjust your chair so that it tilts forward slightly, giving your back a slight arch. Problems of skin rashes from the static charge surrounding VDTs can be minimized by using an electrostatic shield. Eye complaints can usually be ameliorated by finding out whether special eyeglasses are needed to accommodate the requirements of the "middle distance" of the screen. Neither a reading lens nor a distance lens, as combined in bifocals, is a suitable solution. For women over 40, when focusing begins to become a problem, testing for new glasses to be worn at the VDT is recommended. The likelihood of eye discomfort is also significantly reduced if the screen is movable so that it can be adjusted to a comfortable angle.

The results of a six-year study undertaken by NIOSH and published in the *New England Journal of Medicine* in March 1991 indicate that pregnant women who work all day at VDTs are at no greater risk of miscarriage than pregnant women who work at similar jobs that do not involve the use of a terminal. This study is by no means accepted as conclusive. The National Institute of Child Health and Development has sponsored the first study of whether VDTs pose any risk to *early* pregnancy. Unlike the NIOSH study, this later one by the Mt. Sinai School of Medicine is examining the possible role of stress. Other researchers recommend that pregnant women take the special precaution of arranging for half-time work during the first trimester.

Among the many factors responsible for stress-related health problems in VDT operators and professionals who use VDTs are the speed with which the technology is changing and the difficulty of mastering it, inadequate training, and electronic monitoring.

Electronic monitoring in the form of surveillance to evaluate an employee's speed and general performance has been going on for some time. With advances in technology, evaluation has been transformed into spying. By scanning E-mail and computer files as well as checking voice-mail messages, a supervisor can gain access to many aspects of the employee's personal life and opinions. So far, most of this spying is legal. The only relevant restrictive law is one that forbids the employer from knowingly listening in on a worker's personal phone calls. Both government and nongovernment agencies, such as unions and other advocacy groups, have been trying to address the stress effects of electronic monitoring. Congressional interest in privacy for workers has been expressed in bills introduced for consideration since 1987 without success. In 1994, for example, Senator Paul Simon (D-Illinois) proposed a Privacy for Consumers and Workers Act, which would require that all employers inform new workers that they will be monitored, describe the type of monitoring, its frequency, and how it will be used. Both "9 to 5" and the Service Employees International Union have developed standards to put an end to monitoring abuses affecting millions of women. Invasion of privacy on a level heretofore impossible has created an atmosphere of anxiety and tension affecting health and job performance. Women who would like to urge their company to create an official policy on this matter, agreed to by a consensus of management and employees, can receive guidance from the American Civil Liberties Union's National Task Force on Civil Liberties in the Workplace (212-944-9800 ext. 416) or the Job Survival Hotline (800-522-0925) operated by "9 to 5."

For the reduction of psychological stress, an adjustable work schedule has been suggested. NIOSH also recommends job rotation and rest breaks for the reduction of fatigue, irritability, and anxiety: operators with moderate visual demands should take a 15-minute break every two hours; those with heavy demands, a similar break every hour. These recesses should be spent away from the work station with the option of resting, walking about, having refreshment in the cafeteria—whatever is most relaxing. During work breaks, stress management skills such as breathing exercises, meditation, and time alone in a quiet environment (even for 5 minutes), can help maintain equilibrium when pressures accumulate. (See "Alternative Therapies.")

PHOTOCOPIERS

Almost all offices are equipped with photocopiers, and although they are a boon to modern business, care should be taken with their use. A particular problem is carbonless copy paper (CCP), which is still being used in spite of worldwide health complaints attributable to it. Reactions range from itching and rash to hoarseness and coughing. The ingredient in CCP responsible for these reactions is alkylphenol novolac resin. Women showing signs of sensitivity to CCP when handling it should discuss the problem with superiors in terms of its potential dangers.

The following recommendations should be followed to ensure safety when working with copiers:

- Don't try to save time by ignoring the manufacturer's recommendations for safe use.
- Always keep the document cover down, and never look directly at the light, even if you're only making a few copies.
- Make sure that the machine is installed in a well-ventilated area. No one should be expected to use a copier in an airless cubbyhole.
- If you handle quantities of electrosensitive paper, protect your hands and fingers with disposable surgical gloves.
- No one should be expected to sit in the path of the chemical exhaust from a copier. These fumes are a serious health hazard and should be properly vented.

NOISE

An excessively noisy working environment is by no means limited to factories. Many women who work in offices, airports, and retail stores complain of the disastrous effects of ringing bells, clacking machines, loud voices, and the sound of piped-in music. Many unpleasant physical symptoms—rise in blood pressure, increase in sweating, "jumpy" stomach—are attributable to unacceptable noise levels. And when the sounds not only produce headaches but interfere with the ability to think straight, the secondary effects are likely to be general irritability and anxiety.

Because some of your coworkers may not know the extent to which the noise level is affecting their health and job performance, you might discuss the problem with them and try to present a list of practical suggestions for improvement: better soundproofing, phones that light up instead of ringing, sound-absorbing drapes and carpeting, and a lower sound level for the canned music.

STRESS

The previously mentioned NIOSH study found that in addition to secretaries and especially VDT operators, women's high-stress jobs are (listed alphabetically): bank teller, computer programmer, dental assistant, hairdresser, health technician, practical and registered nurse, social worker, teacher's aide, and telephone operator.

Health authorities are concerned about the increasing prevalence among working women of stress-induced aches and pains, sleep disorders, indigestion, eating problems, and loss of sex drive, not to mention the alarming rise in alcoholism and the abuse of legal and illegal drugs. One cardiologist (Dr. Robert S. Elliot at the University of Nebraska) has remarked on the growing number of heart attacks among the "superwomen," who are under more stress than their male counterparts.

However, on-the-job stress is not to be confused with challenge, especially the challenge that leads to accomplishment and recognition. No, the women most likely to suffer from stress and its related wear and tear on body and mind are those who

- feel locked into a job situation over which they have no control;
- get no respect or recognition from their superiors;
- have to deal with invasion of privacy and rudeness from men—either their peers, their superiors, or the company's customers;
- find their work boring *and* exacting;
- fear the prospect of unemployment because of increasing age;
- anticipate the negative aspects of automation;
- spend eight hours a day, five days a week, in an environment that is too noisy, badly ventilated, unsuitably illuminated, and too cramped for comfort.

Dealing with life's inevitable stresses is easier when you're in good health. While many of the stressful circumstances of your job may be out of your control, you *can* be in charge when it comes to eating the right foods, getting enough physical exercise, and setting your priorities so that you have some free time that belongs only to *you.*

If you have to do a lot of standing, be sure you're wearing shoes that fit properly. Have your eyes checked regularly, especially if your job makes special demands on your vision. If you feel that tinted glasses would reduce the discomfort of glare, see about getting them. If the job involves lots of bending and lifting, learn how to perform these tasks efficiently with a minimum of back strain. If you have to sit still for several hours at a time, do suitable stretching exercises during your midmorning and midafternoon breaks. At convenient intervals, practice some meditation techniques.

In many instances, solutions to job stress can be worked out by group action that is friendly rather than combative. Informal meetings with supervisors or with the boss can result in practical solutions to problems that actually interfere with efficiency and productivity. If you can take this point of view rather than proceeding from an adversary position, you may actually alert your employer to conditions that he or she wasn't even aware of.

More and more large organizations have inaugurated workshops in stress management. In some instances, these endeavors may have been an offshoot of an alcoholism treatment program; in others, they may be part of the company's overall employee health program. Companies both large and small are sponsoring Employee Wellness Programs that include dietary counseling, nutrition education, and physical fitness seminars. L.L. Bean in Maine has inaugurated an annual cholesterol and blood pressure check; other family-run enterprises are offering weight-control workshops and are making changes in the foods offered in employee cafeterias. (See also the chapter on "Alternative Therapies" for stress management through the arts, exercise, meditation, and the like.)

SEXUAL HARASSMENT

In the Military:

In emotional, sometimes halting voices, the one officer and three enlisted women, representing each of the military services, told the House Armed Services Committee that they had endured unwanted sexual advances and lewd remarks before turning to military authorities for relief, only to be disdained, ostracized, and, in some cases, transferred to dead-end jobs (*New York Times* 3/10/94).

The Navy has prepared a new 64-page manual on how to recognize, prevent, and deal with sexual harassment. It is a compendium of orders and memorandums Navy leaders have issued since dozens of women were assaulted at the Tailhook Convention of naval aviators in Las Vegas in 1991. Using these new orders and regulations, the Navy has dismissed 89 officers and sailors for sexual harassment since 1991 (*New York Times* 4/10/94).

"I felt that if I didn't make it off the floor, I was sure I was going to be gang-raped," said former Navy lieutenant Paula C. Coughlin, describing the scene at the 1991 convention of the Tailhook Association, an independent group of retired and active naval aviators (New York Times 10/4/94). The former lieutenant was awarded $6.7 million in punitive damages from the hotel where the gathering took place.

In the latest embarrassment for the Navy, a senior admiral has been demoted and forced to retire after being found guilty of sexually harassing a woman who worked for him. . . . The case is another disheartening signal that even at the highest levels, the message has not got through (New York Times 12/9/95).

IN THE LEGAL PROFESSION:
A San Francisco jury has hit the world's largest law firm, Baker & Tindal, with the largest-ever sexual harassment award. Rena Weeks, a secretary who objected to the bawdy remarks and crude gropings of a high-powered partner, stands to collect $50,000 for emotional distress—and $7.1 million in punitive damages (New York Times 9/12/94).

IN THE CORPORATE WORLD:
Faced by a suit containing allegations from 15 secretaries that the company's CEO sexually harassed them at work, Del Laboratories, a cosmetics and pharmaceutical company on Long Island agreed to pay $1.185 million in punitive damages, the biggest settlement ever obtained by the Equal Employment Opportunity Commission in a sexual harassment suit. The most money previously obtained by the commission was $577,750 in a Minnesota case in 1993. The women in the Del Labs case were limited by law to $300,000 each in punitive damages and had asked for back wages as well (New York Times 8/4/95).

Ever since the 1991 testimony of Anita Hill at the Clarence Thomas confirmation hearings conducted by the Senate Judiciary Committee, the subject of sexual harassment in the workplace has continued to make national headlines. In the United States Army and the United States Navy, where women's work often involves putting their lives on the line, it is now known that sexual harassment frequently becomes sexual assault. Careers in the fighting forces, in politics, and in the corporate world have been affected. Women keep saying, "Men just don't get it," and the serious students of human behavior ask whether sexual harassment, like date rape, is inextricably woven into the fabric of American society—an expression of the power men have over women rather than an expression of erotic passion.

Many misunderstandings and ambiguities complicate the relationship between the sexes in the workplace. Some are the result of differences in ethnic traditions; others are caused by socially conditioned generational differences.

Many mixed messages are transmitted by people who are out of touch with their feelings. An increasing number of women, and especially women executives, are now involved in new situations that make both sexes uncomfortable. Many men in their 50s and older have the greatest difficulties in dealing with women who are their professional peers. Many men of all ages feel ill at ease about going to another city to attend a convention with a female coworker. Many women aren't sure about how to entertain male customers or clients. And because no one wants to be accused of sexual bias or sexual harassment, it often becomes even more difficult to spell out the nature of the problem. But unless such problems are anticipated and aired for discussion, mutually satisfactory solutions can't be achieved.

What a woman perceives as sexual harassment depends to some extent on how she sees herself in relation to men. However, offensive, unwanted, and uninvited attention in the form of a day-in, day-out barrage of off-color jokes, sneaky pats and squeezes, and outright "propositions" can become so stressful that they affect a woman's health and competence. Such behavior becomes most threatening and difficult to deal with when it is an expression of power. Even after Senator Bob Packwood was driven from his office by his peers because of his egregious behavior, he continued to be bewildered by the charges against him, saying that some women "did not complain at the time and continued to work" for him.

A typical traditional occurrence: in spite of appropriate behavior on your part, your superior takes advantage of his position and makes it clear that your work status, training, and advancement depend on the extent to which you grant sexual favors. A more recent scenario: with more and more women entering trades and professions previously considered male preserves, sexual harassment becomes an expression of hostility on the part of male peers. This form of angry aggressiveness is likely to be encountered in widely different groups—for example, among resident doctors in hospitals, among police officers and firefighters, and in unionized skilled trades—where the message being conveyed is "No Women Wanted Here." In every occupation, when women become a competitive threat, sexual comments (both verbal and visual) become one of the power ploys for trivializing women and "putting them in their place" as no more than sex objects. An example of a situation now considered justifiable cause for complaint and corrective action: a secretary is expected to spend time in the mailroom several times each day to instruct mailroom employees on how to handle particular packages. The walls of the room are covered with obscene and pornographic pinups. In 1991 a federal judge ruled that such pictures were a form of sexual harassment because by presenting women only as sexual objects, they did not recognize women as competent coworkers. It is therefore the legal responsibility of company management to remove these images.

Many men have been raised in a tradition that has led them to believe that ogling, whistling, joshing, and patting are ways to flatter women, and they are truly astonished when they are told that many women find such behavior insulting and unacceptable. A department manager, male or female, can usually cool escalating antagonisms by having a talk session during which grievances are expressed and the perpetrators are made to understand the nature of the problem: not that *they* are objectionable, but that their behavior is. The essence of sexual harassment is that it is *unwanted*.

In its more extreme expression, sexual harassment usually consists of an escalating series of acts that can be grouped in one of two categories: the first consists of sexual actions that are an invasion of privacy, such as physical molesting, dirty jokes, and overt "propositions" that occur so frequently and are so unnerving that they interfere with the woman's competence and even her safety on the job. The second category of actions typically occurs as a form of revenge and retaliation for a rejection of the sexual offers, especially if the woman has complained. If the rejected person has the power to do so, he will proceed to undermine the woman's confidence by openly and severely criticizing everything she does and by depriving her of possibilities for adequate training and advancement.

As the stress grows, the woman may ask for a transfer, or she may be fired "because she can't handle interpersonal relationships." Or she may quit, knowing that she'll have to find another job without being able to get a recommendation from her former boss. One of the most destructive aspects of such situations is the woman's feelings of guilt—that she is somehow at fault for being a victim.

SEXUAL HARASSMENT AND THE LAW

Public attention began to focus on this problem in the 1970s, when investigations were conducted by various women's groups. Reports indicated that significant numbers of women who rejected sexual advances on the job not only were being deprived of advancement and raises but were also suffering from health problems induced by stress. In a 1976 survey of *Redbook* magazine readers, unwanted sexual attention in their work situations was reported by 88 percent of the 9,000 respondents. In a U.S. Merit Systems Protection Board report called *Sexual Harassment in the Federal Workplace*, it was estimated that this problem resulted in job turnover, absenteeism, and the use of health benefits that cost taxpayers $189 million over a two-year period.

Women who were denied job advancement or were fired because they rejected the sexual advances of a superior started to take legal action. Rulings by federal courts began to pile up in favor of the claimants, who based their cases on the view that sexual harassment was a violation of the antidiscrimination laws spelled out in Title VII of the 1964 Civil Rights Act. By 1980 the Equal Employment Opportunity Commission issued a series of guidelines that stated:

"Harassment on the basis of sex is a violation of Section 703 of Title VII. Unwelcome sexual advances, requests for sexual favors, and other verbal or physical conduct of a sexual nature constitute sexual harassment when (1) submission to such conduct is made either explicitly or implicitly a term or condition of an individual's employment, (2) submission to or rejection of such conduct by an individual is used as the basis of employment decisions affecting such individuals, or (3) such conduct has the purpose or effect of substantially interfering with an individual's work performance or creating an intimidating, hostile, or offensive working environment . . ."

The regulation holds the employer or its agents or supervisory employees responsible for acts of sexual harassment in the workplace and concludes: "Prevention is the best tool for the elimination of sexual harassment. An employer should take all steps necessary to prevent sexual harassment from occurring, such as affirmatively raising the subject, expressing strong disapproval, developing appropriate sanctions, informing employees of their right to raise and how to raise the issue of harassment under Title VII and developing methods to sensitize all concerned."

Six years later, in 1986, the U.S. Supreme Court ruled that sexual harassment in the workplace was a form of sex discrimination under Title VII of the Civil Rights Act of 1964 and was therefore illegal. It was this decision that finally led many companies that had been somewhat remiss in handling the issue to hire consultants, show videos, and conduct workshops to generate discussion and clarification. What usually needs to be clarified is the difference between a warm, friendly environment and one in which sexual innuendos and pressure are making some people very uncomfortable. To implement the Supreme Court ruling further, large organizations have issued policy and procedural statements to supervisory personnel. In many cases the company's guidelines are spelled out in employee handbooks.

In spite of these provisions, however, many women are reluctant to appear to be "troublemakers" or to take steps that seem to indicate that "they can't handle the situation on their own." Procedural red tape takes a long time to unwind, and besides, in smaller offices, a woman may be summarily fired. Also, women whose jobs involve direct contact with customers—waitresses, showroom personnel, and the like—may be flatly told that being nice to the customers goes with the territory.

The bottom line appears to be that until all levels of society—from United States senators to the messengers in the mailroom—understand what the victim means by sexual harassment, a large part of the efforts to reject it in the workplace will continue to be unsuccessful.

SOME PRACTICAL SUGGESTIONS

Early in the 1980s Dr. Mary Rowe, a labor economist at the Massachusetts Institute of Technology, wrote an article for the *Harvard Business Review* in which she proposed a letter-writing strategy for dealing with sexual harassment. She has since monitored more than 700 cases in which the letter produced the desired results. "The typical reaction was no reaction. It just stopped. In eleven years of working with the problem," said Dr. Rowe (in a *New York Times* interview, 4/11/83), "I've found the letter to be the most effective way to get harassment stopped at no cost to the offended person."

Here's the kind of letter Dr. Rowe recommends:

1. The first paragraph describes the offensive conduct in detail. ("Dear Mr. ____: Last month, your hand went from your lap to my lap to my knee and made its way under my skirt to the inside of my thigh. Several times since then, you put your arm around my shoulders and your hand ended up on my breast. The other afternoon, you suggested we 'make a motel date for an evening fling.' ")
2. The second paragraph describes the writer's feelings about this behavior. ("I've been so upset by these unwarranted sexual advances that I haven't been able to sleep. My work is beginning to suffer because you've made me so nervous.")
3. The letter should conclude with an unambiguous statement about what the writer expects in the future. ("I would appreciate your treating me with professional courtesy and discontinuing all personal remarks from now on.")

Such a letter serves several purposes. First, it enables the woman to make a statement, thus giving her the feeling that she has some control over the situation. It also tells the perpetrator in no uncertain terms that the woman is serious in her rejection of the sexual advances. (This is no small matter. Many men have been socially conditioned to believe that when a woman says "No" she really means "Yes," and all they have to do is to keep trying.)

The letter should be brief, polite, and clear in its message. If possible, it should be hand-delivered by a messenger, with a signed receipt requested, or it should be sent by certified mail. A copy should be kept in the event that the harassment continues or escalates. If this should occur, the next step may be a meeting with the person in charge of hearing such grievances. Sometimes a transfer to another department can be arranged. If the recommended alternative is filing a formal complaint, the machinery for a hearing is then put in motion.

If your immediate boss or the personnel manager shrugs off your complaint and you're not sure of how to proceed, you can turn to other sources for practical help. A dependable counseling resource is the "Y," many of whose branches sponsor "rap" sessions and strategy guidance by professionals. The local office of the Equal Employment Opportunity Commission is the official agency for dealing with such complaints. And if you wish to get advice from a private lawyer, you can use the referral facilities of the Women's Bar Association of your city or state.

Women who belong to unions (not only those in industry but nurses, teachers, laboratory workers, and many secretaries) can press for clearly spelled-out clauses in their contracts.

If you are on the verge of quitting a job or have had to quit because of sexual harassment, you should find out promptly whether your state is one of the many that now guarantee unemployment benefits for such cases.

PREGNANCY

After many years of litigation over an employer's right to exclude women from certain jobs based on a policy of "fetal protection" and to exclude them during their childbearing years, whether pregnant or not, from jobs involving exposure to low levels of lead, the Supreme Court handed down a historic decision in 1991. Justice Harry A. Blackmun's majority opinion, joined by Justices Marshall, Stevens, O'Connor, and Souter, declared in part, "Decisions about the welfare of future children must be left to the parents who conceive, bear, support, and raise them rather than to the employers who hire those parents." The five justices took the most sweeping view of the issue by declaring that the Civil Rights Act prohibited all fetal protection policies and noting, "Women as capable of doing their jobs as their male counterparts may not be forced to choose between having a child and having a job." It has been estimated that 20 million jobs for women were at issue, and it has also been pointed out that exposure to some of the toxic substances in question could be as damaging to male sperm as to female ovaries.

Four years earlier, in a 1987 ruling, the Supreme Court had already established that from a legal point of view pregnancy leave be considered a right and not a privilege. However, this ruling is based on the concept that a woman's pregnancy is a "disability" comparable to a man's broken leg or some other temporarily incapacitating condition. It does not take into account either the pregnant woman's need for prenatal and postnatal care or hospital delivery costs, all of which should be, and now in many cases finally are, covered by medical insurance.

Working women have been slow to insist on their rights as they relate to reproduction, childbearing, breast feeding, and parenting, not to mention day care centers, provided free by the employer in practically all other industrially advanced countries. More and more concerned groups are pressing for the extension of maternal benefits, and in this connection it should be noted that forward-looking employers have been providing on-site day care facilities, while government employees on various levels, teachers, and workers with strong unions have achieved many parental benefits that are still out of reach for most women employees nationwide.

There was a time when women who became pregnant while they were working had to educate their doctors about some relevant circumstances. Nowadays, physicians are more knowledgeable about pregnancy and work and more involved in helping their patients resolve their interrelated work and pregnancy care needs. This is partly because employers are making it necessary for them to do so and partly because their patients are asking questions, just as we urge you to do. The American College of Obstetrics and Gynecology has published guidelines on this subject, and physicians are finding them to be helpful.

- After a consultation on the subject with your doctor, you and the father-to-be can make an informed decision about the most practical time to begin a maternity leave.
- If you stay on the job after your condition becomes obvious, you may have to deal with some good-natured and not so good-natured teasing from your male colleagues and/or customers, clients, etc. Keep your responses cool! "I happen to need the money." "I enjoy my job as much as you enjoy yours." "The boss wants me to stay until the last minute because my work is essential." Write your own script and use it as necessary.
- If it's possible to do so, rearrange your work schedule so that you can avoid traveling during rush hours.
- Backaches are more common than ever, so be sure that your chair gives

you the right support. Never sit on a chair that teeters or wobbles. If your usual chair is somewhat rickety, have it replaced.

- If your job normally requires long hours of standing (as it does for bank tellers, waitresses, saleswomen, and teachers, for example), request a stool of the right height so that you can sit occasionally without decreasing your efficiency. (Women who stand at their jobs for five to six hours increase the risk of premature delivery.)
- If you sit at a desk most of the time and your ankles are beginning to swell, provide yourself with a small footstool so that you can keep your feet raised under the desk.
- Don't feel embarrassed or apologetic about having to use the bathroom more often than usual.
- "Morning sickness" may strike at any time of the day, especially if you work in a poorly ventilated environment. For some women, an extra snack, such as a dry biscuit, is helpful.
- If you think air pollution is the problem, try to find out what the offending substance might be and discuss the situation with your doctor. Normally, the nausea that accompanies pregnancy subsides altogether by the eighteenth week.
- Be sure you're taking care of your extra nutritional needs by drinking milk during your "coffee break" and bringing chunks of low-fat cheese for midafternoon snacking.

BABIES AND YOU: A WORK-SITE PRENATAL HEALTH PROGRAM

Several employers and unions are participating in a work-site program developed in 1995 by the March of Dimes Birth Defects Foundation as part of the organization's Campaign for Healthier Babies. The purpose of the campaign is to create awareness about the connection between prenatal care, positive life-style behaviors, and the birth of a healthy baby. Many employers find it to their advantage to promote this campaign because it can significantly reduce health insurance costs. (Physician and hospital charges for the protracted care of low-birth-weight babies range from 3 to 10 times as much as for normal babies.) Educational materials can be requested from the March of Dimes for distribution to interested workers and their families. Educational seminars conducted by trained health professionals can be arranged to suit workplace convenience: during the lunch break or after hours so that family members can attend. The seminars include informative videos and discussions.

Among the topics discussed are the supportive role of family, friends, and colleagues; alcohol and tobacco during pregnancy; exercise; stress management; and genetic defects and who should consider genetic counseling.

FOOD AND DRINK ON THE JOB

Many women find it difficult to maintain decent nutritional standards at work, especially if outside eating facilities are either unavailable or too expensive and the company cafeteria offers an unsatisfactory choice of food. Pregnant women may have to work out special solutions for the essential between-meal snacks and extra milk recommended by their doctors. Here are some ways in which *all* women can achieve a wholesome diet during working hours:

1. If the assortment of foods offered by the company cafeteria is inadequate when judged by current nutritional standards and if there is no access to outside eating facilities, bring your own lunch from home. This can include a thermos container of hot soup for a midmorning snack.
2. Instead of overloading on caffeine, sugar, and doughnuts or Danish pastry during your coffee break, choose milk, a bran muffin, fresh fruit, yogurt, or soup.
3. In workplaces that have vending machines offering only candy, junk food, and carbonated beverages, make a group request for machines that sell milk, pure fruit juice, bags of unsalted peanuts, boxes of raisins, and the like.
4. If there is no eating facility on the premises, ask the management to install a small refrigerator for storing food and a hot plate or microwave oven for preparing meals. In some offices the preparation of "group soups" has become a standard procedure.
5. If you and some of your coworkers would like to have breakfast together, find out whether it's possible to have the company cafeteria open at least one hour before the workday begins.
6. Women who have been led to believe that "drinking with the men" is essential to getting ahead should give some serious thought to the negative aspects of this type of socializing, including sexual harassment and the problem of alcohol addiction as it affects their male colleagues. Any woman can firmly and politely refuse to become an off-hours "drinking buddy."

KNOW YOUR BENEFITS

If your employer or your union offers a pension plan, examine the advantages of maximum participation and be sure you understand what happens to your contributions if and when you decide to leave the job before retirement.

Income from a pension can eventually make the difference between economic independence and poverty.

If you haven't done so already, find out exactly what your medical benefits are. Your policy should spell this information out in detail, but if you still have questions, they can be answered by the personnel director, your union representative, or your boss.

If you're planning to quit your job, be sure that you know whether and for how long your medical coverage will continue between jobs. And when you start a new job, find out how soon your benefits begin.

When you're interviewed for a new job, find out what the health benefits are. (The variation from job to job and from state to state is very wide. Some benefits include abortion as well as all costs connected with pregnancy and delivery. What about psychiatrists' fees? What about dental surgery? Does your policy cover dependents?)

Do you have a doctor who is sympathetic about your on-the-job health complaints? Are you offered practical suggestions for how to deal with them? If Valium is prescribed as an all-purpose solution, don't think about changing jobs; consider changing doctors.

The organization 9 to 5 publishes "The Working Woman's Guide to Office Survival," available to members, and also provides its members with newsletters and fact sheets covering all developments that affect women's well-being on the job.

DISABILITIES

The Americans with Disabilities Act has opened up a whole world of employment opportunities for people with disabilities (as well as a Pandora's box of litigation problems). Legislation had already required that properties open to the public be made accessible to disabled people, and by January 1992 buildings and businesses with more than 25 workers were required to make a good faith effort to remove barriers to the disabled. As far as jobs are concerned, employers may not discriminate against qualified disabled individuals in hiring, advancement, compensation, or training, and are required to adapt the workplace if necessary. Companies with 15 to 24 employees were expected to comply with this law by July 1994. There are 14 million Americans with mental or physical handicaps who are of working age, and it is estimated that less than 14 percent have been gainfully employed. Faced with this federal mandate, more than half a million employers are expected to offer people with physical or mental impairments the same opportunities as other employees as long as they are qualified to handle a particular job. If disabilities are obstacles, employers are expected to provide whatever practical adjustments are necessary: ramps, special furniture, flexible working hours, instructing supervisors in sign language. The question that will have to be settled case by case in the courts is at what point these adjustments impose "undue hardship" on the employer.

If you are a woman of working age who is collecting disability insurance because of hearing or sight impairment or who must use a wheelchair because of a chronic joint disease, you are entitled to enter or reenter the workforce on the basis of your job qualifications. Explore your options with a sympathetic and well-informed employment agency and meet the challenge provided by this legislation.

HOME-BASED WORKERS

Women have been making a living in some part of the home for a long time: think of dressmakers, voice teachers, freelance artists, piecework typists, not to mention legitimate child care providers. What's new is the home office, and since most people can't afford to turn a whole room over to this requirement, the "office" is usually confined to an area in the dining room, bedroom, or den; or a guest room may be partially transformed for double duty.

Thanks to the advances in microelectronics, it has become possible for anyone to work anyplace where there is a power supply and a phone line. The Link Resources Corporation, a research and consulting firm that conducts annual national work-at-home surveys, reported that in 1994 over 43 million Americans (roughly one-third of the workforce), were working at least part of the time from a home office. The number of home-based workers is expected to reach 57 million by 1997, and of that number, at least 20 million will be women. The specialty known as telecommunicating currently accounts for the 7 million women working at home for banks, insurance companies, and government agencies, and the number of "telecommuters" is growing more rapidly than any other type of home worker. All it takes is a personal computer, a fax machine, and a cellular phone. And for all types of home-based operations, the office furniture industry has been keeping pace, providing ingenious wall arrangements, dual-purpose surfaces, and computer storage units.

The woman whose work is home-based should plan her work area very carefully, with physical comfort a top priority. A sturdy, ergonomically designed chair is an important investment: the seat height should be adjustable; the back rest should provide firm support for your lower back, and for the chair to be stable, it should be supported by a five- (not four-) pronged safety base. Good light is essential; make sure there's no glare reflected on your screen. Books, reference materials, files, phone, should all be within easy reach. Good ventilation is a must. If you're working in a basement or a garage, check air circulation so that you don't suffer from the symptoms of sick building syndrome in your own home. If like at least half the women working at home, you have children under age six, you may have thought that you would be spared the expense of child care, but studies indicate that practically all professional and clerical workers have to rely on child care to get their work done properly and without undue stress.

Whether you're a computer whizz, a copywriter, a graphic designer, or you're on the phone most of the time, whatever the nature of your work, if it's sedentary, try to establish a regular exercise routine to prevent "office slouch" and pains in your back and neck. You might also find out whether your community offers a convenient daytime exercise class, letting you combine some desired social contact with a fitness session. Above all, learn some of the techniques of stress management so that you can handle the multiple roles of home-worker, homemaker, and parent without losing your cool. (See "Alternative Therapies" for suggestions.)

BUSINESS TRAVEL AND HOTEL SAFETY

According to the United States Travel Data Center, 40 percent of all business travelers are women. Although efforts have been made to improve safety and security, many women whose work takes them on frequent trips think that a great deal still has to be done, and not only in economy accommodations. In the recent past, security lapses have resulted in a highly publicized rape, a murder, and the Tailhook sexual assault case, costing the hotels involved millions of dollars in damage settlements. Of special concern as safeguards against becoming a crime victim are an effective key control system, efficient locks, bright lighting in public areas, and strategically placed security guards. Here are some suggestions offered by experienced solo travelers: When you make your reservation on the phone, ask whether the establishment offers individualized electronic room keys, and get a description of the door locks. When you check into your room, make it clear that you expect to be accompanied by a porter or some other staff member who will make sure no one else is in the

room by checking the closet and bathroom and looking behind the shower
curtain and under the bed. You can also take safeguards on your own. If you're
sitting alone in the lounge, don't accept the offer of a drink from a stranger,
and after a conference or a meeting, don't invite anyone—male or female—to
your room.

$\mathcal{A}$GING HEALTHFULLY— YOUR BODY, MIND, AND SPIRIT

Helene MacLean

Medical Writer and Editor; Author, *Caring for Your Parents, Relief from Chronic Arthritis Pain*; Coauthor, *Recovering from a Hysterectomy, Migraine: Beating the Odds*

Maureen Mylander

Author and writer/editor, National Center for Research Resources, National Institutes of Health, Bethesda, Maryland

Adapted from a chapter in an earlier edition by

Barbara Gastel, M.D., M.P.H.

Formerly of National Institute on Aging, National Institutes of Health, Bethesda, Maryland

Older people—and older women in particular—are far healthier than prevailing myths would have us believe. About 7 in 10 persons age 65 and older describe their health as "good" or "excellent" if asked to compare themselves with others of their own age, according to the U.S. Census Bureau. Death rates of the older population, especially of women, have fallen considerably over the past 40 years. Yet these decreases do not mean that all who live longer enjoy better health. In fact, hand in hand with women's increasing longevity goes the problem of increased and extended periods of chronic ailments. Fortunately, more and more doctors are trained in the health concerns that afflict the elderly. In 1982, Mount Sinai Medical Center in New York City was the only teaching hospital in the U.S. with a department of geriatric medicine. By 1992, 17 teaching hospitals had AMA-accredited residency programs in geriatrics, and according to the American Hospital Association there were more than 1,200 geriatric clinics nationwide, including those with acute-care units. Is there any medical school nationwide that includes in its curriculum a course on the special health problems of a majority of the over-65 population, namely women? Not yet. The Association of American Medical Colleges says that as of 1996, 13 schools give separate *required* courses in geriatrics, up from only 8 in 1990. It can be assumed that the others give required courses in pharmacology, family and community medicine, and so on that include information on the older patient.

The good news for all women, however, is that, as a result of years of lobbying and the compelling evidence before Congress that women have been given second-class treatment as coronary, cancer, and other types of patients, the legislature enacted a law creating a new arm of the National Institutes of Health known officially as the Office of Research on Women's Health. We can only hope that the medical establishment will produce fewer doctors inclined to ascribe older women's complaints to the post-menopausal syndrome or to hypochondria or to the inevitable crankiness of old age. But since there are still too many doctors who don't know about treating older women, the final responsibility for guarding your health as you grow older is your own. Aside from counting on a good genetic inheritance, the healthy aging woman should be able to depend on the accumulated benefits of long years of good habits and well-informed self-care.

AGE-RELATED CHANGES IN PARTS OF THE BODY

Healthful aging requires attention to the various parts of the body, to particular disorders, and to general well-being.

SKIN

Neither beauty nor health is skin deep, but healthy skin can contribute greatly to both appearance and comfort in the later years of life. With age the skin becomes less elastic, its glands lubricate less effectively, and cells controlling its color often start to malfunction. Thus, wrinkles and "age spots" frequently occur. Although some age-related changes in the skin seem to be inevitable, others can be prevented or delayed.

Long hours of exposure to the sun, often called "the skin's worst enemy," accelerate aging of the skin and increase the risk of skin cancer. To prevent sun damage it is necessary either to avoid the sun or to guard the skin. If properly applied, creams, oils, and lotions known as sunscreens help to protect the skin. A brimmed hat should also be considered indispensable for the beach and summer country hikes.

Several other factors also can make the skin appear older. In winter, cold weather and freezing winds, dry and overheated rooms, and even the use of electric blankets can make the skin scaly and inelastic. In summer, air conditioning can have similar effects. Excessive alcohol intake and poor diet also damage the skin. In addition to the really deadly harm they are inflicting on themselves, women who smoke are likely to have many more wrinkles than women who don't.

Although nothing can completely arrest or reverse age-related changes in the skin, it is still possible to have attractive, healthy skin. One's own outlook is essential to others' perceptions. Aged skin does not mean lack of beauty. Many women feel that they are no longer attractive or even worthwhile once physical signs of aging begin to appear. However, attitudes are changing. As the population ages, so does our ideal of beauty. Among women considered beautiful, Jessica Tandy, who died at the age of 85, was an inspiration throughout her final years; Lena Horne, born in 1917, continues to be a dazzling beauty; and Angela Lansbury, now in her seventies, is a favorite host for Hollywood and Broadway events. With women achieving more varied roles in society, other criteria are becoming more important than a youthful appearance.

Several mechanical procedures, including dermabrasion, chemical peel, collagen injections, and face lift, which can help to correct some types of age-associated skin damage, are discussed in the chapter on "Cosmetic Surgery." Simpler approaches, including the use of "wrinkle creams," skin lighteners and bleaches, make-up, and moisturizers, can also improve or conceal the appearance of aged skin. Wrinkle creams generally contain both oil to smooth the skin and an irritant to cause slight swelling and thus fill out small lines and creases. Skin lighteners and bleaches can help to fade darkened areas of skin; as with medications, they must be used only as directed.

Moisturizers, among the most popular products for aging skin, temporarily improve the texture and appearance of skin and help to relieve dry, tight, itchy sensations. For moisturizers to be most effective, water should be patted onto the skin before their application. Generally, the effectiveness of a moisturizer is unrelated to its cost; many women find inexpensive products satisfactory, and moisturizers of different prices actually may contain similar ingredients.

Itching is a common problem in older persons. Several measures can help to relieve dry, itchy skin on the body. When bathing, use only mild soaps or cleansers, apply soap only to areas that need especially thorough cleansing (the underarms, pubic and anal areas, feet, hands), use warm rather than hot water, avoid long baths, and pat the skin dry gently instead of rubbing it briskly. After the bath, bath oil or another moisturizer should be applied to the moist skin. Addition of oil to the bath water is unwise, as the tub can become dangerously slippery. Humidification of the air, use of soft cotton flannel sheets, and addition of a small amount of bath oil to water used to rinse laundry also can be helpful.

Severe or persistent skin conditions such as rashes, sores, and unmanageable itching should be seen by a doctor. Some of the conditions may be relieved by locally applied measures, and others may be the first noticeable signs of a disease that affects the entire body and requires treatment. Growths on the skin should receive prompt attention to determine if they are malignant. The early removal of skin cancers almost always results in cure.

EYES

Visual impairment becomes more common with age. Of the estimated more than 500,000 Americans who are legally blind, nearly half are above age 65. However, conditions affecting the eyes of older persons often can be treated successfully, and many special aids and services are available to individuals with irreversible visual impairment.

Even before middle age, the lens of the eye starts to become less elastic. By age 40 the reduced elasticity produces in most people a condition called presbyopia, or difficulty in focusing on objects at close range. Most persons over 40 require reading glasses or bifocals. Trifocals are preferred by some women who don't want to keep changing glasses for their various visual needs, especially if they need correction for the middle distance—when playing the piano, looking at art on the walls of a museum, or viewing a computer screen. (Trifocals enable the viewer to see the painting clearly *and* to read the text that accompanies it *and* to recognize a friend from a distance of 20 feet who has just entered the gallery.) It takes some patience and practice to grow accustomed to wearing multifocal glasses, but in terms of eventual convenience, the time is well spent. Glasses in which the separation between the lenses is invisible are more attractive but may cause more difficulties during the early weeks of wear; persistence is usually rewarded.

Another condition affecting the eye is cataract, in which the lens becomes opaque or cloudy and thus vision becomes unclear. Although 95 percent of persons over 65 may have some degree of cataracts, in only a small proportion is the condition severe enough to interfere significantly with vision and require treatment. At present, surgery to remove the cataract is the only treatment available, and it is successful in 90 to 95 percent of cases. After surgery, replacement of the function of the individual's own lens is necessary, and special glasses or contact lenses are usually prescribed. A relatively new alternative to eyeglasses or contact lenses is the placement of a permanent plastic lens inside the eye during cataract surgery. The long-term safety and effectiveness of this procedure are still being evaluated. Since it is now known that constant exposure of the eye to the ultraviolet rays of the sun can cause cataracts to develop prematurely, protective measures are essential at the beach. (See SUNGLASSES.)

Glaucoma, a condition characterized by increased pressure within the eye and loss of visual function, is the leading cause of blindness among the aged. In the most common type of glaucoma, medication can usually control the pressure and prevent visual loss if the condition is detected early. However, surgery may be needed in some cases. All adults aged 40 and over should therefore have a glaucoma check once a year and, if there is a family history of the condition, twice a year.

Diabetes, especially if present for many years, can damage the retina of the eye. The condition is known as diabetic retinopathy and necessitates careful, frequent eye examinations. A treatment called photocoagulation, which uses a laser beam, can help to destroy abnormal tissue and blood vessels in the retina and thus preserve sight in some patients.

Senile macular degeneration, a poorly understood deterioration of the part of the retina responsible for sharp, clear color vision, affects about 10 percent of persons over 70 years of age and appears to be more common in women than in men. Individuals with this condition generally retain some vision and thus can continue to care for themselves. However, as senile macular degeneration produces a large blind spot in the middle of the visual field, it interferes with such activities as reading, sewing, watching television, and driving. The condition is associated with abnormal blood circulation to the retina, and photocoagulation may prove useful in some early cases, although this treatment has not yet been fully evaluated. Special low-vision aids, including magnifiers, telescopic lenses, and closed-circuit television that projects printed matter onto a screen, can allow some people with macular degeneration to continue many normal activities.

Whatever the state of one's vision—and most older women can see very well if they are wearing the proper corrective lenses—the eyes should be treated with special consideration. Regular checkups by an ophthalmologist are essential. Any sudden variation in vision should be diagnosed at once because the condition of the optic nerve is an indicator of certain neurological problems. Tinted prescription lenses should be worn to protect aging eyes against strong sun, especially when driving on bright days.

Numerous public and private organizations assist the sight-impaired of all ages. The federal government and each state and territory have offices to provide and coordinate such services, and the American Foundation for the Blind is a major nongovernmental source of information. Aids available to the visually impaired include large-type books, magazines, and newspapers; recorded literature; counseling; at-home instruction; special Social Security benefits and income tax concessions; and devices to facilitate daily living. (See "Directory of Health Information.")

EARS

Ability to hear declines with age. Although often the loss is too slight to interfere with ordinary activities, an estimated one-third of all persons over 65 have significant difficulty hearing. Hearing loss is more common in men, perhaps in part because of greater occupational exposure to noise. Although little is known about prevention of age-related hearing loss, avoidance of excessive noise is advisable.

A wide variety of hearing deficits occur in the aged, but certain features are especially common. The elderly often have the most difficulty perceiving high tones. In addition, speech can sound loud enough but nevertheless seem unclear. Thus, older persons may say that others are mumbling and may remark, "I can hear you all right, but I can't understand what you're saying."

The first step in managing a hearing impairment is identification of the specific problem. A general physician can examine the ears, perform basic tests of hearing, and manage some hearing disorders. For additional evaluation and treatment, the patient may be referred to an otorhinolaryngologist (an ear, nose, and throat specialist), otologist (a physician specializing in the ear), or audiologist (a nonphysician specially trained to diagnose and manage hearing problems).

Often the diagnosis is presbycusis, which means hearing loss associated with aging. Although this condition cannot be cured, approaches such as hearing aids and special training can be very helpful. Otosclerosis is a condition in which one of the three bones of hearing, the stirrup, becomes immobilized by bony deposits. It can sometimes be corrected by surgery. In other instances a reversible condition may be discovered. For example, treatment of an unsuspected ear infection or removal of wax clogging the ear canal can improve hearing.

Many older men and women find that hearing aids enable them to maintain satisfactory contact with family and friends and achieve maximum pleasure from lectures, concerts, and favorite radio and television programs. Individuals are advised not to buy a hearing aid without consulting a physician or audiologist, who can help select the most appropriate device and give advice about its most effective use. Hearing aids make sounds louder, but they cannot correct hearing as precisely as glasses correct vision. A period of adjustment is often necessary, and sometimes a hearing specialist can help a patient to obtain hearing aids for trial periods of a few weeks each until a satisfactory device is found. Persons with conditions such as arthritis or stroke may find the small parts of hearing aids difficult to handle. Special hearing aids that compensate for some of these problems are available. A hearing-impaired woman who is comfortable with computer technology can take advantage of communicating via e-mail.

Aids that may be especially helpful to hearing-impaired persons who live alone are attachments for telephones and televisions to amplify voices and devices that flash on a light when the doorbell or telephone rings. The American Humane Association trains "hearing dogs," which aid the deaf in somewhat the same way that seeing eye dogs help the blind.

Special training can help the hearing-impaired to make the most of their abilities. For example, "lip-reading," sensitivity to facial expressions and gestures, and use of appropriate questions can help the individual with a hearing loss to take an active part in conversation. Both individual instruction and classes in these skills are available in many communities. Family members, close friends, and employers may find attending such sessions along with the

hearing-impaired individual useful in appreciating and dealing with the problem.

If you have difficulty hearing, the following suggestions may make communication easier.

- Ask people to face you.
- Keep background noise to a minimum.
- Ask people to speak clearly and loudly but not to shout.
- Suggest that someone addressing you get your attention, for example by a
  gentle tap on the shoulder, before speaking.
- Ask to be told what is being discussed if you join a conversation already in
  progress.
- If you do not understand what someone is saying, ask the speaker to
  repeat the statement using different words.
- When you are given important instructions, be sure you have understood
  the message by repeating it to your informant and asking whether you
  have the information right.

Effective management of hearing problems in the elderly has social and
psychological benefits. It helps the individual to retain or regain an active role
in the family and the community. Likewise, it aids in combating the loneliness,
boredom, and depression that can befall those who are unable to take part in
conversation and to enjoy fully many popular forms of entertainment.

TEETH AND GUMS

For years being old meant being toothless, a condition detrimental to nutrition, speech, and appearance. Today, however, increasing numbers of older
persons are retaining their teeth or obtaining satisfactory dentures. Lifelong
care of the teeth and mouth is essential to general health in old age.

With age the mouth undergoes several changes. Although the risk of tooth
decay decreases with increasing age, tooth loss because of periodontal disease
(disease of the gums and other tissues surrounding the teeth) becomes more
common with age. Gum recession may loosen teeth and expose tooth roots that
are then more susceptible to decay and do not hold fillings well because their
softer dentine is not covered by enamel. In addition, age-related changes and
certain medications can cause the mouth to become dry. Dryness causes discomfort, fosters decay, and makes dentures more difficult to retain. Because of
factors such as tooth loss and a diminished sense of taste, many older persons

choose soft, sweet diets, which promote root decay. Age-related bone loss can make old dentures uncomfortable and new dentures difficult to fit.

Throughout life and particularly in old age, prevention of dental disease can be effective and more economical than treatment. Regular checkups, which should include detection of signs of local and systemic disease, prompt treatment of abnormal conditions of the teeth and mouth, and instruction in proper techniques of oral hygiene are essential, although unfortunately not covered by many insurance programs. Daily mouth care, generally including both brushing and flossing, also is necessary. Devices such as electric toothbrushes and long-handled toothbrushes may help persons partially disabled by arthritis and other handicaps to maintain good oral hygiene. A well-balanced diet that provides plenty of chewing, is low in sugar, and includes sufficient fluid also promotes oral hygiene. As smoking is the prime cause not only of lung cancer but also of cancer of the mouth, avoidance of this habit is vitally important.

Proper management and suitable diets can help to reverse or arrest incipient conditions that affect the teeth and mouth in later life. For example, prompt replacement of missing teeth helps to preserve oral structures and aids in maintaining good nutrition. Sipping plenty of water with meals and in some cases rinsing with specially prescribed mouthwashes can relieve dryness of the mouth. Because of age-related changes in the mouth and elsewhere in the body, both the older patient and the dentist sometimes need extra patience and effort to achieve the desired results. Just as some dentists specialize in dentistry for children, some are making a specialty of treating older patients. For more information about geriatric dentistry in your area, write to the American Dental Association. (See "Directory of Health Information.")

NERVOUS SYSTEM

Although mental impairment and other disorders of the nervous system are among the most feared conditions of old age, most people maintain a high level of mental competence and neurological function throughout life. Even after age 80, changes normally are slight and of little consequence. The fact that mental decline in very old age is not inevitable is borne out by the late creativity of such figures as Grandma Moses, Martha Graham, Picasso, and George Burns. However, a significant minority suffer from disorders of the nervous system.

Any possible symptom of neurological disease, for example, partial paralysis, numbness, tremor, memory loss, or difficulty with speech, requires medical evaluation. In many cases examination will reveal a reversible condition such as depression, a vitamin deficiency, a side reaction from a drug, overmedication with tranquilizers, or incipient alcoholism. In others, such as stroke, early diagnosis can help patient, family, and medical personnel cope more effectively with the condition. Unfortunately, many neurological problems are poorly understood, difficult to manage, and frustrating to all involved.

An estimated 4 to 5 percent of Americans over age 65 have some degree of serious intellectual impairment. Alzheimer's disease is the cause in about half of these cases, while a number of treatable conditions and stroke each cause about one-fourth. Impairment may be somewhat more common in women than in men, perhaps because women tend to live longer. Such impairment is commonly but rather imprecisely termed "senility," a label that does not denote a specific disease but rather stands for a wide variety of conditions. Technically, dementia is the term for loss of intellectual abilities, such as memory, judgment, and language, without loss of consciousness or alertness. CAT scans, MRIs, and cognitive testing are helpful in ruling out or arriving at some causes of senile dementia, but they are of no use in reaching a definitive diagnosis of Alzheimer's disease.

Alzheimer's disease, a progressive, incurable degeneration of the brain of unknown cause, is believed to affect 4 million Americans. One in three families is touched by it, and it is the fourth leading cause of death in the United States. Recent research indicates that several defects in a particular gene are responsible for an aberration in normal brain chemistry. By studying the stored tissue samples of 31 family members from three generations, researchers have established that every family member who got the disease had inherited the altered gene. Because there is as yet neither a cure nor an effective treatment, doctors have been facing the problem of whether to tell patients and their families that the condition exists. Dr. Barry Reisberg, an Alzheimer's specialist at New York University Medical Center, is of the opinion that knowing of the presence of the disease can help the patient and the family learn how to deal with behavioral and other problems that appear as the disease becomes more disabling. A common early symptom is severe difficulty with short-term memory (not the slight forgetfulness that many people exhibit). Later the individual may have difficulty thinking, undergo personality changes, and become confused. Eventually Alzheimer's disease renders its victims helpless and completely dependent on the care of others. When Ronald Reagan decided to address the public about his affliction at the age of 83, he wrote from his home, "Unfortunately, as Alzheimer's disease progresses, the family often bears a heavy burden," adding that when the difficult times come for his wife, Nancy, "I am confident that with your help, she will face it with faith and courage."

Physicians and other health personnel can help the individual to make the most of remaining cognitive abilities (for example, through the use of memory aids known as mnemonics and through the use of music) and can help the patient and family to cope with the condition. In both the United States and Canada, families of patients with Alzheimer's disease are banding together to share support and information, and many communities have established "Alzheimer's hotlines" to provide family caregivers with referrals. (See "Directory of Health Information.")

Among the elderly, at least one-fourth of all dementia-like or "pseudo-dementia" symptoms are caused by over 100 other conditions, many of them treatable, even curable. Underlying treatable problems that can produce signs and symptoms mimicking those of Alzheimer's disease include depression, drug reactions, alcoholism, infections, heart disease, kidney failure, thyroid disease, head injury, and anemia. Mental impairment due to depression, for example, can be caused by such potentially correctable nonmedical problems as loss of family ties, anxiety over lack of money, and loss of physical independence. Certain medications, including small doses of tranquilizers and even over-the-counter antihistamines, can trigger Alzheimer-like symptoms. Blood clots in the brain, which could be treated by surgery, sometimes cause pseudo-dementia. Elderly patients in nursing homes or similar institutions for more than three months are likely to have symptoms of dementia, as are some people with inadequate nutrition and fluid intake. When these underlying problems can be discovered and remedied, normal mental function may return. Therefore a thorough medical evaluation, including history, physical examination, and laboratory tests, is essential for anyone who seems to have become "senile."

Stroke occurs when part of the brain suffers damage because of insufficient blood supply: blood clots and broken blood vessels supplying the brain can be responsible. Although various symptoms can occur, the most common is paralysis of part of the body, either alone or combined with impaired speech. In time and with promptly instituted, vigorous rehabilitative therapy, improvement often occurs. Special devices can help persons with lasting disability to perform everyday tasks independently.

At least 2 million people now alive in the United States have suffered strokes. They affect approximately twice as many women as men and are the third most common cause of death in this country. However, particularly in the elderly, strokes have become considerably less common in recent years. The cause for this reduction is unknown, but recent strides in controlling high blood pressure, which strongly predisposes to stroke, may be playing an important role.

Although information on how to prevent strokes is incomplete, control of high blood pressure and adherence to the measures recommended in this chapter's section on the heart and blood vessels appear to be wise. "Little strokes" (short periods of partial blindness, speech difficulty, paralysis, or other impairment) warn of the possibility of major stroke and thus demand medical attention. Of course, anyone with symptoms that may result from stroke should seek medical attention promptly. For more information or free brochures on stroke, call the National Stroke Association at 1-800-787-6537.

Parkinson's disease is estimated to affect only 1 person in 1,000 in the general population but 1 person in 40 over age 60. The three most common features of the disease are tremor, rigidity, and a bent posture. This condition's severity and rate of progression vary considerably from patient to patient.

Although the underlying cause of Parkinson's disease remains unknown, the condition is known to be associated with a shortage of dopamine in part of the brain. Since 1970 the drug levodopa, or L-dopa, which helps to replenish the supply of this substance, has been available by prescription. This medication has helped many patients, but it is not totally and permanently effective, and often side effects eventually develop. Scientists are investigating several other agents in search of a medication that has fewer side effects and is more effective. Experimental brain tissue transplant surgery that originated in Mexico City in 1987 and now being performed in the United States has not yet become standard procedure but has produced some promising results. The most promising experimental procedure to date is the implantation of fetal brain cells to replace the dead brain cells responsible for producing the debilitating symptoms. Proof of the effectiveness of this procedure was presented in the *New England Journal of Medicine* (5/95), in which Dr. C. Warren Olanow, professor and chairman of the department of neurology at Mount Sinai School of Medicine in New York, discovered upon the death of a man who had had a fetal cell implant that the implanted cells had grown and made exactly the right connections in the brain and that these connections had been responsible for dramatic improvement in his condition before he died of other causes. However, this study was done in only *one* patient.

Most older persons escape the serious diseases just described, but the nervous system often becomes slightly less efficient with age. Generally, ingenuity and effort can overcome these limitations. For example, the use of lists and other reminders can compensate for minor difficulty with memory, attention to simple safety measures can prevent decreased balance and coordination from becoming hazardous, and a little extra time is often needed to learn complex new tasks. With patience and a positive attitude, knowledge and skills can continue to grow impressively throughout life. "Most notions about aging and the brain are based on folklore rather than fact," according to Dr. Zaven Khachaturian, a director of research at the federal government's National Institute on Aging. "If you really study aging carefully, there is no reason to believe that aging per se leads to a decline and loss of cognitive and intellectual activities" (*New York Times*, 4/16/91).

Indeed, perhaps the best advice for keeping the normally aging nervous system healthy is to keep it active. The individual who remains interested in the world, who continues to use and develop mental and physical skills acquired throughout life, and who continues amassing knowledge is most likely to remain young at heart—and young at nerve and brain. In addition to a lifelong habit of intellectual activity, two other factors that influence good mental function are physical: regular exercise and good pulmonary function.

HEART AND BLOOD VESSELS

Cardiovascular diseases (diseases of the heart and blood vessels) remain the chief cause of death in the United States, as well as the cause of much suffering in the older population. With age the heart muscle thickens and narrowing of the arteries is likely to occur. The healthy aged heart can still perform satisfactorily under normal conditions but is less able to respond to extraordinary stresses. In addition, various cardiovascular disorders, including angina pectoris, myocardial infarction (heart attack), congestive heart failure, high blood pressure, and stroke, become more common with advancing age.

Research has indicated that the risk of cardiovascular disease is increased by smoking, high blood cholesterol levels, obesity, lack of regular exercise, high blood pressure, diabetes, and chronic excessive stress. Thus, not smoking, a well-balanced diet low in animal fat, maintenance of a normal weight, frequent and regular exercise, control of high blood pressure, and avoidance of unnecessary stress are practical ways to reduce the likelihood of heart problems. These preventive measures also help to avoid further, more serious damage in persons who already have cardiovascular disease. None of this is news; however, several developments have caused the medical profession to take a closer look at the ways in which they have been treating women's heart problems in particular and the alternative ways of dealing with heart disease in general.

Extensive studies reported in the *New England Journal of Medicine* in 1991 revealed that women were half as likely as men to undergo common diagnostic procedures to find out how advanced their heart disease was. In the same year the American Heart Association announced that a study of nearly 5,000 men and women treated for heart attacks in 19 hospitals in the Seattle area found a dramatic gender gap in the kind of treatment being administered: only half as many women as men were receiving injections of the newer "clot buster" drugs, and twice as many men as women were having their clogged arteries opened up and cleaned out by angioplasty. Following the negative publicity surrounding these revelations, there has been a flood of books, articles, and statements indicating that more doctors now recognize heart disease as an equal opportunity killer and are treating women's coronary complaints with the attention they merit. Here are some of the facts:

Heart disease is the leading killer of women, as it is of men. Of the 520,000 annual fatalities in the United States, 247,000, almost 50 percent, are women, and more than 88,000 die each year of stroke. On a larger scale, all heart and blood vessel diseases combined claim more than 485,000 women's lives each year. That compares with fewer than 223,000 for all forms of cancer. It has been observed that women are 10 to 20 years older than men when they develop coronary problems; by the time women reach the age of 40, these problems are second only to cancer as the major cause of death, and by age 55 they outdistance it. The revelations that women have been treated like second-class citizens in the treatment and, even more important, the prevention of heart disease have led to a flurry of corrective actions. One of the most important of these was the 1991 federal funding of an extensive long-term study by the National Heart, Lung, and Blood Institute on whether low doses of aspirin protect women against heart attacks. Early evidence suggests that the use of one to six aspirins every week can reduce the risk of a first heart attack by 30 percent. The study is tracking 45,000 nurses of different ages and racial and ethnic origins. Although its main purpose is the evaluation of aspirin in preventing heart disease and strokes, a subsidiary study is measuring the effectiveness of two vitamins—beta carotene and vitamin E—in preventing cancer and cardiovascular disease.

According to Dr. Claude J. Lenfant, director of the institute, these are some of the important differences between men and women in the development and progression of coronary heart disease:

- Women experience painless heart attacks more often than men.
- Women are likely to be 20 years older than men at the time of a first heart attack.
- The first indication of heart disease in women is chest pains from angina; in men, it is a heart attack.
- A first heart attack is more often fatal in women than in men, and their death rate in the first year after a heart attack is higher.

Many researchers have pointed out that one of the main reasons that younger women rarely suffer from coronary disease is that the estrogen produced by the ovaries seems to boost the production of the "good" high-density lipid (HDL) cholesterol. A variable that dramatically increases the risks of heart attack in women is a hysterectomy, even when the ovaries remain intact. Because there is a strong possibility that the hormones secreted by the uterus in post-menopausal women may be a protection against such an attack, the American Heart Association has warned against hysterectomy now that other procedures are available. (See "Gynecologic Problems and Treatment.")

Danger Signals

Angina pectoris, a temporary but recurring chest pain caused by an inadequate supply of oxygen to the heart muscle, is usually a sign that the blood vessels supplying the heart have become narrowed. It tends to occur during exercise, stress, and other situations in which the heart must perform extra work. Anyone with chest pain should consult a physician, who may determine if the condition is angina and, if necessary, prescribe suitable medication. If corrective bypass surgery is recommended, at least one other opinion, if not two others, is indicated, because there is compelling evidence that for a significant number of patients nonsurgical treatment can be equally effective and considerably less costly and less traumatic. (Practically all health insurance plans, including Medicare, usually pay for second opinions when expensive procedures are involved.)

Heart attack, technically known as myocardial infarction, occurs when part of the heart muscle dies because the artery supplying blood to it becomes blocked. Anyone experiencing symptoms of a possible heart attack—pain or pressure in the center of the chest that may spread to the shoulders, neck, or arms and sometimes dizziness, fainting, sweating, nausea, or breathlessness— should receive medical help immediately. With appropriate treatment most people can return to an active life after recovery from a heart attack.

Congestive heart failure, which occurs when the heart does not pump efficiently, can produce shortness of breath and swelling of the ankles. Medically prescribed measures including treatment of any associated heart conditions, drugs such as digitalis and diuretics, and a low-salt diet may provide relief of symptoms. Several drugs are now being prescribed to prevent the development of symptoms. (See "Plain Talk About Medications.")

In addition to medical treatments or as a possible alternative to them, nonmedical nonsurgical programs should be investigated by women who have heart disease or who have survived a heart attack. The program developed by Dr. Dean Ornish, director of the Preventive Medicine Research Institute in Sausalito, California, combines diet, meditation, exercise, and support groups and not only treats heart disease but in some cases reverses it. When the Ornish program was granted insurance coverage in 1993, it was publicized as the first alternative medical technique not taught in traditional medical schools to be approved for reimbursement by a major insurance carrier. Among the reasons for the increasing popularity of the Ornish program is not only its effectiveness but also its cost-effectiveness. (It costs about one-tenth the amount of conventional coronary care.) Clearly inspired by this success, the federal government's Public Health Service has begun to issue guidelines for supervised cardiac rehabilitation programs that offer customized prescriptions for exercise, low-fat diets, stress management, and support for life-style changes such as stopping smoking, which many women cannot manage on their own. About 1,000 such programs have been established in hospitals and medical centers nationwide; more recently they are being offered by individual doctors and community health plans. A typical cardiac rehabilitation program that lasts from 8 to 12 weeks costs from $800 to $1,800. Medicare and most insurance companies cover all or most of the cost. Summaries of the guidelines in English and Spanish may be ordered by telephoning 1-800-358-9295 or by writing to Cardiac Rehabilitation, Agency for Health Care Policy and Research, Publications Clearinghouse, P.O. Box 8547, Silver Spring, MD 20907.

"Silent Epidemic: The Truth About Women and Heart Disease" is an informative brochure offered free of charge by the American Heart Association. You can request a copy from the local chapter of the association listed in your telephone directory, or call 1-800-242-8721 for referral to a nearby source.

High blood pressure, or hypertension, especially essential (no known cause) hypertension, becomes more common with age. Among older persons it is found more frequently in women and tends to be especially common and severe among older black women. Although hypertension itself is painless and generally symptomless, it predisposes to heart attack, stroke, kidney damage, congestive heart failure, and other disorders. Every physical examination should include measurement of blood pressure. In treating hypertension a physician may suggest measures such as those described above, in the discussion of prevention of cardiovascular disease, recommend a low-salt diet, and prescribe specific medications. Although vigorous treatment of hypertension is strongly recommended in youth and middle age, the benefits of treating some types of mild or moderate hypertension in those over 65 without heart disease are uncertain, and therefore less aggressive management may be considered.

Stroke, a cardiovascular disease resulting from insufficient blood supply to part of the brain, has already been discussed in the section on the nervous system.

Perhaps because more people are observing the measures described at the beginning of this section, death rates from cardiovascular disease, including heart attack and stroke, have decreased considerably in recent years.

Other Circulation Problems

Both being female and getting older increase the risk of developing varicose veins, enlarged or distorted veins often visible below the skin surface. Pregnancy leaves many women with this condition. With age the veins tend to become less elastic and the muscles supporting them generally weaken, thus predisposing to this disorder. Although many cases of varicose veins merely are unsightly, others can result in serious complications such as leg ulcers if not properly treated. Therefore anyone who has this condition and experiences leg pain or discomfort should seek medical care. Doctors may recommend various measures, depending on the severity and type of varicose veins. The following suggestions for fostering good circulation are commonly made:

- Avoid round elastic garters, socks with tight elastic tops, and wearing elastic girdles for long periods of time.
- When possible, sit instead of stand. When sitting, do not cross your legs; instead, elevate them on a chair or stool.
- Exercise your legs frequently. Walking and swimming are especially effective.
- When sitting for long periods of time, be sure to stretch your legs every hour or so.

To support the weakened veins, physicians sometimes prescribe elastic stockings or elastic bandages. In other cases they suggest surgery, which may consist of such procedures as removing ("stripping") or tying off ("ligating") damaged veins.

A circulatory disturbance known as Raynaud's syndrome causes the fingertips to turn pale and blue in response to the cold. Numbness and in some cases pain may also result from spasms in the tiny blood vessels at the extremities of the hands. It may take many minutes for the fingers to warm up, at which time the tips become red and tingly. Vasodilator drugs may be prescribed if the condition is chronically painful. The most effective self-treatment is wearing lined ski mittens or thermal gloves during cold weather.

LUNGS

Although respiratory function declines with age, the normally aging lung has sufficient reserve to function effectively under ordinary conditions. However, cigarette smoking increases the age-related changes, often to a dangerous extent. Chronic lung disease, especially if associated with smoking, makes activity and even breathing difficult for many older persons. There is now compelling evidence that exposure to secondary smoke over a long period is a major health hazard.

The chronic obstructive lung diseases, emphysema and chronic bronchitis, are considerably more common among smokers and tend to become evident between the ages of 45 and 65. In emphysema progressive damage to the smaller airways and to the air sacs may hinder the movement of air into and out of the lung and interfere with gas exchange. In chronic bronchitis the lung cannot obtain enough air because its passageways become blocked by swelling and by mucus and other fluids. These and other respiratory diseases, symptoms of which can include a persistent or recurring cough, "tightness" or pain in the chest, and a tendency to tire easily, require prompt medical attention. Measures such as stopping smoking, using appropriate medications, good nutrition, sufficient rest, and practicing special pulmonary exercises (bending with head and chest down to promote lung drainage) can help to control chronic obstructive lung disease.

Lung cancer, mainly a disease of smokers and once largely a disease of men, has become so common among women that women's death rates from lung cancer have more than doubled in the last 15 years and since 1986 have superseded breast cancer as the leading type of cancer death in women.

The message of this section should be clear: avoidance of smoking is one of the most important factors in aging healthfully. Many harmful changes in the lungs, heart, blood vessels, and other parts of the body can be avoided or delayed by stopping smoking. Even in persons who have smoked heavily for many years, lung function often improves or its deterioration is halted or slowed after stopping smoking.

With the accumulated evidence of the dangers of secondary smoke, many states have enacted legislation compelling employers to set aside restricted areas for smokers. Women who themselves have never smoked but have had years of exposure to secondary smoke from family members' cigarettes, cigars, and pipes should urge the smokers to restrict their addiction to the out-of-doors, especially when children are part of the household.

DIGESTIVE SYSTEM

The digestive system usually ages successfully. Digestion of food generally remains adequate, but, as in other stages of life, upset and uncooperative stomachs are common.

In later life many factors can produce gastrointestinal distress. As at other ages, emotional stresses often produce abdominal discomfort and disturbances in bowel habits. Gallstones most frequently occur in women over 40, and cancers of the digestive tract generally become more common with age. Many other conditions, including ulcers, infections, and even back problems, can produce abdominal symptoms.

Because so many conditions can cause similar symptoms, self-diagnosis and self-treatment of digestive problems can be dangerous: self-medication with over-the-counter remedies can intensify some conditions rather than cure them.

"Heartburn," especially at bedtime, is a common complaint of older women, often caused by the protrusion of part of the stomach above the diaphragm. Technically known as a hiatus or esophageal hernia, the discomfort of this condition may be eased by some minor dietary changes and by sleeping with the head raised. In cases of extreme discomfort where less drastic measures are ineffective, surgery may be recommended. An acid backflow or "reflux" into the mouth by way of the esophagus of some of the contents of the stomach is the result of the weakening of the muscular ring known as the esophageal sphincter. When this ring closes properly, it separates the bottom of the esophagus from the top of the stomach. Both the conditions described above are commonly linked together as "acid indigestion" and, in fact, both often respond positively to a change in eating and drinking habits, loss of weight if indicated, and avoidance of heavy meals in favor of more frequent "light" ones.

Constipation concerns many older people, often needlessly, because twice-a-day bowel movements may be as normal for one person as two a week are for others. Constipation is a problem *not* when one's bowels fail to move but when pain or discomfort occurs *because* the bowels have not moved. Although constipation can result in part from age-related changes in the digestive system, life-style seems to be a more important factor. Diets low in fiber and high in fats and refined sugars, anxiety and depression, lack of exercise, overuse of laxatives, inadequate fluid intake, skipping meals (especially breakfast), and repeatedly ignoring the bowel reflex all can contribute to constipation. To prevent or treat this problem, eat a high-fiber diet that includes fruits, vegetables, whole grain cereals and breads, and bran. Make exercise (walking, bicycling, swimming) a part of your life-style, avoid laxatives and enemas in favor of a stool softener, drink lots of fluids (six to eight glasses daily), eat breakfast, drink a warm beverage or prune juice in the morning, and respond to "nature's call" when it comes.

Fiber, a largely undigestible food component that is abundant in bran and in many fruits and vegetables, has received considerable attention in the popular media. While fiber helps to control constipation, it remains unclear whether, as some claim, a diet high in fiber also aids in preventing hemorrhoids, bowel cancer, heart disease, and other disorders.

Anyone with symptoms such as abdominal pain, vomiting, change in bowel habits, or blood in the bowel movements should seek medical attention. In many instances the condition can be treated successfully. For most individuals "an apple a day" and *not* keeping the doctor away when he or she is needed are basic to successful, comfortable aging of the digestive system.

See COLON CANCER and COLONOSCOPY.

URINARY AND REPRODUCTIVE SYSTEMS

In part because of post-menopausal changes in the reproductive system, some types of urinary problems become more common with age. Low estrogen levels may predispose to infections of the urinary tract. Furthermore, weakening of pelvic structures, particularly in women who have borne several children, can produce "stress incontinence," a leakage of urine during such activities as coughing, sneezing, and straining. Special exercises often can help to control stress incontinence, and underwear is now available that has been especially designed to offer protection and assurance to women with this problem. The fact that these garments are widely advertised on television by an attractive well-known older actress is a gratifying sign of the progress that has been made in openly talking about matters once considered too embarrassing to discuss even with one's close friends. A common cause of urinary incontinence among older women is medication: sedatives such as Valium, diuretics such as Lasix, over-the-counter insomnia drugs such as Sominex, and various decongestants. Alcoholic drinks and tea and coffee all can exacerbate an incontinence problem. In most cases, even though the problem cannot be entirely eliminated, it can be treated in various ways that reduce its impact on one's normal life-style. (See "Directory for Health Information" for the names and addresses of helpful support groups.)

Menopause does not end the need for breast and pelvic examinations; their importance may even increase in the later years of life. Because older women no longer have the monthly menstrual reminder to do a breast self-examination, they should choose a specific date, for example, the first day or the day corresponding to one's birthday, on which to do it each month. The indications for special breast examinations, such as mammograms, are discussed in the chapter on "Breast Care," which also deals in detail with breast cancer and the progress that has been made in surgical treatment and reconstruction.

Regularly scheduled gynecologic checkups as well as consultation with a physician whenever problems such as bleeding arise continue to be important throughout life. Although in most cases of post-menopausal bleeding the underlying cause is benign, prompt medical attention is necessary to identify potentially serious conditions while they remain easily treatable. It should be kept in mind that unnecessary surgery is too often performed on older women (40 percent of the hysterectomies done in the United States are considered unnecessary by many reputable authorities). Therefore second or even third opinions should be sought before proceeding with this operation.

BONES AND JOINTS

Brittle bones and stiff joints are common as our bodies age. One condition, osteoporosis, in which the bones become thin and brittle, is mainly seen in women who have passed the menopause. In the United States an estimated 15 million persons, at least 75 percent of them older women, have osteoporosis. At greatest risk are small-boned Caucasian and Asian women as well as those who are addicted to smoking, caffeine, and alcohol, and have been compulsive dieters for most of their lives. Osteoporosis may remain undetected until one of the weakened bones breaks. Fractures of the spine (vertebrae) and the hip (neck of the femur) are the most common. Or the condition may become apparent with the gradual compression of the spine, the loss of as much as 2 inches of stature, and the development of a conspicuous curvature of the spine that causes the head to fall forward. Other indications of osteoporosis are persistent lower back pain and the loss of tooth-bearing bone known as periodontal disease.

Women who show signs of osteoporosis or whose life-style and medical history place them at high risk for developing brittle bones should consult their doctor about scheduling a bone density test. The most popular and accurate test scans the entire body, is painless, and takes about 40 minutes. The procedure is called dual-photon absorptiometry (DPA) and may be done at one of the newer scanning centers or in the radiology department of a hospital.

Early detection of osteoporosis makes it possible to plan a program that can halt and even reverse the condition. Researchers agree that the main cause is post-menopausal estrogen deficiency, and that smoking, heavy alcohol consumption, and physical inactivity are much more important factors in the development of osteoporosis than calcium deficiency. It would therefore appear that taking calcium supplements is effective only when combined with estrogen replacement therapy and regular exercise. If this form of treatment is undertaken, it should be combined with progestin (synthetic progesterone) to prevent endometrial cancer and should be closely monitored for the entire duration of the treatment. Post-menopausal estrogen replacement is contraindicated altogether for women who have had endometrial or breast cancer, stroke, liver disease, or who suffer from coronary artery disease or severe migraine headaches. (For additional discussion of estrogen replacement therapy, see "Gynecologic Problems and Treatment.") A comparatively recent experimental treatment is the administration of the synthetic hormone calcitonin, which in its natural state in the body is thought to promote the storage of calcium in the bones. Originally given by injection, it is now used in the form of a nose spray that appears to cause fewer negative side effects.

About 10.6 million older Americans, most of them women, have arthritis, which is not a single disease but a class of several conditions affecting the joints. Pain, swelling, stiffness, and other joint symptoms demand medical attention because the various diseases in the arthritis family require different treatments. Often the physician can reassure the patient that the symptoms are likely to remain mild and require little or no treatment. In other cases rest, medication (commonly including aspirin), exercise, physical therapy, and sometimes surgery may be necessary to relieve pain and preserve function. Persons with arthritis should be wary of quack remedies and devices that waste money and can cause permanent injury. Because arthritis generally comes and goes, these "cures" often are mistakenly considered effective. Devices such as long-handled combs and kitchen utensils, heightened chairs and toilet seats, and clothes without buttons or snaps can make daily activities easier and preserve independence for those partially disabled by arthritis.

When many people think of arthritis, they think of rheumatoid arthritis, a disease producing inflammation of the joints and swelling of the tissue that lines the joints. Rheumatoid arthritis can also affect the skin, lungs, and eyes.

Although it can strike at any age, it is most often seen in older women. It is best treated by a rheumatologist with a combination of anti-inflammatory drugs, and a regimen including heat, exercise, rest, and, where necessary, surgery to preserve range of motion.

Osteoarthritis, unlike rheumatoid arthritis, is not an inflammatory disease. It is much more common than rheumatoid arthritis, especially among the older population. Aging, irritation of the joints, and normal wear and tear all may contribute to this condition. Other risk factors include overweight, poor posture, injury, and physical strain at work or play. Generally, osteoarthritis is a slowly developing disease and is less severe than rheumatoid arthritis. In fact, most persons with X-ray evidence of the condition have no symptoms from it.

Gout is the best understood and most easily treated form of arthritis. Although most cases occur in men, some women develop gout after menopause. In this condition excess uric acid accumulates in the blood, leading to the formation of sharp uric acid crystals that accumulate in the joints and cause the surrounding tissue to become inflamed. Specific drugs reduce the amount of uric acid in the body and avoidance of foods rich in purines, such as sardines, mussels, anchovies, and liver, can reduce the likelihood of recurrent attacks.

FEET

Throughout life feet bear tremendous burdens. Year after year they support our weight; changing fashions, including towering heels, pointed toes, and tight shoes, create special stresses. Diseases such as diabetes and circulatory impairments increase the risk of serious foot problems.

Some foot conditions require the attention of a physician or a podiatrist (a specialist in foot care). For example, attempting to treat corns, calluses, and ingrown toenails oneself may be dangerous. Experts in foot care offer the following advice:

- Avoid decreasing the circulation to the feet. In particular, do not cross your legs thigh over thigh. Do not sit with one of your legs tucked under your bottom. Never wear a tight girdle, never use round elastic garters, and avoid socks with tight elasticized tops.
- Be kind to your feet by avoiding injuries and never placing them in very cold or very hot water. Test the temperature of the water with your hand before stepping into the bath; do not go barefoot, even at home; and do not apply hot water bottles or heating pads to your feet.

- Wash feet daily in warm, not hot, water and mild soap. Dry feet gently and thoroughly, especially between the toes.
- Inspect feet regularly for redness, rashes, injuries, and other abnormalities. Seek medical attention for such problems.
- Wear well-fitting hosiery and shoes. Shoes should be comfortable and provide both support and protection. In order to avoid irritation of the feet, new shoes should be worn at home for brief periods before keeping them on for longer intervals.
- Exercise your feet. Walking is the best exercise. In addition, doctors may prescribe specific exercises.

Manufacturers are now offering special walking shoes similar in construction to jogging shoes but taking into account the different foot muscles involved in the two activities. If custom-fitted inserts are necessary to balance the feet properly, they can be provided as well (see ORTHOTICS). In addition to walking, exercises may be recommended by a podiatrist or orthopedist if foot problems can be minimized by them.

Because people with diabetes are especially prone to serious foot disorders and must guard their feet carefully, they should obtain specific instructions from their physicians and podiatrists.

DIABETES

Diabetes, a condition in which excess sugar appears in the blood, is more common in later age and affects a greater proportion of older women than older men. Many new cases that occur in later life affect overweight persons, are relatively mild, and can be controlled by diet alone. Because people with diabetes are especially prone to foot disorders, eye problems, infections, diseases of the heart and blood vessels, and other conditions, frequent medical care and attention to one's own health are important. (See DIABETES.)

INFECTION

Infection is another threat to the older population. The usual signs and symptoms of infection may be absent in an older person. For example, an elderly individual with pneumonia may be tired and confused but lack fever or chest pain. Medical attention should be sought for any symptoms, not just the classic indications of infection.

Good general health practices, including sufficient rest, a balanced diet, and avoidance of unnecessary exposure to contagious disease are helpful in preventing infections. As the elderly are especially prone to serious or fatal complications of influenza, annual vaccination against this disease is commonly recommended for persons aged 55 and above: the newly developed "flu shots" are more effective and less likely to cause side reactions than those available years ago. The recently developed pneumococcal vaccine, which helps to protect against some types of pneumonia, also may be advisable for some older persons.

Travelers should take special precautions against gastrointestinal infections caused by bacteria in food and drinking water. Such precautions extend to insisting that bottled beverages be served without ice.

GOOD MEDICAL CARE

Care by health professionals becomes increasingly important in the later years of life. Finding appropriate physicians, home and community services, and nursing homes is of great importance.

Until recently, few doctors in the United States had any training in geriatrics. Today, however, more and more medical students, residents, and practicing physicians are studying the care of the aged. If a nearby medical school has a division of geriatrics, it may be able to recommend physicians who appreciate the needs of older patients. Friends, family, and colleagues also can provide useful recommendations. In choosing a primary care physician, inquire about his or her interest and training in geriatrics and knowledge of the facilities available for the aged. Because many older women are hospitalized at some time, information about the hospital to which the physician admits patients is also important.

Communication is basic to a good relationship with any health professional. A physician should show interest in understanding and helping the patient with her problems, explain illnesses and their treatment, and discuss the patient's role in guarding her own health and safety. A helpful physician must be someone a patient can and will talk to openly about symptoms and problems, who not only listens but really hears what's being said, who answers all questions as fully as possible, who doesn't reach for the prescription pad before the patient has finished talking, and who can be depended on to take complaints seriously rather than dismissing them as a bid for attention.

All patients have the right to be treated with respect and consideration regardless of age or economic circumstance. Unless a woman finds it congenial to be addressed by her first name by the doctor and the doctor's staff while she is expected to address them more formally, she should make it clear that she wishes to be addressed as "Miss" or "Mrs." or "Ms."

In addition to a main physician, older women often need the services of such specialists as cardiologists, neurologists, and rheumatologists. Also, routine care by ophthalmologists, gynecologists, dentists, and other specialists is important. Whether a patient can choose her own specialists depends on the nature of her health care and health insurance arrangements. (See "You, Your Doctors, and the Health Care System.")

Nonphysician services for the ill and disabled also are of great importance to the aged, as they can enable an older person to continue living at home rather than to be prematurely institutionalized. Professional services include those offered by physical, occupational, and speech therapists, visiting nurses and a visiting case worker who evaluates the homebound person's needs on a continuing basis. Other services include Meals on Wheels, homemaker visits, and day-care arrangements. Sources of information about such assistance include physicians and other health professionals, local health departments, government and private agencies concerned with aging, religious and civic groups, and especially the local Area Agency on Aging, mandated by the federal government's Department of Health and Human Services to supply information and referrals to all older citizens and their families regardless of income.

Sometimes health problems become so severe or home services are so limited that nursing home care is the only feasible alternative. About 5 percent of the population over 65 resides in such institutions at any one time, and a much higher proportion of the population spends time in a nursing home at least temporarily during the later years of life. Almost three-quarters of elderly nursing home residents are women. For many older persons, the transition into a nursing home can be highly stressful. Likewise, many families and close friends experience feelings of guilt because they cannot care for an ill or disabled relative or lifelong friend. In many instances good nursing home care truly is in the best interests of the ill elderly individual, the spouse, and the offspring, as well as other family members and friends. Finding a satisfactory nursing home can alleviate much of the stress and guilt.

Concern about good nursing homes should begin early. Attention to the type of care that older or sicker friends and relatives are receiving can be helpful. Interest in volunteer work at nursing homes in one's community both improves the facilities and provides an inside view. Participation in local organizations concerned with the quality of nursing home care achieves similar goals.

The Federal Office of Nursing Home Affairs has prepared an informative booklet, "How to Select a Nursing Home," which concludes with a list of several dozen questions. Among items to consider in choosing a nursing home are:

- Is the atmosphere pleasant and friendly and do the current residents feel free to discuss their feelings about the staff?
- Are the mentally disabled residents separated from the others?
- Do the residents participate in planning activities and do they meet regularly with management and staff to air their complaints and offer their suggestions?
- Is the Patient's Bill of Rights conspicuously posted and is the name and telephone number of the state's Long Term Care Ombudsman (an officially designated functionary as required by federal law) known to the residents and their families?
- Does the nursing home seem to be a pleasant, friendly place to live? What do the current residents say about the home?
- Is the home clean, orderly, well-lighted, well-ventilated, and a comfortable temperature?
- Are residents' rooms attractive, conveniently furnished, safe, and sufficiently private?
- Does the nursing home have the required current license from the state or letter of approval from a licensing agency?
- Is the home certified to participate in the Medicare and Medicaid programs? Are you eligible for such coverage?
- Are necessary services, such as special diets and rehabilitative therapy, available?
- Is the nursing home safe for its residents, including the handicapped?
- What medical and dental services, including emergency care, are available?
- Does a qualified pharmacist supervise the pharmaceutical services?
- Is at least one registered nurse or licensed practical nurse on duty day and night?
- Are meals and snacks nutritious, appetizing, and sufficiently frequent?
- Is there a high-quality program of social and recreational activities?
- Does the nursing home have telephone service and indoor and outdoor recreational areas?
- Do the total estimated monthly costs and general financial policies compare favorably with those of other homes? Is the cost quoted inclusive, or

are there extra charges for laundry, drugs, and special nursing procedures?
- Does the contract specify in detail such important aspects as costs, services, and standards?.

MEDICATION

The 11 percent of the population over 65 uses approximately 25 percent of
all prescription medication dispensed in this country, and the average older
person receives 13 prescriptions, including renewals, each year. Drugs are the
largest out-of-pocket medical expense for older persons.

Because the aging process and age-associated diseases can alter the body in
various ways, reactions to certain medications can change with age. For example, age can affect the rates with which your body absorbs, processes, and
eliminates certain drugs. Thus, the doses required can change, often in a
downward direction. It is only recently and in response to considerable pressure from such advocacy groups as the Older Women's League (OWL) that the
FDA has begun to take the age factor into account when approving recommended doses of drugs. Women especially have been the inevitable guinea
pigs in testing out the cumulative long-term effects of medicines prescribed for
chronic illnesses because they live so much longer than men. Thus, many
women have been taking drugs for heart disease, hypertension, and arthritis
for as long as 30 years.

Older women can also experience side effects from drugs that differ from
the side effects experienced by those who are younger. In addition, medications prescribed for one ailment can intensify or nullify the effects of a medication prescribed for a previous condition. It is especially important to contact
your doctor promptly if a drug produces any unfavorable effects, especially
nausea, drowsiness, or mood swings, or if after taking it for the prescribed
time, it fails to have any effect at all. For a detailed discussion on medicines
and the older woman, see "Plain Talk About Medications."

EXERCISE

Women in their late eighties lifting weights? According to a study published
in the *New England Journal of Medicine* (6/94), after a few weeks of lifting

weights to strengthen their legs, these women were able to get around more quickly, climb stairs, and even dispose of their walkers. Another recommendation for women unsteady on their feet is the practice of t'ai chi. (See "Alternative Therapies.")

Exercise is absolutely key to quality of life for perhaps the majority of older women. If they did not exercise earlier in their lives, then they tend to say it is "too late" to do anything about their frailty. *Not so!* Most older women can enjoy and benefit from frequent exercise. Many communities offer exercise classes for their older members. The decline in physical condition that occurs with age often results in part from lack of exercise. Appropriate exercise can help to prevent or reverse this process. It contributes to muscular function and to the health of the heart and blood vessels as well as to relieving tension and promoting a sense of well-being. Exercise also helps to maintain the figure and to decrease the risk of osteoporosis.

Certain types of exercise are specifically recommended for older women. Brisk walking has been called the safest and best exercise for those with and without heart disease. (Running is considered inadvisable for women over the age of 35 because of the heavy toll it places on the knees.) Because of the support that water provides, aquatic exercises often allow movement of joints and muscles in a manner impossible on land. In order to avoid potentially harmful changes in blood pressure, older women should enter and leave the water slowly. Physicians and physical therapists can prescribe special regimens for women with various disabilities, including exercises for rehabilitating muscles damaged by a stroke or slackened through long disuse following a fracture or for minimizing the crippling effects of arthritis.

Such vigorous activities as bicycling, long-distance hiking, and rowing can be done with friends to combat a disability or as a way of dealing with loneliness. Many women join health clubs that offer a large variety of activities ranging from modern dance classes to individually designed exercise programs. Before embarking on *any* program that makes unusual demands on one's body and stamina, it is essential to consult a physician. In addition to evaluating general physical condition, the doctor may perform tests that measure the heart's response to exercise. Instructions regarding such matters as the maximum amount of exercise to be performed daily and the highest heart rate to be reached should be followed carefully in order to maximize benefit and minimize risks.

Millions of women nationwide are using their local malls for socializing. Malls also have become indoor athletic fields for elderly walkers. A *Mayo Clinic Health Letter* (11/95) suggests ways to maximize the benefits of this popular pastime. Wear lightweight clothing suitable for the indoor temperature; wear shoes that offer good support and traction on slippery floors; walk slowly for the first 5 minutes, and if you haven't been exercising regularly, add additional walking time slowly. Increase your tempo gradually, but not so fast as to interfere with your ability to talk to your companion. Carry a water container and drink a cup of water every 20 minutes or so. Set a goal of 20- to 40-minute walks three times a week to keep your weight down and improve cardiovascular function.

In the belief that most people over the age of 60 are not getting enough exercise, the American Association of Retired Persons (AARP) together with the Travelers Companies and the President's Council on Physical Fitness and Sports produced an illustrated manual called *Pep Up Your Life: A Fitness Book for Seniors.* Included are three categories of exercise: for strength, flexibility, and endurance. Many in the first two categories are appropriate for a person in a wheelchair. This manual is available upon request to all AARP members.

SAFETY

As people age, accidents remain common and become more dangerous. Problems such as impaired eyesight and hearing, poor coordination, weakness, fatigue, and stiffness from arthritis can increase the risk of accidents. Sleepiness from medications and worries about personal problems can lead to carelessness. Accidental injuries often are more serious in the elderly: a minor fall may only bruise a youngster but break an older woman's hip. In addition, older persons often do not recover well from injuries such as severe burns.

Many simple measures can help to prevent accidents. Slowing the pace of our daily activities is one way. Another is to pay special attention to the safety features when moving to a new dwelling or correct the hazards in one's own. It's a well-established fact that there's no place like home—for serious accidents.

Falls are the most common cause of accidental death in those over age 65. To prevent the likelihood of their occurrence:

- Provide good, convenient lighting throughout and around the home.
- Place night lights in bedrooms and bathrooms or install remote-control switches that enable persons in bed and elsewhere to turn lights on and off.
- Light outdoor walkways and stairs.

- Wherever possible, place light fixtures and lamps so that bulbs can be changed without standing on a ladder.
- Pay special attention to stairways. Light steps well and provide light switches at both the bottom and the top of each flight.
- Have sturdy handrails—and use them.
- Use nonskid treads where possible.
- Tack down loose stairway carpeting and replace it if holes or slipperiness present a hazard.
- Place a gate at the top of a stairway if you might walk near it at night.
- If moving, consider a house or apartment with few or no steps.
- Use nonslip floor waxes, avoid slippery throw rugs, and keep floors clear of objects over which a person could trip.
- Install grab bars over the bathtub and near the toilet, and place nonslip rubber mats or nonskid strips in the tub or shower.
- Keep outdoor walkways in good repair.
- Wear proper footwear. Well-fitting shoes with low, broad heels and non-slip soles and heels are best for everyday wear. Keep them in good repair.
- Arise slowly from lying and sitting positions. Otherwise, faintness, dizziness, and falls can result. (Of course, anyone who becomes faint or dizzy often or for more than a moment should call a doctor.)

Burns are especially dangerous in later life. They are most likely to be avoided if you:

- Give up smoking entirely or, if you must smoke, never do so in bed or at any time when you're likely to be dozing off with a cigarette in your hand.
- Wear tailored, close-fitting clothes when cooking. Loose long sleeves of housecoats, bathrobes, and nightgowns are likely to catch on fire.
- Use ranges that have controls that are easy to see, reach, and use and elements or signal lights that glow when burners are in use.
- Set controls on water heaters or faucets to prevent water from becoming hot enough to scald the skin, and check water temperature with the hand before entering the bath.
- Install smoke detectors throughout the house, test them regularly to make sure they're working, and have an emergency exit plan in case of fire.
- Use small, lightweight, easy-to-handle pots and pans for cooking, and discard or repair those with loose handles.

Motor vehicle accidents are the most common cause of accidental death in the 65 to 74 age group and the second most common in older persons in general. Nearly one-fourth of all deaths to pedestrians occur in those aged 65 and over. To reduce this risk:

- At night wear white, beige, or fluorescent clothing or carry a flashlight.
- Give yourself extra time to cross slippery streets in bad weather.
- To allow plenty of time to cross the street, wait for a new green light before starting.
- Always cross at designated pedestrian crosswalks, never cross between parked cars, and be especially careful in walking from your car to your destination after parking in a large shopping mall area.

Whether to continue driving a car and, if so, how to adjust driving habits are important concerns. Age-related changes such as greater sensitivity to glare, poorer night vision, impaired hearing, diminished coordination, slower reaction time, and drowsiness induced by medications can make driving more difficult. Older drivers tend to compensate somewhat for these problems by driving less often and more slowly and by driving less at night, during rush hours, and in the winter. Many older drivers are taking to the road with greater confidence and competence after attending refresher courses offered by the American Association of Retired Persons. Another option is the Mature Drivers Course offered by the American Automobile Association. Those considering stopping or limiting their driving may wish to discuss the matter with their doctors. Because older women sometimes *must* stop driving, any plans to change one's residence should give consideration to easy access to public transportation, availability and expense of taxi services, and community travel companion chauffeuring for elderly nondrivers.

Several precautions should be taken to help prevent falls when using buses and other public transportation:

- Brace yourself when the vehicle is about to stop or turn.
- Because walking forward while the vehicle is slowing down is especially dangerous, move toward the door only when the vehicle has stopped or is moving at constant speed.
- Watch for slippery pavement and other hazards when entering and leaving the vehicle.
- Have fare ready in order to avoid losing your balance while fumbling for money.
- Use the vertical support bars when walking down the center aisle and if you must stand while the vehicle is moving.
- In order to keep one hand free to hold on to entrance and exit railings, don't overload yourself with bundles.

With age the body becomes less able to adjust to high and low temperatures. Therefore it is important to avoid extremes of heat and cold. On hot days you should stay in a cool place and avoid strenuous exercise. If you must be out in the sun, wear a broad-brimmed lightweight hat and carry a fan in your purse. Keep your fluid intake high and don't drink alcoholic beverages.

Exposure to cold or to circumstances that cause body temperature to drop below 95°F can result in the life-threatening condition called hypothermia. People over 65 are at special risk for many reasons, including limited mobility, a slowed-down cardiovascular system, impaired perception of body reactions, and the effects of such medications as antidepressants and barbiturates. The National Institute on Aging and other groups specializing in geriatric health and safety make the following recommendations:

- Set the thermostat at 70°F or higher for the bedroom and one other room, and spend a minimum of time in parts of the house that are colder than that.
- Wear the right clothing indoors and out, awake and asleep. Indoors, put on woolen or part-woolen sweaters and socks, a loose woolen robe, and a knitted cap if necessary. Outdoors, wear layers of clothing, starting with long underwear—either silk or cotton tops and bottoms. *Always* wear a hat, earmuffs if necessary, and water-repellent footwear and outer garments when necessary. At bedtime, have warm milk and honey or cocoa, not an alcoholic drink. Sleep under flannel sheets and several lightweight woolen blankets.

Observing safety "rules" does not necessarily prevent accidental injuries. Emotions are incubators for accidents. People who tend to stumble, scald fingers, and drop heavy objects on their toes may be angry, frustrated, impatient, sad, or depressed. Thus, accidents can best be prevented by anticipating the underlying feelings and behaviors that invite them.

PSYCHOTHERAPY AND PERSONAL GROWTH

Depression not only leads to accidents; it causes enormous emotional anguish. Yet it remains among the most underrecognized and undertreated diseases of humankind, especially among older people. Reactions differ, but most depressed people feel hopeless and withdrawn from others. At all ages, the depressed tend to lose their self-esteem, become anxious and irritable, and have trouble concentrating, reading, conversing, and getting up in the morning. Older people who are depressed often have many physical complaints, especially of pain, and they tend to have poor appetites and lose weight. Yet the depressed, especially older people, receive very little psychiatric care. This occurs because many members of this age group are unaware of the availability and benefits of treatment—which can be delivered on an outpatient basis— with appropriate antidepressant drugs and/or psychotherapy. They grew up in an era when talking openly about feelings of sadness or personal problems, even to friends, simply was not done. Older people, like much of society, tend to accept emotional distress and mental deterioration as inevitable parts of aging. In addition, many doctors are likely to treat depression and other emotional problems of older patients solely with tranquilizing drugs, or the patients themselves may turn to alcohol as a buffer against psychological or physical pain. (Adult offspring of aging parents should be very careful about tossing off such suggestions as "Have a drink, Mom, and you'll feel much better." They should also be alert to signs of the condition known as late-onset alcoholism.)

Until recently, many older people who would have benefited from some form of psychotherapy were discouraged from doing so because of financial constraints, since Medicare covered payments only for psychiatrists, that is, MDs who specialize in the treatment of mental illness and emotional distress. The good news is that since 1990 Medicare payments for psychotherapy have been extended to psychiatric and clinical psychologists and social workers who have the required accreditations and licenses. These health professionals are usually part of a team that includes a physician who can prescribe medication if it is deemed necessary. With the proliferation of outpatient geriatric treatment centers, there are many more psychotherapists of all kinds who specialize in helping older women overcome depression or develop new attitudes toward their potential for enjoyment. While some women benefit most from one-on-one treatment, others thrive in group therapy because they become members of a social group that counteracts the effects of isolation. They learn to interact with others and to solve current problems, often with the help of another group member whose self-esteem is bolstered by being able to help. Rather than analyze childhood experiences or reconstruct personality as therapy often does for younger people, the focus is on immediate concerns. Family members often become part of the therapy counseling as well. Thus, the older patient might deal with grief, sexual and drug problems, fear of physical illness and disability, anxiety about death, and making new starts. One therapist has written that older people are better psychotherapy risks than the young, because the former can better postpone gratifications and acknowledge that one must perform to achieve.

A comparatively new field in psychotherapy is the specialty known as grievance counseling. These practitioners can be very helpful in enabling older women deal with the loss of a spouse, a beloved sibling, or an adult offspring who has been the source of emotional and even financial support. Tragic as the loss of a husband may be, the loss of a child is even greater. It is against the natural order of things for a 70-year-old woman to outlive a 45-year-old son killed by a heart attack or for a 65-year-old woman to lose her daughter to breast cancer. Under such circumstances, a grievance counselor can provide the understanding and coping skills to make adjusting to loss less painful.

Older women in therapy—and their families—should guard against overmedication with tranquilizers and especially with powerful psychotropic drugs such as Thorazine that may be inappropriate treatment for their emotional distress. Many women in their sixties and seventies who exhibit signs of memory loss or mental confusion may be suffering not from various forms of senile dementia but from the effects of having been drugged to the point of mental incompetence.

ADAPTATION

The emotional problems of the elderly and their response to the realities of aging are, in a sense, problems of adaptation. There is literally no end to what an older woman can do for her own well-being and for the needs of her community. How, then, can an older woman direct her efforts to adapt? How, more specifically, can she begin to lead a more rewarding life? The final section of this chapter offers suggestions for income building, learning, travel, sexual needs, shared living, and activism.

EARNING POWER

To ensure an adequate income for old age, many women cannot rely solely on Social Security income or retirement and pension plans. In fact, among retired workers receiving Social Security benefits based on their own work records, women's average monthly payments in 1995 were $538 compared with an average of $858 for men. The sex gap also persists in pension figures. A 1994 census report indicated that the mean private pension for women is $3,940 annually, compared with $7,468 for men. Since both Social Security and most pension benefits are based on the number of years a woman has worked and the amount of annual earnings, many women, especially those who are widowed or divorced, want to extend their work record to the maximum.

In many households where both husband and wife have been working, the question of simultaneous retirement is becoming a matter of contention. The stereotypical image in which the husband joins his wife at home and they both travel, play golf, and spend their declining years in a retirement community no longer reflects reality. Although many working women do join their husbands in retirement, the growing trend indicates that a significant number of couples are out of sync. The men who have been working for 40 years or more are ready to bid farewell to job pressures, but their wives who entered the workplace late because they were raising the children have many reasons for wanting to go on working: they like their jobs, they're still expanding their responsibilities, and they want to assure their economic independence in old age, no matter what happens to their marital status.

Women who have remained in the workplace into their sixties because of economic necessity are likely to have caught up with computer technology. Being computer-literate, they have more options following enforced retirement: they can make a transition to home-based work or they can qualify for part-time jobs. In the absence of computer know-how, ingenuity and resourcefulness are great assets. One 72-year-old woman operated her husband's two-car taxi service after his death nine years earlier. She also served as treasurer for another cab company, was a notary public, and collected rent for several landlords. A widow in Arlington, Virginia, started boarding dogs of neighbors in her home. She then operated a full-time pet hotel business and had all the companionship, human and animal, that she needed. Another woman, lacking job market skills, decided at age 70 to put her culinary talents to commercial use. She cooked a week's worth of dinners at a time for customers' deep freezers.

These days when younger wives and single parents are working from 9 to 5, older women can augment their income and provide an essential lifeline in the form of responsible day care and outings, not only for children but for aged relatives who would like special attention while their family caregivers are away at work.

Older women who have retired on a pension or Social Security payments that scarcely cover necessities might take inventory of their marketable skills, especially those related to homemaking. A woman with an elegant handwriting can make posters and address invitations; talented needlewomen can create crafts and practical items; seamstresses can relieve women with full-time jobs of doing the family sewing. An ad placed in a local newspaper or a flyer posted in a laundromat can bring many responses to offers of house sitting, cat feeding, plant watering, and mail collecting for absent vacationers.

Another avenue to be explored and exploited is skill swapping. It may not increase cash flow, but when properly done, it can save you money and get some things done you might otherwise be unable to afford. For example, you might prepare a week's supply of elegant desserts in exchange for having your piano tuned or give English lessons in exchange for minor plumbing repairs.

In 1974, Trish Sommers, cofounder of the Older Woman's League, created the designation "displaced homemakers" for women who lose their source of economic support through divorce or widowhood. According to Women Work! The National Network for Women's Employment, in the U.S. there are at least 17.8 million displaced homemakers and more than 1,300 displaced homemaker centers and programs that offer personal counseling, career planning, and workshops to teach job-hunting skills. For a list of programs in your state, call Women Work! at 1-800-235-2732.

LEARNING POWER

In spite of some myths to the contrary, current research indicates that, among people who remain physically and emotionally healthy, certain crucial areas of intelligence continue to grow well beyond age 80. There is ample testimony that creativity doesn't diminish with age. Verdi wrote some of his greatest music when he was well into his eighties; the late Agnes de Mille continued to choreograph new ballets after a stroke and into her eighties, and we know that Grandma Moses didn't even discover how creative she was until she was quite old.

As for "going back to school," it is no longer unusual for a parent and offspring to receive an academic degree at the same graduation ceremony. Lifetime learning programs abound; continuing education courses are offered at colleges and universities nationwide; and many women have embarked on a "career" for the first time at the age of 65, as practical nurses, social workers, paralegals, and the like. Many are mastering computer skills so that they can work more quickly on the novel they never got around to writing when they were busy homemakers. Moreover, grandmothers with computer skills can communicate with their grandchildren more often and more easily.

One of the most successful and intellectually rewarding enterprises is the Institute for Retired Professionals (IRP), which was organized in New York City in 1962 and has become a nationwide model for well-educated retirees who enjoy teaching one another about their special areas of expertise. For example, a retired art historian will conduct an informal seminar in Chinese painting that includes slides and a museum trip; a retired music teacher will sit at the piano and enlighten the group about Wagner. Some groups ask a member to conduct a chess or bridge class. Architectural walks and talks, performances, and papers on topics of particular interest are all part of the IRP's activities.

Many women are learning self-sufficiency by taking adult education courses in car maintenance, household repairs, money management, and karate. Some find outlets for creativity at local colleges, senior centers, YWCAs, YWHAs, and other groups that encourage them to write, paint, draw, and sculpt, thereby fulfilling long-postponed desires to express themselves. The roster of women who published their first books or exhibited their first photographs or drawings after age 70 is long and distinguished.

A publication on educational opportunities for older people has been prepared by the AARP. Its title and order number is *Directory of Centers for Older Learners* (D13973). For a free copy, write to AARP Fulfillment, 601 E Street NW, Washington, DC 20049.

ELDERHOSTELING

For more than 20 years, older Americans have been enjoying unusual and inexpensive adventures in learning organized by the nonprofit educational institution known as Elderhostel. Short-term academic programs are hosted by educational institutions in all 50 states and Canada as well as by an international network of 1,800 participating institutions in 45 other countries worldwide, including Indonesia, Israel, Japan, and Ukraine.

In 1995, a quarter million people enrolled in Elderhostel. Individuals 55 years of age and older are eligible. Spouses of any age are welcome; companions of age-eligible participants must be at least 50 years old. Elderhostelers represent a broad diversity of life-styles, ethnic origins, and religions. What they have in common is a lively interest in learning—not only about new academic areas but also, especially in the foreign-based programs, about cultural differences and the varied ways in which people live their lives, prepare their food, raise their children, and celebrate their holidays. All lectures are in English. Efforts are made to match hostelers who have specific disabilities with institutions that can accommodate their special needs. Applications are also accepted for the few scholarships that are available.

A typical program in the United States and Canada is conducted on a college campus or similar educational facility providing simple living arrangements. College-level liberal arts and science courses are taught by top faculty members. Although participants are expected to attend the courses for which they register, no preparatory work is required, there is no assigned homework, and there are no exams or grades. Programs usually begin on Sunday afternoon, include five or six nights, and end Friday afternoon or Saturday after breakfast.

The charge for a typical six-night program in the United States is $340. Dormitory accommodations and meals are included. International Elderhostel programs are usually two to three weeks long and consist of classroom lectures augmented by field trips. Housing may be in a college dormitory or a modest hotel. All major program-related expenses are included in the program charge. Most include international airfare as well as travel costs within the host country, and range from $2,000 to $4,000 for two- to three-week programs. Barge and bicycle programs are available in some countries as well as suitable home-stay arrangements.

You can examine the latest Elderhostel catalogs at your local library. If you want to receive copies of your own, or information about Elderhostel's International video that can be played on your home VCR, write to Elderhostel Inc., 75 Federal Street, Boston, MA 02110-1941 or call (617) 426-8056.

TRAVEL TIPS

Whether you have a chronic health problem or are coping with a disability, you need not deny yourself the pleasures of travel if you plan ahead with caution and good sense. Here are some suggestions:

Be prepared for the unexpected. More and more aging women are venturing abroad for the first time, and with adult offspring scattered worldwide, it's always possible that you may suddenly be expected to turn up in Paris or Paraguay. *Therefore, make sure your passport is always up-to-date.* Check your health insurance to find out whether you're covered when you're out of the country. Find out well in advance of departure whether your protection against polio and tetanus needs updating and whether your destination indicates the need for immunization against cholera and other endemic diseases.

Make sure you know about the seasonal temperatures you'll encounter, and pack only the garments you'll need. Think *layered clothing.* Take comfortable walking shoes and extra pairs of cotton socks. For immediate necessities, a back pack is more manageable than a shoulder bag, and a "belly bag" is a good way to carry valuables and money. Heavy luggage should be on wheels. *Make conservative decisions about food and beverages:* no raw seafood, no undercooked meat, and where public health controls are minimal, no unpeeled fruit or raw vegetables. Stay away from gravies and sauces, avoid dairy products, drink only bottled water or bottled beverages *without ice,* and the less alcohol, the better. If you wear glasses or contact lenses, take an extra pair as well as your lens prescription, and tuck a small magnifying glass in your purse. (The type size in bilingual dictionaries can be very small.) No matter where you're going, pack an insect repellent, and stuff the spaces in your luggage with as many soft packages of tissues as will fit. They're especially useful if you run into a shortage of toilet paper.

If you're planning to go abroad, or if you're taking a long vacation in another state, check the current state of your health and medications with your doctor, and ask for a printout of your medical records. (This information will be indispensable should you need medical care in an emergency.) *If you have a chronic respiratory ailment,* avoid visiting high-altitude areas and parts of the world where smog is a permanent problem. *If you have diabetes,* take an extra supply of insulin, check your blood sugar more often than usual, and get a letter from your doctor to explain to customs (if necessary) why you're traveling with hypodermic needles. *If you have a heart ailment,* plan a vacation that involves very little strenuous activity and very little dashing hurriedly from one place to another.

Make your trip as stress-free as possible by setting your own pace instead of being at the behest of a younger or healthier companion. Get yourself into better shape by scheduling a supervised daily exercise program and staying with it for a few weeks before your departure as well as after your arrival at the journey's end. Don't attempt any unusual activities you wouldn't attempt at home. *If you have arthritis,* a spa vacation either here or abroad is an excellent choice. Otherwise, find out in advance if the hotel you've chosen has ramps, bathtub handrails, reliable room service, and a heated swimming pool. If you're traveling a considerable distance by car, stop often so that you can do some stretching exercises; if you're airborne, get up and walk frequently during the flight. A final note about healthy travel: remember that you can order in advance a low-fat, low-salt, vegetarian, or kosher meal, and of course you're free to bring your own supply of fruit, cheese, and multi-grain bread.

NETWORKING

Many paths besides jobs and education lead to new life for the elderly. Old people, like young, need to replace the loss of loved ones. The distinguished psychiatrist Dr. Ewald W. Busse writes that living alone and losing loved ones do not in themselves produce the social isolation that afflicts so many older women. Instead, it is failure to develop any significant *new* relationships that saps life satisfaction. Thus, no woman need remain socially isolated because of widowhood or living alone.

One solution is to maintain close, emotionally supportive ties to others. The Unitarian Church's system of extended families, whose members act as one another's relatives, provide such ties. The American Association of Retired Persons sponsors Widowed Persons Service Programs in hundreds of communities nationwide. These programs offer practical help to bereaved men and women through a network of locally based religious, social service, mental health agencies, and educational institutions. The AARP also has compiled a comprehensive listing of resources in the United States and Canada for the widowed. A single copy of this directory, *On Being Alone*, is available without charge from the AARP Widowed Persons Service.

One of the most effective advocacy organizations is the Older Women's League (OWL) whose members meet regularly coast-to-coast to discuss ways to improve the lives of older women. OWL membership provides a special comfort to those who are isolated in rural areas as well as an agenda for better pay equity, health benefits, pension programs, job training for displaced homemakers, and decent housing for older women living alone. Older women also need to maintain networks of children, kin, friends, young people, and co-workers as well as members of the same organizations. Throughout life these networks can be an important source of support. They help members find jobs, housing, practical help, companionship, and emotional support. They are a resource, like money in the bank, that women should maintain all their lives.

LOVE AND FRIENDSHIP

An important source of emotional support and pleasure in old age is sexuality. One couple, after 35 years of marriage, moved to an isolated house in the country where they spend most of their time working the garden, swimming, and making love. The 68-year-old woman, in an article in *Ms.* magazine, wrote that she hopes the honeymoon will last forever. "We are always touching. I'm glad I'm not like Mama was—she slept downstairs, Daddy slept up, and they never gave each other a good word."

The late Maggie Kuhn, who at 65 launched an activist career that led to the founding of the Gray Panthers organization, included maintaining an interest in sex and companionship with the opposite sex among her five life-styles for the elderly. She once told of a widow who for five years had been bedridden most of the time in her son's home. One day the widow received a letter from a man she had not seen in years. Next came a phone call. Shortly thereafter she appeared downstairs fully dressed and carrying her suitcase. She told her astonished son and daughter-in-law that she was leaving to be married, gave them her love and a forwarding address, and left for a new life at age 82. She lived with her second husband until her death eight years later. In his book *Retirement Marriage*, Walter McKain wrote that marriage among older people is most likely to succeed when the bride and groom know each other well, when children and friends approve of the marriage, and when both bride and groom own a home, have sufficient income, and are reasonably well-adjusted individuals.

A 1994 population survey by the Census Bureau reported about five times as many widows as widowers in the United States—11.1 million widows and 2.2 million widowers—which means that only a small percentage of older women are likely to remarry. One solution to the shortage of older men is offered by author Anne Cumming in *The Love Habit: The Sexual Odyssey of an Older Woman*. Ms. Cumming advocates "intergenerational love" between older women and younger men—even men in their teens and twenties—and predicts that "my book will be required reading in the schools in 50 years' time."

More than 200 years ago Ben Franklin, who appreciated women until the end of his long life, offered similar advice. Franklin argued that older women (presumably, in those days, in their forties) and younger men (in their twenties) are ideally suited for one another, and that young men "in all (their) Amours . . . should *prefer old women to young ones.*"

There is also unwillingness on the part of many widows to remarry. Marlene Sanders, a television news correspondent, once wrote that she had no interest in remarrying after 25 years of an "egalitarian" marriage. "As widows, women tend to become more independent," she said, "and as widowers, men tend to become more dependent, and that also applies to divorced men. That's not a good mix." Another woman who had been married for 40 years when her husband died, said, "I've always had women friends, but now I realize even more that women can be as interesting, or more interesting, than men. . . . Unless a man is interesting, intelligent, and fun, I'd rather stay home." Other widows speak of feeling grown up for the first time now that they no longer have to rely on a man.

What actually happens to sexual functioning in old age? Basically, women and men experience a decrease in intensity and rapidity of sexual response. For a woman this means that she may take as long as 5 minutes, compared to 15 or 30 seconds in younger years, to lubricate, but clitoral response remains the same. Between ages 50 and 70, the duration of her orgasm gradually declines from 8 to 12 contractions to 4 or 5. But there is no decrease in sexual arousability and frequently there is an increase. More important, women can still have multiple orgasms well into their eighties, an ability few men enjoy at any age.

As for missing sexual intercourse, self-pleasuring is an alternative, but many contemporary older women find it difficult to enjoy masturbation. Their generation tends to feel guilty about it and to believe that sexuality should be shared only with a husband or possibly a partner of long-standing commitment. They also tend to have a culturally induced difficulty accepting masturbation. An even more controversial sexual outlet for older women exists. In addition to those women who have maintained lesbian relationships for the better part of a lifetime, increasing numbers of women are finding physical and emotional fulfillment during their later years by establishing a mutually gratifying relationship with another woman. Such commitments often develop beyond friendship into satisfying sexual and emotional bonds. Many women who create these relationships after a divorce or the death of a spouse have never thought of themselves as homosexual or bisexual. They may, if confronted, refuse to call themselves lesbians, but they will tell anyone who is curious about their way of life that they have a companion whom they love and whose presence brings them great joy. Friendship is possible on many levels and with different people. Some women have a talent for "making friends" easily. Others are very private and see reaching out as a form of weakness. Two valuable brochures titled "So Many of My Friends Have Died or Moved Away" (D13831) and "On Being Alone" (D150) are available from the American Association of Retired Persons. For a free copy, write to AARP Fulfillment, 601 E Street NW, Washington, DC 20049. These publications contain practical suggestions on how to maintain old friendships and—more important—how to develop new ones. One of the most important things to remember is that a difference in age is not an insurmountable barrier to enjoying a warm relationship.

Women have other ways to find emotional fulfillment. For example, low-income men and women over 60 can receive special training to spend 20 hours a week with children who have special needs, such as those who are mentally or physically impaired and have been abandoned by their parents to foster homes and detention centers. Participants in the Foster Grandparents Program receive a small stipend and other benefits, and the time a child spends cuddling on the lap of a foster grandparent provides comfort, security, warmth, and the immeasurable benefits of loving and being loved to both.

Another program, the Retired Senior Volunteer Program (RSVP), is open to any retiree without regard to financial status. Participants can choose activities ranging from visiting the homebound to acting as surrogate grandparents in day-care centers or children's hospital wards to reading to the visually impaired in nursing homes. Many women are enjoying newfound love and appreciation that gives their later years a deeper meaning.

PETS

Women who have always enjoyed involvement with a pet might consider adopting one as they grow older, especially if they live alone. Women who have not yet discovered the many blessings of pet ownership (which more than offset the responsibility and inconvenience involved) could enter a world of new emotional experiences. Specialists studying the beneficial aspects of the interaction between pets and people have written that "when older people withdraw from active participation in daily human affairs . . . animals can become increasingly important. [They] have boundless capacity for acceptance, adoration, attention, forgiveness, and unconditional love. . . . For the elderly, the bond with animal companions is stronger and more profound than at any other age" (*California Veterinarian*, 8/82).

Involvement with a pet can help decrease the stress of depression, anxiety, and isolation as well as stress-related conditions such as coronary heart disease and high blood pressure. Taking care of a pet provides a built-in motivation for taking care of one's self. It is well-known that when pet owners are hospitalized, their recovery is hastened by eagerness to get home to the animal who is being deprived of their loving care.

In choosing a pet for the first time, women should take their individual situation into account. Those who enjoy walking will find a dog an ideal companion. (A smaller breed can be paper-trained as well as house-broken should a spell of bad weather make walking difficult.) Cats are a great comfort and require less care, especially if there are two to entertain each other. Although cats tend to be more independent than dogs, they can give deep affection when treated affectionately. Finicky housekeepers can derive great satisfaction from birds or fish. Whatever the choice, sharing one's home with a pet can open up new worlds of love, companionship, and fun. Involvement with living creatures also provides informal membership in a community of people with similar interests. Dog lovers get to know each other and their pets when they are out walking them or taking them to a nearby park for a romp. Cat lovers are a special breed who can amuse each other endlessly with anecdotes and who share a feeling of superiority to friends who prefer canines. And with a pet of any species, photography becomes a new experience and a new challenge. (See "Alternative Therapies" for additional benefits of pet ownership.)

SHARED LIVING

According to U.S. Census Bureau figures for 1994, 9.3 million noninstitutionalized older people were living alone: 7.2 million women and 2.0 million men, representing 40 percent of older women and 16 percent of older men. Older people living alone increased in number by about 30 percent between 1980 and 1994. Yet while most older people prefer the privacy and independence of living on their own, it is not surprising that group and age-integrated living arrangements are also becoming more popular. Challenging the notion expressed by the sixteenth-century poet that "Crabbed Age and Youth Cannot live together," one elderly woman shared her home with several young medical students who helped her maintain it. This kind of living arrangement redefines the family as a group of people united not by blood or marriage but by mutual needs and interests. Another woman, after her husband's death, subdivided their large old house into six apartments, lived in one, rented out the others to friends, and paid her mortgage and repair bills from the proceeds. Communal living arrangements of several people living together can provide companionship, mutual help, protection from crime, and an alternative to institutionalized living.

Some women live in accessory apartments in underoccupied single-family residences. These apartments have their own kitchen and bathroom and offer total privacy without imposing a sense of isolation. Self-contained units known as "granny flats" are connected by a sheltered breezeway to the main family house. Information about match-up programs that help people locate shared housing is available from county and local agencies on aging or from the National Shared Housing Resource Center, 321 East 25th Street, Baltimore, MD

21218; phone (410) 235-4454. The Center also maintains a directory of over 400 shared housing programs nationwide. Information about both the shared housing programs and the match-up programs in your area is available free of charge on request by phone or letter.

Another alternative is retirement homes, which offer a continuum of care ranging from independent living apartments to skilled health-care facilities such as those found in nursing homes. Additional information may be obtained from the AARP. Ask for "Consumer Housing Information for Seniors" when you write. A growing number of retirement communities are located on or near a college campus. These living arrangements offer the special benefits of excellent medical facilities and a broad spectrum of creative and intellectual possibilities.

A recent development is for women to live together—on the move—in motor homes or trailers. Many who once enjoyed the freedom of the road with their late husbands are joining together for safety, companionship, and new adventures. Those with sufficient funds may share a luxury motor home. For women with limited incomes a trailer offers an economical way to see the USA and visit distant family members.

MORE ABOUT EXERCISE—FOR EMOTIONAL WELL-BEING

Some people become convinced as they grow older that traveling and other exertions are bad for their health. But the human body is a marvelous machine that thrives on use. More than 2,000 years ago the physician Hippocrates suggested that functions that are not used become atrophied—"use it or lose it!" Several hundred years later Cicero listed four factors that adversely affect aging—being barred from useful activity, being weakened physically, being deprived of pleasure, and being aware of the nearness of death. More recent theories of successful aging add lack of proper sleep and diet, smoking, and heavy drinking to the list of harmful factors. Other studies confirm the importance of exercise not only in maintaining physical health but in preventing or relieving depression, possibly because exercise increases one's sense of well-being by releasing the brain's endorphins, potent substances that act as analgesics and can produce a sense of euphoria.

It is never too late to start exercising, although the amount and type of exercise should depend on one's state of health—and nerve. One woman, described by author Jane Howard in her book *Families*, learned to swim at the age of 75 and before long was diving off the high board. Others are participating in special athletic events for seniors—women's jogging competitions, bicycle races, and overnight hiking trips. Women who used to drive to destinations only a few blocks away are discovering the many pleasures of walking—in well-designed shoes. Many communities offer group walking tours that explore historic urban areas, and nature lovers can join bird watchers or wild life preservationists or other special-interest groups on seasonal outings. Physical fitness classes with the focus on the needs of older women are available in most communities, and a membership in a good health club is a rewarding gift to request from a spouse or an offspring.

LIFE WORK

Mental activity may be even more important than physical. Margaret Mead, who remained a working anthropologist until she died of cancer at age 76, used to say, "I know I can't live forever. I'm just not ready to go yet." She kept a journal of observations on the progress of her cancer and remained, until her death, passionately involved in life.

Simone de Beauvoir once said, "The only solution to the problems of old age is for each old person to go on pursuing ends that give existence meaning." One woman decided at age 70 to fulfill a lifelong dream of living in San Francisco. She invested her savings in a bus ticket and, despite a limited Social Security income of $160 a month and a lame leg, successfully settled in a strange city where she had no friends or family. She played in a band at a senior center and walked across the Golden Gate Bridge six times. Another woman at age 72 founded an organization called Neighbors Helping Neighbors in which volunteers provide rides to doctors' offices, hospitals, and clinics for disabled people with no other means of transportation. For eight years she ran this enterprise from her small cottage in Sharon, New Hampshire, before turning it over to a new manager. Looking back, she says, "Who would have thought my seventies would be the happiest years of my life?" In her nineties another woman began to write essays about aging. Asked why she took up writing, she replied, "I'd be bored to death if I didn't have something to do." After the better part of a lifetime devoted to classical Greek scholarship, Edith Hamilton wrote her first book at the age of 62 and continued to write and publish until 1957, when *The Echo of Greece* appeared to mark her ninetieth birthday.

Charles Schulz, creator of *Peanuts*, once suggested in cartoon form another way old people could remain assets to society. Lucy, while reading a composition to her class, concluded:

> "And so World War II came to an end. My grandmother left her job in the defense plant and went to work for the telephone company. We need to study the lives of great women like my grandmother. Talk to your own grandmother today. Ask her questions. You'll find she knows more than peanut butter cookies! Thank you!"*

Lucy, in effect, recommends "life review," an autobiographical process that allows an old person to take pride in the past by talking or writing about it, reading diaries or letters from a former lover, attending a reunion, or visiting one's birthplace. When an older person is encouraged to reminisce, perhaps by a grandchild with a notebook or tape recorder, the listener gains wisdom and experience, and the reminiscer discovers that somebody cares enough to listen.

MAXIMIZING YOUR LATER YEARS

One of the most wholesome developments in contemporary American society is the growing activism of people over 65. About 2.2 million men and women celebrated their sixty-fifth birthday in 1990, and it is anticipated that by the year 2000, the 65-plus age group will represent 13 percent of the population. As the population ages, women increasingly outnumber men: 122 women for every 100 men in the 65 to 69 group; 259 women for every 100 men in the 85 and older group. Because older people vote in larger numbers than any other part of the population, and because their numbers are growing, they have considerably more political clout than in the past. They have also learned a lot about group activism, lobbying, and fighting for satisfactory solutions to their particular problems. Women have been playing an outstanding role in these efforts, whether banding together as displaced homemakers or making their voices heard in Congress for better medical care, adequate housing or income, or greater rights for grandparents.

It is encouraging indeed that increasing numbers of old people are making themselves heard as members of such activist groups as the AARP, Older Womens' League, and Gray Panthers, a coalition of young and old who oppose age discrimination, age stereotyping, and other dehumanizing forces in our society.

* Text from PEANUTS by Charles M. Schultz; © 1976 United Features Syndicate, Inc.

Women in rural areas are beginning to join together to seek better solutions to problems of isolation, economic depression, and hard, underpaid work on the farm. They are holding statewide conferences to establish more effective networking and encourage political activism.

For some women the major adjustment to aging seems to take place following menopause. For others it occurs when the children go off to college or get married and move away from home. For still others the adjustment comes with the retirement of their spouse or, more dramatically, with widowhood. But whether you are adjusting to wrinkles, to a developing disability, to the loss of a spouse, or to a decrease in income, *attitude and adaptability* are coping strategies that can make your later years a time of personal growth in balance with a greater need for dependence on family, friends, and community.

Anticipation is another strategy for coping with the challenges of your later years. Thinking ahead of possible difficulties and preparing for them by talking about them with your spouse, children, or lawyer can lead to enlightened decision-making. Practical guidelines for planning ahead about money, housing, health care, and other concerns appear in the American Association of Retired Persons publication *Tomorrow's Choices: Preparing Now for Future Legal, Financial, and Health Care Decisions.* It is available to AARP members by written request to AARP Fulfillment, 601 E Street NW, Washington, DC 20049.

A final way of exercising power, in this case over yourself, is through living wills, which give you legal control over your own and your relatives' bodies. These documents enable you to decide, while you are still healthy and legally competent, whether you wish others to prolong your life by artificial means and heroic measures despite the indignity of deterioration, dependence, and pain. The growing movement toward hospice care, in the same vein, promises to provide a pain-free, humanistic environment in which to experience a terminal illness.

Society continues to view old people, even while they are still healthy, more as a problem than as a valued social, economic, and political resource. Dr. Robert N. Butler, former director of the National Institute on Aging, once commented on the survivorship of the old: "I for one am somewhat tired of hearing about the 'aging problem.' We are talking about a major human triumph in this century." Despite the problems an older woman faces, she has great strengths and potentials. For example, she has the opportunity to:

- Become, perhaps for the first time in her life, an independent being, undominated by others and in full control of her life.
- Guard her physical and mental health.

- Fulfill her own expectations, not those imposed by society.
- Enjoy good friends and leisure pastimes.
- Exercise to keep physically fit.
- Continue to discover and use her talents.
- Remain curious and eager to learn.
- Remember that what is frowned upon in a girl of 20 is applauded as "character" in a woman of 80.
- Remain passionately involved with life, enjoying each day as it comes.

The older woman who does even a few of these things will begin to see a different person when she looks in the mirror—not a wrinkled facade but a successful individual who knows there still is work to be done, dreams to be dreamed, pleasures to be enjoyed. Older women who can view the aging process in this manner serve as role models for women now in their fifties, forties, thirties, and even twenties. The women most likely to adapt successfully to the stresses of old age will be those who have adapted well to stresses of equal or greater severity throughout their lives. What is past is prologue.

LOOKING AHEAD

The 50-year-old woman of today has not been hardened to adversity like the 80-year-old who learned in the Great Depression to deal with problems similar to those encountered in old age. Yet these younger women have more education than ever before, and when they reach age 70 and beyond, they will have more earned pensions and financial resources of their own. They will have children and grandchildren to support them economically and emotionally in old age. Family ties will be extended, with parent-child bonds lasting 50 years or more and grandparent-grandchild bonds 30 years or more. In sum, women now in their fifties and younger are almost certain to experience old age differently than the women who preceded them, and the experience will, on balance, be better.

$\mathscr{P}$LAIN TALK ABOUT MEDICATIONS

Helene MacLean

Medical Writer and Editor; Author, *Caring for Your Parents, Relief from Chronic Arthritis Pain*; Coauthor, *Recovering from a Hysterectomy, Migraine: Beating the Odds*

As the century draws to a close, women's health issues are beginning to receive the special attention previously denied them. At long last, with the establishment of the Office of Research on Women's Health as part of the National Institutes of Health (NIH), the federal government has officially recognized that many *"diseases, disorders, and conditions are unique to, more prevalent among, or more serious in women, or for which there are different risk factors or interventions for women than for men."* In practical terms, this means that the NIH, which is the major funding agency of biomedical research in the United States, has set new guidelines to ensure that these gender-specific problems are adequately addressed and that women from all age groups and different ethnic origins are sufficiently represented in clinical studies for new treatments, especially in clinical trials for new medications.

Another recent development with the same focus is the recent compendium from the publishers of the authoritative *Physicians' Desk Reference*. Called *The PDR Family Guide to Women's Health and Prescription Drugs*, it concentrates on the medications available for conditions and health problems that are the exclusive concern of women, concerns ranging from contraception to fertility

problems, premenstrual syndrome to menopause, as well as the various gynecological infections and cancers. Special attention is given to the latest medical
treatments for heart ailments as they specifically affect women—an area of
diagnosis and treatment in which women's problems had been neglected for
too long.

This spotlight on women's health problems is not only the result of the
highly publicized backlash against the male medical establishment; it also
comes at a time when many women have been turning to alternative therapies
with the goal of taking as few medicines as possible, hoping to achieve and
maintain good health through better nutrition, regular exercise, and changes in
life-style. Women of all ages and different ethnicities are exploring the many
techniques for managing stress without turning to cigarettes, alcohol, and tranquilizers, and for dealing with pain in ways that don't produce undesirable side
effects. These efforts have been receiving support from many primary care
physicians, especially from the proponents of preventive health care.

Of course there's a critical difference, frequently a life-saving difference,
between taking fewer medicines and taking none at all. Rejecting the major
accomplishments of medical science out of hand is one of the sure signs of the
medical quack. After all, contraceptive pills and abortion pills are medical
treatments; vitamin therapy is a medical treatment, and so is every immunization that protects us during our lifetime from devastating diseases. Antibiotics,
chemotherapy, new drugs for diabetes, new drugs that compensate for bone
loss all play an essential role in promoting well-being. What is as essential as
the medication itself for the woman who wants to be an active participant in
self-care is the *information* to make informed choices when presented with
different treatment options.

It is hoped that the various aspects of medication discussed in the pages that
follow will enable you to approach all drugs—both prescription and nonprescription—with greater confidence in your own judgment. It should also be
emphasized that while your doctor is responsible for answering your questions
about the medications being prescribed or recommended, *you have the final
responsibility for using the medication according to directions.* If you intend to
do otherwise, your responsibility extends to informing the doctor of your
intentions.

AVOIDING MISUSE AND DRUG ABUSE

Because prescription tranquilizers, sleeping pills, and antidepressants (as well as a number of painkillers) have a high mood-altering potential, they are easily misused. With some women, misuse can imperceptibly slide into abuse. In other words, the gradual use of the drug in greater amounts than prescribed, or for purposes other than those for which it was originally intended, can lead to the development of a psychological and/or physical dependency. In more extreme cases, the woman may seek prescriptions from as many different doctors as she can convince that her need for the medication is legitimate.

Because these drugs are not life-saving in the same way as an antibiotic that prevents death from pneumonia, the benefits of relieving the symptom—anxiety, sleeplessness, mild depression—have to be weighed against the side effects and hazards. This evaluation is different for each individual. In the case of a woman whose alcohol consumption is out of control, the risks involved in taking any mood-altering drug are very great. Not only is dependency on yet another substance an important consideration; the combination of alcohol and sleeping pills has resulted in more than a few "accidental" deaths. A physician confronting a woman with an alcohol problem has to take the responsibility of withholding the drug in favor of recommending treatment for alcoholism, at the same time suggesting some possible alternative therapies for stress management. In another instance, for a woman who has undergone surgery, the benefits of controlling postoperative pain with powerful narcotics far outweigh the risk of the patient's becoming a drug "addict."

TRANQUILIZERS

There are two kinds of tranquilizers: antianxiety drugs (or minor tranquilizers) and antipsychotic drugs (which are or should be prescribed only for severe mental illness). Minor tranquilizers are properly prescribed for the temporary treatment of anxiety and the relief of stress caused by cumulative emotional conflict or by a sudden trauma, such as the death of a parent, child, or husband; an unexpected request for a divorce; or, for a single working mother, the dislocation of having to move her family to another city in order to keep an important job. Under these and similar circumstances, the use of a minor tranquilizer is best viewed as temporary or, if advisable, as a transitional bridge to counseling or therapy.

All of us feel anxious, tense, and excessively stressed from time to time. Unfortunately there is a seductive philosophy that has convinced too many Americans of the possibility and desirability of achieving a life free of any distress. For those who are seduced into believing that growth and development can be achieved without experiencing pain and unhappiness, relief from these feelings can be just a pill away. The fact that too many doctors have been promoting this view accounts for the billions of tranquilizers (notably Valium) and sleeping pills consumed each year. Recently, however, with the increasing awareness that irresponsible pill-popping creates new problems rather than solving old ones, more women are coping with anxiety-producing circumstances with such alternative methods as behavior modification, marriage counseling, exercise, support groups, meditation and massage, and assertiveness training.

If you're feeling apprehensive about going on a job interview, for example, there are several things you might do: you might talk about it with friends, ask a former colleague to put you through a tough rehearsal with a barrage of likely questions, or imagine the worst-case scenario and brace yourself for it by figuring out the next step. Although you may still be anxious when you turn up for the interview, afterward you're likely to feel somewhat hopeful and to have made several important discoveries: it wasn't as difficult as you anticipated; nothing terrible happened and you didn't disgrace yourself; there were some aspects of the interview you handled very well and some things you'll know how to handle more effectively next time. Overall, you should feel pleased with yourself for having met the challenge, and you'll be less anxious the next time around. But suppose you pop a couple of tranquilizers before the interview. You haven't really learned much about yourself in trying circumstances. By denying yourself the experience of being able to function well even though anxious, you haven't coped with anxiety, and you'll need the pills so that you can manage to face the next interview. The credit for getting through these experiences doesn't bolster your self-regard; the credit goes to the pharmaceutical company.

The effect of tranquilizers on the brain is similar to that of alcohol. Low doses make you feel pleasantly relaxed while higher doses can be intoxicating. Of the millions of women who have used tranquilizers since their appearance almost 40 years ago, the majority have used them safely, if perhaps often unnecessarily. Some, however, found that as frequency of use increased, they were in a catch-22 situation in which their anxiety mounted as their dependency grew. A woman in this situation is similar to a woman increasingly dependent on alcohol. She is unable to control her use. She is frightened and ashamed of what's happening to her. She feels she should be able to stop. She tries. She can't. She feels even more ashamed. When she does stop for a while, she experiences severe anxiety, jitteriness, and insomnia. She may even have a convulsion. She needs help desperately and finally must seek professional intervention.

Women who do manage to kick the tranquilizer dependency after long use report withdrawal symptoms ranging from moderate to severe. A significant percentage of women in this category have had to deal with extreme emotional distress, dizziness, restlessness, headaches, and gastrointestinal upsets, as well as heightened anxiety—all considerably more unpleasant and immobilizing than the symptoms for which they took the medication in the first place.

When Betty Ford publicly announced her dependence on alcohol and tranquilizers and her determination to deal with her substance abuse problems, she not only saved her own life but also established a commendable precedent enabling many women, both public figures and private citizens, to admit they needed help. Nowadays there is no shame attached to seeking treatment at a local hospital facility or at the Betty Ford Center, a deserving monument to a brave woman.

SLEEPING PILLS

There is an ongoing debate among doctors specializing in sleep problems about whether sleeping pills are the best way to treat insomnia. Fortunately, there is now general agreement that barbiturates, once widely prescribed with little regard for their addictive properties and negative side effects, are the worst possible treatment. For short-term need where undisturbed rest is essential for healing—for example, in a hospital after surgery or at home during postoperative convalescence—sleeping pills, properly monitored, have a limited use. But for chronic insomnia, many physicians have concluded that they can do more harm than good.

Sleeping pills act by chemically shutting down some areas of the brain. They work very effectively over a short period; however, because the brain adapts rapidly to the drug action, the same dose no longer has the same effect after a few days. Thus the use over an extended period results in three main problems. The first and most common is that although the drug is no longer having a pharmacological effect, it becomes incorporated into the nighttime routine. For many of us, the behavior patterns involved in preparing for sleep are so unchanging as to be more of a ritual than a routine. Disturb one aspect, and falling asleep becomes difficult. The second and more dangerous problem is that of having to increase the dose to achieve the same effect. Increasing the dose increases the risk of dependency. As the dose goes up, the brain adapts to the new dose, so the next dose has to be higher to be effective. The third problem of long-term use is connected with the special nature of the newer drugs. Because they remain neurochemically potent over a longer period, they produce increased undesirable side effects during waking hours. These effects can include not only a decrease in attention and a carryover of drowsiness but also subtle disorders of thinking and judgment, any of which can have disastrous consequences.

Many women have discovered that there are various alternatives to medical treatment for their insomnia. Some of the causes that interfere with their ability to get a good night's rest can be eliminated by changes in diet, exercise, and erratic sleep routines. Training in relaxation techniques, including imaging, and massage combined with aromatherapy can also be effective. If these treatments fail to produce the desired results when combined with behavior modification, consultation with a sleep specialist may reveal the presence of a treatable medical cause.

What You Should Know about Halcion

In spite of a history of negative publicity, Halcion continues to be the world's best-selling sleeping pill. It is a member of the benzodiazepine class of drugs, which includes Valium, and when it was introduced in 1983, it was advertised as promoting sleep without producing daytime drowsiness. From that time to this, the pharmaceutical company (Upjohn) that produces Halcion has been the target of considerable criticism for originally withholding important information about its adverse effects. The drug has been banned altogether in Great Britain, and in the United States its manufacturer continues to be the target of hundreds of lawsuits because of these effects. The suits have been categorized as "the drug made me do it" cases, in the most extreme of which Halcion has been held responsible for producing psychotic behavior resulting in murder. No one knows how many of these suits have been settled out of court. Following the British ban, Upjohn changed its labeling, shortened the recommended length of treatment from no more than a month to 7 to 10 days, and warned of reports that tied Halcion to "suicidal thinking and bizarre behavior." Originally sold in 1 milligram form, it is now packaged in ½ milligrams. Some countries, France, for instance, require that it be sold in ⅛ milligrams. Halcion has received full approval of the FDA, and most people who use it *for the short-term treatment of insomnia* have reported no untoward effects. But various well-known individuals have said that it made them "crazy" and caused them to become severely depressed, to suffer from amnesia, and to be at the mercy of suicidal thoughts. Fainting has also been reported, as well as increased anxiety during the day.

Extreme caution should be exercised when combining Halcion with other drugs, and its effects should be monitored by the doctor who prescribed it before the prescription is renewed. If Halcion has been used for more than a few weeks, discontinuation should be gradual and embarked on under the guidance of the prescribing physician to avoid acute withdrawal symptoms.

Is Melatonin a Treatment for Insomnia?

Melatonin is a hormone secreted by the pineal gland located deep within the brain. One of the functions of this hormone is the regulation of the sleep-wake cycle by suppressing the electrical activity of the brain, thereby producing a sedative effect. Through the recommendation of some alternative therapists, melatonin has achieved widespread popularity as a substitute for conventional sleeping pills. It is also being recommended among friends and in some women's magazines as an effective way of dealing with jet lag when doses are carefully timed.

According to FDA regulations, melatonin can be promoted only as a "dietary supplement," and as such, it is sold over the counter along with vitamins and minerals in health food stores and pharmacies. It is packaged in 3 milligram capsules (some capsules contain an additional 6 to 10 milligrams of vitamin B_6). Although all labels suggest that one tablet be taken before bedtime, the instructions about how long before bedtime range from 20 minutes to 2 hours. Warnings vary as well: *Do not combine with a tranquilizer. Should not be taken by adolescents, pregnant women, or lactating women. Do not take this product when driving a motor vehicle or operating machinery. As a dietary supplement, take one capsule before bedtime, but do not take more than one in a 24-hour period.*

If you decide to try melatonin to help you overcome insomnia, you're on your own. Doses have not been officially arrived at through clinical trials, nor is there an accumulation of reliable information about side effects resulting from long-term use. (See also MELATONIN)

PROZAC AND OTHER ANTIDEPRESSANTS

Prozac came on the market with deafening fanfare in 1988, and by 1994 it had been prescribed for more than six million Americans, most of them women between the ages of 20 and 50. Although it is considered safe and generally nonaddictive, very little is known about its long-term effects, and already there are reports of loss of sexual competence, insomnia, and suicidal impulses similar to the claims made against Halcion. There is also considerable concern that Prozac is being widely prescribed and inadequately monitored by primary care doctors who are not specialists in treating clinical depression. At many colleges, for example, it has become the panacea for complaints about depression, and it is especially popular among some female undergraduates because it appears to help them deal with bulemia, an obsessive-compulsive eating disorder.

Prozac was the first of the most recent group of antidepressants, which achieve their feel-good results by enhancing the action of serotonin, a chemical transmitter of messages between brain cells. Among the other new drugs in this category are Zoloft, Paxil, and Effexor, with more on the way when the FDA approves them. According to the manufacturers of Effexor (Wyeth-Ayerst Laboratories), it is effective with some people unresponsive to Prozac because it enhances not only serotonin, but also norepinephrine, a second neurotransmitter. The popularity of these newer drugs is explained by the fact that they avoid some of the more unpleasant side effects (dry mouth and eyes, blurred vision, weight gain, sensitivity to bright light, and sexual difficulties) of two earlier groups of antidepressants, known as tricyclics (Elavil, Pamelor, Tofranil) and monoamine oxidase (MAO) inhibitors (Nardil). Also, because the newer drugs are less toxic, they are less likely to be used successfully in suicide attempts.

Many psychiatrists, however, believe that the older drugs may continue to be the choice for patients suffering from immobilizing clinical depression. Now that they are available in generic form, the older drugs also have an enormous price advantage, as the more recent antidepressants cost about two dollars per pill wholesale. The managed care industry has already begun to require physicians to get special authorization before prescribing the newer drugs. Dale Kramer, pharmacy director for the Kaiser Foundation Health Plan, this country's largest health maintenance organization has said, "These things are relatively new. Sometimes it takes a number of years before the real bad stuff comes to light." Sidney Wolfe, director of the Public Citizen Health Research Group, a consumer advocacy group based in Washington, warned against "popping a pill instead of helping people cope with underlying causes of depression . . . I see this as a 1990s version of Valium. These drugs are being used in an overly broad fashion just as the tranquilizers were."

A woman suffering from immobilizing clinical depression can benefit from the guidance of a doctor trained in the treatment of this illness. The advantages and disadvantages of various antidepressant medications suitable for her situation should be discussed so that she has the option of making the decision in terms of side effects, likely benefits, and cost. The doctor should monitor both the side effects and the effectiveness of the drug and, where indicated, switch to a different one for better results. The use of the drug may or may not be discontinued as soon as the patient is ready for a type of therapy suitable to her situation—grievance counseling, marriage counseling, family counseling. As for the millions of women who manage to function responsibly even though they feel rotten a lot of the time or at different times of the year or because of different circumstances, pills are available at a price, but consideration should also be given to other types of therapy: light therapy for the winter blahs, exercise, massage, meditation, various types of stress management, even informal group gab sessions where blowing off steam can decrease the pressure.

ANTIBIOTICS—RIGHT WAY, WRONG WAY

One of the leading concerns of medical science is the increase in bacterial resistance to the effectiveness of antibiotics. Especially worrisome is the development of strains of drug-resistant bacteria that cause gonorrhea, tuberculosis, and some types of pneumonia. Patients and doctors alike appear to be responsible for compromising the dependability of the "miracle" drugs through indiscriminate and excessive use.. The result is a race between tougher new bacterial strains and the development of new antibiotics that can successfully outwit them.

The findings of a Gallup poll released by the American Lung Association in 1995 indicated that most patients are poorly informed about the role of antibiotics and the correct way to use them. This widespread misinformation is one of the main reasons that more people are dying of infections that were once easily cured. You can promote your own well-being and safeguard the vital role of antibiotic medicines by observing these rules:

- Do not ask your doctor to prescribe an antibiotic for symptoms of a cold or the flu. Antibiotics are effective only against bacterial infections and are useless in the fight against viruses.
- Do not insist on an antibiotic prescription during a viral illness as a way of preventing an ear infection or bronchitis.
- If an antibiotic is about to be prescribed, be sure to tell the doctor about adverse reactions to any antibiotics in the past.
- Always take a prescribed antibiotic according to the doctor's instructions. This means taking *all* the doses even if you've begun to feel better and in spite of the inconvenience.
- When you have an antibiotic prescription filled, ask the pharmacist whether an information sheet is available to go with it.
- Call the doctor promptly about unpleasant reactions to an antibiotic, especially if you develop a rash.
- To counteract the occurrence of vaginitis caused by an overgrowth of yeast during antibiotic therapy, take three acidophilus capsules with meals or apply plain yogurt made with live lactobacillus cultures directly to the vagina several times a day with a tampon.
- Doubling up on a dose to make up for a dose you've forgotten doesn't do any good. To jog your memory, set an alarm clock or post a chart on the refrigerator door or the bathroom mirror.
- If a few pills remain after you've completed the prescribed amount, throw them out so that neither you nor anyone in the family will be tempted to use them in the future.
- Learn to tell the difference between symptoms of a virus infection and a bacterial infection: infection with a flu virus is characterized by running nose, scratchy throat, minor aches and pains, slight headache, coughing that produces clear watery phlegm, a feeling of fatigue, and a light fever. These symptoms last for about a week. Respiratory bacterial infection is characterized by a painfully sore throat, severe headache, breathlessness, chest pain, fever of 101° F or above, and continual coughing that produces yellow, green, or rust-colored phlegm.

"A Common Sense Guide to Antibiotics" is a helpful brochure produced by the American Lung Association. For a free copy, call 1-800-LUNG-USA (586-4872).

SORTING OUT NONPRESCRIPTION PAINKILLERS

Confronted by shelves and shelves of analgesics, and bombarded by what seem to be conflicting claims on television commercials about the latest the best the most effective the strongest the least harmful painkiller, it has become increasingly difficult to choose between this one, that one, and the other one. Adding to the complications of choice is the fact that some of the more effective products combine two ingredients, one of which might produce undesired results. It should therefore be helpful to sort out the current crop of nonprescription painkillers and examine them one at a time. Let's begin with the oldest and best known:

ASPIRIN (brand names: Bayer, Empirin, Ecotrin, and others)

The first and still one of the cheapest of all painkillers in the nonsteroidal anti-inflammatory drug (NSAID) category, aspirin continues to be widely used to alleviate headache, toothache, the aches of arthritis, and menstrual discomfort. It is also used to reduce fever, and it may be recommended in small daily doses to reduce the likelihood of stroke as well as the onset or recurrence of a heart attack. It should never be given to children under age 18 without a doctor's approval, nor should it be taken during late pregnancy or when nursing.
How to take aspirin: To reduce stomach irritation, take it with milk or food. Do not combine it with alcoholic drinks. If you are especially sensitive to aspirin, choose a coated brand such as Ecotrin. If you are taking insulin, steroids, blood thinners, diuretics, or antiasthma drugs, check with your doctor about taking aspirin at the same time.
Possible side effects: Gastrointestinal upset, heartburn, interference with blood clotting, bleeding, ringing in the ears; use over along period may result in hearing loss. Coated aspirin (Ecotrin) reduces stomach discomfort. *(Some recent analgesics without anti-inflammatory effects have added aspirin as a component. This is yet another reason for reading all labels carefully.)*

ASPIRIN/CAFFEINE (brand name: Anacin)

All information as above plus the side effect of wakefulness.

ACETAMINOPHEN (brand names: Tylenol, Panadol, Aspirin-free Anacin, Aspirin-free Excedrin, and others)

Tylenol, the best known of the acetaminophen drugs, is effective for the relief of some headaches, minor muscle pains, and menstrual cramps. It reduces fever, but *it is not an anti-inflammatory drug* and is therefore less effective for arthritis than drugs in the NSAID category. Because acetaminophen does not interfere with blood clotting, it is used instead of aspirin to treat mild post-surgical pain.

How to take acetaminophen: Instructions for dosage should be followed very carefully. Recommended days of use for adults and children should not be exceeded without consulting your doctor. This category of painkiller is an inappropriate choice for anyone with impaired liver function, especially impairment caused by heavy drinking or exposure to toxic substances. Combination with other prescription and nonprescription drugs should be discussed with the doctor. Pregnant women should ask the doctor about taking this drug.

Possible side effects: Although acetaminophen does not cause stomach irritation, overuse may produce liver and kidney damage. If an allergic reaction causes a rash, hives, or breathing difficulties, discontinue use immediately. Accidental overdose may result in nausea, vomiting, and exhaustion.

ACETAMINOPHEN/ASPIRIN/CAFFEINE   (brand name: Excedrin)

Users of this popular painkiller should be aware not only of the positive effects of its three components, but of the negative ones as well.

IBUPROFEN   (brand names: Advil, Nuprin, Motrin, Rufen, Cramp Relief Formula B)

Ibuprofen, like aspirin, belongs in the NSAID category and is therefore a popular treatment for the stiffness, swelling, and pain associated with arthritis. Ibuprofen is also used for menstrual cramps and muscular discomfort associated with overexercise. It is less irritating to the stomach than aspirin, but more so than acetaminophen.

How to take ibuprofen: Take with food or milk to reduce stomach irritation. Never take larger than recommended doses, especially NOT in combination with alcohol. This combination has been known to produce stomach and intestinal bleeding severe enough to require emergency hospitalization. The doctor should be consulted about using ibuprofen in combination with any other drugs being taken for other conditions, especially for high blood pressure. Pregnant women should not take ibuprofen without the doctor's permission.

Possible side effects: Nausea, dizziness, problems with vision, fluid retention, ringing in the ears, serious adverse effects on already impaired kidney and/or liver function. At the first signs of a serious allergic reaction, discontinue use and consult your doctor.

NAPROXEN   (brand name: Aleve)

For 10 years before 1994, the year that it became an over-the-counter contender in the painkiller competition, naproxen was one of the leading prescription NSAIDs. Presented in recent years directly to consumers as Aleve, it is used to relieve the joint pain, swelling, and inflammation of arthritis as well as the soft tissue inflammation associated with bursitis and tendinitis. The special appeal of Aleve is its long-term action. One dose is said to provide relief for up to 12 hours, making it a suitable choice for chronic low back pain or menstrual cramps.

How to take Aleve: Follow the dose instructions on the label exactly. If a dose is accidentally missed, do not take a double dose to make up for it but continue with your regular schedule. To avoid stomach upset, take Aleve with food or an antacid plus a glass of water. *Never take it on an empty stomach.*

Possible side effects: Anyone who has had previous allergic reactions to aspirin or ibuprofen may react similarly to Aleve. Taking Aleve on a regular long-term basis should be monitored by a doctor because of the possibility of developing ulcers. Other side effects include dizziness, nausea, headache, and ringing in the ears. Consult your doctor about using this drug if you have liver or kidney disease or if you are pregnant.

KETOPROFEN   (brand name: Orudis)

Orudis is one of the most recent additions to the list of NSAIDs being sold without a prescription. Like the other drugs in this category, it lowers fever and reduces inflammation, swelling, and pain. The 25 milligram (mg) version known as Orudis KT is advertised as being as effective as 400 mg Motrin, 440 mg Aleve, and 1000 mg extra-strength Tylenol. It is therefore possible that the side effects may be especially troublesome.

How to take Orudis: Take according to label instructions or as advised by your doctor. To reduce stomach upset, take with food, milk, or an antacid. For the relief of chronic arthritis pain, it should be taken on a regular basis, even during periods of remission.

Possible side effects: If Orudis is being used over a long period of time, the patient should be monitored for anemia and bleeding ulcers. Other side effects may include changes in kidney function, diarrhea, constipation, headache, and sleeplessness.

SUMMARY of practical considerations that should affect your choice of painkillers:

- One particular type is not the best solution for all types of pain. Be aware of the difference between those that offer short-term relief and those that are best for a chronic condition.
- Be sure to remember previous adverse reactions to a particular category and try an alternative.
- Review the state of your health and the drugs being taken for problems other than pain. It is especially important to make a choice that will not increase gastrointestinal problems or liver and kidney disabilities.
- In trying to find the best pill for your particular pains of the moment, take into account such descriptions as "extra-strength," "one-a-day," "maximum strength," "coated," and "buffered."
- In the interest of economy, compare the prices of the various products in terms of the number of pills in the bottle, the amount of medication in each pill, and the daily dose required for pain relief.
- When you have specific questions, don't hesitate to discuss them with the pharmacist. If you're still uncertain, call your doctor.
- Look for the generic version of the painkiller that suits you best. The label will simply say "aspirin" or "acetaminophen" or "ibuprofen."
- Prices vary widely for different brands and even for the same brand at different times. Watch for special sales at your local pharmacy and for discount coupons in your local newspaper.

THE MENOPAUSE INDUSTRY AND ESTROGEN REPLACEMENT THERAPY

Some significant events:

- Hormone replacement became popular for the first time in the *early 1960s*. The slogan was "Young Forever," but because the result of taking large daily doses of estrogen significantly increased the risk of uterine and endometrial cancer, the treatment lost its appeal.
- *In 1982* Dr. Wulf H. Utian, professor of reproductive biology at Case Western Reserve University School of Medicine, opened the nation's first menopause clinic in Cleveland, Ohio.
- *In the mid-1980s* hormone replacement therapy was revived with a changed regimen that combined lower doses of estrogen with progestin.
- *In 1989* the North American Menopause Society was formed under the

leadership of Dr. Utian to serve the professional interests of doctors, nurses, and other health specialists in this field. .

- *In 1991*, yielding to pressure from female health professionals, the Older Women's League, and the Congressional Caucus for Women's Issues, Congress held the first subcommittee hearing on the health problems of older women, especially the problems relating to menopause.

- Under the new directorship of Dr. Bernadine P. Healy, the NIH embarked on a nationwide comprehensive 10-year study of these special concerns. A federal appropriation of $25 million was set aside for this study. In launching this long-term project, Dr. Healy noted: "Physicians still do not have enough scientific information to respond to a woman's questions about post-menopausal hormone replacement therapy."

- *In 1992*, when the first phalanx of baby boom women began to move into the 45 to 54 age group, it was calculated that the menopause population would increase from 13 million to 19 million within the next 10 years.

- *In 1994* the first issue of *Menopause*, the journal of the North American Menopause Society, was published by Lippincott-Raven Press. Contributors to this bimonthly journal are among the most prestigious biomedical scientists in the field.

- *By 1994* Premarin, the estrogen replacement medication of choice, had captured 80 percent of the $750 million market.

Ever since the female baby boomers began to reach middle age, there has been an unprecedented number of books, magazine articles, TV specials, and radio talk shows on the subject of menopause. From the tone of some of this material, it might be concluded that this generation of women is not only the first to discover menopause but that some of them are determined to reinvent it as a major disaster.

Of course younger women who remember what older female kin had to say about "the changes" have always had to sort out myth from fact, pay attention to or discard the folk remedies used by their forebears, and when necessary, seek the guidance of the family physician. But matters have become more complicated since estrogen replacement therapy was hailed as a way of "treating" menopause. And complications are compounded by the different points of view within the medical profession. Here, for example, is the prevailing attitude of many doctors, expressed by Dr. Clark Gillespie, a professor of obstetrics and gynecology at the University of Arkansas School of Medicine. In his book *Hormones, Hot Flashes, and Mood Swings: Living Through the Ups and Downs of Menopause*, he summarizes his approach in the following statement: "Menopause and the years that follow have been clearly established as an endocrine-deficiency state—a disorder worthy of, and indeed almost always requiring, comprehensive treatment." The point of view that a natural occurrence experienced by all women all over the world is a *disorder that must be treated* is certainly open to question. The women who experience very little discomfort during menopause, never suffer a broken hip, don't have to deal with clinical depression, and live to a ripe old age are not part of the menopause misery statistics because they don't seem to need "treatment." On the other hand, there is compelling evidence that for a significant number of women, the benefits of combined hormone replacement therapy do outweigh the risks. It then becomes the doctor's responsibility to take into careful consideration each patient's personal medical history, her family's medical history, her life-style, medications taken regularly for chronic conditions, and her particular complaints relating to menopause. On the basis of this information, the doctor can then inform each patient about the benefits and risks that relate to her particular case. (For example, unsuitable candidates for estrogen replacement include those with a history of breast cancer, gall bladder disease, and clotting disorders.) When the doctor takes the time to answer the inevitable questions about this comparatively recent therapy, the patient can become an informed participant in deciding how to proceed in her own best interests.

Benefits:

- Hot flashes and night sweating are eliminated.
- Insomnia is decreased.
- Sexual comfort is restored.
- Contributes to prevention of osteoporosis.
- May diminish the likelihood of heart disease.
- Energy is increased.
- Mood swings are diminished.
- Tooth loss may be decreased.
- Concentration may improve.
- Longevity may be extended.

Risks and Drawbacks:

- Increased likelihood of cancer of the uterus (endometrial cancer) with long-term use or large doses of estrogen.
- Possible association with breast cancer.
- Continued bleeding.
- Unpleasant side effects.
- Expenditure of time and money involved in treatment, cost of medication, monitoring and changing doses.

Alternative Ways to Reduce Menopausal Discomfort:

- To reduce night sweating, use bed linens and sleepwear made of natural fibers—cotton or linen rather than synthetics.
- Reduce caffeine intake or eliminate it altogether.
- Treat vaginal dryness with vitamin E oil and comfrey ointment.

HOW ESTROGEN REPLACEMENT THERAPY IS PRESCRIBED

The medication of choice is Premarin, known generically as "conjugated estrogens." It is usually prescribed in capsule form in low doses to be taken daily for 20 days, followed by a 10-day rest period. Premarin is also available as a vaginal cream. The tablets are prescribed to counteract unpleasant menopausal symptoms, especially hot flashes and night sweating. The cream lubricates dry, itchy genital skin and reduces vaginal irritation.

Early in this treatment, monitoring for dosage changes is usually scheduled every three months. One of the advantages of Premarin is its availability in a wide variety of doses. The average time that women continue this therapy is approximately nine months (which is the average time for the duration of hot flashes and night sweating). The doctor who hopes to maximize the benefits for each patient should monitor doses carefully and adjust them to reduce unwanted side effects.

Estrogen may also be administered by the Estraderm patch, which delivers a continuous amount of estrogen through the skin. The site of application of the patch may be the torso, abdomen, or buttocks. Once applied, it is not affected by contact with water when swimming or showering. The site of the application has to be rotated in such a way that an interval of at least a week must occur before the same site is used again. Unpleasant side effects are less likely to occur, but the patch is considered of less benefit in protecting against heart disease than estrogen taken orally.

UNDERSTANDING PRESCRIPTION NOTATIONS

Rx	quantity	gt	drop
aa	equal amounts of each	l.a.s.	label as such
ac	before meals	mg	milligrams
ad lib	whenever you wish	pc	after meals
b.i.d.	twice a day	p.r.n.	as needed
cc	cubic centimeter	qd	every day
d.a.w.	dispense as written (to prevent	qh	every hour
	generic substitution)	qs	as much as is sufficient
ea	each	q2h	every 2 hours
extr	extract	Sig	directions for taking
gm	gram	t.i.d.	three times a day

GETTING DOWN TO SPECIFICS

WHY ARE PRESCRIPTION DRUGS SO EXPENSIVE?

In 1993, responding to consumer complaints about the rising cost of prescription drugs, a congressional committee studied the matter and found that an average of $359 million is spent to develop each new drug that reaches the market. This outlay covers the expense of researching and developing not only the drugs that eventually get to the consumer, but also those that never go beyond the laboratory. One of the most extravagant aspects of this research is the three- to four-year period devoted to experimental testing with animals. Whether this use of animals is morally justifiable is open to question. What seems unreasonable is the obsession with "secrecy" that causes the world's major pharmaceutical companies to refuse to share the results of experiments, which are duplicated over and over by the different manufacturers—experiments for which consumers eventually have to pay.

Drugs that pass the laboratory tests are then subjected to "clinical trials" on humans, both healthy volunteers and patients suffering from the condition for which the only available medicines are an unsatisfactory treatment. (It is only in the last few years that women of different ages have been included in these trials.)

The various phases of the trials are supervised by the FDA and usually continue for an average of six years. During Phase I, the safety and side effects are evaluated. If it is generally agreed that the drug is safe enough to warrant closer scrutiny, the process passes to Phase II, during which potential toxicity is further tested. When the drug enters Phase III, the clinical trials become more extensive in order to arrive at the most effective doses with the fewest undesirable side effects for patients categorized by age, sex, previous conditions, pregnancy, and the like. (Most drugs are never tested on pregnant women for fear of potential liability.)

On completion of the trials, the FDA schedules a final review, which may be completed within a few months or may take a few years. During this time the federal agency assembles an advisory board of specialists for every step that will be taken to bring the drug to the consumer: how it is manufactured, labeled, marketed, and advertised. The exclusive right to manufacture a drug that has been developed in this way lasts for 20 years, during which time the long-term investment must be recouped and a profit must be made. After exclusivity comes to an end, other companies can develop generic versions of the drug and sell it for considerably less.

In spite of the time-consuming and costly testing procedures designed to assure the medical profession and consumers that new medications are safe and effective, liability lawsuits claiming payment for unanticipated damages seem to be inevitable. These payments, often reaching millions of dollars, are also figured into the final cost of the drug to the consumer.

SOME WAYS TO SAVE MONEY ON YOUR MEDICATIONS

- Many drugs previously available only by a doctor's prescription are being sold over the counter. Make sure your doctor is aware of this change (which usually represents a considerable saving).
- Large retail outlets for over-the-counter drugs usually market the more popular ones under their own house label at a much lower price. When you compare the list of active ingredients in both versions, you'll find that they are identical.
- When a drug is prescribed for a specific condition, ask whether an alternative therapy might be just as effective. Exercise, a change in diet, various nonmedical ways of dealing with pain and stress cost much less than sleeping pills and antidepressants.
- When your doctor prescribes a drug and says it's new, find out whether it

costs more than the one already on the market for the same condition. Unless you're given a convincing reason, ask that the less expensive drug be prescribed.

- If you're given a prescription for a drug you've never taken before, ask that a minimum amount be prescribed until you find out whether you're having severe negative reactions to it. (There's no reason to pay for and be stuck with 30 expensive pills if you react badly to the first three.)
- Ask your doctor whether the drug is available in generic form. If it is, have the prescription indicate that the generic version is wanted. (In some states the pharmacist is required by law to provide the generic version unless the physician indicates that the brand name is wanted.)
- Surveys indicate that prices for the 20 most prescribed drugs can differ by as much as 75 percent. Shop around at the larger drug chains for the best deal during any given week.
- Check your health insurance coverage for all or part of your drug costs, and find out which pharmacies offer the best drug plan arrangements.
- Take advantage of the best discounts for Medicare or Medicaid recipients.
- If you're taking a drug on a regular basis for a chronic condition, the price per dose may be considerably less if you order a year's supply by mail. Make sure the expiration date extends well beyond the time you'll be taking the last remaining dose.

Warnings:

—Remember that when you fill your prescriptions in many different pharmacies, you lose the advantage of having all your prescribed medications computerized under your name in one place. You are therefore deprived of the guidance of one pharmacist with whom you can discuss the possible dangers of combining a newly prescribed medication with the ones already listed on your computerized record.

—Don't look for bargains from abroad. Quality controls in some countries are not sufficiently rigorous to ensure the safety of some products.

—Don't be misled by "specials" offered by the self-styled "pharmacy" counters in health food stores, where prices for vitamins, mineral supplements, and such items as acidophilus pills are likely to be considerably higher than the prices at large discount drugstores.

INFORMATION INSERTS: LESS THAN ADEQUATE

For about half of the more than 900 new prescriptions written every year in the United States, no package information is provided for consumers about side effects and dangerous combinations. (When such package inserts *are* provided, they are frequently unreadable even with a magnifying glass and unintelligible even with the help of a dictionary.) In the same way that the FDA has been able to simplify food labels (see chapter on "Nutrition, Weight, Body Image, and Eating Disorders"), the agency is trying to do the same for all prescription drugs, claiming that because patients are not given enough clear and simple information about their medications, the treatment of people who take them incorrectly costs the nation about $20 billion a year. As of 1996, the FDA requires only about 40 or so drugs, mostly those with the most severe and life-threatening side effects, to be accompanied by package inserts. As for the other thousands of prescription drugs, the FDA has proposed that by the year 2006, pharmacists provide 95 percent of their customers with the necessary information, and should they fail to meet this requirement voluntarily, it would become mandatory. To pharmacists who object that it is too complicated and cumbersome to maintain filing cabinets full of informational brochures to distribute with each drug, the FDA points out that all this information is available by computer and can be printed out as necessary.

GET THE FACTS AND WRITE THEM DOWN

The first person to answer your questions about a medication is the doctor who hands you the prescription. Nowadays, many women find it helpful to keep a notebook devoted entirely to the medicines they take. It is especially useful to maintain a written record of the questions asked and the answers given so that the information is available as needed instead of having to make repeated phone calls to clear up uncertainties. Also, when seeing the doctor for a checkup or for diagnosis of a particular problem, *bring along a list of all the medicines in current use*—and "all" means not only drugs previously prescribed by this and other doctors, but also over-the-counter drugs taken with some degree of regularity, for heartburn, constipation, headaches, insomnia, allergies, weight loss, and so on. Although the pharmaceutical company and the pharmacist are responsible for supplying you with essential information on a particular prescription drug, neither source can account for all the possible combinations of medicines users are likely to take.

Questions to Ask

- How is the name of this drug spelled and what is the generic name?
- Exactly what is it for and what effect will it have on my condition?
- Would it be possible to achieve the same results by losing weight or by a change in diet or through exercise?
- What side effects does this drug usually produce?
- What are the risks of combining this drug with any of the ones I usually take, including nonprescription drugs for allergies or headaches?
- Should any foods be avoided when I'm using this drug?
- Should alcohol be avoided altogether, or may I have an occasional beer or glass of wine?
- Should the medicine be taken before, with, or after meals?
- Can it be taken first thing in the morning or just before I go to bed?
- Is it all right to continue normal activities such as driving?
- What should I do if I accidentally skip a scheduled dose?
- Do I have to take the prescribed number of pills or doses even if I'm feeling better?

SOME SPECIAL GUIDELINES

For Pregnant Women

Most substances, including drugs such as alcohol and nicotine, pass from the mother's blood supply to the fetus. The doctor will therefore insist that every effort be made to stop drinking and smoking altogether. Of all the drugs on the market, 85 percent have not been tested for safe use during pregnancy; many are known to be potentially harmful, and some have a well-documented history of producing birth defects. It is therefore important for the mother to find out whether any medications she takes or might be taking are likely to be harmful to the fetus. The doctor should be consulted about all drugs—prescription, nonprescription, and "recreational"—as well as about those taken regularly for a chronic condition such as diabetes. Most doctors permit the use of Tylenol for the relief of cold symptoms, minor back pain, or headaches. Any condition that produces a fever of more than 100° F should be brought to the doctor's attention. Absolutely do not self-medicate with aspirin because it interferes with blood clotting. Depending on the mother's diet, the doctor may prescribe iron and vitamin supplements, especially folic acid.

A woman who is trying to become pregnant should discuss this intention with her doctor since it may affect the kinds of drugs prescribed for various disorders.

Mothers Who Are Breast-feeding

To minimize the infant's unwanted exposure to a drug that is essential for the mother's well-being and that is likely to come through in the milk, the prescribed doses should be taken directly after nursing rather than before.

For Older Women

Because the aging process and age-associated diseases can alter the body in various ways, reactions to certain medications can change with age. For example, age can affect the rates with which the body absorbs, processes, and eliminates certain drugs. Thus the doses required should be changed, often in a downward direction. It is only recently and in response to considerable pressure from such advocacy groups as the Older Women's League that the FDA has begun to take the age factor into account when approving recommended doses of drugs. This aspect of medication is also a concern of the Office of Research on Women's Health. Over the years, because women live longer than men, they have been the guinea pigs in finding out about the cumulative long-term effects of medicines prescribed for chronic illnesses. Indeed many women have been taking drugs for hypertension, heart disease, and arthritis for as long as 30 years. Also, older women are likely to experience different side effects from those experienced by younger women; in addition, medications prescribed for one ailment can intensify or nullify the effect of a medication prescribed for a previous condition. It is therefore especially important to contact the doctor promptly if a newly prescribed drug produces nausea, dizziness, or mood swings, or if it fails to have any effect at all on the condition for which it was prescribed.

Too many older women are in the habit of self-medication with high-dose supplements of various vitamins and minerals in the hope of preventing or curing a disease or slowing the aging process. This practice can be a waste of money or, worse, a threat to health. Large amounts of some of these nutrients usually pass out of the body, but sometimes they can build up to dangerous levels; excess vitamin A, for example, can cause headaches, nausea, diarrhea, and eventually bone and liver damage. Foods and drugs can interact negatively. Frequent use of mineral oil as a laxative can hinder the absorption of vitamin D and other nutrients. Diuretics, commonly prescribed for older heart patients, can result in the loss of essential potassium. (The body's supply can be replenished by eating such foods as bananas, tomatoes, oranges, raisins, prunes, and potatoes.)

Although many older women have been trying to prevent increasing osteoporosis by a regimen of weight-bearing exercises, hormone replacement, and calcium supplements, they have not been sufficiently alert to the fact that certain medications contribute to bone loss. The greatest offenders in this regard are the useful and widely prescribed synthetic versions of the glucocorticoids, the steroids produced by the adrenal glands. Among the best known are cortisone, hydrocortisone, prednisone, and prednisolone. These and others in the same group are often prescribed to treat arthritis, asthma, allergies, and various types of cancer. Effective as they may be in reducing inflammation and autoimmune disorders, they also interfere with the absorption of dietary calcium and in large doses can cause a level of bone loss that almost inevitably leads to fractures. High doses of thyroid hormones and anticonvulsants like Dilantin, prescribed for epileptic seizures, can also cause brittle bones. The National Osteoporosis Foundation also wants women to know that many over-the-counter antacids they take for gastrointestinal distress (Maalox, Gelusil, Gaviscon, and Rolaids) contain large amounts of aluminum, and that aluminum can replace the calcium in their bones. A better solution, the foundation suggests, is a change in diet, a switch to Alka-Seltzer or Tums, or a doctor's recommendations.

DRUGS FREQUENTLY RECOMMENDED OR PRESCRIBED FOR

COMMON CONDITIONS

allergies:	Hismanal (astemizole), Phenergan (promethazine hydrochloride), Seldane (terfenadine)
anxiety:	Atarax (hydroxyzine hydrochloride), Ativan (lorazepam), BuSpar (buspirone hydrochloride), Miltown (meprobamate), Valium (diazepam), Xanax (alprazolam)
arthritis:	Anaprox (naproxen sodium), Ansaid (flurbiprofen), aspirin (OTC), Feldene (piroxicam), Lodine (etodolac), Mo-

                    trin (ibuprofen over-the-counter), Naprosyn (naproxen), Relafen (nabumetone), Voltaren (diclofenac sodium)

asthma: Azmacort (triamcinolone acetonide), Medrol (methylprednisolone), Proventil (albuterol sulfate), Theo-Dur (theophylline)

bacterial infections: Amoxil (amoxicillin), Augmentin (amoxicillin and clavulanate potassium), Ceclor (cefaclor), Ceftin (cefuroxime axetil), Cipro (ciprofloxacin hydrochloride), Duricef (cefadroxil monohydrate), Suprax (cefixime)

diabetes: Glucotrol (glipizide), Micronase (glyburide), Orinase (tolbutamide)

diarrhea: Imodium (loperamide hydrochloride over-the-counter), Lomotil (diphenoxylate hydrochloride and atropine sulfate)

fungal infections: Diflucan (fluconazole), Micatin (miconazole nitrate), Nizoral (ketoconazole)

heart disease: Calan (verapamil hydrochloride), Cardizem (diltiazem hydrochloride), Lanoxin (digoxin), Lopressor (metoprolol tartrate), Procardia (nifedipine)

herpes infections: Zovirax (acyclovir)

high blood pressure: Capoten (captopril), Cardizem (diltiazem hydrochloride), Dyazide (triamterene with hydrochlorothiazide), Lasix (furosemide), Lopressor (metoprolol tartrate), Lozol (indapamide), Vasotec (enalapril maleate), Zestril (lisinopril)

parkinsonism: Artane (trihexyphenidyl hydrochloride), Cogentin (benztropine mesylate), Eldepryl (selegiline hydrochloride), Sinemet CR (carbidopa and levodopa)

ulcers/acid reflux: Axid (nizatidine), Cytotec (misoprostol), Pepcid (famotidine), Prilosec (omeprazole), Propulsid (cisapride), Tagamet (cimetidine), Zantac (ranitidine hydrochloride), and an ever-growing selection of over-the-counter antacids, including Alka-Seltzer, Bisodol, DiGel, GasX, Gaviscon, Gelusil, Maalox, Mylanta, Rolaids, and Tums.

urinary tract infections: Macrodantin (nitrofurantoin)

vaginitis and yeast infections: (see *fungal infections*)

RULES TO FOLLOW

- Read the instructions on the label, and if they differ from your doctor's instructions, call the doctor for clarification.
- Never take someone else's prescription medicine and never offer yours to anyone else.
- Keep every prescription medication in its original container and dispense from the container as needed. This rule especially applies if you're taking different drugs at different times of the day.
- When you're traveling, take the drugs in their original containers. DON'T empty a weekend's supply of all your medications into a pillbox.
- Always complete the full course of a medication as instructed even if you're beginning to feel better.
- You have the right to refuse to pay for a filled prescription if the expiration date on the container does not extend beyond the time when you'll still be taking the drug.
- If you have a hard time opening a container with a safety cap, ask the pharmacist for a screw-on cover.
- If you have trouble swallowing pills, drink some water first, and drink at least half a glass of water with your pill.
- Don't take medications when you're lying down. Sit up straight, or better still, stand up.
- Store drugs according to instructions. If you're told to store it in a cool dark place, don't keep it on a sunny kitchen windowsill.
- Check the expiration dates on all the drugs in your medicine cabinet. Those too old to be effective should be flushed down the toilet.
- NEVER give children candy-coated medication.
- Children and grandchildren should have no access to the contents of the medicine cabinet.

CONCLUSION

Pharmaceutical companies can create useful medications, doctors can write prescriptions for them, and pharmacists can advise you about the possible dangers of mixing them, but none of the above can force you to stop smoking, eat properly, exercise regularly, and reduce your alcohol consumption. What has come to be known as "life-style" is now given its due recognition as the crucial ingredient in achieving and maintaining good health. And doctors who are practitioners of preventive medicine can be depended on to support those patients who want to be active and responsible partners in this enterprise. Seeking out such a doctor doesn't mean seeking out a crank or a quack or a "holistic healer" who doesn't "believe" in medicines. Obviously, there are those critical moments when the right medicine administered at the right time can save your life, or those later years when a chronic disability has to be faced, and the newest effective medication for heart disease or arthritis is the boon that makes normal activity possible.

Apart from emergencies or life-threatening conditions, the role of medication on a day-to-day basis is a matter of attitude. What a comfort to know that it's available when you need it! But before you ask your doctor for a prescription for a tranquilizer or a stronger antacid or something to alleviate shortness of breath, it might not hurt to consider what steps you could be taking on your own behalf to make yourself feel better.

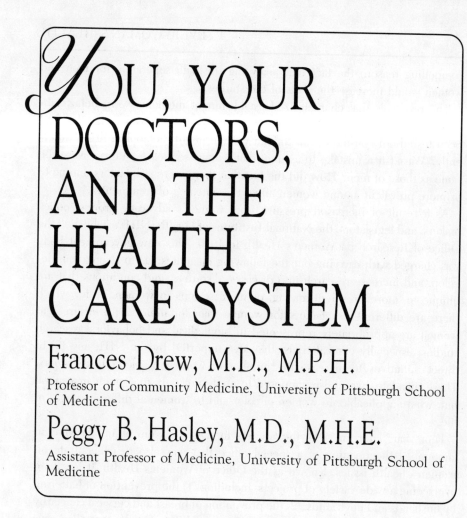

YOU, YOUR DOCTORS, AND THE HEALTH CARE SYSTEM

Frances Drew, M.D., M.P.H.

Professor of Community Medicine, University of Pittsburgh School of Medicine

Peggy B. Hasley, M.D., M.H.E.

Assistant Professor of Medicine, University of Pittsburgh School of Medicine

As recently as the end of the 1980s, most of what was known about preventing diseases was learned mainly from studying healthy men between the ages of 18 and 55. Scientists admitted that relatively little was known about whether women differed from men in their disease patterns and their response to treatments, because *as a general rule, women of no matter what age or ethnicity had not been included in clinical studies.* There were many explanations for this policy of exclusion: the danger that an experimental drug or vaccine might harm the fetus during the first weeks of pregnancy when the woman might not know she was pregnant; the belief among scientists that the changes in reproductive hormones experienced by women during the menstrual cycle would complicate the design of the study; and (probably the most compelling reason) the fact that analyzing the data separately for men and women would increase the costs of the studies.

The protocols that characterized establishment medicine were being subjected to mounting criticism. Why were women being given drugs that had been tested only on men even though women might metabolize drugs differently? Wasn't it a mistake to assume that women's disease patterns were the same as those of men? How did the fact that there were risk factors unique to or more prevalent among women affect the outcome of treatment?

As a result of increased pressure from women's advocacy groups, policy makers, and legislators, the National Institutes of Health (NIH) established the Office of Research on Women's Health in 1990. This new government body was charged with carrying out the following mandates: (1) to strengthen, develop, and increase research into diseases, disorders, and conditions that are unique to, more prevalent among, or more serious in women, or for which there are different risk factors for women than for men; (2) to ensure that women are appropriately represented in biomedical and behavioral research studies, especially clinical trials, that are supported by the NIH; and (3) to direct initiatives to increase the number of women in biomedical careers. These mandates were also supposed to apply not only to women in general but, where applicable, to women of color and to women at different stages of life.

Four years later, in 1994, the Centers for Disease Control and Prevention announced the opening of a special office that was also to concentrate on women's health issues. Known as the Office of Women's Health, it has been overseeing a wide variety of projects, including (1) the prevention of battering by husbands and boyfriends; (2) the prevention of breast and cervical cancer by promoting early screening and testing; (3) research into female-controlled contraception, both for birth control and for preventing the spread of AIDS; and (4) the prevention and treatment of sexually transmitted diseases before they result in sterility. At the time this office was opened, Bill Grigg, a spokesman for the federal Department of Health and Human Services, was quoted as follows in the *New York Times* (7/14/94): "The office is part of a government response to years of criticism that women's health has been underfunded and ignored."

As far as women are concerned, the health care system today neither begins nor ends with physicians. The vastly improved health education offered daily in all media has drawn us, the patients, the public, the "consumer," into an awareness of and responsibility for our own health. Dr. Benjamin Spock's book on babies began an ever-expanding "do-it-yourself" movement. The women's movement produced *Our Bodies, Ourselves* and its successor, *Ourselves Grow-*

ing Older, books empowering women through understanding of how our bodies work and how to keep them working well. All of the women's magazines have columns about health maintenance and health problems, and their informational quality is generally high. Most newspapers have both a "Dear Abby" and a "Dear Doctor" letter-answering column. Television is producing some excellent documentaries, and every major network has a reputable medical consultant who does not participate in the fictional features about how hospitals function. Many books have been written for the lay public, running the gamut from excellent and informative to tedious and overtechnical to downright quackery. Clearly, this torrent of information is responding to a perceived public interest, spurred on by the complexities, inadequacies, and above all, the costs of the health care system.

Not only have words tumbled forth. Numbers of self-help groups have arisen, whose goals are to alert people to their own ability to cope with illness. Women's cooperative clinics are one fine example; a group like Reach for Recovery for mastectomy patients is another. The patient is acquiring a growing sophistication about health, which is all to the good.

The result of all these trends is a new participation by the patient in a system that used to operate on a strictly authoritarian basis. Sensing a mounting backlash against the entire profession, doctors are responding (in many cases grudgingly) to the increasing independence of women so that a partnership is established in which both parties profit from the circumstance that the well-informed patient is healthier, recovers faster, and is more gratifying to treat.

Furthermore, this trend puts more pressure on women to accept responsibility for their own health. The list of life-style–related diseases grows each year: cancer, heart disease, hypertension, alcoholism, obesity—all in some degree are under the control of the patient, who can prevent the disease or alter its outcome. More and more, physicians expect patients to take this responsibility rather than to ask for a magic medicine that will "do it for me." Roles are changing. The physician increasingly teaches as well as prescribes, and patients listen and learn.

Doctors have been learning too. Thanks to pressures from consumer advocates, from the legal and counseling professions, and as a result of the rapid growth of specialists with credentials other than an M.D., physicians have been learning about subjects that were all but ignored in medical schools. Courses in human sexuality and sex therapy were not part of any medical school curriculum until the advent of Masters and Johnson. Except for a nod at deficiency diseases and special diets for particular gastrointestinal problems, nutrition was not seriously examined until more and more women concerned themselves with healthful diet rather than constant dieting. Interns can now recognize battered children when they are brought into the emergency room as "accident" cases. The concept of substance abuse is no longer limited to opium derivatives as doctors learn more about alcoholism, nicotine dependency, and addiction to some of the drugs they themselves prescribe. Death as a subject for discussion was ignored; now most reputable medical schools conduct seminars in dying, death, and bereavement, and they also examine the increasing number of questions that come under the heading of medical ethics, hoping to instill wisdom as well as knowledge in the men and women who play such a crucial role in all our lives.

One of the most significant developments in the past decade is the increasing respect for alternative therapies, not only for stress management and pain control but for augmenting more conventional methods of dealing with illness. (See "Alternative Therapies.")

Doctors are not only learning new information; they are also learning to listen to what their patients are saying to them. One of the most important developments in doctor/patient relationships is a new concern on the part of the medical establishment about the way interviews are conducted. A study in 1991 of more than a thousand letters from dissatisfied patients at a large midwestern health maintenance organization revealed that the most common complaints were that physicians had conversational habits that would be considered rude in anyone else. Their physician made them feel humiliated, used medical jargon that was confusing, and cut them off when they asked questions. Other researchers found that physicians constantly interrupt patients and disrupt their efforts to finish a thought. When doctors dominate the medical interview, patients don't do as well as when the patient exerts more control. The new research suggests that doctors would do well to listen more and talk less.

As a result of these and similar findings, many medical schools have been introducing new courses on how to conduct patient interviews. Equally important is the fact that several residency programs require that new doctors check into the hospital as patients to experience for themselves what it feels like to be treated as a customer rather than a patient. One of the most innovative and effective programs on communication has been the hiring of professional actors to impersonate patients with a variety of complaints and illnesses that medical students must deal with. At the end of the sessions (which are videotaped) the fake "patient" writes an evaluation of the behavior of the young doctor-to-be.

Such efforts at improving communication are a response to mounting concerns that today's doctors are much more effective in the use of procedures, technology, and jargon than they are in expressing human interest and genuine feeling. When the young medics see the tapes, they are surprised and humbled. They say, "Do I always have that expression on my face? Am I that harsh?" It's hard for some of them to acknowledge their behavior. But if they don't face it as residents, when are they going to face it?

The other half of the communication falls to the patient, who should make the most of a visit to the doctor by speaking up and asking the right questions. Consumer advocates advise patients to write down their questions beforehand and find out all they can about recommended procedures and medications after they have been examined. (See "Plain Talk About Medications.")

As for our competence in caring for ourselves and others, there was a time when women shared a body of practical and useful information—how to deliver a baby, how to feed the family, how to raise the children, how to care for the sick. But male "specialists" undermined women's authority and competence in these matters. For good or ill, Dr. Spock replaced the wise grandmother; the male obstetrician replaced the female midwife. But women in our culture still usually plan the meals, make the major decisions about the lifestyle of the household, and are, even when they work outside the home at a fulltime job, the custodians of the "nurturing" skills: nursing the sick and caring for the children and the elderly. In mastering this knowledge of preparing healthful meals, helping the helpless, recognizing the signals of substance abuse, women seek an ally they can trust.

How does the woman of today find a physician—for herself, her family, her child—who will both teach and treat her? How can she get the best available care? This chapter will attempt to serve as a guide to our present health care system.

CHOOSING YOUR DOCTORS

On the assumption that you are in a position to choose your own doctor (many women can no longer do so because of the nature of their own or their spouse's health insurance coverage), it is important that you make your selection with care and enlightened concern. There are women who have lived to regret a decision to go to a particular physician because he was charming at a PTA meeting, or because she wrote a best seller, or because a friend found this wonderful M.D. who provided her with any number of amphetamines to help her lose weight.

Not only is it estimated that as many as 28,000 people may be practicing medicine and treating tens of thousands of patients each year even though they hold no licenses and have had little or no medical training but also, when the Department of Health and Human Services conducted its first comprehensive survey (1986) of medical discipline and peer review, results indicated that although the majority of American doctors are well qualified, 20,000 to 45,000 licensed physicians are likely candidates for some kind of discipline. These figures are derived from statistics on the prevalence in the profession of alcoholism, drug abuse, and mental illness. Other studies indicate that charges requiring some kind of disciplinary action include not only substance abuse but unnecessary surgery and sexual molestation of patients.

One of the most important steps ever taken by the federal government to protect patients from incompetent doctors and other licensed health practitioners was the establishment in 1990 of a single computerized data base to identify them. While the information contained in the data bank is not available to the public, it has the effect of motivating hospitals to take and report disciplinary action against incompetent staff physicians because hospitals that fail to do so are subject to penalties under the law as well as to lawsuits from other hospitals. Since 1994, consumers have had access to a toll-free number through which a doctor's credentials can be verified. When you call 1-800-776-2378, an operator can tell you whether the doctor in question is certified by the American Board of American Specialists, and, if so, the field of certification, and the year in which it was obtained. This information can also be supplied by directories in your local library. Others required by law to report disciplinary action against doctors of medicine and osteopathy, dentists, and other state-licensed health providers, including psychotherapists, are state medical and dental boards, professional societies, and HMOs, as well as individuals or organizations making a payment on behalf of a doctor to settle a malpractice claim. State boards vary widely in the frequency and the type of discipline they mete out to practicing physicians, depending on their state laws and investigative resources. It is good news that according to the Federation of State Medical Boards, the number of doctors being disciplined nationwide has increased sharply. In 1994 this number was 11.8 percent higher than in 1993 and 40 percent higher than in 1990. The federation pointed out, however, that this figure represented a tiny fraction—only 0.6 percent—of the 615,854 physicians licensed to practice medicine. Complaints in greater numbers leading to discipline had been coming not from patients (why not?) but from other medical professionals and insurance companies. Punishments range from mild reprimands to revocation of licenses for major infractions. Although there has been no statistical breakdown of the nature of the offenses, some few physicians lose their licenses for defrauding Medicaid and Medicare or for having been the cause of wrongful death; many more are disciplined for sexual misconduct, substance abuse, or providing controlled substances to their patients.

Of course, most doctors are honest, competent, hardworking, and uphold the standards of their profession. But it does no harm to be aware of the pitfalls in making your choice. The following pages discuss some important considerations to review when deciding on a primary care physician.

GEOGRAPHY

While the doctor closest to your home may not be the top-of-the-list choice, it isn't practical to have to travel for more than an hour to reach the doctor you may have to visit regularly. If you live in a semirural or rural area, you may not have much choice. Know where your nearest hospital is located, and try to connect with a physician on the staff. While doctors on the staff of a teaching hospital (one attached to a university medical school) are usually well qualified, you can check out any doctor's background by calling the county medical society or by checking the medical directory at the reference desk of your local public library. Some cities have computerized 800 number directories of physicians.

If you live in a metropolitan area, your choice widens considerably. You may wish to get your care from a university complex; you may have strong preference for one or another hospital because of friends who have been there. The next step is to call either the hospital or a county medical society and ask them to give you the names of physicians in a given discipline on the staff of that hospital. You can then look them up in the telephone book and make inquiries about how soon you can have an appointment as a new patient. Keep in mind that many hospital physicians are not in private practice. Also remember that there is no connection between a doctor's personal religious affiliation and the fact that he or she is on the staff of a hospital with a denominational adjective in its name.

QUALIFICATIONS

When you call for the first time, you have every right to ask about the doctor's credentials if you haven't been able to find out about them on your own. Nearly every physician under 60 today is board certified in some discipline. Certification in either family practice or internal medicine indicates that the physician provides primary care rather than concentrating on the treatment of specific conditions.

FEES

Before you make your appointment, don't hesitate to ask about fees. If you have insurance coverage, ask whether you must pay the fee and wait for reimbursement or whether the doctor applies for reimbursement. If you're on Medicare, find out whether the doctor accepts assignment, and if the reply is "No," you'll have to decide whether you want to find a doctor who does.

When you ask about fees, find out if full payment for a first visit is expected before you leave the office, and if it is, ask whether a personal check or credit card payment is acceptable. Above all, find out what the cost of a first visit will be and how long you can expect the visit to take. Because many if not most health-related bills are paid by insurance companies, it is important to determine how much of each office visit will be covered by the insurance company.

STYLE OF PRACTICE

If you are satisfied with qualifications, the next question might be whether the office is a group or solo practice. If it is a group, you should determine whether it is a group of physicians with the same type of practice (i.e., family practice, internal medicine, etc.) or a multispecialty group in which a large number of physicians representing a broad spectrum of specialties work together (internal medicine, surgery, obstetrics, pediatrics, etc.). Group practice of the latter type is an outgrowth of the continuing trend toward specialization. It has been inevitable because the increased amount of information and the proliferation of technical procedures in all aspects of medical science can scarcely be mastered by a "general" practitioner.

Most younger physicians, whatever the nature of their practice, are unwilling to go it alone for a number of reasons, one of which is the demanding nature of solo practice in terms of time and effort; another is the prohibitive cost of equipment and office staff. The pattern of group practice, therefore, continues to grow. Practically all groups have a patient-admitting arrangement with a nearby hospital.

Apart from the advantages to the physician, there are many to the patient. In an office with several physicians someone is almost always available. It may not be the person you see regularly, but your records are easily accessible when they are needed. If the group is a fairly large one, it is likely to include an internist (who may be a subspecialist in cardiology or geriatrics), an ophthalmologist, an obstetrician/gynecologist, a pediatrician, and a general surgeon. There will be a contract with a radiologist, and there will be specific referrals to such other specialists as orthopedists, neurologists, and psychiatrists. The fact that your records are probably computerized means that they are promptly available, thus sparing you from being a completely "new" patient over and over again.

AGE, PERSONALITY, AND SUBCULTURE

Patients are as varied as physicians, and no one is equally comfortable with everyone. Much has been written about why patients choose a particular physician and one of the most readable, accurate, and interesting studies is Earl Lomon Koos's *The Health of Regionville*. The author looked at a town in upper New York State in which five physicians practiced, asking patients of different backgrounds why they preferred a particular physician. The reasons given were that their physician (1) had served the family in the previous generation, and they saw no reason to change; (2) was known to them socially; (3) was recommended by a relative or friend; (4) was generally known in the community as a "good doctor"; (5) made home calls; (6) was "willing to spend time with you"; (7) didn't press for payment; (8) charged moderate fees; (9) was "just liked as a person"; (10) was "the most available"; and (11) had "good equipment."

You will recognize some of these reasons as topics already discussed, but there is no gainsaying that past commonality of experience may make both the physician and the patient more comfortable and their interaction more effective, particularly if social or family pressures are contributing significantly to the ill health. You may need only technical expertise in a one-time visit to a specialist, but you should give extra weight to compatibility if your psychological as well as physical needs are to be met. For example, a 60-year-old woman may be initially uncomfortable discussing her psyche or her sexuality with a 30-year-old man. A teenager may be seriously mismatched on these same topics with a physician her grandmother's age. The physician's expertise and attitudes can sometimes overcome these initial obstacles, but time is lost in the process. The intelligent, informed patient is impatient with the physician who simply expects orders to be carried out and refuses to give answers of substance to questions, and the patient who expects authoritative treatment is equally put off by a physician who says, "I don't quite know what is wrong with you, but let's start here."

The only way to establish whether or not you trust and are comfortable with a physician is to try the relationship out. If you find yourself ill at ease or lacking in confidence, pay your bill and find someone else.

GENDER OF THE PHYSICIAN

Some women prefer male physicians, some are indifferent, and some vastly prefer a woman. Preferences are apt to be particularly strong in seeking an obstetrician/gynecologist. It is estimated that two-thirds of all women use their gynecologist as their primary care physician, and studies indicate that over 80 percent of all women say they would prefer a woman gynecologist. While recent years have brought a sharp increase in the number of young women in all specialties and especially in family practice, the medical world is still predominantly male. Although only 17 percent of the doctors now in practice, women are making their presence known in the area of doctor/patient relationships, which has been attracting so much attention. Studies have shown that female physicians spend more time with their patients than men do, interrupt them less often, and more willingly treat the poor. Of greater significance is the fact that according to a study published in the *New England Journal of Medicine*, women who get their care from female doctors are about twice as likely to receive a Pap smear to check for cervical cancer as those with male doctors and are about 40 percent more likely to receive a mammogram screening for breast cancer.

LESBIANS AND DOCTORS

Lesbians who live and work in large urban areas or university towns can usually find a sympathetic primary care doctor through networking or through their community grapevine. Those in rural areas or small towns may be less fortunate in their options. According to a study by Dr. Katherine A. O'Hanlan, a gynecological cancer surgeon at Stanford University Medical University, lesbians are placed at a greater risk for various life-threatening diseases than other women because of the insensitive treatment and flagrant prejudice of doctors. The bias they are likely to experience results in their having fewer checkups than they should; the fact that they fail to get important screening tests like Pap smears, mammograms, and cholesterol measurements on a regular basis means that cancer and heart disease are not diagnosed in the early treatable stages as they are likely to be with heterosexual women. In a *New York Times* interview (10/11/95), Dr. O'Hanlan, a former president of the Gay and Lesbian Medical Association, compares this circumstance to the medical profession's documented bias against blacks, gay men, and other minority groups. It is widely recognized, she said, that groups facing discrimination are more likely than the general population to suffer from cancer and heart disease and to die from these illnesses because they don't see doctors as often. When Dr. O'Hanlan's study was published in 1995, it was the first broad review of research on lesbian health, incorporating data on 13,543 women who participated in seven health surveys. In one of these surveys, 80 percent of gay and lesbian doctors said they had seen colleagues either deny care to gay and lesbian patients or give them substandard care; 88 percent had heard colleagues joke about these patients. Some erroneously told the women they did not need Pap smears. In another survey included in the study, 72 percent of lesbian patients said their doctors made derogatory remarks about them or ostracized them in some way, with the result that 84 percent said they hesitated to return to their doctors for treatment of new ailments. Instead, Dr. O'Hanlan found that they turn to chiropractors and other practitioners of alternative medicine who are more sympathetic, even if their remedies are not scientifically acceptable.

Reacting to these studies and to the pressure exerted by gay and lesbian doctors, the American Medical Association issued a policy statement urging doctors to be more sensitive to homosexual patients and to cultivate a "nonjudgmental attitude" toward their sexuality. In addition, in line with the goal of making patients more comfortable and more aware of their sexuality as it relates to their health, the American College of Obstetricians and Gynecologists has been including information on lesbian health in its updated brochures. Further efforts in this direction are being made by the American Academy of Family Physicians, which has been sponsoring forums for doctors on gay and lesbian health issues.

Lesbians who would like to have access to a more congenial and understanding physician in their area can write to the Gay and Lesbian Medical Association for information. The association has a membership of 1,800 doctors nationwide and can be reached at 211 Church Street, Suite C, San Francisco, CA 94114; phone (415) 255-4547.

THE FIRST VISIT AND THEREAFTER

Once you have selected a physician, there are several things you need to do and/or find out at your first visit.

- Go when you're healthy and have a complete checkup so that the doctor has a norm against which to measure any future problems. Make a list of your questions in advance of the visit.
- Bring *all* your medications with you in a plastic bag. "All" means prescription *and* nonprescription drugs. If you're given a prescription, ask what the drug is supposed to do, what are the side effects, and what food, drink or activities should be avoided while taking it. (See "Plain Talk About Medications.")
- Find out about office hours and whether any specific time is set aside for telephone consultation. Under what circumstances does the doctor make house calls, if ever?
- Who covers for the doctor during times of unavailability, especially on weekends and during vacations?
- More and more women who are meeting a doctor for the first time ask the staff to arrange that this meeting take place in the doctor's office when both doctor and patient are fully dressed *people* rather than in the examining room when the doctor is fully clothed as an authority figure and the woman is the disrobed powerless patient.
- When you see a physician for the first time, take a copy of your medical records and your family history with you. You should be asked for the following information in the first interview; be sure to provide it honestly: the nature of your job if you work outside the home and how you feel about it, your current living situation, how often you exercise, how much leisure time you have and how you spend it, how much alcohol you consume regularly (this includes wine and beer as well as "hard" liquor), what your regular diet is like, how much caffeine you consume, whether you smoke, and whether you are regularly exposed to secondary smoke.
- If you expect your primary care doctor to perform the functions of a gynecologist, make sure that this is considered part of a regular checkup procedure. If it is, you should expect to be asked questions relating to your sexual health, such as the nature of your sex life, the number of partners, whether you have ever been treated for a sexually transmitted disease, and the like. If the doctor doesn't ask about your sexual practices

and you feel somewhat uncomfortable about initiating such a conversation, the first moments of embarrassment are more likely to be overcome if you write down questions in advance about your special concerns in this area. Some relevant questions are: Will you do any tests for reproductive tract infections? How often should I have a Pap smear? I have a new sex partner and I'd like to know whether oral sex is safe. (See also "Sexual Health," "Gynecological Problems and Treatment," and "Sexually Transmissible Diseases.")

CHANGING DOCTORS

Everyone knows that marriage is easier than divorce and that many marriages are sustained on inertia rather than on compatibility or love. The same is true of doctor-patient relationships, and the techniques of "divorcing" your doctor are nearly as awkward as divorcing your husband. It can be done and in the long run should be, and, if we continue the analogy to marriage, annulment is easier than divorce. The sooner you get out, the better off you are.

If you are moving to another city, the situation is easy. The most comfortable solution is to choose a physician in your new locality (Dr. Y) and then write your former physician (Dr. X) asking to have all your records as well as X-rays and other diagnostic materials sent to Dr. Y. (Fax machines and computers accomplish this transmission within minutes if necessary.) If Dr. Y requests the record from Dr. X, you will be asked to sign a waiver. An even simpler way is to ask Dr. X for your records and take them with you to Dr. Y. Again, you will probably be asked to sign a release. This process is often facilitated by a conference with Dr. X before you move, in which you ask about physicians near your new residence. Each specialist is apt to have a list of all members of that specialty board in the United States, giving age, university, perhaps even residency training sites, and from this you can together cull some likely names.

If you want to change physicians within a group or go to a new office, embarrassment may glue you to the chair. If you are enrolled in a group practice, you are apt to have seen more than one primary care physician over time because of vacations, on-call schedules, and the like. If Dr. A was your original physician, but the last time you had the flu you saw Dr. B with whom you felt more comfortable, you need only make your next appointment with Dr. B through the secretary. If you happen to be seeing Dr. B, you can easily say that you would really prefer to continue this relationship, and Dr. B can then manage the problem in the office with no fuss at all. Occasionally Dr. A may be upset and face you with your decision. Your only course then is to persevere with whatever diplomacy you can muster because your future comfort in your medical relationship is at stake.

You encounter only slightly more difficulty in changing completely to another office. Here the routine is exactly the same as when moving to another town. You choose your new physician, say that you have been seeing Dr. A who has your records, sign a waiver, and let Dr. B request them from Dr. A. If your only contacts with Dr. A were for routine checkups or upper respiratory conditions, the record will contain very little important information and you can forget about asking for its transfer. On the other hand, if you have had any chronic or complicated condition or much laboratory data has accumulated about changes in your cholesterol levels and the like, your new physician needs and deserves to know all of these facts. No amount of embarrassment should prevent you from getting this information into the hands of your new physician.

HOSPITAL OUTPATIENT DEPARTMENTS

The word *clinic* (unless labeled Mayo, Menninger, Lahey, or Joslin) used to conjure up an image of crowded benches, offhand care, and interns as the only doctors. Today the facts are quite different.

Many university clinics are run in tandem with private doctors' offices and there is no way of telling who is the public patient and who the private. If you go to a clinic for your general medical care, it is certainly likely that you will have more than one physician over a five-year period, because much of the care is provided by residents. It is also true that you are apt to encounter an intern first. But a few facts should be taken into account before anxiety takes over.

Approximately 80 percent of visits to physicians are precipitated by either self-limiting illness (flu) or problems easily diagnosed and easily treated (rashes, sprains, headaches, ulcers, hypertension). Even when surgery is required (gallstones, appendixes, hernias, hemorrhoids), the procedure is usually a straightforward one. Appreciating this, recognize that the chairperson of medicine is as powerless to treat flu as is the medical student—aspirin, bed rest, and plenty of fluids to tide you through are still the best treatment. However, if you should acquire a complex disease such as leukemia, you can be certain that you will be seen by the chief of hematology in that institution and you can't improve on *that* quality of care. If you need surgery, you can sleep quietly through the anesthetic knowing that while the scalpel may be held by the chief resident in surgery, that resident has had five years of postgraduate training and a faculty member is scrubbed and standing by to supervise. In short, while it is difficult to consider a clinic as "your doctor," the care provided is of the highest quality. You have the advantage of continuity of records, and referrals are available to all specialties.

While a number of nonuniversity clinics are excellent, particularly in hospitals that have family practice programs or are situated in areas distant from an urban center, there is nonetheless a wide variation in quality. If you have a choice in a large, metropolitan area, choose a clinic associated with a medical school. You can then be confident that there is an approved residency training program, which means that there are an adequate number of appropriately trained faculty members to supervise. If you must choose between two community hospitals, phone and ask whether their residency training program is approved in medicine, surgery, or whatever. If it is not, go elsewhere, because the clinic is likely to be staffed by hospital personnel who will consider it a chore to treat you and will dispose of your problem as rapidly as possible.

In recent years the term *clinic* is frequently encountered in connection with outpatient services that require facilities, technological advances, and team treatment beyond the scope of the private practitioner. Among these outpatient clinics, many of them connected with prestigious medical centers, are orthopedic clinics, psychiatry clinics, headache clinics, pain clinics, sex therapy clinics, alcoholism treatment clinics, rehabilitation clinics, and geriatric clinics.

OUTPATIENT SURGERY

A new and growing development in outpatient procedure is the surgical operation performed without necessitating an overnight stay. The hospital recuperation once associated with tonsillectomy, gallbladder removal, and cataract removal is no longer necessary in many cases, thanks to improved technology, less invasive procedures, and advances in anesthesia. In 1992 the American Hospital Association reported that of the 22 million operations performed in community hospitals in 1990, for the first time more than half (51 percent) were done on an outpatient basis that did not require an overnight stay. That same year, Johns Hopkins Medical Center in Baltimore dedicated a new Outpatient Center to accommodate not only the traditional procedures but especially the more than 39 percent of all surgery performed on a same-day basis. What you have to be wary of as a potential patient is that, although

80 percent of outpatient surgery is still being performed at hospital-related sites, non-hospital-owned surgical clinics are setting up shop nationwide and doing an increasing percent of the business without proper licensing or certification. Many of these clinics are owned and operated by individual doctors and groups of surgeons and are not regulated through hospital affiliation or Medicare certification. Nor are they accredited by professional groups that set standards for equipment, emergency care, resuscitation procedures, and the like. Should you be referred to an outpatient clinic for a same-day surgical procedure, be sure to find out about the qualifications of the staff and the professional accreditation of the establishment itself.

CHOOSING A SPECIALIST

A specialist is a physician who has had intensive training in one particular area of medicine and is usually certified by the national board of that specialty. Many are not in solo practice but share offices and facilities with others in the same specialty. Some accept self-referred patients, others accept patients only when referred by other physicians, and many are associated with health maintenance organizations. If you are a member of such an organization, you are expected to use the specialist who is also a member.

Almost every primary care physician establishes personal patterns of referral to known and trusted specialists. If you happen to have heard that Dr. Gray is a fine dermatologist and you ask to be referred, your physician has two choices: immediate agreement, even though this is not the usual pattern, or another suggestion may be offered. Many interpretations can be put on this latter action: your physician may know that although Dr. Gray is "nice," his competency level is not very high; Dr. Gray may simply be unknown, whereas other physicians in the usual office referral pattern are both known and competent. What is fairly certain is that if your physician is competent and you have chosen well in the first place, your specialists will in turn be chosen well for you.

Your relationship to a specialist need not be as close as to your primary physician unless you anticipate that your condition will require a great deal of interaction over a long period. We all would prefer dealing with congenial people at every turn of the medical road, but if you need a fracture set or a mole removed, you need technical skill more than congeniality. Your physician can and should be asked, "What kind of a person is Dr. Brown?" The honest reply may be something like, "Well, not very attractive, a little gruff, but superb in the operating room." If you know that much, you are likely to accept a less than prepossessing manner because you are assured that this is the best person to deal with your problem. In short, if you are confident in your choice of primary physician, you can let the choice of specialists be part of your doctor's responsibility to you.

An area deserving comment is that of gynecology and obstetrics. While a woman might tolerate a patronizing physician in some limited specialties, such types (almost always men) represent a particular hazard in a specialty that by definition places a woman in a physically unique and dependent examination position that often includes discomfort as well. A pelvic examination should not be accompanied by small talk and should not be prefaced by "Now, honey, just relax." Enough indignity is associated with having one's legs in stirrups; you need not tolerate verbal indignity as well. Nowadays, most male gynecologists conduct their examinations in the presence of a female nurse as a guarantee against a possible charge of sexual molestation. In addition, the physician should spend time with you both before and after the examination when you are fully dressed. If you are not comfortable with your physician, seek comfort by discussing your concerns or change physicians.

We conclude this discussion with some information that appeared in a *New York Times* story (4/28/92) under the headline "As Doctors Become More Specialized and Numerous, Turf Wars Erupt Over Body Parts." It appears that with the increased use of new technologies for getting a closer look at body parts, radiologists are in competition with neurologists and cardiologists who have installed their own scanning machines, and with obstetricians who are doing their own ultrasound procedures. A cosmetic surgeon complains that dermatologists are now doing procedures previously considered the exclusive province of plastic surgeons. And because there are too few neurosurgeons and (it would seem) too many orthopedists, the orthopedists are accused of moving into peripheral nerve work.

Your primary care physician should convince you that you need a specialist in the first place and, if you do, should guide you to the one most appropriate for your needs.

GETTING A SECOND OPINION

Second and even third opinions are far more frequently sought when surgical intervention is an issue than when medical treatment alone suffices. In the surgical world, second opinions are either sought by patients for their own satisfaction or mandated by third-party payers. If the patient has a particular physician in mind, the surgeon inevitably acquiesces and arranges for the consultation. If no name surfaces, the surgeon will suggest someone who is competent in the field. This choice may be another physician in the same group or it may be a physician in another group or another hospital.

A referral is usually made when a physician who practices away from a metropolitan area has a patient with particular complications or a particularly difficult diagnosis. The patient is then referred to someone on the staff of a large medical center whose name is known to the referring physician because it has received publicity in the media and/or because this particular physician is well respected by colleagues because of contributions to a relevant area of research. This is a combination consultation and second opinion. Occasionally such patients are self-referred because the physician has seen one of their friends. In either case, unless the patient is in an emergency situation, there may be a considerable wait for a consultation.

Finally, there is good and sufficient reason for getting more than one opinion about an impending operation, especially if it comes under the heading of elective surgery. Experts agree that a significant percentage of all gallbladder removals, hysterectomies, cesarians, and coronary bypasses are unnecessary, and that alternative treatments and less radical procedures may be just as effective. It would appear to be a basic assumption that where there are more surgeons, there is more surgery. In this connection, many corporations are asking the companies that provide health insurance for their employees to submit information that will make it possible to evaluate the competence of the doctors and hospitals with which it deals. Thus, it can determine which doctors are performing too many operations or are charging too much for them. In any case, corporations want the medical community to conform to standards. They want to know, for instance, why hysterectomies are performed seven times more often in one community than in another and how this variation relates to the prevalence of uterine cancer where the operation is performed less frequently. (See "Suggested Health Examination Schedules for Women" in the Appendix.)

HEALTH CARE PLANS

Until the United States Congress enacts a health plan providing universal coverage, we remain the only industrialized nation without this essential safeguard. As of 1996 the elderly have the increasingly uncertain and partial protection of Medicare, and eye care, dental care, and long-term care have never been covered. The poor have some protection (very little in many areas) through Medicaid benefits. But although a few states have made some progress in providing decent coverage, we are still waiting for a federal plan similar to the one that prevails in Canada, not to mention Great Britain, France, Germany, and the Scandinavian countries. While wrangling continues among legislators, lobbyists, insurance companies, the medical profession, and consumer advocates, many Americans remain uninsured. Some women stay in unrewarding jobs because they happen to provide excellent health benefits; women who are newly divorced or widowed have to figure out what to do now that they are no longer participants in the family health plan provided by their husband's employer.

Choosing a health plan is a major decision complicated by a lack of reliable information. Women who have done their own research about comparative costs and effectiveness of treatment (known as "outcome data") are bewildered by the conflicting claims of various HMOs and other managed care plans. According to Dr. David Eddy, a physician and statistician who has been specializing in managed care research, "It will be five to fifteen years before sophisticated comparative data come out" (*New York Times*, 1/14/96).

In the meantime, accreditation surveys are conducted by impartial voluntary professional organizations that evaluate a plan's services, doctors, responsiveness to members, and other aspects of care. Evaluating boards are composed of representatives of employers, unions, managed care plans, and consumers. By early 1996 the nonprofit Washington-based National Committee for Quality Assurance had evaluated about half of the nation's managed care plans, and of these, only one-third were given full three-year accreditation. To find out whether the committee has accredited a specific health plan, consumers can call (202) 955-3515. A brochure containing advice on how to go about selecting a health plan can be obtained by writing to the National Committee for Quality Assurance, 2000 L Street NW, Suite 500, Washington, DC 20036.

Regional editions of *Health Pages* magazine have been issuing health plan report cards. These can be obtained by writing to 135 Fifth Avenue, New York, NY 10010. Locations covered include Columbus, Cincinnati, and Dayton, Ohio; Atlanta, Denver, Phoenix, Los Angeles, Pittsburgh, South Florida, St. Louis, and the states of Vermont and New Hampshire.

HEALTH MAINTENANCE ORGANIZATIONS (HMOs)

HMOs are prepaid health care plans whose membership, originally restricted to the gainfully employed and their families, has grown to about 50 million Americans. Since 1985 Medicare recipients have also been included in their services. In fact, responding to aggressive advertising and promotion of desirable services, far more Medicare recipients than anticipated have become HMO participants. By 1995, the total exceeded 2.5 million.

Basically HMOs combine the functions of an insurance company with those of a doctor/hospital by providing health care for a prepaid annual premium. There are two types of HMOs: the group practice that is connected to a particular hospital and is located in a central "service" area and the "individual practice" that includes doctors who enroll in the HMO and who limit their private practice so that they can accept patients assigned to them by the organization. In exchange for cutting down on their income from private fees, they receive a guaranteed amount of money each month for the patients assigned to them, and they also receive a share of the organization's profits.

You or your spouse may be a member of an employee group that offers prepaid medical care as a fringe benefit or you may live in a community that has a prepaid plan open to the public. You are also likely to have a choice among groups offering such plans. Many women, especially single parents, prefer prepayment, assuming that the physicians offering it are of high quality, because it is easier to budget for a fixed sum each month than to worry about the cost of seeing a physician if a medical problem arises. A number of studies have shown that illnesses are seen earlier and treated more effectively when money is not an obstacle.

Here are some guidelines you can use if you're shopping for a health care plan or if you'd like to switch to another one. If you have trouble getting the information you want in the promotional literature or on the telephone, request an appointment for clarification. If you're given the runaround, you might be well advised to continue looking elsewhere.

- Find out what percentage of the HMO's physicians are board certified.
- If the HMO has been reviewed by the National Committee for Quality Assurance, ask whether it has been certified.
- Do primary care physicians have to get permission from the HMO before a referral can be made to a specialist? Does this restriction apply to referral to a gynecologist?

- Is the physician practice "capitated"? In other words, do the physicians in the practice have a financial incentive to avoid testing, hospitalization, or referral to the care of a specialist?
- What is the procedure for filing an appeal if medical treatment is denied?
- Does the plan cover preventive care in the form of immunizations, including shots that might be necessary for foreign travel?
- If you're taking a prescription drug on a regular basis for a chronic condition, ask whether it is included in the plan's list of medications approved for payment.
- What authorization procedure is required for hospitalization?
- Does the plan cover treatments by alternative therapists such as chiropractors or acupuncturists? Are some treatments excluded because they are considered too "experimental"?

BLUE CROSS/BLUE SHIELD AND OTHER HEALTH INSURERS

If your employee benefits include or you have Blue Cross/Blue Shield, Aetna, or other health insurance coverage as an alternative to a prepaid plan, read the insurance contract carefully, compare the benefits, and estimate what your out-of-pocket costs would be for an ordinary illness. With any such insurance plan you are free to continue with your own physician, but many office charges may not be covered. For covered procedures the insurance carrier may be billed by your physician's office and its payment accepted as full payment. If you have a high income you may be charged an extra amount. If your physician does not participate in Blue Shield or has no mechanism for accepting third-party fees, you will be reimbursed directly by the insurance carrier and are then responsible for paying the bill. Be sure to check any insurance policy as to whether you are covered if traveling outside the United States. All carriers cover costs incurred within the United States.

If your health insurance contract includes "major medical," you have a bolster against catastrophe. If you or a family member is disabled, there are other sources of payment. The important point to remember is to read your contract carefully so you are not taken by surprise by deductible amounts or items not covered. Hospitals, clinics, and group practices all have someone available to explain the variations of coverage and will help you in wending your way through the complications. You can also consult your State Insurance Department for additional information and clarification.

Having established exactly what your coverage includes, you should discuss with your physician or someone in the office what additional charges may occur and under what circumstances. You must not be embarrassed to ask exactly what your care will cost you for a routine visit, for laboratory tests, for a house call. If you know these facts, you will avoid the irritation and dissatisfaction of receiving a "surprise" bill far higher than you expected, even though your expectation may have been unreasonable.

Recently a great deal of publicity has appeared about insurance companies that cancel contracts or escalate rates if a patient is found to have a serious illness. Recourse through complaints to state commissioners have been variable and often ineffective. Before taking out a health care policy, you should not fail to ask whether it is cancellable and, if so, under what conditions.

MEDICARE

If you are eligible for Medicare or if you are within a year of eligibility, inform yourself of the current nature of your entitlements. Fee structure is now based on the evaluation of the work done by a specialist, the costs of the particular practice, and the length of training involved. As a result of proposed budget cuts, Medicare is expected to undergo many changes.

While the new "relative value" scale has been endorsed by the American Medical Association, there is a growing resistance on the part of individual doctors to accept the fee structure, and Medicare patients are finding it increasingly difficult to locate physicians willing to accept them for treatment on the basis of assigned fees. An increasing number of older Americans have therefore been signing up for managed care.

Although doctors increasingly emphasize the importance of preventive health measures, Medicare is prohibited by law from paying for any procedures not mentioned in the Medical Act. In response to unremitting criticism, the act was amended to include coverage for Pap smears for the early detection of cervical and uterine cancer and mammograms every other year for the detection of breast cancer.

If you have any problems finding a doctor who accepts Medicare payments, consult your local Social Security office, and while you're there, be sure to pick up the most recent brochures relevant to your particular situation so that you'll know exactly how the system has been changing. And if you're traveling outside the United States, remember that Medicare does not cover any costs incurred abroad.

MEDICAID

The same legislation that created Medicare in 1965 created Medicaid to provide health insurance for poor people. In theory, coverage is available for all those who meet the eligibility requirements, but these requirements vary considerably from state to state. States receive federal support according to the state's per capita income; thus the poorer states receive a larger share of federal funds.

Although Medicaid was originally intended to provide health care for welfare recipients, it has been expanded to include some children who live below the poverty line, as well as some blind and disabled people, some pregnant women, and many nursing home residents. In 1995, of the nearly 37 million individuals covered by Medicaid, about half were children. Federal guidelines for coverage include inpatient and outpatient hospital services, doctors' services, laboratory and radiology procedures, nursing homes and home health care, diagnosis and treatment for children under age 21, family planning, prenatal care, and rural clinics. Whether Medicaid can pay for abortions for poor women under the family planning coverage has become a matter of partisan politics, turning this service into a class privilege rather than a legal option.

Because Medicaid reimburses physicians at an even lower rate than Medicare does, individuals eligible for the services of a private doctor often have to end up in the outpatient department—or often in the emergency room—of a municipal or county hospital. (In many states, private or community hospitals refuse to accept Medicaid patients.)

You can find out about your current eligibility for Medicaid services by consulting the state's Department of Social Services. If you are seeking this information on behalf of a parent who is entering a nursing home, consult the Area Agency on Aging in your vicinity.

EMERGENCY CARE

Suppose you are ill in a foreign country. What do you do? You know no one; you are unfamiliar with the hospitals and perhaps even the language. Possibly you will turn to the hotel manager, who will supply the name of a physician. If your problem is a simple one, this may suffice. If it is serious and requires hospitalization, you can call the American Embassy if you are in a nation's capital, or the American Consulate if you are in a smaller city. Another option is to ask to be taken to the university hospital if there is one, unless you have had the opportunity to call your personal physician long-distance and a better solution is forthcoming. This at least assures the highest quality of care in that community. Once in the emergency room, you will be seen first by a resident who will assess the situation and perhaps say that you need to be seen by a surgeon. Your next question should be "If you needed a surgeon for your daughter in this hospital, whom would you call?" This question is entirely different from "Whom would you suggest?" because if the resident happens at that moment to be rotating through the service with Drs. A, B, and C, it is likely that one of them will be named. However, all residents know well who are the competent (and incompetent) physicians in that hospital in their discipline; each hospital has at least one "doctor's doctor" who somehow has all the medical and nursing staff families as patients because they know who is the best. If you ask the right question, you'll find that person and that's who you want.

But suppose you are in an automobile accident and find yourself in a hospital in a community you know nothing about. You are there not by your own choice, but because that is where the ambulance driver took you. Immediate care will lessen the urgency—bleeding will be stopped, intravenous fluids begun, some assessment of the gravity of the situation will be made. If the hospital is small and rural, it will be ill prepared to deal with serious injury of the head, chest, or abdomen, and once your medical condition is stabilized, the staff is likely to arrange for transfer to a more appropriate facility. Here again, you will be offered some choices, and if you are too far away from your own physician and hospital, the wisest decision is to request transfer to the nearest university health center complex. Some hospitals other than university centers provide excellent care for the most complicated problems, but you have no way of knowing which they are, and you certainly wish to avoid a second transfer later.

If you have a condition that requires ongoing therapy, such as diabetes, allergies, or epilepsy, make sure that you *always* wear an identification tag, such as the Medic-Alert emblem, which gives the diagnosis and a collect call telephone number for additional information. (Write Medic-Alert, Turlock, California 95380, for further information.) An unconscious person cannot give a history, and your prior illness may be either the cause of your admission or may be seriously complicating it.

One last word about emergencies—they occur at home as well. If an accident happens or a family member suddenly becomes acutely ill, do not bother to telephone your physician. This will take costly minutes and the physician

will almost certainly say, "Go immediately to the emergency room at the hospital." You should save the time of the call and go directly there by ambulance
(call 911). An ambulance is a far better choice than a private car or taxi because
the ambulance is staffed by a trained crew of life-saving medical technicians. If
possible, call or have someone call ahead to the emergency room to tell them
you are coming and let them know the problem. Your physician knows, and
you should know, that in an emergency a house call would do little except
waste time. What is needed is immediate access to an X-ray machine, intravenous fluids, medications that a physician is unlikely to carry, and sophisticated
equipment available only in a hospital.

HOSPITALS

To many people, a hospital is a frightening place. It has unfamiliar machines
and smells; it contains seriously ill and dying people; it is impersonal; it is
above all mysterious. Processions of people in different uniforms troop through
your room, each punching or poking or stabbing you for a different reason,
until finally you lose track and simply submit. Once you submit, you have
accepted your own depersonalization. If you are seriously ill, this matters very
little, but if you are comparatively well, it disturbs you. What are your defenses?

YOUR RIGHTS AS A PATIENT

In 1973 the American Hospital Association published a Patient's Bill of
Rights to which all accredited hospitals must accede. The following is an expanded updated version typical of those supplied to patients on admission to
most hospitals across the country.

Quality Care for All Patients

You have the right to receive the best inpatient, outpatient or emergency
treatment and access to programs that we can provide without regard to race,
color, sex, age, religion, national origin, handicap, veteran status or source of
payment.

Information

You have the right to know the name of the physician responsible for your care and to receive from your physician complete current information concerning your medical problems, the planned course of treatment, the probable length of hospitalization and the prognosis or medical outlook for the future, in terms you can be reasonably expected to understand. If your physician thinks that it is not medically advisable to give such information to you, it will be made available to an appropriate person on your behalf.

You have the right to participate in decisions that affect your care and treatment.

You have the right to consult with other physicians or specialists provided they have hospital staff privileges.

You have the right to know the name and function of each staff member who attends to you and who will perform any procedure or treatment.

Because this is a teaching institution, affiliated with a wide range of educational programs, you will meet doctors, nurses and students-in-training for other health care professions. Many of them will be involved in your care, assisting in the 24-hour, seven-day weekly services you need while hospitalized. They are taught to function as a team in patient care interests, and are under expert professional supervision. We believe that our patients benefit from the extra attention of these professionals and paraprofessionals in training.

Giving Consent

You have the right to receive from your physician information necessary to give informed consent prior to the start of any operation, procedure and/or treatment. Except in emergencies, this explanation must include the risks that may be involved, the probable chance of success, the effects of the tests or treatment, the amount of pain or discomfort that may be entailed, and how long this may be expected to last. You must also be told if there is more than one medically acceptable way to treat your illness and the risks and benefits of alternative treatments.

You have the right to read and to be given a complete explanation of any consent form you are asked to sign, and to question and modify, with your physician, any part of the form that does not apply to your consent before you sign it.

Declining Treatment

You have the right to decline further treatment. In taking such a step, consider your decision carefully and discuss it with your physician and family so that you understand the full extent of the consequences to your health.

Leaving Against Medical Advice

You have the right to leave the hospital against your doctor's advice unless you cannot maintain your own safety, as defined by law, or have an infectious disease hazardous to others. If you do leave against your doctor's advice the hospital will not be responsible for any harm this may cause you, and you will be asked to sign an "Against Medical Advice" form.

Privacy

You have the right to every consideration of both your personal privacy and the privacy of your medical program. Case discussions and consultations are confidential. Your permission will be requested if you are to be presented at any conference or teaching exercise at which personnel other than those directly involved in your care is present.

Confidentiality

You have the right to confidential medical records.

No person or agency outside of those taking care of you can see them unless authorized by you, or by law. Under certain insurance programs, such as Medicare, your records may be reviewed before payment is approved.

Transfer to Another Institution

You have the right to expect that within its capacity the hospital will make reasonable response to your request for services. The hospital must provide diagnostic evaluation, necessary medical care, and, if necessary, arrangements

An unfortunate result of the computerization of hospital records (as well as other medical records) has been the selling of patient information by unscrupulous health providers to drug companies, HMOs, insurance companies, and even prospective employers. In spite of some restrictive federal and state laws, these records have even been crossing state lines. In many states, patients who have never asked to inspect their records may be totally unaware of the misinformation they contain and that this misinformation is finding its way into the wrong hands.

Federal legislators have made an attempt to safeguard the privacy of medical records by proposing the Medical Records Confidentiality Act. Introduced in the Senate with bipartisan support in 1995, it makes it a crime for health care providers to release data without patient consent or to condition medical service on the granting of this consent. It also guarantees every patient's federally protected right to inspect and copy personal health records and to compel corrections of inaccuracies.

The bill as originally conceived has been strongly opposed by civil libertarians, many medical ethicists, and most advocates of patients' rights. Among the reasons for the opposition is that it does not require patient consent when hospitals turn records over to nationally computerized data bases, and it also permits law enforcement agencies to search medical records even if they do not know the name of the individual whose records they are searching.

If you're interested in protecting the privacy of your hospital records, you can follow the progress of this bill during hearings and pay attention to whether it is supported as originally proposed or whether it is being amended. You can write or call your representatives in Congress to let them know how you feel about this legislation, which may affect your insurance rights and your employment.

for your transfer to another health facility when medically permissible. You have the right to receive information and explanation concerning the needs for and alternatives to such a transfer. The health facility to which you are to be transferred must first have accepted you for transfer.

Participation in Research

You have the right to be told if the hospital plans to use experimental procedures or drugs during your care and to choose whether or not you will participate. You have the right to ask how your participation will help you and/or others. Your refusal to participate in research will not prejudice your continued medical treatment at the hospital.

Payment

You have the right to receive a bill itemizing hospital charges related to your care and are encouraged to examine it and to ask questions about any portion that you do not understand.

You have the right to ask for information and help in receiving financial benefits, for which you may be eligible, to help pay your hospital bills.

Complaints

You have the right to voice grievances to our staff, our governing body and the State Department of Health without fear of reprisal.

Participation in Your Health Care

Your active participation will help us render better health care to you. Give accurate and complete information about your past illnesses, about other times you have been hospitalized, about medications you are taking, any allergies you may have, and other matters relating to your health.

Be sure to keep your appointments. If you cannot, notify the doctor, hospital or others who are concerned. Follow instructions carefully. Let the doctor or nurse know if you do not understand any part of them.

If you feel you cannot follow the instructions, say so. If you have any problems at home that may interfere with your carrying out your doctor's orders, a social worker may be able to help you. The nurse will call one for you. Follow your health care plan carefully once it has been agreed upon. Notify your doctor or nurse promptly of any sudden or unexpected change in your health.

Your Responsibilities as a Patient

Following hospital rules and regulations will help the hospital ensure your safety and comfort and that of other patients.

You are asked to respect your roommates' rights to privacy and quiet; to use radio, television and lights in a manner that will not disturb others. Remember, many patients need a lot of rest.

You are asked to limit your visitors to two at a time during visiting hours, and to ask them to maintain a quiet atmosphere and observe smoking regulations which are posted throughout the hospital.

You are responsible for using hospital supplies and equipment carefully in order to assure that they will be available for future patients.

You are requested to provide information for insurance processing of your bills, to pay them promptly, and to ask any questions you have about them as soon as possible.

ADDITIONAL SAFEGUARDS

In a growing number of states, patients now have the legal right to see their hospital records in spite of the opposition of many doctors who say that patients would not understand the meaning of the entries.

A recent development is the presence in a majority of hospitals in the United States of a patient advocate, also known as a patient representative who has nothing to do with caregiving. These intermediaries are on the hospital payroll, in some cases assisted by a volunteer staff, to restore the personal touch, to bend some of the rules to accommodate a patient, to explain some of the doctor's orders and procedures when the doctor is too busy to do so, to arrange for special payment plans, and to provide emotional support for the family. (When you are admitted to a hospital, if you aren't given the patient representative's name along with the Patient's Bill of Rights, ask whether the hospital has such a staff member and get the phone number.)

Every state has passed advance directive legislation, either in the form of a Living Will or Medical Power of Attorney. If you have signed such a document, ask to have it attached to your hospital chart. If you have not signed such a document and you wish to do so as a patient, make your wishes known to the patient representative. If you have any questions about this procedure, you can call the office of Choice in Dying, 1-800-989-9455.

A recent addition to the staff of most reputable hospitals is a specialist in medical ethics. Medical ethicists, also called bioethicists, attempt to help resolve the moral and legal problems raised by technological advances in genetic engineering, third-party reproductive procedures, organ transplants, and the like. Although the ethicists refrain from making decisions, their role is to analyze problems, clarify information, and suggest principles to be considered in arriving at a course of action. The positive results, according to Dr. Arthur Capalan, director of the Center for Biomedical Ethics at the University of Minnesota, is that physicians are more truthful in telling patients exactly what the diagnosis is and what to expect; they exercise more care in getting informed consent for treatment; and they have begun to see the patient not as a passive client but as an important participant in the healing process, a person who sets goals and can select different options.

If you and your family can profit from consultation with a medical ethicist because of confusion or conflict about treatment, be sure to ask whether such a specialist is available on the hospital staff, and, if not, find out how to reach one.

YOUR COMFORT AS A PATIENT

The cost of a private room in most hospitals is very high and is not covered by insurance, so you are likely to have a roommate. By and large this contributes to your comfort and decreases your anxiety. You have someone to talk to; you have a mutual aid source; you have company. The drawbacks come when your roommate is a chronic complainer, entertains a constant parade of noisy guests, has the television turned on from 6 A.M. to bedtime whether she's in the room or not, or keeps you awake at night by groaning or snoring. Under any of these circumstances you should speak with the head nurse and ask to be moved to another room. Discharges occur every day, and within a reasonable time you should be relocated. Such requests are not unusual nor, if done with courtesy, are they interpreted as griping.

Your phone and your visitors maintain your connections with the outside world; you will gradually sort out the staff and greet some of them with pleasure and enthusiasm; you will begin to understand the routines. All these lessen your anxiety and improve your state of well-being. Because most hospital stays last less than a week, you will not have suffered inordinately and your next admission will be fraught with considerably less apprehension. If your condition or treatment requires a longer hospitalization, you will find that you adapt quite well to the restrictions imposed on you by the hospital.

At the time of admission for more serious conditions, many patients and families worry about whether they should engage a private nurse. Will the floor nurses come when one rings the bell or will they be too busy? Can the nursing station down the hall respond adequately to the patient's personal needs? The way to find this out at admission is to ask the doctor under whose auspices you are admitted and (if surgery is involved) the surgeon assigned to your case. The extent of nursing required will be a large factor; the number of patients on the floor, another. In most situations there are enough nurses to meet all the needs of the patients, and they are highly skilled in dealing with the equipment and procedures required for the specialty clustered on that floor. If for any reason you feel that extra care is needed, the hospital has a roster of both registered nurses and licensed practical nurses who are available for special duty. If you feel you can afford a nurse for only a total of three 8-hour shifts, decide whether you would prefer to have around-the-clock attention by three differ- ent nurses for the 24 hours after you come out of the recovery room, or the same nurse for the same shift (say, the 8 A.M. to 4 P.M. shift) three successive days in a row.

The intensive care unit (ICU) can be the most distressing area for patients and their families. Patients are likely to be attached to tubes and other equip- ment, sleep is disturbed by constant monitoring, privacy is nonexistent, and relatives usually may visit only five minutes at a time. Families wonder what they will find and what to say, and often the patient is too ill to know or care whether someone visited an hour ago. The visiting rules were made to ensure optimal care and to limit the number of people hovering around a bed when patient monitoring must be done repeatedly. If the unit is comparatively quiet, the nurse may allow you to stay longer than the five minutes if it will comfort the patient.

If you will need further help or treatment at home, ask to see a member of the Social Service department or the Home Care department. You may be entitled to the services of visiting nurses several times a week for the period specified by your doctor. Depending on your condition, you may also be vis- ited by a team of rehabilitation specialists. If you will need a part-time home attendant or a part-time housekeeper, the hospital social worker will be famil- iar with your Medicare entitlements, other insurance coverage, and the re- sources offered by your community.

COOPERATIVE CARE UNITS

In April 1979, University Hospital of the New York University Medical Center reinvented a pattern of cooperative care long used in third-world coun- tries as well as in many industrialized nations—a facility combining patient education and family participation in medical care. Since that time, similar facilities have become available in a number of hospitals and medical centers nationwide. Typical units have the appearance of motel suites and provide accommodations for patients and partners of their choice—spouse, adult offspring, close friend. The partner, who is housed and fed without charge for the duration of the stay, agrees to spend from 4 to 24 hours a day with the patient and is taught to perform many tasks traditionally performed by nurses and nurses' aides. To qualify for such an arrangement where it is available, the patient must be able to walk independently or with a cane or to get around in a wheelchair. Typical patients are those who enter for chemotherapy or are sufficiently ambulatory to be transferred from another part of the hospital, or suffer from heart disease, vascular disorders, or have orthopedic problems.

Hospital services remain in place, and the patient does the walking, with or without the companion to the various treatment rooms, radiology department, nurses' station, dining room, and lounges. The patient is also given the prescribed supply of medication, and the companion is taught how to administer the drugs and how to keep a detailed chart.

This arrangement has many advantages, both for the hospital and the patient. The average cost is 40 to 45 percent lower than it would be for the same number of days in a traditional setting. As for the patients, they have the comfort of a close ally and are encouraged to participate in their own care and maximize their role and the family's role in recovery. Everyone's dependence on the hospital is reduced. In addition, the creation of a "wellness" environment has a strong positive effect on the patient's morale, which in turn affects the progress of recovery.

YOU AND YOUR PHYSICIAN

Of course you expect your physician to provide good medical care. But you probably have other expectations as well, some you may not consciously recognize and others that may be unobtainable.

WHAT YOU HAVE A RIGHT TO EXPECT FROM YOUR PHYSICIAN

Above all, you want *help.* If you are threatened with a serious illness, you not only want to be confident that you have been referred to the most competent specialists; you also want some time to discuss the threat as well.

Let us assume that you have just discovered a lump in your neck and your doctor has confirmed that indeed it is a cause for further investigation, probably surgery. These are the facts, but many other things are whirling through your mind. Benign or malignant? How much surgery? How many hospital days? How much time off work? Who will look after the children? Will I have a disfiguring scar? Why do I have a lump at all? How much will it cost and how will we find the money? If I am hospitalized for a long time, what will it do to my marriage, my relationship? Who will look after me as I convalesce? If it is a malignancy, how will I face it?

Your physician owes you reassurance and help just as much as you are owed laboratory results, and you have every right to discuss all of these questions. It may well be that the schedule is too tight at that moment to cover the ground, but you should ask whether you can make another appointment in the very near future only to talk. Often you can be immediately reassured that the overwhelming odds are against malignancy and that, if the growth is benign, surgery is simple and hospitalization short. But the "ifs" still lurk in the back of your mind and should be handled with an immediate biopsy if possible.

Of course, many of your questions are not for the physician to answer. No matter how frankly you have discussed your marital situation, no other person can predict how your spouse will react or can tell you how to find money or a babysitter. But you can, and should, have every question answered about the medical situation. If and when surgery turns out to be agreed on, you can then be referred to a social worker or a community agency to help in arrangements for children and for convalescence.

Once you enter the hospital for surgery, you will be expected to sign an "informed consent" document. The surgeon *must*, both legally and morally, describe to you the procedure anticipated, its probable outcome and complications, the period of convalescence you may have to anticipate, and possible alternatives. Multisyllable medical jargon should not be accepted. You have the right to understand exactly what will happen to you as far as the surgeon knows. The occasional rare complication cannot be envisaged, but the usual procedure and its course can be. You should be quite clear that you understand as much as a layman can about what will happen to you. In advance of the surgery, you have the right to ask for control over painkillers for the first few days after the operation. Your physician will undoubtedly come to see you frequently when making rounds and, because of personal knowledge, will be able to allay any new anxieties as well as interpret any findings that other physicians have left unexplained. There will have been discussions with the surgeon and a plan of action for the future will have begun to unroll.

Now let us suppose that you have a malignancy, that the surgery was far more radical than anticipated, the hospitalization longer, the cost greater, the scar wider, and the convalescence more stormy and fraught with new symptoms from X-ray or chemotherapy. The worst has happened and more decisions must be made. There will be conferences between your physician, the surgeon, and the radiologists and a plan of medical action will be formulated; the social service department will assist in sorting out the family and financial problems. Even so, your anxiety about *you* is high. What can you expect then?

You can expect, and should receive, comfort and honesty. Any question that you ask about your future should be answered. That last sentence is very carefully worded, and the appropriate analogy is to the sex education of a child. There is substantial agreement that in childhood, sexual questions should not be answered before they are asked because the child's unconscious or preconscious adapts the question to the amount of information that can be assimilated. Similarly, in questions of malignancy and death the patient virtually always asks the questions she wants answered, and no others. If your physician tells you that today most malignancies are treatable and many curable, you are not being conned: this is the truth. You should not dwell on all the frightening things that may or may not happen; you must participate actively in your own recovery. On the other hand, active participation depends on full information, so you will be told, for instance, that you should not return to work while getting radiation because you will probably be nauseated for a few weeks. The path of your immediate future can be accurately charted, but you cannot expect to be told what will happen in two years because no one knows. You and your doctor will be a team for that period, making decisions as you go in light of what is known about medicine and about you. Even while you're still in the hospital, you may be visited by a member of a support group who is a "survivor" and who can offer many life-enhancing suggestions.

While one example does not cover all circumstances, it should indicate the dimensions of your physician's responsibility to you under the worst eventuality and you can then figure out what you should expect in other, less dire situations. Without question your physician should accept with grace any request for a second opinion; in difficult cases such a consultation usually is welcomed as either a new slant on the problem or confirmation. Any situation that offers a choice of therapies with different risks and side effects must be completely discussed: this is the essence of "informed consent." If a new approach to your problem is available only in another city, your physician should give you an objective evaluation of the treatment, refer you to lay literature in which it has been discussed, and if you wish it, refer you to that site. Such a referral assumes that a complete record of your illness and laboratory findings will be sent prior to your appointment.

You also have every right to expect complete confidentiality from your physician, and this includes responsibility not to discuss anything in your record without your permission, even with your family. There will, however, be times when you will not only allow such a family discussion but should ask to have one. If, for instance, you will have to restrict your activities, it is important that your family understand why this is so and exactly what you can and cannot do. Their cooperation will be more complete if their information is first hand rather than through your interpretation. Furthermore, you may not be a reliable informant, because you may want to spare your family the extra tasks and responsibilities. However, it can't be said too often that successful treatment is the result of "team" participation. When those who are close to the patient become actively involved in performing the day-to-day chores that are part of the prescribed regimen, the probable outcome is vastly better. You also have the right to ask about the role of alternative therapies in your recovery and about pain control through biofeedback training or hypnosis. You should also expect guidance about nutrition and how to deal with the negative side effects of your medication.

You have a right to expect that the doctor or the doctor's nurse will return your phone call within a reasonable length of time when a message has been left with an answering service or on the telephone recording tape.

You have one further right—dignity. To be called "honey" or "dearie" is to be robbed of your identity. To be called by your first name without your permission is to establish a relationship in which you have been immediately cast as the docile child who obeys orders. Some patients prefer being called Mary rather than Mrs. Brown, but the initiative should rest with the patient. State your preference but beware of an office in which first names are bandied around by physician and staff alike.

A word about doctors who overbook patients so that appointment times don't mean very much. If on several occasions (once is excusable) you arrive well in advance of your scheduled appointment time and have to spend the next two hours reading old magazines and listening to music not of your own choosing before you are directed to an examining room and then have to spend another half-hour waiting for the doctor with your clothes off (and, worse still, in a "robe" made of paper) you have every right to inform the doctor that your time is valuable too and that you resent having to waste it in the waiting room. There are, in fact, some patients whose time is worth as much money as the doctor's, and a few of these have sent bills accompanied by letters explaining that they expect to be paid for time lost.

WHAT YOU SHOULD NOT EXPECT FROM YOUR PHYSICIAN

Your physician is neither your parent nor your best friend, even though you have often confided more intimate facts than you have to anyone else. To survive as a good physician objectivity must be maintained. You have no right to expect "love," in the sense of protection from all evil, nor should you ask advice on personal matters. Whether you should break off a relationship with your alcoholic lover or husband, whether you should buy a house instead of renting, or whether you should change your job—these are your decisions. Granted that these problems may cause you anxiety that affects your physical condition, the physician has only two responsibilities: to advise you to see a psychotherapist or direct you to various community resources if your way of dealing with stress and conflict is to drink too much or hit the children or gobble pills, *and* in acute situations, such as death in the family, to prescribe a tranquilizer or a sleeping pill to tide you over. But you should not press to continue such drugs indefinitely. Supportive drugs not only postpone solutions; they can become problems in themselves.

Some patients feel that they have a right to manage their own illnesses and demand treatments that they have read about—multivitamins, chelation, the newest diet. These therapies may be pharmacologically innocuous even though ineffective and costly, but they may, as well, be particularly contraindicated in your case. Your physician can and should explain to you why such treatment will not be prescribed for you. Even generally well-informed patients may try to pressure a physician into prescribing antibiotics so that they can feel that something is being done, even though, as in viral infections, antibiotics are ineffective, involve needless costs, may have unpleasant side effects, such as allergic reactions or digestive upset, and through overuse, prove ineffective when really needed. On the other hand, your physician should be aware of the latest treatments and the most effective new medications described in the professional literature, especially the *New England Journal of Medicine* and the *Journal of the American Medical Association.*

Nothing irritates and embarrasses a physician more than to be asked to play a collusive role in some questionable enterprise: to provide a medical excuse for an irresponsible child who played hookey, to improvise an acceptable reason for your having failed to show up at work when the truth was that you had a hangover, to lie on your behalf in filling out an insurance form. Responsible adults don't ask friends to lie for them, and you certainly shouldn't expect your doctor to do so.

Each physician has a few patients whose "demands" are a way of life. Often they are rich enough to take the position that if they "pay" they can "demand." Implicit in this behavior is the assumption that the physician is their servant. These patients have no insight into their infantile behavior, or that they are making a profession of being "ill" in order to manipulate their environment, whether this be the physician or the spouse or the children. They disrupt office routine; they cause the physician to groan when their name is on the day's appointment list; they are the ones who are visibly offended at being referred to a psychiatrist. When they have used up the tolerance of one physician, they move to the next. Their charts are thick; their bathroom cabinets full of pills; they frequently see more than one physician at a time without revealing this. Unwittingly, they are receiving the worst possible medical care because they will not accept better care.

WHAT YOUR PHYSICIAN HAS A RIGHT TO EXPECT FROM YOU

A doctor-patient relationship is most effective when responsibilities are shared. At its best, the relationship is between allies: you are partners in dealing with problems about which you have unequal information but in which you both have rights.

Patient responsibilities include a number of niceties that you would never ignore with a friend but are often ignored in physicians' offices. If you cannot keep an appointment, phone as far ahead as you can so that another patient can be scheduled for that time. If you must be late because the babysitter didn't come, phone the office before leaving home to find out if the doctor will still be able to see you or if it would be better to reschedule.

There was a time when it could be assumed that a doctor would send the patient a bill for services rendered and most of the time the bills got paid. Nowadays, unless third-party assignment is accepted or you are a participant in managed care, it is usually expected that the fee for the visit be paid in cash or by check before the patient leaves the office.

Another area of patient responsibility, rarely emphasized though exceedingly important to all physicians, is compliance to a therapeutic regimen. You should never lie to a physician about pills you have not taken or procedures you have failed to carry out. Nor should you withhold information about visits to another doctor who has made other recommendations and prescribed other medication or a nonmedical treatment such as a change in diet or acupuncture. Several things may result from such deception. The physician may assume that the regimen has failed and change course to a different, probably less appropriate one when you do not appear to be responding. Or if you found that the medication produced unpleasant side effects and you stopped taking it without saying so, you have kept information to yourself that might be of use to another patient taking the same drug.

THE COMMUNITY OF HEALTH CARE

The physician is not the only source of health care: the network of health services stretches far beyond the physician's office and may provide as much as 90 percent of the total care. One good example is in the area of vision. You see an ophthalmologist who tells you that your child has amblyopia, a condition of muscle imbalance of the eyes that interferes with efficient focusing. If this condition is of moderate extent, surgery will not be suggested, but you will be referred to a clinic where special muscle exercises are taught and progress checked. The ophthalmologist will check the status of the condition in six months, but in the interim you will be receiving excellent and important health care continuously.

Take a more serious situation. You have diabetes, and your ophthalmologist has told you for a number of years that your retinae are deteriorating; you obviously know this because your vision is decreasing. There comes a point when you can no longer manage your job or your housekeeping or your transportation. The physician has done everything known and is powerless, but the resources of the community haven't yet been touched. Referral to a center whose entire purpose is the retraining of the blind should be made. Often physicians are ignorant of community facilities, and you may have to seek these out on your own or through a social service organization. Once you are appropriately linked up to a group, a program, or an institution, you will embark on an educational experience of which your physician does not know the details or the techniques but only knows the results and the availability.

The number of paramedical services is so vast that it is the rare physician who is aware of them all. The accident or stroke victim who requires months of rehabilitation deals almost entirely with physical, occupational, and speech therapists under a doctor's supervision; a woman who has had a mastectomy gains more ongoing help from Reach for Recovery than from her surgeon; the multiple sclerosis victim is bolstered by the MS Society and its members though her physician is supervising her medications. In any of these areas your physician's responsibility rests with knowing what facilities relate to your problem and then referring you to the proper ones.

Another resource available in nearly every community is the Visiting Nurse Association. This group offers a variety of nursing services, from skilled nurse to homemaker, that may provide a much-needed respite for the family member responsible for a chronically ill patient. All too often physicians take for granted that if you are looking after your bedridden parent, no other caregiver is needed. If they have never had such a responsibility, they cannot conceive of the daily drain, of your need to get out of the house two or three times a week to walk in the park or go to a movie or visit a friend. (Many communities also offer respite services for long-term caregivers.)

The group whose responsibility it is to know *all* of these resources is the social service department of a hospital or community. If you are coping with a chronic illness or if you are the caregiver of a patient with one, it is well worth exploring these resources as a means of making daily life more manageable. If the caregiver or the recipient of the care is over 62, the other source is the local Area Agency on Aging.

Over the past decade a number of new categories of health practitioners have appeared, and one, the nurse-midwife, has reappeared. She is the prototype for the others, a professional taught to deal competently with normal pregnancies and to recognize those abnormalities that should be referred to a physician. Physicians' assistants, pediatric and adult nurse practitioners, while doing different tasks, have the same orientation. Well-child care, monitoring of chronic disease, treatment of minor complaints, carrying out assigned tasks that they have been specially taught to perform—these are some of the ways in which they function as physician extenders. The school nurse, the industrial nurse, the "medic" are examples that come readily to mind. Many clinics and group practices include one or more such professionals and you should not feel that you have been cheated if you see them and not the physician during a routine visit. However, at times when you want to discuss a particular problem in detail with the doctor, you need not accept the services of an intermediary.

Other professionally trained people who use such procedures as biofeedback, hypnosis, acupuncture, and meditation are increasingly found to benefit certain patients and certain diseases, and physicians frequently refer suitable patients to such health care professionals. (See "Alternative Therapies.")

CONCLUSION

Many women are intimidated by physicians and the world of illness and hospitals and, thus, they forget that this territory may have its uncertainties and frustrations, but one need not add to the vicissitudes by ignorance or false expectations. If you ask questions and follow directions carefully and intelligently, you have every right to expect the best of medical care.

ALTERNATIVE THERAPIES

Helene MacLean

Medical Writer and Editor; Author, *Caring for Your Parents, Relief from Chronic Arthritis Pain;* Coauthor, *Recovering from a Hysterectomy, Migraine: Beating the Odds*

Reflexology and Rolfing, tai chi and shiatsu, New Age medicine and ancient Asian remedies—alternative therapies of every sort are receiving more and more attention at the same time that we are learning about laparoscopies, magnetic resonance imaging, and bioengineering. What's going on? As great advances continue to be made in high-tech medical practice, alternative therapies have grown to the point where they represent an industry amounting to about $27 billion a year. This development didn't occur overnight, although it is only recently that it has begun to attract attention not only from national media but from traditional medical practice as well.

In 1992 Congress passed legislation that resulted in the establishment by the National Institutes of Health of the Office of Alternative Medicine. In 1993 a major breakthrough occurred when the *New England Journal of Medicine* published the results of a national survey indicating that the use of "unconventional therapies is far higher than previously reported" and concluded that therefore "doctors should ask about their patients' use of unconventional therapies whenever they obtain a medical history."

At the same time, medical schools attached to prestigious universities began to offer courses in unorthodox medicine, and by now many of these institutions have established a department of alternative medicine.

What accounts for the fact that in the year covered by the survey, Americans "made approximately 425 million visits to providers of unconventional therapy" compared with 388 million visits to primary care physicians? When did this backlash against the medical establishment begin? And more specifically, what accounts for the gradual loosening of the bond between women and their male doctors?

GROWING INTEREST IN ALTERNATIVE THERAPIES

The exploration of what have come to be known as alternative therapies or alternative medicine began in the 1960s, when many people became increasingly disenchanted with what they perceived to be the dehumanizing results of science and technology. Not only did they seek to broaden their perceptions beyond the rational through the use of mind-altering drugs, but many undertook a journey of enlightenment into the wisdom of the East with the guidance of a guru. We began to hear about Zen Buddhism, the Japanese religious sect that seeks enlightenment through meditation. Relaxation was accomplished through the discipline of yoga or through chanting a mantra. Parents worried about their young adult offspring who, although they required a proper diet for bodies that hadn't finished growing, were seeking spiritual purity through macrobiotic diets that seemed to consist of nothing but brown rice and tea. Although for several preceding decades a number of forward-looking physicians had been practicing what they called psychosomatic medicine, in which the mind-body connection in sickness and in health was taken for granted, trendier practitioners at all levels of competence and incompetence were beginning to refer to themselves as "holistic healers." There was a tendency at that time—and the tendency persists—to refer to these approaches to well-being as New Age medicine, whereas in fact they were attempts to find in the traditional skills, procedures, and folk remedies of older civilizations a viable substitute for prescription medicine.

The early 1960s also saw the publication of Betty Friedan's *The Feminine Mystique,* the book that for many women provided the rallying cry of the consciousness-raising movement that led to a new feeling of competence and empowerment. Ten years later, in 1973, the Boston Women's Health Book Collective published *Our Bodies, Ourselves,* which fueled the desire of many women of all ages to take charge of their own well-being through education and a better understanding of how their bodies functioned. More and more women were feeling shortchanged by the patronizing attitudes of male doctors who did everything but snicker when their patients told them about the effectiveness of yogurt or cranberry juice in clearing up a vaginal yeast infection. Women were especially distressed at the medical profession's wholesale handing out of Valium prescriptions to the point where it was becoming a scandal.

It was in this spirit—and with the desire to redefine the doctor-patient relationship as a partnership in which they could play an active role in their own preventive health care—that more and more women turned to alternative practitioners. They sought out homeopaths, chiropractors, herbalists, nutritionists; spent lots of money, not always wisely, in health food stores; and became increasingly involved in physical fitness regimens. They looked for help in giving up smoking and drinking and faulty eating habits without depending on tranquilizers or diet pills. Hypnosis and acupuncture were found to be effective procedures for some; relaxation techniques and breathing exercises were effective for others. Medication was spurned in favor of membership in self-help groups, hundreds of which were formed to meet special needs. It was unfortunate that some women who looked on conventional physicians as their enemy ended up as the victims of scam artists, while others failed to get proper treatment for diseases incorrectly diagnosed by a healer without any credentials.

THE MIND-BODY CONNECTION

At the same time that this backlash against conventional medicine was gaining momentum, a significant development occurred in the scientific community. A 1974 best-seller by two highly respected cardiologists, Drs. Meyer Friedman and Ray Rosenman, suggested that personality traits of impatience and irritability increased the risk of a heart attack. In *The Relaxation Response,* published in 1975, Harvard cardiologist Dr. Herbert Benson showed that meditation can lower heart rate and blood pressure. These studies led to his creating the Mind/Body Institute at the Deaconess Hospital in Boston, where his relaxation techniques help treat such conditions as chronic pain and cancer. By 1993 Bill Moyers hosted a five-part television series called *Healing and the Mind,* accompanied by a book of the same name, which presented convincing evidence of the profound relationship between psyche and soma and concluded that conventional Western medicine can learn a great deal from less orthodox methods.

In the intervening years, a major area in which alternative therapies have achieved establishment recognition is in the treatment of chronic pain. Research in the 1970s on the nature of pain led to the recognition of the syndrome known as intractable pain, a condition that is a problem in itself, separate from the circumstances that are the original cause. It has been estimated that 50 million Americans suffer from intractable pain. An increased understanding of the mechanism that produces it and the challenge of how to deal with it led to the introduction of alternative therapies into the bastions of traditional medical practice. Practically every prestigious medical center nationwide, from the Mayo Clinic to Columbia Presbyterian Hospital, established a multidisciplinary pain treatment center where, in addition to surgery and medication, therapies previously considered to be outside the mainstream began to be used routinely—hypnosis, biofeedback training, meditation, visualization—for behavior modification and for easing the withdrawal symptoms of patients who had become addicted to powerful prescription painkillers.

Alternative therapies have become especially popular among people suffering from lower back pain. They seek out specialists in body realignment who use the Alexander Technique or Rolfing or other practitioners who claim that faulty posture is the cause of most bodily discomfort.

With the rapid rise of musculoskeletal problems associated with the workplace and the epidemic in sports injuries, practitioners of unorthodox methods of body manipulation as well as conventionally trained physical therapists are very much in demand as an alternative to strong analgesics. Some may work with patients under the guidance of a medical specialist known as a physiatrist (pronounced fiz-e-AT-rist), who specializes in physical medicine and rehabilitation. Physiatrists emphasize prevention and treatment of disabilities secondary to injuries, and in devising a program for the rehabilitation of a patient who has had a ski accident, they are likely to recommend an unconventional exercise program as well as a series of acupuncture treatments to minimize pain.

The area in which alternative therapies are currently having a conspicuous success is stress management. For baby boomers now coping with teenage children or an aging parent with Alzheimer's disease, for single mothers working at two jobs, overextended corporate executives, men with migraine, women running for political office, life in the 1990s is no picnic. Stress can be pleasant, as in planning a daughter's wedding or preparing for a first trip to Paris; it can be so demanding as to be immobilizing, as in taking on an assignment with an impossibly tight deadline; or it can be self-generated by neglecting to meet one's own needs in fulfilling the needs of others. Instead of turning to sleeping pills or tranquilizers for a quick fix or counting on alcohol or cigarettes when they feel stressed beyond endurance, women are exploring the effectiveness of breathing exercises, meditation, Swedish massage, herbal infusions, aroma therapy, or visualization as a means to relaxation.

The scientific community admits that it has no unassailable explanations for the positive results achieved by many of the alternative therapies discussed in the pages that follow. It is increasingly recognized, however, that an optimistic *attitude* plays a critical role in the effectiveness of the treatment. It is also assumed that the expectation of a cure produces the placebo effect in which sick patients actually show improvement when they are led to believe that the sugar water they have been given is really a wonderful new medicine. And nobody really knows by what mechanisms the powerful "feel-good" substances called endorphins are released in the brain. The woman who tells her tai chi instructor that "just thinking about coming to your class makes me feel better" may have triggered something in her brain that really does diminish her bodily aches and pains.

Dr. Jerome D. Frank, professor emeritus of psychiatry at the Johns Hopkins School of Medicine, points out, "The profound implications of mind-body relationships in illness and healing have not been fully accepted by most Western physicians. Often they fail to recognize that a positive mental state, encouraged by the actions or words of a doctor or nonmedical healer, can promote healing, while a negative mental state can diminish or destroy a patient's faith in the healer as well as his expectation of cure. . . . Western doctors, captivated as they are by medical technology, often lose sight of the fact that, in the final analysis, the success of a cure depends on the healing powers within the patient. . . . They should focus more on how they can exert positive influences on the patient's mental state in order to promote his physical well-being."

At the forefront of research into the connection between the mind and the body's susceptibility to disease is Dr. David Felten, professor at the University of Rochester's School of Medicine and recipient of a MacArthur fellowship. His studies have revealed the network of communication between the body's immune and nervous systems, a network in which the neurotransmitters, immune cells, and hormones act as messengers between our feelings and thoughts, on the one hand, and our immune defenses, on the other.

From mounting anecdotal evidence and the amount of time and money being spent, the therapeutic accomplishments of body manipulation for musicians, of light therapy in counteracting winter depression, of support groups for cancer patients, and of pet therapy for practically everyone are compelling evidence that alternative treatments are playing an important role in reinforcing the mind-body connection.

CHOOSING AN ALTERNATIVE THERAPY

Before proceeding to a detailed examination of some of the more popular alternative therapies, it should be pointed out that they don't necessarily relate to each other. Some, like acupuncture and herbalism, have their beginnings in ancient Chinese medical practice. Some, like the Alexander Technique and Rolfing, are of comparatively recent origin and owe their acceptance to the crusading efforts of the founders whose names they bear. Chiropractic is very widely practiced, while reflexology is known to only a limited number of adherents. It should also be noted that most are noninvasive, so that even if they are not helpful, they are essentially harmless. However, some alternative therapies should be approached with caution. A well-meaning herbalist may recommend a concoction containing ingredients to which a small number of people may be seriously allergic. An overenergetic Rolfer might cause a great deal of physical pain to no purpose. In general, however, alternative therapies represent an expanded terrain of preventive and healing practice well worth exploring. Some have a do-it-yourself appeal that accounts for their widespread following. Several alternative therapies require the services of a trained practitioner or qualified instructor.

As you seek out practitioners, beware of extravagant claims, don't trust an alternative therapist who is unwilling to work with your primary care provider, check credentials and professional licensing or certification where relevant, don't be shy about discussing money, and be sure to be clear about your health insurance coverage. If your primary care physician is open-minded about the value of alternative procedures, discuss your intention to investigate them as a possible option that will eliminate the need for taking painkillers or tranquilizers. Many doctors now recommend not only psychologists and physical therapists but also chiropractors and acupuncturists. A referral to a properly accredited therapist usually entitles you to partial coverage under most health insurance policies. Even if you have a quarrel with conventional—or conservative—medical practice, don't fail to protect your well-being by scheduling regular checkups, including standard blood and urine tests, blood pressure readings, Pap smears, and mammograms.

A SAMPLING OF ALTERNATIVE THERAPIES

The therapies described below have achieved a broad acceptance not only among many women, but also among many physicians who recommend them as supplements, if not substitutes, for more traditional treatments. (See "Directory of Health Information" for listings of relevant organizations.)

ACUPRESSURE (or shiatsu)

This hands-on therapy is a type of Asian massage similar to acupuncture except that it uses finger pressure instead of needles to stimulate or, if necessary, to arrest the flow of vital energy along the channels delineated in acupuncture charts. The procedure, which originated in ancient Japan as a form of family treatment for aches and pains, has become increasingly popular in the United States. There are two types of acupressure: in one, several fingers are used simultaneously to massage specific parts of the body; in the other, one finger applies firm pressure to one or more acupuncture points. While acupressure can be learned as a self-help skill, it is advisable to test its effectiveness for a particular problem by visiting a skilled practitioner. Many women claim to have been relieved of headaches, muscular tension in the neck and shoulders, chronic leg cramps, and back discomfort after a series of 45-minute sessions. Claims are also made for the effective treatment of asthma, bronchitis, and some circulatory ailments. Shiatsu practitioners may combine their hands-on treatments with counseling on nutrition and stress management through relaxation techniques. Most licensed physical therapists include acupressure in their arsenal of treatments.

ACUPUNCTURE

Acupuncture is a technique of treating illness that originated in China perhaps as long ago as 3000 B.C. It is based on the theory that there is a neural connection between the organs of the body and certain specific areas on the body's surface. A tenderness in any of these areas, codified long ago as acupuncture points, indicates the presence of disease. In current practice, stainless steel needles as fine as hairs are inserted at these predetermined points—

by no means identical with the source of the pain—and twirled very quickly by hand or by electrical current. The needles may be left in place for only a few seconds or for as long as five minutes. Because they are inserted only a few millimeters into the skin, the procedure is not painful.

The traditional Chinese explanation for the effectiveness of acupuncture can be summed up as follows: The hundreds of acupuncture points are classified into 12 groups, and the points that are part of one of these 12 groups are connected by an imaginary line on the surface of the body. This line is called a meridian. The 12 most important meridians control most of the body's organs. The body's life forces are said to circulate along these meridians, and all diseases are ascribed to a disturbance in this process. The rotating needles are presumed to release energy that has been blocked, thereby restoring the body's recuperative balance.

Although there is no irrefutable scientific evidence to validate the physiological presence of acupoints or meridians, several important research efforts into the nature and mechanism of pain have pointed out that there is a remarkably high degree of correlation between acupuncture points and the trigger points for pain. Although the acupuncture points were discovered and labeled centuries ago, and the trigger points as recently as the 1970s, many researchers feel that they represent the same phenomenon, explainable by an underlying process of the nervous system. Several decades ago, investigators into what makes acupuncture work as a treatment for pain proposed that the action of the needles stimulated the release of endorphins. It has also been proposed that acupuncture activates a particular part of the brain that has a powerful inhibitory control over the pathways along which pain signals are transmitted. While acupuncture has been achieving some success as a treatment for addiction to nicotine and other drugs, there is little doubt about its effectiveness in alleviating pain originating in a variety of conditions. Success rates in cases where other methods have failed, or where patients prefer not to be treated with strong medications, range from 50 to 80 percent. Facial pain (trigeminal neuralgia), low back pain, some types of arthritis, tension headaches, dysmenorrhea, and postherpetic neuralgia (the acute pain that follows a shingles attack) are among the conditions in which varying degrees of success have been reported.

Because acupuncture is an invasive technique, it is extremely important to seek out a well-qualified practitioner, preferably a physician who uses disposable needles rather than needles that are sterilized and reused. Cases of bacterial infection and hepatitis B transmission have been reported, and the transmission of the AIDS virus is an ever-present risk. Each state has its own regulations governing the practice of acupuncture by physicians and nonphysicians. To locate a practitioner with proper credentials in your area, call the pain treatment center or the department of physical medicine and rehabilitation at the nearest teaching hospital, or write to the National Commission for the Certification of Acupuncturists, 1424 16th Street, NW, Washington, DC 20036; telephone (202) 232-1404.

ALEXANDER TECHNIQUE

The Alexander Technique is an educational discipline that teaches more effective use of the body by changing faulty posture habits. The change is accomplished through the student's recognition of inefficient movements that lead to fatigue and tension. The technique was developed in the 1890s by an Australian actor, F. Mathias Alexander, during a period when he was losing his voice. By standing in front of mirrors and taking a critical look at the way he had been moving his head, neck, and shoulders during stage performances, he realized that his tense and artificial postures were destroying his ability to produce his voice. From these beginnings on behalf of his own career, he went on to develop the technique that since the beginning of the century has been helping students to improve muscular coordination and eliminate body tension. Where the technique is successful, the result is greater ease and freedom of movement and a release of energy. In some cases the technique can lessen pain caused by incorrect posture. In the early days of his practice, Alexander himself taught the discipline to George Bernard Shaw and John Dewey. Today it counts among its enthusiasts prominent actors and musicians and is part of the curriculum of such institutes as the Juilliard School in New York, the American Conservatory Theatre in San Francisco, and the Royal College in London.

The Alexander Technique is not a series of treatments or exercises. It is usually taught in private lessons during which the teacher analyzes the way the student moves when sitting, walking, bending, reaching, lifting, and so on. With the verbal and hands-on guidance of the teacher, the student learns to identify faulty postural habits and to replace them with patterns of movement that reduce and eventually eliminate muscular tensions causing fatigue and pain. Students learn that in order to correct how they move, they have to think consciously about what they are doing that's wrong. In addition to individual instruction, some teachers conduct group classes and workshops. Fees range from $25 to $75 depending on the length and type of session. Practitioners of the Alexander Technique are trained and certified in schools both here and abroad, but since they are not state licensed, their fees are not likely to be covered by your health insurance provider. To locate a certified teacher in your area, consult the North American Society of Teachers of the Alexander Technique, PO Box 112484, Tacoma, WA 98411-2484; telephone (206) 627-3766.

AROMA THERAPY

Since time immemorial, folk medicine has claimed that certain aromatic oils derived from plants have curative powers, not only to heal the ills of the body but also to soothe and heal the troubled spirit. Depending on the nature of the problem, an oil derived from the roots, bark, leaves, or flowers of a plant is massaged into the skin. Or it may be swallowed or inhaled in the form of a vaporized mist. There is ample evidence in the literature of the ancient Egyptians, Greeks, and Romans that aroma therapy was an indispensable part of medical practice, and there are countless references in their writings as well as in the Bible to the restorative effect of fragrant oils on the soul in distress.

During the Middle Ages and through the eighteenth century, aromatics continued to be used as remedies, but eventually, with the development of the science of chemistry, many of the age-old practices were discarded in favor of medicines synthesized and standardized in the laboratory. It was not until 1920, when a Frenchman coined the term *aroma therapy* and wrote a scholarly book on the subject, that it began to be taken seriously, especially in France, where 40 years later another Frenchman wrote about his successful use of aromatic oils during World War II to hasten the healing of wounds and minimize scars. (In France today, the cost of aromatics used therapeutically is reimbursable by the government's health insurance.)

Since the 1960s aroma therapists have been attracting a growing number of adherents, and together with herbalists they now offer a codified pharmacopoeia of oils said to alleviate PMS, stress, sinus congestion, arthritic pain, depression, and chronic fatigue. At the same time that a growing body of anecdotal evidence is available to substantiate the effectiveness of aroma therapy, scientific investigators have discovered that some aromas lower blood pressure, others change brain wave patterns, and in specific instances where sporadic memory loss has become a pathological problem, certain smells associated with the patient's past can trigger a normal response. At the Memorial Sloan-Kettering Cancer Center in New York, a recent study of patients who were anxious about undergoing MRI procedures indicated that 75 percent were calmed by the scent of sweet vanilla. Researchers at Duke University

Medical Center reported that a mixture of five floral fragrances relieved tension and anxiety in a group of menopausal women between 45 and 60.

A popular application of aroma therapy is in body massage. Serious practitioners whose purpose is to alleviate pain or to promote a feeling of relaxation and well-being use hot compresses to open the pores of the skin for the penetration of the oil of choice during energetic manipulation of a particular part of the body.

One of the most attractive aspects of aroma therapy is that it can be a do-it-yourself adventure. But keep in mind that because pure aromatic oils are very expensive, only small amounts find their way into even the most expensive bath oils and soaps. By trial and error you can experiment with the various naturally scented oils now available in body and bath shops as well as in well-stocked health stores. For their use in curing bodily ills, you can find "treatment" charts in naturopathic shops that sell natural oil blends.

ART THERAPY

In the clinical sense, art therapy is one of the means through which individuals can express psychological distress, resolve unconscious conflicts, and convey their concerns about a life-threatening illness. Art therapy may or may not be used in connection with psychotherapy to foster self-awareness. Following such catastrophes as the Oklahoma City bombing, when people, especially children, may be at a loss for words, they are encouraged by trained counselors to relieve their stress by creating pictures that convey their feelings. A woman so traumatized by rape that she can scarcely speak can be guided to externalize her feelings of rage and humiliation through drawings. Participants in alcohol rehabilitation programs may be encouraged to free-associate through art therapy in order to cast some light on the damaging experiences of their early years that have caused their self-destructive behavior. Art therapy is also used to clarify some of the emotional problems that beset couples and families.

Art therapy had its origins more than 100 years ago when the connection between art and mental health gained recognition through the striking images created by institutionalized adults. By the 1960s spontaneous art expression had become a medium through which trained therapists could evaluate and consequently treat their patients. In 1969 the American Art Therapy Association was established as a membership organization. It sets standards for the profession, approves education and training programs, and maintains a list of members who qualify as registered art therapists. It also publishes two journals. Of the 4,000 members, 2,250 are registered by the association. Their professional qualifications, which include graduate studies in both psychology and art, as well as a supervised internship, entitle them to practice in psychiatric centers, drug and alcohol rehabilitation centers, prisons, residences for the mentally impaired, and hospices for the terminally ill.

If there is a need for a qualified art therapist in your community, or if you would like additional information about this profession, contact the American Art Therapy Association, 1202 Allenson Road, Mundelein, IL 60060; telephone: (708) 949-6064.

A spin-off of the formalized discipline of art therapy is the generalized concept of art *as* therapy. Art classes conducted in the evening for working women at the local "Y" or in adult education programs provide a means of self-expression that may be denied them on the job. Homemakers who have lost their sense of purpose when the nest is empty can find a new identity in creating drawings or paintings that reveal a talent never before expressed. At day care centers for the elderly, women who might otherwise be watching television are rejuvenated when they learn how to use art materials under the encouraging supervision of an art teacher.

Most of us can testify to the therapeutic value of going to museums, not only as an escape from the compelling routines of daily life but as a motivation for opening our eyes to the splendors of nature and to the infinite variety in the faces and forms of the human race. After looking and looking at great art, some of us have been inspired to become Sunday painters, and many family photographers have developed into high-level amateurs who are proud to show their work at community centers or libraries.

BIOFEEDBACK TRAINING

The term *feedback* entered the language in the early years of radio technology to refer to an information loop designed in such a way that the results of an activity are "fed back" to the point of origin for modification. The term is now widely used metaphorically when we want another person's reaction to our behavior so that we can suitably modify it.

The term *biofeedback*, which came into the language in the 1970s, is defined in the tenth edition of *Merriam-Webster's Collegiate Dictionary* as "the technique of making unconscious or involuntary body processes (as heartbeat or brain waves) perceptible to the senses (as by the use of an oscilloscope) in order to manipulate them by conscious mental control." Originally used in dream-sleep research during the early 1960s to teach subjects how to produce the alpha waves associated with a state of relaxed alertness, this technique has become a component in the treatment of such stress-related disorders as migraine headaches, insomnia, and asthma, as well as the rehabilitation of damaged muscles. It is estimated that there are currently 10,000 practitioners in the United States.

Biofeedback training, which may be conducted in a hospital, laboratory, or private practitioner's office, consists of the use of sophisticated equipment involving electrodes and oscilloscope screens. This equipment does not stimulate the brain or directly affect muscle relaxation. Through electrodes attached to various parts of the patient's body, muscle tension, hand temperature, heart rate, or brain waves are monitored, and the information is translated into visible signals on a screen or audible signals that the patient can hear. With the guidance of a trained therapist, the patient learns how to alter the signals little by little in order to gain conscious control over involuntary processes that have been the cause of headaches or asthma. The fact that this procedure puts the patient in control has a positive effect: it enables her to see herself not as the victim of an ailment but as someone who is gaining mastery over it by her own effort. When the training is successful (this may be a matter of 8 or 10 sessions along with practice at home), the patient learns how to control the body processes without the use of the biofeedback equipment. It turns out that with the right training, most of us are capable of what used to be thought achievable only through the lifelong discipline of yoga—the ascendancy of mind over matter!

Biofeedback training is being used with notable success in gaining control over migraine headaches and Raynaud's disease, in which the fingers become extremely painful when exposed to cold. Many women suffering from this ailment have learned through biofeedback training to improve the circulation in their hands. The training is usually conducted by licensed psychologists or physicians and is covered in part or in full by most health insurance providers. For a referral, consult your primary care physician or the roster of the nearest teaching hospital.

CHIROPRACTIC

To the many age-old methods of relieving bodily ills through hands-on manipulation was added the discipline known as chiropractic (the Greek word *cheir* means "hand"), which originated in 1895 with a Canadian healer, David

Palmer. We are told that he was able to restore the hearing of a workman who had been deaf for 17 years by manipulating the vertebrae in his neck. Palmer based his system of healing on the belief that all bodily ills resulted from misaligned spinal vertebrae, which he called subluxations. The therapeutic effect of his system of manipulation was the realignment of the vertebrae so that they no longer impeded the free flow of nervous impulses essential for physical well-being. In his most famous case, he manipulated the misaligned vertebrae in a way that reestablished the free flow of the impulses carried by the auditory nerve from the upper spine to the brain.

Following the news of Palmer's accomplishment, chiropractic attracted many adherents, and from that day to this it continues to inspire enthusiastic support and strong opposition. Even though establishment medicine views its more extravagant claims with disbelief, Americans hand over about $2.4 billion annually to chiropractors, with 1 in 20 people nationwide consulting a practitioner at least once a year. About half of all visits are for the alleviation of back pain.

Of the approximately 45,000 licensed chiropractors now in practice, there are only a few who cling militantly to the "single cause single cure" principle of the founding father, taking an adversarial stance toward accepted medical practice. This small but highly vocal hard-core group has given chiropractic a bad name among those who refuse to accept the claim that spinal manipulation can cure everything from bronchial asthma to cancer. There are also many chiropractors who call themselves "holistic" practitioners, functioning essentially as primary care health providers. For a devoted following, they make recommendations about nutrition, vitamins, stress management, and preventive health practices. They also recommend regular checkups so that any vertebrae that have gradually become misaligned without causing symptoms can be manipulated back into their proper place before the situation deteriorates. But no matter what principles they follow, chiropractors may not prescribe drugs or perform surgery, nor may they present themselves as diagnosticians who can treat diseases.

Today most chiropractors concern themselves with alleviating musculoskeletal problems whose solution lies in finding where in the spine the problem originates and, by manipulation, bringing the vertebrae into realignment. In addition to the hundreds of thousands of people they treat for chronic back pain, practitioners are busier than ever because of the increase in two categories of patients: women who sustain injuries during participation in active sports and women who are suffering from on-the-job repetitive stress injuries.

During a first visit the chiropractor usually listens to your complaint, takes a medical history, conducts a hands-on examination of your spinal column from your neck to your coccyx, makes a detailed analysis of your posture, tests your reflexes, and takes a series of X-rays and perhaps even an electrocardiogram. Manipulation, which may or may not be painful, proceeds on the basis of evaluating all this information. You have to be the judge of the improvement in your condition after two or three visits. If you are consulting a chiropractor through a referral, your primary care doctor should receive a detailed report about the results. Whatever the reason for your initial visit, be wary of extravagant claims, extensive X-rays, and the need for prolonged treatments.

If you connect with a chiropractor on your own or visit someone through a friend's recommendation, find out about credentials. There are at least 20 colleges of chiropractic nationwide that offer a broad-based curriculum in addition to concentrated training in manipulation skills. These colleges offer the degree known as doctor of chiropractic. If a practitioner's name is followed by a long string of letters, ask what they stand for. The designation D.C. after the name is the only one that's relevant. You can find out whether the practitioner is licensed to practice in your state by asking to see his or her license or by calling the state licensing board. Visits to a chiropractor are covered by worker's compensation in all states, by Medicaid and Blue Cross in most states, and partly covered by Medicare. Private insurance coverage varies from state to state. If you have any difficulty connecting with a properly accredited D.C., request a referral from the American Chiropractic Association, 1701 Clarendon Boulevard, Arlington, VA 22209.

DANCE/MOVEMENT THERAPY

Body movement is recognized universally not only as the way to celebrate major events and to strengthen community bonds, but also as a powerful medium through which the troubled mind and ailing body can be healed. The ancient ritual of dancing oneself into a trance to receive a divine message or to exorcise evil spirits continues in our own times among various religious sects. Some cultural historians believe that dance was the original inspiration for all other forms of creative expression, especially for music and the rhythmic verbal chanting that evolved into poetry.

The development of what has come to be known as dance/movement therapy (DMT) originated in the years following the First World War, when all forms of expression were concerned with providing an outlet for previously unexpressed deep emotions. In the modern dances created during the 1920s and 1930s, choreographers broke away from the formalism of traditional ballet and the wholesome patterns of folk dancing to externalize feelings beyond the scope of verbal expression.

By the 1940s Marian Chace, a dance teacher in Washington, D.C., noticed that emotionally disturbed children in her classes were deriving therapeutic benefits from this wordless form of expression. Psychiatrists who became aware of Chace's accomplishments invited her to work at Washington's St. Elizabeth's Hospital with patients who were too mentally ill to participate in any group activities. At about the same time, the internationally known dancer and mime Trudi Schoop volunteered to introduce noncommunicative patients in a California state hospital to the healing benefits of dance/movement therapy.

With increasing recognition of the benefits of this form of treatment, the American Dance Therapy Association was established in 1956. It now has a membership of more than 1,100 members, publishes a journal, creates the guidelines for graduate education, and monitors the standards for professional practice. The association also maintains a registry for therapists indicating their level of training and experience in clinical work. The accreditation DTR (Dance Therapist Registered) indicates a master's degree and 700 hours of supervised internship; the designation ADTR (Academy of Dance Therapists Registered), awarded on completion of twice that amount of supervised clinical work, qualifies the dance therapist to teach, supervise, and conduct a private practice.

Dance/movement therapists work with a broad range of patients, from disturbed and traumatized children to withdrawn elderly women in nursing homes who suffer from an absence of stimulation. Through guided body movements, therapists help psychiatric patients express their fears and anxieties, form emotional attachments, and develop a healthier self-image. Severely disturbed women may be encouraged to clap their hands and stamp their feet without the guidance of music so that they can discover their own body rhythms. Dance and movement therapy are also the means for promoting the physical coordination of people with neuromuscular disabilities, thereby bolstering their self-esteem and overcoming their fear of social situations. This therapeutic mode is also used to hasten the healing of muscles and joints whose function has been impaired by a serious accident or injury. Recent studies indicate that in changing how people move, whether individually or in a group, dance/movement therapy provides a healthy outlet for emotional expression, thereby fostering keener self-awareness and promoting more positive social attitudes. It has been shown to decrease depression and bodily tension, to reduce pain, and by stimulating the circulatory and respiratory systems, to promote physical healing.

Most of us have experienced the positive effects of dance and movement without the guidance of a professionally qualified therapist. Classes in social dancing can overcome shyness and develop one's social skills. Participation in aerobic dance groups can increase physical fitness, and folk dancing can promote mutually supportive group solidarity. But these activities should not be confused with the professional accomplishments of dance/movement therapy.

If your community needs a professionally accredited dance therapist for an adult or children's day care center or a nursing home, or if you would like to locate such a therapist in your area for private consultation, call the psychiatric or rehabilitation department at your local hospital, or write to the American Dance Therapy Association, 2000 Century Plaza, Columbia, MD 21044; telephone: (410) 997-4040.

GARDENS AND GARDENING AS THERAPY

You'd never guess it from the media's catering to the male obsession with sports, but the most popular leisure pursuit in the United States is gardening. Making things grow satisfies a wide range of emotional, physical, and practical needs, and for many of us it has a spiritual component not easily put into words. A recent arrival from an Irish farm connects with her new urban environment by creating a "kitchen garden" of herbs in her tenement window boxes; a city-bred woman enjoys her suburban life because it provides better opportunities not only for growing children, but also for satisfying a passion for nurturing a rose garden. Childhood memories of seasonal flower beds are revived by re-creating these plantings on a smaller scale. Women who sit in an office all day consider the physical demands of gardening their most productive form of exercise: they gain not only food and flowers, but also fitness from stretching, bending, and working the soil. In an ethnically and economically diverse neighborhood, planting an urban garden unites residents who hold widely divergent opinions about practically everything else. Through the ongoing project of providing an oasis for young and old alike, they have learned to work together for the common good.

The therapeutic power of gardens and gardening has recently been rediscovered by hospitals and rehabilitation centers nationwide, from the haphazard plantings attached to Bellevue Medical Center in New York to the two-acre meditation garden at the Norris Cancer Center in Los Angeles. In a 1994 *New York Times* interview, Dr. Sam Bass-Warner, a professor of environmental studies at Brandeis University, observed that throughout history the idea of gardens and gardening as therapy has waxed and waned. He points out,

"Wherever medicine has no magic—for AIDS or cancer or mental illness—gardens reappear. When we think science can do it all, they vanish."

The ancient Greeks as well as the men and women in medieval cloisters recognized that walking or meditating in a garden was a source of comfort and solace for the distressed spirit. But as medical science advanced and the antiseptic principle was enthroned in a sterile environment, involvement with nature was no longer considered a relevant aspect of healing.

"Would you rather be in a sterile hospital room squeezing a rubber ball, or in that hospital's greenhouse trimming a boxwood or working with a bonsai?" asks Steven H. Davis, executive director of the American Horticultural Therapy Association, whose 750 members promote the use of plants and gardening as part of a patient's psychological and physical treatment plan.

The Rusk Institute for Rehabilitation Medicine in New York City has been at the forefront of the integration of horticulture and health care. Early in 1970 the institute, which is part of the New York University Medical Center, provided a garden where patients and visitors could spend time with each other in an atmosphere of peace and quiet. Patients could also ask to be transported to this tranquil environment in their wheelchairs, if need be, in order to enjoy the solitude and natural beauty of the garden as a relief from the germ-free environment of their rooms. More recently, the area has been considerably enlarged to accommodate a raised enclosure where wheelchair-bound patients recovering from a stroke or a debilitating injury are guided by horticultural therapists in the cultivation of their own plot of soil. This method of improving motor skills and coordination, as well as increasing physical endurance, reducing pain perception, and hastening recovery, continues to be very popular with patients and staff alike.

We all know that there is a long tradition of humanizing a hospital room with gifts of flowers and plants. What is less well known is that there are impressive figures indicating that a patient whose bed is next to a window with a view of attractive landscaping is likely to make a speedier recovery than a patient who faces a wall.

If your community has a health care facility—a general hospital, nursing home, day care center for the elderly or children, or drug and alcohol rehabilitation clinic—its volunteer workers and professionals can contribute to everyone's well-being by promoting the use of horticulture on a small scale, by showing children as well as recovering substance abusers that they have the power to make things grow. Another possibility is to initiate a community fund for creating a hospital garden, benefiting patients and their visiting friends and families.

HERBALISM

Herbalism is the belief that for practically every ailment or injury there exists a green plant or some part of a green plant that provides the proper treatment. Roots, leaves, flowers, and bark have been used in medicinal preparations throughout the ages to maintain health, cure sickness, and heal the disturbed spirit. They have also been the effective means for contraception and abortion. Herbalism has been and continues to be the foundation of folk medicine historically as well as currently in most of the preindustrialized world. The World Health Organization estimates that four billion people—80 percent of the planet's population—use herbal medicine for some aspect of primary health care. It has also attracted countless adherents in the West among people who are opposed to the use of synthetic medicines because they contain "chemicals" or because medicines made in a laboratory aren't "natural."

To begin with, all substances are made up of chemicals, no matter whether created in a laboratory or found in nature. But more important still is the fact that Mother Nature is by no means dependably benign. There are many obvious examples of her double-dealing. She gives us aloes to soothe the skin and poison ivy to irritate it; some chrysanthemums yield the ingredients for aromatic tea, and others are the source of pyrethrum, the active poison in many insecticides. Although individually monitored amounts of digitalis, which is extracted from the foxglove, keep many heart patients alive, an overdose is fatal.

This underlines one of the chief dangers of herbalism as currently practiced and promoted. Although an herbal compound might be helpful in the right amount or over a limited amount of time, prolonged use or use in excessive amounts can be life-threatening. A second danger is that many of the companies that produce and package herbal preparations are not properly monitored for the purity and potency of their products. Experts at the Nutrition Information Center of Cornell Medical Center in New York have pointed out that some herbs that are edible when immature are poisonous at maturity. Growing conditions, harvesting time, and storage practices can yield highly variable results. Nonetheless, there are many herbal remedies that can be helpful without being risky at all. Feverfew, traditionally used to reduce fever and alleviate cold symptoms, now has the approval of many physicians as an effective treatment for migraine headaches. Ginger root, long recommended to settle an upset stomach, has been shown to minimize motion sickness. Clinical studies indicate that preparations derived from licorice root are effective treatment for some cases of tuberculosis. Garlic shows up in the pharmacopeias of practically all folk medicine. Concentrations have been shown to cure amebic dysentery, and laboratory studies claim that garlic juice has a strong inhibitory effect on many bacteria.

The first international symposium on the health effects of drinking tea, especially green tea, was conducted in New York in 1991 under the auspices of the American Health Foundation, an independent nonprofit research organization, and two groups representing the tea industry. Reports of the health benefits of drinking tea, the world's most popular beverage, were based on research with laboratory animals, as well as on the disease rates among tea-drinking people in various countries. Preliminary findings that are being subjected to close scientific scrutiny report that tea, which is processed in three types—black, green, and oolong—contains various chemicals that may block the actions of many carcinogens, inhibit the growth of malignant tumors, lower blood pressure and cholesterol levels, and kill decay-causing bacteria. To date, most studies have been based on green tea, the type most popular in Japan, where heavy consumers of green tea have lower death rates from all types of cancer than the general population. What is involved in these studies is *real* tea, which comes from the plant *Camellia sinensis*, and not any of the concoctions known as herbal teas.

By far the most exciting development in herbalism was the subject of another symposium organized in January 1992 by the New York Botanical Garden's Institute of Economic Botany and the Rain Forest Alliance, a nonprofit conservation organization. At the same time that medical researchers in the United States have been turning in ever-increasing numbers to plants in the hope of finding cures for cancer, AIDS, and heart disease, many plants are disappearing faster than they can be investigated because of tropical deforestation. The Rain Forest Alliance was formed to halt the transformation of tropical forests into farmland and to provide economic motivation for preserving them. The alliance is made up of major pharmaceutical companies, conservationists, research scientists, and traditional healers, as well as the governments and entrepreneurs of developing countries. Plant prospectors are spurred on by knowledge of the discovery in the 1930s of the curare plant, which provides an effective muscle relaxant; the discovery that the rosy periwinkle can be used to treat childhood leukemia; and most recently the isolation of a cancer-fighting compound derived from a tropical tree. In some efforts governments are hiring local people familiar with the forests and training them to learn the various plants on which to base research. In 1994 the government in Belize in Central America approved the formation of the 6,000-acre Terra Verde Medicinal Plant

Reserve, dedicated to the preservation of medicinal plants. Traditional healers are permitted to harvest these plants and to teach students at the reserve how to prepare and use them.

Among the many pharmaceutical companies who are exploring herbal cures is the appropriately named Shaman Pharmaceuticals, whose president says, "We are driven exclusively by ethnobotany," a strategy that enabled the company in only 18 months to isolate from a medicinal plant in South America the compound that it claims can actively fight a number of viruses, including those of the flu and herpes. Under the auspices of the National Institutes of Health, the U.S. government has provided grants for the study of endangered plants to university researchers, environmental organizations, pharmaceutical companies, and government agencies in the hope of finding treatments for AIDS and cancer. More than 20 organizations are participating in this effort, which unites American scientists with their counterparts in Argentina, Cameroon, Chile, Costa Rica, Mexico, and Suriname.

Ethnobotany is the current designation for these studies of the traditional ways in which different races or groups of people use plants, and we can expect to hear a great deal more about it in the future. Of course, herbalists can claim that they already know all about it.

NOTE: The dangers of self-treatment with herbal remedies received nationwide attention in 1995, when the *Journal of the American Medical Association* published a report by doctors at the University of Chicago Hospital that described a case of kidney and liver destruction caused by the herbal remedy known as chaparral. The patient had been increasing her doses of a preparation made from the leaves of this plant in the mistaken notion that it would cure her coronary artery disease. Although in 1992, because of reports of its toxic effect on the liver, chaparral had been removed from the FDA's list of substances "generally recognized as safe," it was still easily available in the Chicago area. (The patient's survival was made possible by a liver transplant.)

The same issue of the AMA journal contained a list of many herbal products said to be toxic to the human liver. Among the substances listed were comfrey, pennyroyal, and maté tea. Hepatitis is also said to be caused by a Chinese product called Jin Bu Huan.

Because herbs are officially categorized by the FDA as foods rather than drugs, they are not subject to the agency's rules on safety, effectiveness, and side effects. While many herbs sold in health food stores and pharmacies may be harmless in small doses, others contain ingredients that, if ingested in large doses, can cause stroke, arrhythmias, and other life-threatening conditions. They may also result in sleep disorders, anxiety, and general listlessness.

If you are in doubt about an herbal remedy, call the Herbal Research Foundation (1-800-748-2617).

HOMEOPATHY

Homeopathy is a system of treatment developed in the nineteenth century by a German physician, Dr. Samuel Hahnemann, who was reacting against such barbaric "cures" as bloodletting and purging. It is based on four principles: (1) Substances that produce symptoms similar to those experienced by the patient will cure the patient. (Hahnemann called this the Law of Similars.) (2) Only one dose of the substance is needed. (3) A minimum dose is the most potent dose. (4) In order to attain homeostasis—a relative state of equilibrium within the body—the patient must be relied on to set in motion dynamic vital forces.

Translated into practice, homeopathy uses extremely diluted natural substances derived from plants, animals, and minerals. If these substances were taken in large quantities, they would cause the condition to worsen, but in diluted form they are said to stimulate the body to heal itself. Homeopathic "medicines," which are used by practitioners and are also sold in health food stores and many old-fashioned pharmacies, are produced in the following way: An extract of the substance recommended by the approved Homeopathic Pharmacopeia of the United States for a particular condition is combined with water or water and alcohol in dilutions ranging from 1 part in 10 to 1 part in 10,000. The mixture is shaken vigorously for a specified time, then diluted in the same proportions and shaken again. This procedure of diluting and shaking continues until it seems unlikely that even a vestige of the original extract remains. The explanation for the curative power of the diluted substance is that the shaking safeguards the "molecular memory" necessary to effect the cure.

Although there is a vast amount of anecdotal evidence to support the effectiveness of homeopathic cures and occasionally a success (that turns out to defy duplication) is reported in scientific journals, homeopathic results are dismissed by conventional physicians because the procedures used don't meet scientific standards. At best they can be attributed to the placebo effect.

This negative attitude is less widespread in other parts of the world. In France, 32 percent of family physicians use homeopathy; in Great Britain, 42 percent of physicians refer their patients to homeopaths. And in this country, as yet another aspect of the movement toward alternative therapies, there has been a resurgence of interest in homeopathy. The homeopathic drug industry has become a multimillion-dollar enterprise. These drugs, now recognized and regulated by the FDA, are manufactured by established pharmaceutical companies under the guidelines laid down in the homeopathic pharmacopeia. They are available not only in health food stores but also in many reputable pharmacies.

There are currently more than 3,0000 homeopathic practitioners in the United States licensed according to state-by-state "scope of practice" guidelines. Under these guidelines, a wide range of health providers may be entitled to practice homeopathic medicine, ranging from M.D.s, dentists, and chiropractors, to nurse practitioners and acupuncturists. At present, only Arizona, Connecticut, and Nevada have specific licensing boards for homeopathic physicians.

While a visit to a homeopathic practitioner for a minor ailment such as an allergy or persistent cold can do little harm, such conditions as a chronic cough or immobilizing headaches might require sophisticated diagnostic procedures to exclude the possibility of tuberculosis or a brain tumor.

The professional organization to consult for information about self-help, training courses, and referrals is the National Center for Homeopathy, 801 N. Fairfax Street, Alexandria, VA 22314; telephone: (703) 548-7790. This organization does not provide any free information. It does offer a comprehensive kit that costs about six dollars. Your local library may provide much of this information free of charge.

HYDROTHERAPY

Hydrotherapy is the use of water and steam to promote well-being and to cure various ailments. Most of us are the beneficiaries of hydrotherapy in one form or another: a relaxing end-of-the-day soak in a perfumed bath for the relief of mental stress or muscular discomfort; the use of a humidifier for a sore throat, of a Jacuzzi for sore feet, of the health club pool for an invigorating early morning swim. Women are especially aware of the soothing effects of water and the special advantages of underwater exercise.

A permanent testament to the curative powers of taking "the waters" is the ancient town of Bath in England, originally a miniature Roman city built around the hot springs presumed to be both medicinal and sacred. During the years of the Roman occupation, invalids came to this sanctuary from all over Britain and from overseas to enjoy the benefits of its bubbling natural waters. Although the town of Spa in Belgium, which specialized in drinking cures, not in bathing, has deteriorated since its nineteenth-century renown, it has become the generic term for vacation retreats that specialize in hydrotherapy. In many parts of the United States, Mexico, and South America, these retreats have been proliferating. Depending on the range of services and specialties offered, they range from the affordable to the last word in luxury. Spa vacations have become increasingly popular because their varied water treatments not only have a healing effect on lower back pain, overworked muscles, and arthritic joints, but also wash away the debilitating effects of daily stress. The pleasant surroundings and agreeable personnel who make an effort to pamper the women in their charge have immeasurable positive effects as well.

In addition to special "cleansing" diet plans, exercise routines that include outdoor hikes, meditation sessions, and health-oriented lectures, here are the hydrotherapy procedures offered by most spas:

Underwater massage, during which you lie in a bath while your weightless body is "massaged" by strong jets of pressurized water.

Aerated baths, in which the constant bubbling produces the relaxing effect of a foam bath without the use of a detergent.

Needle sprays, in which very fine sprays of alternating hot and cold water stimulate the circulation.

Also popular are *algae and seaweed wrappings* followed by an aromatic massage; *salt rubs,* in which the body is completely and energetically rubbed with salt and then hosed down with cold water from a distance of five feet; *Turkish baths,* which produce the beneficial results of heavy sweating.

At most traditional German and Italian spas, as well as at our own time-honored Saratoga Springs in New York and Hot Springs in Arkansas, drinking the healthful "mineral waters" has always been an essential part of "taking the cure." Many of these establishments also continue to offer the traditional "cleansing" procedure known as *colonic irrigation,* in which the large intestine is thoroughly washed out with slightly pressurized water. In the United States, this ancient practice, frequently performed by naturopathic practitioners, is currently embroiled in a legal dispute attempting to limit it to licensed physicians.

Many women, recognizing that two weeks at a spa may be as expensive as a year's membership in a local health club, opt for the latter, where hydrotherapy in its many forms is one of the chief offerings. In shopping around for a health club that best satisfies your needs in terms of convenience and price, it is important to get as much information as possible in advance about the facilities and qualified personnel. If a request to inspect the premises before you pay for a membership causes any problems, it is advisable to look else-where.

Most economical and convenient of all the ways to enjoy the advantages of hydrotherapy is to turn your own bathroom into a private spa. This can be accomplished at very little expense by investing in a portable "bathtub spa" that provides whirlpools, bubblers, and water jet attachments—none of which need to be built into bathroom fixtures. Although hardheaded consumer advocates and many physical therapists do not believe that home spas are therapeutically superior to a warm bath or a bracing shower, they generally agree that bathtub spas provide excellent treatment for an aching back, tired feet, and arthritic joints. Another positive effect: the privacy and easy accessibility of hydrotherapy at home help you handle the stressful demands of daily life.

CAUTIONARY NOTES: Since the combination of water and electricity can be extremely dangerous, the manufacturers of home spa equipment have tried to ensure that safety devices are built into the design of their products. It is equally important that users pay the strictest attention to instructions for safe operation.

Women who are pregnant or those who have diabetes or some other chronic condition should not use bathroom spa equipment until they have consulted their doctor.

HYPNOSIS

Gone are the days when the mention of hypnosis conjured up scenes of demonic control by one person over another, of a Hollywood heroine "put into a trance" by a maniacal villain. A majority of medical and dental schools now teach hypnosis technique, and there are about 15,000 health professionals who use it to help their patients stop smoking, overcome fear of flying, and, most frequently, control sensations of pain. (The use of hypnosis by psychiatrists as what was presumed to be a reliable method of helping their patients recall the traumatic experiences of childhood is now being widely attacked because it appears to be encouraging many women to fictionalize their early years.)

The origin of hypnosis goes back to ancient rituals of religion and healing, rituals that to this day continue to be practiced in many parts of the world, including the United States. An eighteenth-century physician, Dr. Franz Mesmer, believed that the hypnotic state could be induced through what he called "animal magnetism" and promoted it as a scientific cure for a long list of mental and physical ailments. Hence the term "to mesmerize."

As the practice of medicine became more scientific, hypnotism was discredited. Over many decades it remained the province of theatrical entertainers and a number of diehard enthusiasts, among whom were nonmedical "healers" as well as reputable psychiatrists who found it a productive tool in patient treatment. In 1958, largely through the efforts of this latter group, the American Medical Association acknowledged its usefulness as therapy. Twenty years later, in 1978, hypnotism had moved sufficiently into the medical mainstream that chronic pain patients at the Veterans Administration Hospital in San Francisco underwent a hypnosis training program during which they were taught the techniques for controlling pain perception. By 1980 it was reported that hypnotherapy was being used for more than half the patients being treated at the pain clinic of Walter Reed Army Medical Center. Nowadays, the procedure is widely used not only for pain management, but also to allay anxiety, eliminate warts, reduce the discomfort of allergic reactions, and control bleeding during dentistry.

It turns out that the critical component in achieving the hypnotic state is the patient's ability to remain alert in order to focus intently on the hypnotist's suggestions instead of focusing on the sensation of pain. Here are some of the experiences the patient undergoes as the hypnotic state deepens: At the same time that there is a loss of awareness of the immediate surroundings, there is increased awareness of such body functions as breathing and pulse. Openness to the hypnotist's suggestions is heightened so that if, for example, she tells the patient that his right arm—which has been extremely painful—is cool because it is immersed in cold water, he focuses on the sensation of coldness rather than on the sensation of pain. Or if, for example, a patient's reason for consulting a hypnotist is her desire to stop smoking, she will be instructed to focus on images of herself without a cigarette or tossing an unopened package of cigarettes into the trash.

Levels of suggestibility vary from person to person. It seems that the best subjects enjoy a vivid fantasy life and are capable of sustained visualization. A leading expert in medical hypnosis, Dr. Herbert Spiegel, has introduced the concept of measuring the patient's trance capacity so that treatment strategy can be properly planned. He has created a five-minute hypnotic induction test that measures the patient's hypnotizability on a scale of 1 to 16. Those on the high end of the scale can eventually learn how to achieve the trance state on their own after a few sessions with the therapist, thereby gaining control over pain perception, anxiety about flying, or other negative aspects of their lives.

If you would like to investigate hypnosis as an alternative to heavy medication or as an aid to behavior modification, ask your doctor for a referral to a psychiatrist or a licensed psychologist trained in the technique. Since many states have no licensing requirements for those who practice hypnotism, beware of flashy advertising or "holistic specialists" without reputable credentials. A reliable source for a referral in your area is the American Society for Clinical Hypnosis, 2200 E. Devon Avenue, Des Plaines, IL 60018-4534; telephone: (708) 297-3317.

LIGHT THERAPY

The feelings of depression that set in for millions of Americans, especially women, as the days grow shorter and the weather grows drearier are no longer known as "the winter blahs." They have been tagged with the designation SAD, an appropriate acronym that stands for seasonal affective disorder, for which the remedy is one or another form of light therapy. Women who suffer from SAD usually live in the northern states, and as winter approaches, they begin to manifest the same set of symptoms: they feel increasingly lethargic, can't seem to get enough sleep, even with afternoon naps, and want to eat a lot more than usual, especially carbohydrates. One woman known to be a powerhouse during the hottest weather said that when daylight saving time came to an end, she would become "all fat and grumpy and lazy like a bear."

When a three-year study of 160 women suffering from SAD was undertaken in 1982 by the National Institute of Mental Health, Dr. Norman Rosenthal, the research psychiatrist who directed the study, found that, in addition to overeating and oversleeping, these women lost interest in sex, social activities, and work. In another study of the same problem undertaken more recently by the New York State Psychiatric Institute at Columbia-Presbyterian Medical Center, it was reported that SAD patients didn't improve without treatment until March or April, when the days become significantly longer.

The treatment that eliminated most SAD symptoms for both groups of women was two hours a day of light therapy from fall until spring. Light therapy consists of exposure to 10,000 lux of white fluorescent lights usually contained in a box. It is possible to sleep through the therapy because the light, which is as bright as sunlight at sunrise, can reach the retina through closed eyes. Dr. Michael Terman, who originated the winter depression program at Columbia-Presbyterian Medical Center and continues to be its director, says, "The best studies show 75 to 80 percent clinical remission of winter depression. We're talking about days before you see clinical benefits, rather than weeks or even months with proven medication for depression."

This type of light therapy is also being used successfully to treat insomnia, jet lag, and the body-clock disturbances associated with working the night shift.

If you think you're a candidate for light therapy, the first thing you should know is that you can't make up the deficiency of exposure to natural sunlight by sitting under a sun lamp or using a reflector to benefit from the sun's ultraviolet rays. This kind of exposure puts you at risk not only for skin cancer but for cataracts as well. Among the commercially available lights recommended for use in treating SAD are Vita-Lites and the Ultra-Bright 10,000. The latest development in home equipment is the Bedroom Illuminator created by the same company that manufactures Ultra-Bright. The new equipment consists of a "sky cover" programmed to grow dimmer as you go to sleep and to provide full sunrise at the time of awakening. When you wake up at the dawn signal, the light therapy session is over for the day.

MASSAGE

Massage therapy is the scientific manipulation of the soft tissues of the body with the goal of promoting the body's ability to heal itself. It is one of the oldest health care procedures, advocated in 4,000-year-old Chinese medical tracts and in continuous use in the Western world since the time of Hippocrates.

Scientific massage therapy was introduced to Americans in the 1850s by two physicians, the brothers Charles and George Taylor, who during their studies in Sweden were impressed by the health-promoting aspect of systematic body manipulation. After the Civil War, when the Swedish Health Institute was opened in Washington, D.C., it enjoyed the regular patronage of President Ulysses Grant and President Benjamin Harrison, as well as members of Congress.

Massage therapy continued to be a popular aspect of health care until the medical profession, including nurses and physical therapists, abandoned it in favor of more "scientific" cures. A small number of therapists, mainly European practitioners who settled in the United States, kept the tradition alive. It wasn't until the 1970s that the growing interest in healthier life-styles and alternative treatments resulted in a proliferation of massage therapists nationwide. By 1993 it was estimated that 20 million Americans had received massage therapy, and along with relaxation techniques and chiropractic, it has become the most widely used type of alternative treatment for 34 percent of the population. The popularity of massage therapy is based on its cost effectiveness in treating pain, reducing anxiety, and promoting relaxation.

Of the approximately 80 different methods now classified as massage therapy, only a small fraction can be described as traditional. The greater number date from the comparatively recent explosion of interest in alternative therapies of all kinds, during which new practitioners have developed methods based on healing traditions from other cultures, adding their own creative spin to ancient hands-on techniques.

Touch is the essential ingredient in all methods of massage. The effective practitioner not only applies pressure; her fingers must be sensitive enough to locate muscle tension and to know how much pressure is suitable for each individual. Excessive pressure causes the body to defend itself by flexing already tense muscles, thereby increasing rather than diminishing the tension. Methods in current use are divided into two categories:

Traditional European methods, of which Swedish massage is the main example, use these categories of soft tissue manipulation: gliding strokes, kneading, rubbing, and percussion.

Contemporary Western methods, which go beyond traditional methods and goals, include deep tissue massage, manual lymph drainage, neuromuscular massage, myofascial release (see "Rolfing"), and other touch techniques said to promote the emotional release essential for achieving a healthy balance of mind, body, and spirit. It has become increasingly popular to combine aroma therapy with massage to enhance the effects of both.

Although the services of a masseur or masseuse are offered by all spas, most local health clubs, and a growing number of comprehensive beauty salons, not all these practitioners are qualified health professionals. However, with the continuing growth of the massage therapy profession, a system of credentials has been put in place. As of 1994, it is estimated that there are approximately 50,000 qualified practitioners in the United States. Nineteen states have licensing requirements. Licensing is based on the completion of 500 hours of education in a recognized school program and passing a licensing examination. The American Massage Therapy Association is the primary sponsor of national licensing and accreditation programs. For referral to a fully qualified massage therapist in your area, or for additional information about massage therapy, contact the association at 820 Davis Street Suite 100, Evanston, IL 60201-4444; telephone: (708) 864-0123.

MEDITATION

Meditation as a discipline has been practiced for centuries as a way of purifying the mind and achieving a higher level of consciousness. More recently it has attracted the attention of many health professionals who are recommending it as a way of managing stress, relieving insomnia, controlling pain (especially of migraine headaches), and even overcoming mild depression. What once seemed to some people a questionable pursuit of the 1960s is now attracting followers in increasing numbers because they find it an effective alternative to tranquilizers, sleeping pills, and painkillers. Also, once the technique is mastered, it offers a reliable sanctuary where one can escape—if only for 15 minutes—from the excessive demands of one's daily routine.

There are no hard-and-fast rules for learning how to meditate effectively. Find a place that's free of distracting noises and disturbing interruptions. If you think soothing sound would be helpful, you can make a selection from a wide assortment of tapes or records marketed for this purpose. In choosing a position, find one in which you are relaxed and comfortable but also alert. Some women choose to lie on the floor; some prefer to sit in a chair that has a back support, with their legs together and their hands lying lightly in their lap. Others like sitting on the floor with their back straight against the wall, legs stretched out, and ankles crossed. For those who know yoga postures, the lotus position seems most suitable. Having arrived at a relaxed posture that enables you to take full breaths, close your eyes and concentrate on breathing deeply and slowly, taking air in through your nose and exhaling through your nose or mouth. You can count with each breath, concentrating on the rhythm as it becomes slower and more regular. This concentration on a single physical event enables you to empty your mind. These are the two phases of meditation: the body sufficiently relaxed so that the mind is focused and empty. When the technique is mastered, the result should be a feeling of tranquility and a state of well-being.

The first few attempts to achieve this calm may be hampered by mental habits that are hard to break. Instead of fighting the ideas and images that flit into and out of your consciousness, continue to focus attention on your breathing. Some women find that focusing on a candle flame, the repetition of a single sound, or the repeated sound of a musical phrase produces the desired result. With practice, most women can learn to meditate and achieve an oasis of calm.

MUSIC THERAPY

The ability to create music and enjoy it is surely one of the blessings of humanity. Beyond the pleasures of music, however, is what can only be called its magical power to alleviate sorrow and pain and to promote healing. The role of music as therapy has been recognized throughout history, and every culture is replete with myths and metaphors that pay tribute to this power.

It is assumed that hand-clapping and foot-stamping with or without chanting were used by tribal members and witch doctors to exorcise a sick person's demons. (This tradition continues into the present among many religious cults.) We know from the text of the Old Testament that "when the evil spirit from God was upon Saul, David took up a harp and played with his hand, so Saul was refreshed, and was well, and the evil spirit departed from him." And our own culture has been enriched by the spirituals and the blues created by African Americans as a form of self-healing.

Over the past century, there have been many books and academic studies attesting to the curative role of music for the very old, the very young, and the very ill. But only recently have scientific studies revealed that music memory is stored in a different part of the brain than verbal memory. This explains the fact that people who cannot be reached by words as a result of a stroke or a brain injury or who are suffering from mental illness or Alzheimer's disease can respond to songs that trigger musical memories. Music therapists point out, "Songs are not just songs; they embody life experiences, bringing back memories of childhood games, participating in a school glee club, a courtship, a wedding, war experiences." In fact, the profession of music therapy began when the Veterans Administration hospitals incorporated music into the program for rehabilitating soldiers who were returning from the battlefields of World War II. It is now widely used in psychiatric hospitals, mental health facilities, residences for people with developmental disabilities, nursing homes, rehabilitation programs for substance abusers, and prisons. The therapist is trained to assess the physical, mental, and emotional capabilities of each individual so that an appropriate program can be devised. Such a program might include improvising songs, moving alone or in a group to music, pounding on a drum, playing an instrument, or after listening to music, discussing one's fantasies in a one-to-one session with the therapist.

Many studies continue to document the therapeutic role of music: it promotes quicker recovery by diminishing stress following a heart attack; when used to relax patients before and after an operation, it reduces the need for heavy doses of tranquilizers and painkillers. It is especially helpful in energizing elderly patients so that they are distracted from pain and concentrate on their rehabilitating exercises. Then comes the news from an article in the *Journal of the American Medical Association,* which concludes that many surgeons do a better job when they are operating to the accompaniment of music of their own choosing! (Some like rock and roll; others prefer opera.)

Every woman has her own stories to tell about the important role of music in fostering her emotional and physical health from childhood on: one will talk about the comforting memories of her mother's lullabies; another remembers that joining a church choir helped her overcome her depression; still another says she was finally able to stop smoking when she began to play the flute.

If your community would benefit from the services of a qualified music therapist, or if you would like to arrange for a consultation with a board-certified private practitioner for yourself or a member of your family, consult the National Association for Music Therapy. Established in 1950, the association sets the professional standards for education, training, internship programs, and ethical procedures. There are more than 5,000 music therapists (RMTs) in the association's registry. For a referral, write to the National Association for Music Therapy, 8455 Colesville Road, Silver Springs, MD 20910; telephone (301) 589-3300.

NATUROPATHY

Naturopathic medicine is a distinct system of health care that treats and restores well-being through the use of a variety of "natural" alternative therapies. It originated in the United States over 100 years ago, and by the early 1900s most states were granting licenses to naturopathic practitioners whose treatments relied mainly on herbal remedies, hydrotherapy, and body manipulation. With advances in public health measures, pharmaceutical drugs, and immunization, naturopathy as a medical discipline went into almost total eclipse until the 1960s. During the decades that followed, the growing interest in healthier life-styles and in the contributions of other cultures to healing brought about a revival of naturopathic practices. In addition to the procedures used by the founders of naturopathy, current practices now include acupuncture, nutrition recommendations (with a special emphasis on vitamin and mineral supplements), stress and pain management through skills derived from Chinese and Indian disciplines, and behavior modification. Hypnosis and biofeedback training may be used to achieve desired results. Naturopathic doctors attend to the needs of pregnant women and supervise "natural" delivery in a birthing center rather than in a hospital. They may also perform minor surgery under a local anesthetic.

The principles that guide naturopathic doctors are:

1. Recognize and respect the inherent ability of the body to heal itself.
2. Identify and treat the cause of the ailment rather than suppress its symptoms.
3. Treat the whole person.
4. Practice preventive medicine by promoting a healthy life-style and controlling risk factors.

Although it is difficult to estimate the number of self-styled "natural" or "holistic" or "naturopathic specialists" nationwide, there are in fact only about 1,000 *licensed* naturopathic doctors (N.D.s) in the United States today. Credentials for licensing are achieved by successfully completing a course of study at either of two accredited naturopathic medical schools—one in Oregon and the other in Washington State. A third institution, located in Arizona, began to give classes in 1993. Practitioners who fulfill the requirements of these institutions receive the degree of N.D. (not M.D.) and are currently licensed to practice in Alaska, Arizona, Connecticut, Hawaii, Montana, Oregon, and Washington.

If you would like to explore the advantages of having a naturopathic doctor as your primary health care provider, be sure that the practitioner of your choice functions within the limitations of his or her training and will refer you to better-qualified conventionally trained specialists when necessary. Also make sure that your health insurance provides coverage for naturopathic treatments.

You can get additional information about naturopathy and a referral to a qualified practitioner in your area by writing to the American Association of Naturopathic Physicians, 2800 East Madison, Suite 200, Seattle, WA 98112; telephone (206) 323-7610.

PET THERAPY

The many blessings of sharing one's life with a pet are well known to those of us who don't mind sweeping up cat hair or walking the dog in rotten weather or cleaning the canary's cage. Companionship, unquestioning trust, an expectant creature eagerly waiting for the sound of the key in the door, and social interaction with other people who share our passion for the same species or the same breed—these are a few of the rewards. There's also the fun of taking photos and showing them, and collecting anecdotes to swap at work and at dinner parties.

It's true that bonding with a pet is a responsibility, an expense, and a limitation on one's freedom to come and go as one pleases. But the benefits in terms of physical and emotional health more than make up for the costs. Researchers have studied the positive role of pets in restoring self-esteem and building self-confidence for women who have suffered the rejection of a divorce or the loss of a job. They have documented the fact that pet owners take better care of their health so that they can be there for the creatures whose well-being depends on them. A study of nearly 1,000 Medicare patients at a Los Angeles health maintenance organization found that pet owners paid significantly fewer visits to doctors than those who lived alone. Dr. Judith M. Siegel, a University of California professor of public health who conducted the study, pointed out: "We know from social research that people go to the doctor for a variety of reasons besides physical ailments. Psychological distress and lack of companionship seem to influence perceptions of health and are associated with more frequent contact with physicians."

The therapeutic aspects of people-creature relationships have been under investigation for several decades. It has been noted that when there's an aquarium in a doctor's waiting room, patients mesmerized by the movements of the fish experience a drop in blood pressure. Stroking a cat and hearing it purr can reduce the pain of arthritic fingers. One of the earliest and most significant developments in pet therapy was discussed in an article entitled "Animals in Long-Term Care Facilities," which appeared in the Winter 1984 *Journal of Long-Term Care Administrating.* In the introduction to the article, the editors point out that "bringing animals into long-term care facilities where they can be petted, hugged, and loved by residents is an innovative program for reaching withdrawn and lonely residents. But they are not the only ones well served by pet therapy; staff members benefit as well."

Since that time, visiting and resident pets have become part of therapeutic programs—both physical and emotional—not only in nursing homes, but also in children's hospitals, psychiatric clinics, rehabilitation centers, prisons, and residences for developmentally disabled adults. One of the most important of these enterprises is the Pet Partners Program created by the nonprofit Delta Society in the state of Washington with the cooperation of local affiliates of the American Society for the Prevention of Cruelty to Animals (ASPCA). Companion animals that successfully complete health exams and skills training and pet owners who complete volunteer training are registered as a team. By the end of 1995, the society had about 2,000 registered teams nationwide. On the level of training for the Animal Assisted Activities (AAA) program, the team visits various community facilities on an informal basis to get people talking, laughing, and reminiscing. In the more specialized Animal Assisted Therapy (AAT) program, the pets are incorporated by a professional health care provider into the patient's goal-directed treatment plan, such as rehabilitation of muscles through brushing a cat or a more positive outlook through the bonding of a depressed patient and an affectionate dog.

If you would like to participate in these volunteer programs with your pet, additional information is available through your local ASPCA office, or call the Delta Society toll-free at 1-800-869-6898.

REFLEXOLOGY

Reflexology, sometimes called zone therapy, is a healing method based on the application of pressure to designated areas of the bottom and top surfaces of the hands and feet that are believed to correspond to specific interior organs. Stimulation of these areas by a knowledgeable therapist is said to promote health, reduce stress by relaxing muscles, and further the body's ability to heal itself. Traditionally used with acupuncture by Chinese healers, reflexology began to attract a Western following through the efforts in the 1930s of the practitioner Eunice Ingham, who created what is called the Ingham Reflex Method of Compression. This method claims that widely separated areas of the body share the same sensory receptors below the skin's surface. When the receptors are stimulated by pressure, they send messages along the afferent (inward-carrying) fibers of the peripheral nervous system to the spinal cord, thereby producing changes that dilate or constrict blood vessels, contract or relax muscles, or reduce the perception of pain. Practitioners do not claim to be qualified to diagnose and treat specific ailments, nor do they prescribe medication. Their prime goal is to facilitate healing.

Although some people say that practically anyone can learn this discipline quickly, trained reflexologists insist that positive results can be achieved only through "well-educated" fingers. While different therapists may use different foot maps, the procedure is essentially the same. The therapist holds the bare foot in one hand as the thumb and fingers of her other hand move slowly along the top, bottom, and sides, stroking, pressing, and rotating as they go. When a tender spot is discovered, the therapist keeps returning to it, increasing the intensity of the pressure until the tenderness disappears.

There is an impressive body of anecdotal evidence that corroborates the claims of reflexologists in alleviating headaches, asthma, allergies, digestive disorders, insomnia, back pain, and PMS. As a noninvasive method, it has a loyal following and is especially popular among dancers and active sports participants. Of the 75,000 trained reflexologists nationwide, many work with chiropractors, and many are on the staffs of full-service spas. For a qualified practitioner in your area or more detailed information about the technique, consult the International Institute of Reflexology, 5650 First Avenue N., St. Petersburg, FL 33733; telephone: (813) 343-4811.

ROLFING

Rolfing is a method of manipulating parts of the body in order to break down obstructive connective tissue and free muscles from tension and pain. The theory on which this procedure is based presumes that when muscles of the neck, torso, lower back, and legs are freed by deep massage from lifelong patterns of tension, the body is no longer based *against* gravitational pull, thereby permitting gravity to produce a more natural realignment and balance. Rolfers believe that when this change is brought about, the person not only moves more efficiently but also enjoys greater mental focus and alertness.

The system that now bears her name was developed by a biochemist, Dr. Ida Rolf, who called it Structural Integration. After studying osteopathy and the Alexander Technique, she came to the conclusion that when one part of the body is tense, the whole body is thrown off balance. Unnatural posture when the body is moving or at rest causes muscles to contract in an unnatural way, and these contractions lead to an overgrowth of the connective tissue that binds muscles to bones. By the 1950s, Rolf had developed the deep and energetic hands-on massaging that reestablishes muscular efficiency and was teaching it to therapists here and abroad. In 1970 the Rolf Institute of Structural Integration was established in Boulder, Colorado, to promote research and training and to formulate standards for practitioners.

Among enthusiastic supporters of Rolfing are many athletes, dancers, and people who have been relieved of acute neck and back pain by this system of manipulation, which in itself can be extremely painful during treatments. Those who get themselves "Rolfed" regularly insist that when they step off the treatment table, they are completely free of pain and totally reenergized. Women being treated for osteoporosis should consult their primary care doctor about the advisability of being Rolfed. Unwanted fractures may be the result of the energetic pounding and pummeling. To find out more about this alternative therapy or to connect with a qualified practitioner, write to the Rolf Institute, PO Box 1868, Boulder, CO 80306. Your telephone directory may also contain listings for local Rolfers. Keep in mind that these treatments are not likely to be covered by your health insurance provider.

TAI CHI

Officially designated as one of the martial arts, this Chinese system of physical and mental discipline is formally known as tai chi chuan, which means "Supreme Ultimate Power." It is considered the most meditative of the martial arts, and its chief purpose is to stimulate the flow of energy (chi) through the body by coordinating movements in a slow but steady manner.

Like the other martial arts, it originated in ancient ritual dances celebrating seasonal changes, folk heroes, and totemic animals. By the second century, these dance movements were systematized by a Taoist physician into a health regimen. It was his theory that his system of 13 body movements enhanced both physical and spiritual well-being. These movements, which are supposed to flow without a break from one posture to the next, were increased to 24 in a standardized version promoted by the Chinese government in 1956. Current enthusiasts give it high marks for easing muscle strain, reducing stress, and increasing the fitness and stamina of older people. A special advantage for the elderly is that by promoting good body balance, tai chi exercises reduce by 25 percent the risk of hip fractures and other serious injuries caused by falls, according to the results of a study published in the *Journal of the American Medical Association* (5/95). Of all the exercise programs that were tried, tai chi proved to be the most effective in achieving better stability for people who wobble and totter when they walk either because of the infirmities of age or simply because they don't walk often enough.

Many women in all age groups prefer the slow, almost dreamlike movements of tai chi to more energetic forms of exercise. The controlled slow motion can be achieved even when the body is fatigued or when arthritis is a constant problem because it is an underlying principle of tai chi that the mind must be permitted to control the body. Those who constantly feel rushed and stressed in the performance of their jobs and family responsibilities claim that they look forward to their tai chi classes because, by the end of a session, they feel relaxed and invigorated at the same time. It is also recommended by physical therapists for women recovering from surgery or in need of rehabilitation following an accident.

Women interested in the self-defense maneuvers of tai chi can look for a class that teaches not only the slow movements of the basic form, but also shows how these movements, when speeded up, result in the martial chops, kicks, and other actions that can ward off a physical assault. Many women feel that by mastering these skills, they achieve a self-confidence they might otherwise not have.

When shopping around for group that meets your requirements in terms of time and money, the following guidelines are suggested:

1. Find a teacher who specializes in tai chi and who can explain the purpose of each movement.
2. Don't make a financial commitment until you've been permitted to visit a class as an observer. This is the only practical way of finding out if there is a good interaction between the teacher and the class members, and if the physical setting is comfortable.
3. Be wary of a teacher who makes exaggerated claims for the curative powers of tai chi, and look elsewhere if you're expected to invest a large sum of money in special clothing. All you need for tai chi exercises are loose garments and comfortable shoes.
4. Find out in advance how large your class will be to make sure you can get personal attention when you need it. A group of no more than 20 members provides the best individual results.
5. Before you sign a contract, read it carefully at home and make sure you understand the terms of the agreement: how many classes the fee covers; what happens if you have to miss a class because of illness or a conflict of responsibilities; whether you will be entitled to a partial refund if circumstances beyond your control make it necessary to quit before completion of the course.

VISUALIZATION

Visualization, also called guided imagery, is a technique in which the patient is helped to achieve a relaxed state by imagining herself floating on a wide expanse of calm water or lying alone in the sun on a sandy beach. As a state bordering on a trance is achieved, the therapist then suggests positive imagery suitable to the patient's needs: athletes, musicians, or actors suffering from anxiety or stage fright are guided to visualizing themselves as performing with assurance and distinction; a patient whose teeth are suffering from neglect because she's terrified of visiting the dentist is guided to seeing herself lying comfortably in the dentist's chair, her body so relaxed that she can concentrate on the music coming from the radio rather than on expectations of pain.

Many studies indicate that there is a direct relationship between imagining bodily change and actually experiencing the bodily change. Like biofeedback and self-hypnosis, it appears to have the capability of altering heart rate, blood pressure, skin temperature, and the like.

Psychologists and psychiatrists who specialize in cognitive therapy and behavior modification find visualization a useful tool in helping patients rid themselves of self-defeating attitudes. Practicing visualization on your own is like self-hypnosis in that you can learn to concentrate on the positive aspects of an experience in order to meet its challenge with confidence rather than apprehension.

YOGA

As practiced in India for thousands of years, yoga is a way of life that includes ethical guidelines, dietary regimens, and specific exercise routines. The goal is the achievement of an exalted state of consciousness that promotes physical and spiritual well-being. This achievement is based on the assumption that because mind and body are inextricably bound together, it is possible to control bodily responses through mental discipline.

In the Western world, yoga has had a cult following for many years, and it was especially popular with the antiestablishment young during the 1960s. But more important is the fact that since then the claims of yoga practitioners have been subjected to thousands of rigorous scientific studies with the purpose of validating their therapeutic usefulness. These studies have shown that with the proper training, an individual can learn to control blood pressure, skin temperature, brain waves, and other body processes previously believed by the medical establishment to be beyond conscious manipulation.

With the growing acceptance of the physical and psychological benefits of yoga, doctors are beginning to incorporate some of its disciplines into their practice. Yoga for stress control is combined with meditation, dietary recommendations, and moderate aerobic exercise in the widely publicized "alternative" program devised by Dr. Dean Ornish of the Preventive Medical Research Center in California for the reversal of coronary artery disease. Yoga is increasingly used in treating chronic pain and controlling asthma symptoms. It has become part of fitness programs for athletes and for professionals in the performing arts. There are yoga instructors at many spas, and for those who

can afford it, there is a yoga "camp" (more properly called an ashram) beauti-
fully situated in the Bahamas, where participants follow the precepts of the
founder, the late Swami Vishnu Devananda.

The following aspects of traditional yoga practice have been adapted to fulfill
our desire to learn how to relax and to manage stress as well as to foster bodily
well-being:

- the postures, or asanas, of hatha yoga designed to stimulate circulation in
  particular parts of the body and thereby increase the health of individual
  organs
- the breathing techniques of pranayama yoga
- meditation, or "the stilling of the mind," during which external stimuli are
  blocked out in order to achieve a higher level of consciousness

Yoga classes vary widely in the seriousness with which they apply all the
philosophical aspects of this approach to total physical, mental, and spiritual
health. Those conducted by teachers who received their training from traditional Indian practitioners are likely to include not only the yoga exercises, but
also dietary recommendations and other health-promoting behavior modifications. The most popular classes are those that concentrate on the postures, or
asanas. These classes are given by various community groups, including the
"Y" and health clubs. Local classified telephone directories are another source
of information about yoga centers.

CONCLUSION

This overview of alternative therapies is by no means comprehensive. Serious examination of the healing arts of other cultures and of the folk and past
treatments of our own continues to yield useful remedies and techniques—
some previously scorned, some discarded. Here are some special examples:
Consider the reappearance of the medieval remedy of leeches, now being used
to drain excess blood following such microsurgical procedures as the reattach-
ment of fingers and toes. This worm has also attracted the attention of bioengi-
neers who hope to re-create its saliva, which contains an anticoagulant, a local
anesthetic, and an antibiotic! To some doctors, aromatherapy may seem a form
of sybaritic self-indulgence, but others, especially those in France, where national health insurance covers it as an authentic treatment, accept the scientific
evidence that certain scents can reduce blood pressure, alter the heart rate,
and affect brain-wave patterns. The marriage of current technology and the

ancient activities of tai chi and yoga has resulted in attractive videos that provide self-instruction at home at the user's convenience.

It is hoped that readers will inform themselves about alternative therapies and discuss them as viable alternatives with their health providers when the more orthodox methods and medications don't alleviate stress or the usual run of aches, pains, and minor ailments.

As scientists learn more about brain-mind function and its intimate connection with the body, we can expect the emergence of new therapeutic disciplines and the reemergence of very old ones.

Part Two

ENCYCLOPEDIA OF HEALTH AND MEDICAL TERMS

Abdominal Pain • Acute pain or persistent ache in the region between the chest and the pelvis is a symptom that may be difficult to diagnose. Because the abdominal cavity contains the stomach, liver, spleen, gallbladder, kidneys, appendix, intestines, ovaries, and during pregnancy the expanding uterus, a disorder or infection of any of these organs may be the source of the discomfort.

Pain that disappears within a few hours and doesn't recur may be due to indigestion. If it is accompanied by nausea and diarrhea and subsides within a day or two, it may be due to a comparatively harmless virus infection of the intestinal tract.

Among possible causes of severe upper abdominal pain are the onset of a heart attack or food poisoning, both of which require emergency medical treatment. The formation of gallstones leading to gallbladder inflammation will produce pain ranging from mild and recurrent to acute enough to require hospitalization. When gallbladder inflammation affects the liver, symptoms of jaundice and hepatitis may produce pain when pressure is applied to the upper right side of the abdomen.

Colitis is likely to produce abdominal cramps and attacks of diarrhea; a peptic ulcer manifests itself in a burning pain a few hours after meals. Gastritis, an inflammation of the stomach wall, may be a temporary condition caused by stress, too much spicy food, caffeine, and/or alcohol. Its characteristically severe pain may subside when a new regimen is established.

Cramps in the lower abdomen sometimes occur immediately before or during the first day of menstruation, and for some women menstrual pain may spread to the back and down the leg. Among other causes of lower abdominal pain are endometriosis or endometritis (disorders of the uterus), infection of the fallopian tubes, ectopic pregnancy, and intestinal obstruction.

Persistent pain localized in the lower right part of the abdomen is a characteristic signal of the onset of appendicitis.

Abscess • An accumulation of pus in an area where healthy tissue has been invaded and broken down by bacteria. An abscess may form anywhere in the body that might be vulnerable to bacterial infection—around a hangnail or splinter, around an infected tooth, in the breast, in the middle ear, in the lung. Many abscesses can be cured with antibiotics, but some require surgical incision and draining.

A simple abscess beneath the skin may break through the surface, drain, and heal itself. A skin abscess should never be squeezed or cut open by an untrained person. A doctor or the emergency services of the nearest hospital must be consulted at once if the redness that surrounds an abscess begins to travel in a visible line toward a lymph node.

A tooth abscess is not only the cause of pain, but can also lead to a serious systemic infection if the bacteria get into the bloodstream. Prompt surgical treatment combined with antibiotics is essential. *See* LYMPH NODES and "Plain Talk About Medications."

Abuse • *See* "Domestic Violence, Sexual Abuse, and Rape."

Acetaminophen • The generic name of a nonprescription drug that relieves pain and reduces temperature. It is especially useful for those with a low tolerance for aspirin, but, unlike aspirin, acetaminophen is not an anti-inflammatory drug and therefore is not effective in treating arthritis. *See* "Plain Talk About Medications."

Acidophilus Pills • A dietary aid to the restoration of intestinal bacilli destroyed by antibiotics. Unless this restoration takes place, the change in intestinal flora can result in a yeast infection. Acidophilus pills are sold in health food stores as well as pharmacies and are a convenient alternative to yogurt, which is also an effective dietary supplement when taking antibiotics.

Acne • A skin disorder occurring mainly in association with the hormonal changes of adolescence, although women may experience it for the first time when they are in their 20s or 30s. The increased amounts of androgen produced by both the male and female sex glands stimulate the sebaceous (oil) glands of the hair follicles to produce an increased amount of the fatty substance called *sebum* that is normally discharged through the pores to lubricate the skin. The overproduction of sebum results in oily skin. The characteristic pimples, pustules, and blackheads of acne are formed when the pores become plugged by the sebum that has backed up, mixed with the skin pigments, and leaked into surrounding areas.

Acne is not caused by junk food or faulty hygiene: the chief cause is the onset of puberty combined with the hereditary factors that govern the oiliness of the skin. Mild cases usually clear up by themselves, especially when the affected areas are kept free of oily cosmetics by regular cleansing. Nonprescription products containing benzoyl peroxide are helpful, and, for more stubborn cases, vitamin A acid cream (Retin-A), sun lamp treatments, and tetracycline pills may be beneficial.

If acne has left scars and blemishes, a dermatologist can be consulted about the advisability of removing them by dermabrasion. *See* "Cosmetic Surgery."

Acquired Immune Deficiency Syndrome (AIDS) • A condition, usually fatal, in which the body's immune system becomes incapable of warding off diseases and infections that would normally be overcome. AIDS is caused by a virus that is sexually transmissible. At greatest risk have been homosexual males and intravenous drug abusers, who spread the disease through contaminated needles. The latter spread the disease to women who in turn infect their newborn infants. Also at risk are hemophiliacs requiring frequent blood transfusions and women who have sexual intercourse with bisexual men. The disease continues to spread among heterosexual males and females, including teenagers, who have many sexual encounters without regard to safe sex practices.

Major efforts are being made worldwide to develop a vaccine against AIDS, but until such protection becomes available, the condom is promoted as the most practical safeguard against sexually transmitted infection. *See* KAPOSI'S SARCOMA, PNEUMOCYSTIC PNEUMONIA, MENINGITIS, "Sexual Health," "Sexually Transmissible Diseases," and "Substance Abuse."

Acute Symptom • A symptom of a disorder that has a sudden onset and runs a comparatively brief course such as an "acute" asthma attack as opposed to a persistent, or chronic, manifestation of a disorder. "Acute" should not be confused with "life-threatening."

Addiction • A compelling physical need for or psychological dependence on a drug or chemical substance such that its habitual use must be maintained no matter how self-destructive the results. In recent years, the term has been more loosely applied to certain types of compulsive behavior such as overeating, gambling, and overspending so that the techniques successfully used by Alcoholics Anonymous can be duplicated by other self-help groups. *See* "Substance Abuse."

Addison's Disease • (adrenal insufficiency) A rare disorder whose immediate cause is failure of the adrenal gland cortex. The glandular underfunction is sometimes the result of tuberculosis. Other causes may be a tumor, hemorrhage, or any injury that interferes with hormone production. Addison's disease, once fatal, is now treated with cortisone and other forms of hormone replacement therapy in the same way that diabetes is treated with insulin.

Adenoma • A usually benign tumor composed of glandular tissue.

Adhesion • The union of two internal body surfaces that are normally separate

and the formation of the fibrous, or scar, tissue that connects them. The scar tissue that forms around a surgical wound during the healing process may cling to adjoining areas causing them to fuse. Although most adhesions are painless and without consequence, they may occasionally cause an obstruction or malfunction that requires surgical correction. The incidence of postoperative adhesions has dramatically diminished as a result of early ambulation after surgery.

Adoptive Pregnancy • (donated embryo or embryo transfer) The transfer of an embryo, a few days after conception, (or a month or two if frozen after conception) from the uterus of a fertile woman to the uterus of an infertile woman with a synchronous menstrual cycle so that the pregnancy can continue in the infertile woman. *See* "Infertility" and "Directory of Health Information."

Adrenalin • One of the hormones produced by the medulla or inner core of the adrenal glands; also known as epinephrine. This hormone maximizes the body's physiologic response to stress by increasing heart rate and blood pressure. By transforming the glycogen in the liver into glucose, adrenalin also provides the muscles with a quick source of energy so that they can perform effectively without suffering fatigue. Adrenalin dilates the pupils of the eyes for more effective vision and expands the bronchial tubes for more effective respiration. When the body sustains a wound, adrenalin increases the clotting capacity of the blood.

Agoraphobia • Literally, "fear of the marketplace." For those who suffer from this phobia, a panic attack occurs when they venture into public places or open spaces. This distress causes the victim to circumscribe activities and to refuse to leave the safety of home. Anxiety in this form is likely to be accompanied by hyperventilation, which in turn produces dizziness, sweating, weakness, and a sense of impending disaster. Agoraphobia, even in a mild manifestation, should be treated by a professional therapist. *See* "Alternative Therapies."

AIDS • *See* ACQUIRED IMMUNE DEFICIENCY SYNDROME.

Air Sickness • *See* MOTION SICKNESS.

Alcohol • Any of a group of related chemical compounds derived from hydrocarbons. Ethyl alcohol, also called ethanol or grain alcohol, is the intoxicating ingredient of fermented and distilled beverages. Methyl alcohol, also known as wood alcohol or methanol, is widely used in industry as a solvent and a fuel. Taken internally, it is a poison that can lead to blindness and death. Rubbing alcohol, used on the skin as a cooling agent or disinfectant, may be ethyl alcohol made unfit for consumption by the addition of chemicals known as denaturants (denatured alcohol) or it may be another compound called isopropyl alcohol.

Alcoholic Beverages • Drinks that contain ethyl alcohol, the substance that results naturally from the fermentation of carbohydrates (sugars, such as those in grape mash, molasses, and apples, or starches, such as those in wheat, rice, barley, and other grains). Hard cider, beer, and ale contain about 3 to 5 percent alcohol; table wines about 10 percent; fortified wines like sherry about 20 percent. Beverages of higher alcoholic content, such as vodka, bourbon, and brandy, are called liquors or "hard" liquors and are produced by distilling the alcohol from the fermented mash. Liqueurs like Benedictine or Cointreau may contain as much as 35

percent alcohol, and whiskey and rum as much as 50 percent. The concentration of alcohol in a beverage is usually given in terms of "proof." Half of the proof number is the percentage of alcohol by volume; thus a 90-proof vodka is 45 percent alcohol, with the remainder made up of water, flavoring, and other ingredients. In assessing alcohol intake, it should be kept in mind that a 12-ounce can of beer contains four-fifths as much alcohol as a 1½-ounce jigger of 80-proof whiskey, 6 ounces of wine equal 1½ ounces of vodka, and 6 ounces of sherry contains almost twice as much alcohol as a 1½-ounce jigger of whiskey.

All states have a law defining the minimal age for drinking alcohol legally, whether in a bar or at home. Driving when intoxicated (DWI), especially by teenagers, is a major cause of automobile accidents, many of them fatal. Thanks to the efforts of Mothers Against Drunk Driving (MADD), greater numbers of intoxicated drivers have been convicted and greater vigilance on the part of law-enforcement agencies has reduced the number of fatalities.

The U.S. Surgeon General has warned that pregnant women should abstain from all alcoholic beverages because there is no definitive information about a safe level of alcohol in the blood that would not cause damage to the fetus. Mounting evidence of serious birth defects resulting from alcohol consumption during pregnancy (fetal alcohol syndrome) resulted in the passage of a law in 1989 requiring that all alcoholic beverages have warning labels alerting women to the dangers of drinking during pregnancy. Such warnings must also be posted in a conspicuous place wherever alcoholic beverages are sold. There has yet to be an extensive study of the effects of excessive alcohol consumption on the male sperm and consequent effects on the development of the fetus.

Anyone on a weight reduction diet should cut down on or eliminate alcohol: a glass of whiskey contains 120 calories with no nutritional value, and alcoholic beverages simultaneously increase the appetite and weaken the will to diet. Alcohol in any form generally should not be given as a first aid measure or as emergency treatment unless a doctor has issued the instruction. *See* "Pregnancy and Childbirth" and "Substance Abuse."

Alcoholism • *See* "Substance Abuse."

Allergy • Hypersensitivity to a substance such as food, pollen, cosmetics, animal dander, or medicine, or to a climatic condition such as sunshine or low temperature that in similar amounts is harmless to most people. An allergic response can occur anywhere on or in the body: on the skin, in the eyes, lungs, gastrointestinal tract. While an allergy may develop at any age, symptoms experienced in childhood have a tendency to abate with time, and some disappear altogether. A tendency to allergic response is inherited, although the nature of the allergy itself may differ from one generation to another. Why a particular allergy develops remains a medical mystery.

Allergies are essentially the result of a faulty response by the body's immune system, which reacts to an allergen by manufacturing antibodies as if the substance were a dangerous invader. In this process chemicals known as histamines are released into the bloodstream, and these chemicals are the immediate cause of the allergic symptoms. Histamine can produce two main effects: first, by increasing the permeability of the small blood vessels, it causes the fluid portion of the blood or serum to leak into the tissues; second, it causes spasm of particular muscles, especially in the bronchial tubes. The first condition produces swelling, blisters, and irritation of some tissues such as the eyes, nose, and skin; the second produces labored breathing and asthmatic episodes. In extreme cases hypersensitivity to penicillin or nonhuman antitoxin serum or to the venom in an insect sting produces sudden shock (anaphylactic reaction) that can be fatal.

Most allergies are treated by identifying the offending substance and avoiding it. In many instances, however, identification can be extremely difficult. Specialists have evolved various scratch tests and patch tests that are painless, time-consuming, and not always helpful.

For cases in which avoidance is not possible and relief from symptoms is necessary there are desensitizing treatments that can build up a resistance to the allergen once it is identified. Medicines may be effective in controlling the symptoms and reducing discomfort. Self-medication with any drugs prior to identifying the problem is always inadvisable. *See* ANTIHISTAMINE and ASTHMA.

Alopecia • *See* BALDNESS.

Amebiasis • An infection caused by an ameba that invades the colon, resulting in diarrhea and bloody, mucoid stools. Amebiasis is one type of "traveler's diarrhea" and is also sexually transmissible. *See* "Sexually Transmissible Diseases."

Amnesia • Loss of memory. Amnesia may be partial or extensive, temporary or permanent. With total amnesia (very rare), practically all mental functions would necessarily cease. Memory loss may result from brain damage caused by injury, tumor, arteriosclerosis, stroke, Alzheimer's disease, or alcoholism. It may also be caused by the psychological mechanism of repression. Amnesia following an accident or acute emotional shock may cause the victim to black out and forget the event itself but remember all details leading up to it. Except for the amnesia associated with senility, memory loss that wipes out past identity occurs more frequently in fiction than in fact.

Amnion • The tough-walled membrane that forms the protective sac in which the embryo is contained within the uterus during pregnancy. *See* "Pregnancy and Childbirth."

Amphetamine • A category of drugs, including Benzedrine, Dexedrine, and Methedrine, that act as stimulants to the central nervous system. *See* "Substance Abuse."

Amyotrophic Lateral Sclerosis • (also called Lou Gehrig's disease) A progressive and eventually fatal disease of the nervous system characterized by muscular weakness of the extremities and increasing loss of function and mobility. Typical victims of this neuromuscular disorder are males over the age of 40. Physical therapy on a regular basis can slow down muscle atrophy. Some progress is also being made in finding substances that will help regenerate damaged nerve cells responsible for this disease.

Analgesic • Substance that temporarily reduces or eliminates the sensation of pain without producing unconsciousness. *See* ANESTHESIA, PAIN, "Plain Talk About Medications," and "Alternative Therapies."

Analysis • *See* PSYCHOANALYSIS.

Androgynous • Having both male and female sex characteristics. True androgyny is extremely rare and can be corrected in part by a combination of hormone therapy and surgery.

Anemia • A condition in which there is a deficiency in the number of red blood cells, hemoglobin, or the total amount of blood. Anemia, whether acute or chronic, is not a disease in itself but rather the result of an underlying disorder: chronic malnutrition, industrial poisoning, bone marrow disease, heavy bleeding, intestinal parasites, kidney disease, or a defect in the body's ability to absorb iron. It is also a sign of colon cancer. Because treatment varies according to the cause, accurate diagnosis is extremely important. The symptoms of a mild deficiency may be vague: listlessness, general lack of vitality, and fatigue following little effort. When the condition is more severe, the inability of the anemic blood to supply oxygen to body tissues can result in shortness of breath, rapid pulse, and the sensation that the heart is working harder or faster.

Anemia should never be self-diagnosed for the purpose of self-treatment with tonics, vitamins, pills, or herbal remedies. It is a specific condition that can be diagnosed accurately only by laboratory analysis of blood samples.

There are several types of anemia. The most common form, iron deficiency anemia, is a deficiency of iron essential for the body's manufacture of hemoglobin. It may result from insufficient iron in the diet or from chronic blood loss from excessive menstrual flow or internal bleeding due to an ulcer or some other gastrointestinal disorder.

Pernicious anemia, also known as Addison's anemia, is a serious disease characterized by a breakdown in the mechanism of red blood cell formation, usually traceable to a deficiency of vitamin B_{12}, although this is rare because the amount required by the body is easily obtained from small amounts of animal products. It may sometimes occur among the strictest vegetarians unless their diet is supplemented by the vitamin in capsule form.

Hemolytic anemia results from the destruction of red blood cells, which may occur because of Rh incompatibility, mismatched blood transfusions, industrial poisons, or hypersensitivity to certain chemicals and medicines.

Aplastic anemia is caused by a disease of the bone marrow, the part of the body where red blood cells are manufactured. While some cases result from bone marrow cancer, others follow excessive radiation exposure or contact with a long list of substances that have the same destructive effect (the chemicals in certain insecticides, antibiotics, medicines containing bismuth and other heavy metals).

Hemoglobinopathies are forms of anemia of genetic origin. Included in this category are sickle-cell trait and anemia, thalassemia (Cooley's anemia), and hemoglobin C disease. When such a congenital trait is known to exist, genetic counseling is advised before pregnancy. *See* "Nutrition, Weight, and General Well-Being."

Anesthesia • Partial or total loss of sensation or feelings. Analgesia, one category of anesthesia, refers specifically to loss of sensation of pain. The great advances in surgery have gone hand in hand with modern methods of anesthesia and the discovery of a variety of anesthetics. The study of these substances and their application is known as anesthesiology. An anesthesiologist is a doctor who specializes in this branch of medical science. An anesthetist is not a doctor but usually a nurse with advanced training.

The following are among the procedures that produce anesthesia and analgesia. They may be used separately or in combination. Intravenous injection of sleep-producing drugs such as sodium pentothal produces light anesthesia. The injection of light anesthetics often pre-cedes the use of longer-lasting methods when major surgery is involved. Inhalation of gases is used to anesthetize the whole body. Spinal injection of one of the cocaine derivatives deadens the nerves in a specific part of the body. Rectal administration by a light enema or paraldehyde, a sleep-inducing drug that is quickly absorbed by the body, is used for patients who are especially difficult to deal with, such as alcoholics, psychotics, or those who are extremely apprehensive. More limited procedures are local freezing, nerve block, such as the injection of procaine for dental surgery, and surface or topical analgesia, such as the use of cocaine-related drugs for eye surgery. Hypnosis is being used successfully in situations such as childbirth and pediatric dentistry. Acupuncture is being evaluated scientifically for its analgesic applications. *See* "Alternative Therapies."

Aneurysm • An abnormal widening or distension of an artery or vein, forming a sac that is filled with blood. Aneurysms may be congenitally caused by a deficiency in the vessel walls or they may be acquired through injury or disease, especially atherosclerosis. The condition may exist for many years without any symptoms and may be detected only as a result of an X-ray taken for some other reason. Aneurysms in the arteries of the brain or in the aorta may make themselves known by pressure in the surrounding area, for example on the optic nerve or on an organ in the chest. Diagnosis of an aneurysm may also be confirmed by a CAT scan or sonography.

When the swelling is detected in a small artery or vein, the vessel can be tied off so that the flow of blood is redirected to healthier channels. The repair of larger vessels has recently been made possible by organ banks that provide vascular replacements, both plastic and those available from smaller mammals. Rupture of an aneurysm requires emergency hospitalization and treatment.

Angina Pectoris • Literally, pain in the chest and the signal of an interference (generally reversible) with the supply of oxygen to the heart muscle. The pain is rarely confused with any other; it characteristically produces a feeling of tightness and suffocation beginning under the left side of the breastbone and sometimes spreading to the neck, throat, and down the left arm. Angina pectoris is more common among men than women, but women, especially in their late fifties and sixties, may suffer from the condition, especially if they smoke or are overweight, hypertensive, or diabetic.

The onset of an angina attack is likely to follow strenuous exercise, exposure to cold and wind, eating and digesting a heavy meal, or the emotional stress of a quarrel or a frightening dream. In such circumstances the heart works harder and pumps faster and therefore needs an extra supply of blood and oxygen. When circulation is impaired in any way, especially by atherosclerosis, the blood supply does not reach the heart muscle cells quickly enough. The resulting lack of oxygen is the immediate cause of the pain.

Recent research supports the contention that angioplasty is a more effective treatment than medicine alone for chest pain originating in uncomplicated heart disease. It is only recently that the medical profession is being urged to recognize that chest pain in women should be taken as seriously as it has been in men. Angina in women should not be dismissed as "merely" a sign of anxiety or stress. When it occurs, it should be evaluated as a possible warning of life-threatening heart problems to come. Coronary bypass surgery, which replaces damaged coronary arteries, does not necessarily guarantee greater longevity than treatment by other means.

Angiography • A diagnostic procedure in which radiopaque substances are injected into the blood vessels so that any abnormalities or displacements are visible on an X-ray film. This type of radiological picture is called an angiogram.

Angioplasty • A procedure for widening diseased arteries severely blocked by atherosclerotic plaque. A catheter with a balloon-like tip is threaded through the artery, and when it reaches the blocked area, the tip is inflated, thereby flattening the fatty deposit and enlarging the arterial passage. Angioplasty does not involve surgery and is usually done with local anesthesia. It may be recommended as a cheaper and less invasive alternative to coronary bypass surgery as well as for the treatment of blocked arteries in other parts of the body. Women are still less likely than men to be offered the diagnostic benefits of angiography and the treatment benefits of angioplasty.

Animal Bites • Any animal bite, even by a family pet, that breaks the surface of the skin requires attention. It should be washed at once with soap under running water. Medical attention should be sought for deep or severe bites and for any bite by a wild animal, especially if rabies is a problem in your area. Not only dogs and cats but squirrels, horses, mice, bats, foxes, and other warm-blooded animals are capable of spreading diseases through bites. For any bite that breaks the skin, the victim should go at once to a local doctor or hospital emergency room for diagnosis and treatment. *See* RABIES.

Ankles, Swollen • The tissues around the ankle may swell for various reasons: heart disease, kidney or liver malfunction,

ANGINA PECTORIS

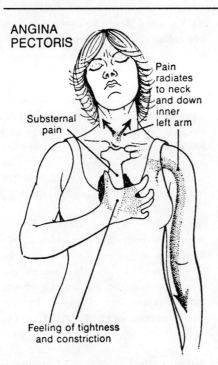

Substernal pain

Pain radiates to neck and down inner left arm

Feeling of tightness and constriction

for stimulating the stomach to secrete additional acid.

Antibiotic • A chemical substance produced during the growth of various fungi and bacteria that has the capacity to kill or inhibit the growth of other bacteria or fungi. Since the discovery of penicillin in 1929, literally thousands of antibiotic substances have been isolated and studied. As disease-causing bacteria develop strains resistant to a particular antibiotic, new drugs are developed to counteract the adaptation. See "Plain Talk About Medications."

Antibody • A component of the immune system produced by cells called plasmacytes in the presence of an antigen (any substance foreign to the body) to destroy or neutralize that antigen: a specific monoclonal antibody is produced for each antigen. This specificity is the basis of immunization by vaccination: the introduction of a controlled amount or variety of a disease-producing organism stimulates the plasmacytes to develop the antibodies necessary to fight the organism in advance of an uncontrolled invasion of the body. See IMMUNITY AND IMMUNIZATION.

Antidepressant • A class of mood-changing drugs that counteract some of the immobilizing effects of depressive illness. See "Substance Abuse" and "Plain Talk About Medications."

Antidote • Any substance natural or synthetic that counteracts the effect of another substance, usually a poison. There are very few specific antidotes, and because ridding the body of a poison is a complicated matter, a local poison control center should be consulted immediately for emergency care. See "Directory of Health Information."

pregnancy, or an injury. Women who spend lots of time on their feet, such as salespeople, artists, waitresses, hairdressers, and full-time homemakers are especially susceptible to this complaint in hot weather, not because of disease but because of insufficient venous return. When the puffy condition persists in spite of sitting with the feet extended and raised or a warm bath before bedtime, a doctor should be consulted.

Antacid • A substance that, by neutralizing the acidity of stomach juice, relieves heartburn and gastric distress. In choosing a nonprescription antacid among the different types on the market, keep the following in mind: some have significantly more salt than others, those in liquid form may be more effective even though less convenient, and the calcium contained in others may be responsible

Antigen • Any substance that stimulates the production of antibodies. Antigens are present in bacterial toxins, pollens, immunizing agents, blood, and other substances.

Antihistamine • Any of various drugs that minimize the discomfort of hay fever, hives, and other allergic reactions caused by the body's release of chemicals known as histamines. Depending on the nature of the allergy, antihistamines may be prescribed in the form of drops for the nose or eyes, a salve or topical ointment to be used on the skin, or pills to be taken orally. They may also be a remedy for motion sickness. However, they may reduce the effectiveness of birth control pills, and they should not be used by pregnant women to relieve the discomfort of "morning sickness."

Continuous and indiscriminate use of these drugs may have unpleasant effects and should be avoided. Widely advertised over-the-counter sleeping pills containing antihistamines are not consistently effective and are likely to produce "morning-after" dizziness, memory lapses, and coordination problems resulting in falls, especially in older people. Antihistamine pills may also trigger or intensify an asthma attack.

Antiperspirant Deodorants • A mixture of chemicals including aluminum chlorohydrate that diminish the amount of perspiration reaching the skin and reduce the rate of growth of the odor-creating bacteria. Because antiperspirants are considered drugs, their ingredients must be listed on their containers, and because they may contain irritants to the skin, it may be necessary to experiment with different brands to find one that does not produce a rash. Those packaged in spray cans may contain propellants harmful to the lungs and should be rejected in favor of a cream or roll-on product.

Antiseptic • A substance that inhibits or slows down the growth of microorganisms; in more recent usage the term means a substance that kills bacteria. Disinfectants are included under the general heading of antiseptics, although they are too strong to be applied to body tissues and are meant to make surfaces germ-free in kitchens, bathrooms, and sickrooms.

Antitoxin • A type of antibody that neutralizes the specific toxin released by a disease-causing agent. Antitoxins may be manufactured by the body's immune system or they may be injected as a defense against diseases such as tetanus, diphtheria, or botulism. *See* IMMUNITY AND IMMUNIZATION.

Anxiety Attack (also called panic attack) • In the clinical sense, an abnormal feeling of apprehension and fear in which the threat is not easy to identify. This condition of internally generated stress is typically accompanied by hyperventilation, rapid heartbeat, and sweating. An alcoholic hangover can be accompanied by such an attack; an excessive intake of caffeine can trigger an anxiety attack. Frequent episodes of this kind can lead to agoraphobia resulting in immobilization. Anti-anxiety drugs are recommended for short-term use only in order to reduce agitation and make psychotherapy possible. *See* "Alternative Therapies," "Substance Abuse," and "Plain Talk About Medications."

Aorta • The largest and most important artery carrying blood from the heart to be distributed throughout the body. *See* "The Healthy Woman."

Apnea • *See* SLEEP APNEA.

Appendicitis • Inflammation of the appendix, the 3- to 6-inch appendage or sac that lies in the lower right portion of the abdominal cavity at the junction of the small and large intestine. Appendicitis accounts for at least half the abdominal emergencies that occur between the ages of 10 and 30. The critical aspect of an attack of acute appendicitis is that the inflammation may result in a rupture leading to peritonitis (infection of the abdominal lining). When some undetermined element plugs up the tubelike appendix and hinders normal drainage the likelihood of bacterial infection increases. If the body's defenses do not stop the multiplication of colon bacilli and streptococci, inflammation results, causing three main symptoms: pain in the lower right side, nausea or vomiting, and fever. If one or all of these symptoms persist, see a doctor promptly.

If no doctor is available, call an ambulance to take you to the nearest hospital's emergency room. Under no circumstances should anything be taken by mouth without professional instructions: no food, no fluid, no medicines, and especially *no laxative or cathartic*. Self-treatment with an enema or a hot-water bottle is equally ill-advised.

An appendectomy performed under the best medical conditions has a very low mortality rate. Even when postoperative complications occur, they can be overcome with antibiotics.

So-called chronic appendicitis is a designation with little medical validity. Constant complaints of discomfort in the lower right part of the abdomen should be investigated for the correct cause.

Arrhythmias • Abnormalities in the rhythm of the heartbeat due to disturbances in the electrical impulses that trig-

APPENDICITIS

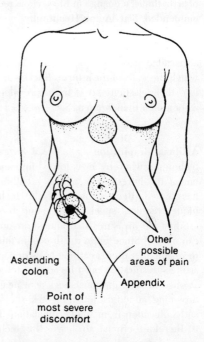

Other possible areas of pain

Ascending colon

Appendix

Point of most severe discomfort

ger the pumping of the heart muscle. The most common of these disturbances is a rapidly racing and pounding heart, called palpitations. Other abnormalities include excessively slow rate (below 60 beats a minute) called bradycardia, premature contractions of one or the other heart chambers sometimes caused by anxiety or too much caffeine or heavy smoking, and ventricular tachycardia in which an excessively rapid beat is accompanied by dizziness and chest pain.

Treatment depends on the circumstance. Artificial pacemakers correct a sluggish beat that deprives the heart of sufficient oxygen; medications such as digitalis and quinidine slow the heartbeat and reestablish a normal rhythm when fibrillation occurs. Beta-blocking drugs and calcium-channel blockers are also prescribed for treating disturbances in heart rhythms. When stress and/or alcohol, coffee, and cigarettes are the obvious cause of arrhythmia, a change in life-style is recommended. *See* "Aging Healthfully."

Arteriosclerosis • A disease of aging, also called hardening of the arteries, in which the walls of the arteries thicken and lose their elasticity. It is more prevalent among men than women. *See* ATHEROSCLEROSIS.

Artificial Respiration • Any of several techniques whereby air is forced into and out of the lungs when natural breathing has ceased. Because none of the techniques requires special equipment, they are first aid measures that almost anyone can master. Since brain death occurs four to six minutes after breathing has stopped, artificial respiration must be administered at once in such circumstances as a near-drowning, an almost lethal electric shock, and suffocation from smoke inhalation. It is therefore crucial to learn the techniques *before* the need arises in order to function swiftly and competently. Local Red Cross chapters or other community organizations should be contacted for information about courses that cover instruction in first aid for common emergencies.

Asbestos • A group of fibrous minerals of unusual strength, flexibility, and durability, characterized by resistance to heat and corrosion. Asbestos has been widely used to insulate buildings, as a fire-retarding component in construction materials, and as a protective covering against electrical damage. It is now known to be as deadly as it is useful if it is inhaled or (less likely) swallowed.

The submicroscopic silica-like fibers are responsible for the lung disease asbestosis and where exposure is combined with smoking, the result is almost always a fatal lung cancer. Other types of cancer,

especially mesothelioma, a deadly malignancy of the lining of the chest and abdominal cavity, have been traced to inhalation or swallowing of asbestos dust more than 40 years after the exposure. In 1989 the Environmental Protection Agency imposed a gradual ban on virtually all products made of asbestos. This ban will not protect people who were previously exposed, but it will prevent otherwise healthy people from future exposure. Exposure in the past now causes an estimated 10,000 deaths each year in the United States. The government agency emphasized the fact that this ruling does not affect asbestos materials already in place in older buildings. Owners must seek professional advice about whether it is safer to leave the asbestos where it is rather than to risk releasing the fibers into the air by removing it. Anyone who becomes aware of the presence of asbestos in a dwelling or in the workplace should contact the local EPA office about safe procedures to follow. Vigilant parents have increasingly refused to send their children to schools in which faulty repairs or negligence put them at great risk of inhaling the harmful dust.

Aspirin • Common name for the pure chemical acetylsalicylic acid; originally the brand name invented by the Bayer Drug Company but now a generic term. Aspirin is always aspirin no matter what company packages it. Therefore, there's no reason not to buy the least expensive brand. Aspirin is one of the greatest discoveries of all times because of its many benefits. It is a painkiller (analgesic); it lowers fever (antipyretic); it reduces some of the destructive consequences of arthritis (anti-inflammatory); and its role in controlling the mechanism that causes blood to form clots (anti-coagulant) has made it an effective medication in preventing heart attacks and strokes.

The addition of certain chemicals to aspirin may be profitable to the manufacturer but of questionable value to the consumer. Aspirin combined with caffeine? It probably costs less to have plain aspirin with a cup of coffee. With phenacetin? In large doses this is an ingredient likely to produce stomach upsets and kidney problems.

Aspirin itself can be a stomach irritant and should be avoided by anyone with ulcers or gastritis. It can be "buffered" by combining it with an alkalizer such as a bicarbonate of soda pill or a half glass of milk. When aspirin causes an allergic response, acetaminophen (Tylenol or other aspirinlike analgesics) should be substituted. Women in the last three months of pregnancy or those who are nursing are also advised to avoid using aspirin.

Headaches, ringing in the ears, and drowsiness are signs of aspirin overdose. Severe cases of aspirin poisoning, with symptoms of vomiting and delirium, require emergency treatment.

There is compelling evidence that aspirin can increase the risk of Reye's syndrome, a little-understood, life-threatening disease associated with some viral infections of childhood, especially chicken pox. See "Plain Talk About Medications."

Asthma • A chronic respiratory disorder in which many different kinds of "triggers" cause the bronchial tubes to go into spasms, resulting in inflamed airways that tighten and fill with thick sticky secretions. Because the narrowing of the airways makes it difficult to get enough oxygen into the lungs, breathing is a daily struggle that, if not correctly dealt with, can become life-threatening.

No one knows why there has been a sharp increase in the number of asthma cases in recent years. It is the leading cause of chronic illness among all children and claims 12.4 million adult sufferers. It is an exploding problem among African-Americans, with the death rate nearly three times the death rate for whites. Contrary to popular belief, childhood asthma is not outgrown even though it may go into remission for years at a time. Where it is an early-onset condition, it persists into adulthood in 86 percent of women and 72 percent of men. Among the more common circumstances and substances that can produce the characteristic wheezing and gasping are smoke, pollen, molds, chemical air pollutants, animal dander, cold air, exercise, and stress. Specific allergies can be demonstrated in 75 to 85 percent of asthma patients.

Recent studies sponsored by the American Lung Association indicate that people with asthma have airway walls that are three times thicker than normal. Thus even a normal response to an irritant can cause the walls to come together more easily and cause a significant reduction in airflow. People at risk for a fatal asthma attack can be identified by undergoing an MRI procedure.

The federal government has been conducting a National Asthma Education Program urging doctors to treat the condition through the periodic use of various anti-inflammatory agents, recommending that bronchodilators be used only for the alleviation of symptoms. Supportive therapy in the form of stress management can also reduce the severity of attacks. See "Alternate Therapies."

Astigmatism • A defect in the curved surface of the lens or the cornea that results in blurred vision. When the refracting surface is not truly spherical, rays of light coming from a single spot are not brought into sharp focus. Astigmatism is a common disorder of vision that is easily corrected with properly fitted eyeglasses or hard contact lenses.

Atherosclerosis • A thickening and decreased elasticity of the arteries combined with the formation of fatty deposits (plaques) on or beneath their inner walls. When these plaques become large enough to block the flow of blood, the tissue beyond the block dies (infarcts). This blockage of blood flow is what causes the brain damage in most strokes and the heart muscle damage (myocardial infarction) in most heart attacks. Similar blockage may occur in other blood vessels, resulting in such conditions as kidney failure and gangrene in the legs.

The causes of atherosclerosis are not sharply defined. Because the disease is rare in undernourished populations, some specialists blame overeating, especially of animal fats. Because the disorder is not a major problem in agricultural countries, other specialists blame the stresses of industrial society.

Smokers of both sexes are at higher risk for developing cardiovascular disease because the tars and nicotine as well as the gases in the smoke itself combine to increase the plaque deposits within the arterial walls.

A recently developed diagnostic procedure for assessing arterial disease is angiography. *See* ANGIOGRAPHY, "Nutrition, Weight, and General Well-Being," and "Aging Healthfully."

Athlete's Foot • *See* FUNGAL INFECTIONS.

Autoimmune Responses • The body's production of antibodies against its own tissues. The autoimmune mechanism is thought to be responsible for such diseases as lupus erythematosus, Crohn's disease, rheumatoid arthritis, multiple sclerosis, AIDS, and probably many other diseases and phenomena.

Autopsy • Examination of body tissues and fluids after death. Autopsies permit precise identification of the cause of death and can sometimes identify genetic disease, which it is important for surviving family members to know about.

AZT • A drug (also called zidovudine) developed in 1987 that prolongs the life of some HIV-positive patients. It is also recommended as a prophylactic treatment for the fetuses of HIV-infected pregnant women.

Backache • The discomfort of backache can in many cases be reduced by appropriate exercises and by rectifying such causes of the problem as poor posture, overweight, ill-fitting shoes, high-heeled shoes, or an improper mattress. Upper back pain can often be traced to stress and to osteoporosis of the spine in older women. Lower back pain may be caused by arthritis, diseased kidneys, premenstrual pressures, or a sedentary job during which too many hours are spent in an improperly designed desk chair. Most cases are caused by strain on the muscles and connective tissues surrounding the spinal column. With increasing age, these muscles can be strengthened by exercises so that the back is properly supported. Good posture when sitting and standing as well as a firm mattress when sleeping can minimize lower back problems. *See* "Fitness," "Health Safeguards for Working Women," and "Alternative Therapies."

Bacteria • Single-cell microscopic organisms, essentially a form of plant life without chlorophyl, that occur everywhere in nature. Some bacteria are harmless, many are useful, and some cause disease. Bacteria are classified by their shape: bacilli are rod-shaped, spirochetes spiral, vibrios hooklike, and cocci round. Cocci are also classified by the way they are grouped: diplococci occur in pairs, streptococci run together in a chain, and staphylococci are clustered.

The development of antibiotics was based on the observation that there are substances in nature, produced by microorganisms and fungi, that can destroy disease-producing bacteria. However, a major concern of health professionals is the speed with which new strains of treatment-resistant bacteria are now emerging as a result of the excessive and inappropriate use of antibiotics.

Bacterial Endocarditis • A serious infection of the lining of the heart. The internal chambers and valves of the heart are lined with a delicate tissue called the endocardium. Normal endocardium is usually resistant to bacterial infection, but where valve abnormalities exist, either congenital or caused by rheumatic fever, valve replacement, or mitral prolapse, the danger of endocarditis is a particularly serious threat. Women with such a heart disability should discuss prophylactic antibiotic therapy with their oral surgeon before a tooth extraction and with other surgeons before any procedure. Otherwise the bacteria, usually streptococci, that escape into the bloodstream may cause bacterial endocarditis, which can be fatal. The protocol for this therapy is available by calling the local office of the American Heart Association.

Baldness • Loss or absence of hair; technically called alopecia. Although women may temporarily lose hair as a result of an acute fever, anticancer chemotherapy, tuberculosis, thyroid disorder, or pregnancy, they are spared the characteristically male baldness that is permanent. When women's hair begins to thin, estrogen or steroid treatment may be effec-

tive. Although chemicals in hair dyes or constant "permanents" may cause hair to break off, it will grow back unless the root is destroyed.

Barbiturate • A class of potentially habit-forming sedative and hypnotic medicines derived from barbituric acid that have a depressant effect on the central nervous system.

Sedatives and sleeping pills that contain no barbiturates have become available in recent years. See "Substance Abuse," "Plain Talk About Medications," and "Alternative Therapies."

Barium Test • A diagnostic test for the exploration of gastrointestinal disorders by X-ray. Barium sulfate, a harmless chalky substance, is administered to the patient. The opacity of the barium causes the gastrointestinal (GI) tract to stand out in a white silhouette on the fluoroscope or X-ray plate, making visible to the diagnostician ulcers, tumors, and various other disorders of the stomach, duodenum, colon, or intestines.

Bed Sore • Patch of degenerating skin tissue, technically called decubitus ulcer, caused by prolonged and uninterrupted pressure of the bedding on the skin of a patient immobilized during an illness or postoperative convalescence. The ailment also afflicts hundreds of thousands of bedridden women in nursing homes and those restricted to a wheelchair. Elderly women and women with diabetes or heart disease are especially susceptible. The parts of the body most vulnerable are the area over the heels, the shoulders, the elbows, the buttocks, and the ankles. The first symptom of the sore is redness of the skin; continued interference with circulation produces a blue appearance of the affected area and then the formation of ulcers. Preventive measures are advisable as bed sores heal with great difficulty and are susceptible to infection. Bed linens should be soft, smooth, and dry. The patient's skin should be washed and powdered each day and the vulnerable areas cushioned with cotton pads. To promote healing, the bedridden patient should change body position every few hours; sores should be cleaned with saline solutions (not peroxide or Betadine); a pillow should be placed under the legs from midcalf to ankles to keep the heels off the bed; and doughnut-type devices should be avoided since they are more likely to cause pressure sores than prevent them.

Bee Stings • *See* INSECT STINGS AND BITES.

Bell's Palsy • Paralysis of the muscles of one side of the face caused by pressure on the facial nerve that consequently becomes incapable of transmitting impulses. The cause is assumed to be an infection of the ear canal with resultant pressure on the facial nerve. The condition may also occur as one of the neurological involvements of Lyme disease. The muscular paralysis causes loss of the blink reflex, inability to close the eyelids, a flow of tears from the affected eye, and the dribbling of saliva from the immobilized side of the mouth. Recovery occurs without treatment in practically all cases. Electrical stimulation of the damaged nerve is recommended by some doctors; others prescribe cortisone to reduce inflammation. Until the blink reflex is restored, the eye must be protected from excessive dryness and foreign particles. In most cases the condition subsides in a few weeks. At its very worst the deformity caused by Bell's palsy can be partially corrected by cosmetic surgery.

Benzodiazepines • A chemical family of tranquilizers (of which Valium is a member) commonly prescribed as sleep aids on the assumption that they are not dangerously addictive and that lethal overdose is rare except in combination with alcohol. However, because of other damaging effects, these drugs are considered unacceptable by many authorities. In older women, they are known to be a contributing factor to falls because—among other negative effects—they impair coordination and they are among the sedatives that increase the likelihood of urinary incontinence where the tendency already exists. *See* "Plain Talk About Medications."

Beta Blockers • Certain drugs that reduce the activity of the heart and narrow the bronchial tubes by blocking the body's natural flow of epinephrine, the substance that normally increases the heartbeat and relaxes the muscles of the bronchi.

Bifocals • *See* EYEGLASSES.

Biopsy • The microscopic examination of small fragments of tissue cut from an organ of the body.

Most biopsies are performed under local anesthesia in the physician's office. While the procedure is considered essential in order to confirm or rule out a diagnosis of cancer, it may also be scheduled for exploratory purposes when such conditions as infertility or arterial inflammation are involved. *See* "Gynecologic Problems and Treatment," "Breast Care," and "Infertility."

Birth Defect • Any disorder or disease that is either genetically determined (inborn or inherited) or congenitally caused by drugs, including alcohol, caffeine, nicotine, prescribed medications; occupational, residential, or environmental exposure to chemicals or radiation; or

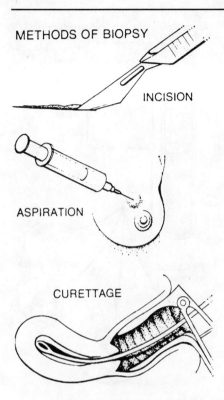

METHODS OF BIOPSY

INCISION

ASPIRATION

CURETTAGE

virus infection, injury, malnutrition, or other aspects of inadequate prenatal care that affect the normal physical and mental development of the fetus before birth. *See* "Pregnancy and Childbirth" and "Substance Abuse."

Bisexuality • Sexual attraction to both men and women. An increase in the number of people who consider themselves bisexual may be due to the fact that more men and women feel free to acknowledge their bisexual feelings. However, the problem of AIDS raises many questions about the vulnerability of women who have sexual relationships with bisexual men. *See* "Sexual Health" and "Sexually Transmissible Diseases."

Black Eye • Discoloration, swelling, and pain of the tissues around the eye, usually caused by a bruise that has ruptured tiny blood vessels under the skin. An icepack or cold compress applied immediately after the blow will slow subcutaneous bleeding, thus reducing the symptoms. A warm, wet compress applied on the following day will help absorb the discoloring fluids. If a blow to the eye is followed by persistent blurring of vision or severe pain, an ophthalmologist should be consulted promptly. If the black eye is the result of physical abuse by one's spouse or some other member of the household, prompt steps should be taken for police intervention to avoid more serious injuries and indignities. *See* "Domestic Violence, Sexual Abuse, and Rape."

Blackhead • A skin pore in which fatty material secreted by the sebaceous glands has accumulated and darkened, not because of dirt, but because of the effect of oxygen on the secretion itself. Blackheads usually accompany the acne of adolescence and may occasionally trouble older women whose skin is oily. Their occurrence may be reduced by keeping the skin clean and dry. When blackheads do appear, the temptation to squeeze them should be resisted in order to avoid infection. *See* ACNE.

Bleeding • *See* HEMORRHAGE.

Blister • A collection of fluid (lymph), usually colorless, that forms a raised sac under the skin surface. A common cause of blisters is friction on the skin. Improperly fitted shoes should be stretched or discarded and gloves should be worn when using tools that may blister the hands. Minor injuries that do not break the skin may rupture a tiny blood vessel beneath the skin and cause a blood blister. Blisters are also associated with allergic reactions to poison ivy, with infections caused by the herpes simplex virus (fever blisters or cold sores), and with fungus invasions such as ringworm.

A large and painful blister may be drained in the following way: sterilize a needle by placing it in a flame, swab the area with soap and water, prick the outer margin of the blister, press the inflated skin surface gently with a sterile gauze to remove the fluid, and apply Betadine and a sterile bandage. Any inflammation or accumulation of pus around a blister that has ruptured is a sign of bacterial infection and should be examined by a doctor.

Blood • The principal fluid of life: the medium in which oxygen and nutrients are transported to all tissues and carbon dioxide and other wastes are removed from tissues. Blood maintains the body's fluid balance by carrying water and salts to and from the tissues. It contains antibodies that fight infection, delivers hormones from the endocrine glands to the organs they influence, and regulates body temperature by dispersing heat in the form of perspiration. Every adult body contains about 1 quart (1,000 cc) of blood for every 25 pounds of weight. About 45 percent of blood composition consists of red cells that contain hemoglobin, white cells that fight infection, and platelets essential for the clotting process. The remaining 55 percent of blood composition is plasma. Blood plasma consists of water (over 90 percent) and proteins, hormones, enzymes, and other organic substances. Dissolved in the plasma are such proteins as globulins, fibrinogen, and albumen. See also The Circulatory System in "The Healthy Female," BLOOD SERUM, HEMOGLOBIN, and blood diseases are discussed under the specific headings: ANEMIA, HEMOPHILIA, LEUKEMIA.

Blood Clotting • The coagulation or solidification of blood during which blood proteins and platelets combine to seal a

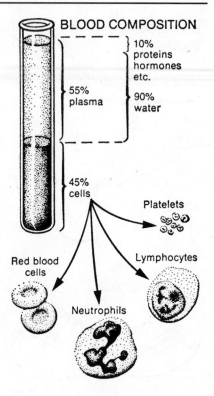

BLOOD COMPOSITION

55% plasma

10% proteins hormones etc.

90% water

45% cells

Platelets

Lymphocytes

Red blood cells

Neutrophils

break in the circulatory system. One of the plasma proteins indispensable in the clotting process, AHF (the anti-hemophilic factor), is missing from the blood of hemophiliacs. Medicines known as coagulants are available to hasten clotting in the case of hemorrhaging; vitamin therapy may be necessary in those cases where diet deficiencies or faulty metabolism interfere with normal clotting. The reason that Tylenol is the preferred analgesic rather than aspirin following all surgical procedures (including tooth extraction) is that aspirin is an anticoagulant and might cause hemorrhaging rather than healing.

Blood clots that form within the cardiovascular system are a major hazard because they impede circulation and can deprive vital organs of oxygen necessary for survival. Anticoagulants are used to counteract the formation of dangerous blood clots that may accompany diseases of the veins (phlebitis) or arteries (atherosclerosis). Heparin, a drug until recently used only in high doses to reduce the possibility of clotting in high-risk patients after surgery, injury, or childbirth, is now being used preoperatively in low doses by some surgeons. In addition to its many other properties, aspirin is an anticoagulant because it depresses platelet activity. *See* "Plain Talk About Medications."

Blood Serum • The clear, yellowish liquid that separates from whole blood when it clots. It contains proteins, enzymes, hormones, and chemicals such as glucose and sodium—all the constituents of whole blood except hemoglobin and fibrinogen. Protein antibodies (gamma globulins) present in the blood naturally or subsequent to active immunization can be fractionated out from serum, concentrated, and injected intramuscularly into another person to provide passive (short-lived, not more than 6 months) immunization against such diseases as hepatitis and measles. *See* GAMMA GLOBULIN

Blood Test • Laboratory analysis of the blood that provides information for the diagnosis of a disorder or disease. If only a small amount of blood is required, it is taken from the fleshy cushion of a finger. When a large amount is needed for several different laboratory tests, blood is usually taken from a vein in the crook of the arm.

A patient entering the hospital for surgery is often given several blood tests. These are necessary for diagnostic purposes as well as to establish the patient's blood type in the event a transfusion is required. Blood tests for hemoglobin, cholesterol, and glucose are among the routine procedures of a comprehensive annual checkup. Such tests can indicate the presence of diabetes, anemia, kidney disorder, glandular disorder, hepatitis, and the presence of antibodies indicating the exposure to such diseases as AIDS. *See* "Suggested Health Examinations."

Blood Transfusion • The infusion of blood into the veins of a patient from an outside source. Transfusions had unpredictable results until the beginning of the twentieth century when blood groups were discovered. The accurate matching of blood is necessary for a successful transfusion.

The replenishment of blood is a lifesaving measure in such circumstances as hemorrhage resulting from accident, tissue injuries caused by severe burns, or blood loss attendant on surgery. While whole blood may be desirable in most cases, it may not be essential in instances of shock when the crucial requirement is blood plasma or serum. These components can be accumulated without regard to type because they are universally compatible. They can be stored frozen in large amounts and drawn on in emergencies involving large numbers of victims such as a plane crash.

Among the recent developments in blood transfusion are two techniques with broad application. *Plateletpheresis* involves taking blood from a healthy donor, removing the platelets that are the component essential for clotting, and immediately returning the remainder—the red cells, white cells, and plasma—to the donor. The transfusion of platelets can extend the lives of patients with certain types of anemia, leukemia, and other malignant diseases for whom bleeding episodes might otherwise be fatal. This procedure in no way endangers the donor's blood supply because platelets in the body of a healthy person are automatically replaced within two days. The second innovation in transfusion is a technique whereby white blood cells can be supplied to cancer patients who are receiving drugs that temporarily suppress the ability of the bone marrow to manufacture them. In this way patients undergoing anticancer chemotherapy are provided with the white cells necessary for fighting infection.

Fear of contracting HIV, the virus that leads to AIDS, causes some patients preparing for elective surgery to bank their own blood in advance should a transfusion be necessary.

Blood Types • For many years it had been observed that some blood transfusions were successful and some were not, but it was not until the twentieth century that the riddle of incompatibility was solved. It is now known that the blood of all humans, regardless of skin color, race, country of origin, or sex, can be classified under four main groupings: A, B, AB, and O. Blood type O (the "O" stands for zero) is composed of red cells that can blend with any type of plasma. Because of this compatibility, a person with O type blood is a universal donor. Conversely, anyone with AB type blood is a universal recipient. Of each 100 individuals, approximately 45 will be type O, 40 will be type A, 10 will be type B, and 5 will be type AB. There are many minor subtypes that are inconsequential for most people.

Body Odors • Natural odors associated with the human body. Fresh perspiration from a healthy body is practically odorless. Most unpleasant body odors are caused by the presence of bacteria or fungi that multiply in areas where perspiration can accumulate, such as the genital area, the armpits, and between the toes, and by stale perspiration absorbed by clothing. Regular scrubbing with soap and water and regular changes of clothes should keep the body clean and free of

offensive odors. It should be noted that vaginal sprays can be quite harmful to the delicate membranes they are supposed to deodorize. *See* ANTIPERSPIRANT DEODORANT and PHEROMONES.

Boil • A painful bacterial infection, usually staphylococcal, of a hair follicle or sweat gland, occurring on the face, scalp, neck, shoulders, breast, or buttocks. The infected lump, technically called a furuncle, may be as small as a cherry pit or quite large. Because the infection can easily spread, a boil should be treated promptly. Moist, hot compresses should be applied several times a day. The boil should then be covered with a topical antibiotic and protected by a sterile gauze bandage. Boils that do not drain naturally following the application of heat and moisture may have to be incised surgically. Those that occur in groups (carbuncles) or that recur may be the result of faulty habits of personal hygiene, low resistance, diabetes, or a strain of bacteria requiring a newer antibiotic. Such cases should be treated by a doctor.

Bone • The hard tissue that forms the major part of the skeleton. The 206 bones in the human body are connected by ligaments at the joints and are activated into movement by muscles secured to the bones by tendons. Bones are covered by a thin fibrous membrane called periosteum that sheathes and protects them and supports the adjacent tendons. The periosteum stops at the joints that are covered by a layer of cartilage. The fibrous layer of tissue directly under the periosteum gives bones their elasticity. Next are the dense hard layers called compact tissue within which are encased the porous materials known as spongy tissue. The innermost cavity of bone contains the marrow, which is the source of red blood cell production. Every layer of bone is crisscrossed by blood vessels. Bone tissue also contains a large number of nerves.

The hardness and strength of the skeleton result from the mineral content—calcium phosphate. This mineral, plentiful in milk, is essential for the transformation of cartilage into the calcified part of bone during childhood and adolescence. Bone tissue, even when fully formed in adulthood, constantly renews itself, but because the rate of renewal slows with age, the bones of the elderly become more brittle as they become more porous and less elastic.

The health of bones may be impaired by dietary deficiency of the mother during pregnancy or of the child during the years of growth, by infectious diseases (osteomyelitis), degenerative diseases (osteoporosis, osteoarthritis), tumors, and a rare form of primary cancer (sarcoma). The most common bone injury is a fracture, and bones may also bleed internally after sustaining a severe bruise. *See* "Aging Healthfully."

Bone Scan • A procedure that aids in the diagnosis of cancer, various degenerative disorders, and injury. The test involves the injection of a radioisotope, which takes several hours to reach the bone. The patient may leave during this time and return for the scan, which is done on an outpatient basis and takes about one hour.

Bone Density Tests • Various scanning procedures that assess the extent of osteoporosis in postmenopausal women. *See* "Aging Healthfully."

Botulism • A form of food poisoning caused by bacteria that produce a toxin that attacks the nervous system. The causative bacterium, *Clostridium botulinum*, thrives in low-acid, low-sugar substances where there is no oxygen. It is typically found in improperly preserved foods, such as canned vegetables, meat, or smoked fish. The contaminated food rarely smells, tastes, or looks spoiled. Diagnosis is simplified by the fact that several people, including household pets, are likely to be affected at the same time.

Nausea and vomiting occur generally in less than 24 hours and may or may not precede the central nervous system symptoms, whose onset usually is from 12 to 36 hours after eating. These symptoms are double vision, puffy or drooping eyelids, and paralysis that impedes swallowing and breathing. The person must be hospitalized at once for treatment to nullify the toxin and to prevent respiratory failure. Anyone who has eaten the spoiled food must be treated without delay with botulinus antitoxin.

Brain • The central organ of the nervous system, interpreting all sense impressions, controlling the activities of over 600 of the body's voluntary muscles, regulating the autonomic nervous system, and through its capacity for storing and recalling the messages received by its billions of cells, functioning as the memory bank that we call the mind.

The human brain is made of soft, convoluted, pinkish-gray tissue that weighs about 3 pounds and fits within the confines of the skull. Enveloping the brain and separating it from its bony encasement are three tough membranes, collectively called the meninges, which also sheathe the spinal cord. Between two of these membranous layers is the cerebrospinal fluid that may be tapped for accurate diagnosis of such diseases as cerebrospinal meningitis. The portion of the brain that has come to be synonymous with the mind is the cerebrum whose outer layer, the cerebral cortex, is fissured, furrowed, and wrinkled into "gray matter." The deepest fissure divides this part of the brain into two distinct halves: the nerves in the right hemisphere control the left side of the body and vice versa. Emerging from the cerebrum at the middle of the skull and extending down the back of the neck into the spinal cord is the brain stem; on either side of the brain stem are the two halves of the cerebellum. The cerebellum is the portion of the brain whose essential function is the coordination of muscular activities.

The brain also functions as a gland, manufacturing substances similar in chemical composition to morphine that have the same effect on the body as synthetic painkillers. These hormonelike substances are called endorphins and enkephalins. The amounts in which they are produced and released are presumed to define the body's sensations of pain and pleasure as well as to account for the symptoms of some forms of mental illness.

Advances in scanning and imaging techniques (CAT scan and MRI) have largely replaced the electroencephalograph (EEG) as a diagnostic tool. These advances have enabled neurologists to "map" the brain, differentiating between the areas that control specific functions, such as memory and language. Recent research indicates that in fact the female brain differs significantly from that of the male. The consequences of these differences have yet to be clearly detailed.

Many brain tumors that were previously untreatable or inoperable can now be reduced by radiation or completely removed due to advances in the techniques of hypothermia and microsurgery. Legal death is now defined not by the cessation of the heartbeat, but by the death of the brain resulting from oxygen deprivation. *See* EPILEPSY, CONCUSSION, and "Aging Healthfully."

Bronchitis • Inflammation of the lining of the bronchial tubes, the air passages that connect the windpipe and the lungs. In its acute form the inflammation may be an extension of an upper respiratory viral infection or may be caused by a bacterial infection following an upper respiratory illness. Such an attack is accompanied by fever and coughing up of the excess mucus secreted by the inflamed membranes. Bed rest and an expectorant medicine that loosens the sputum rather than one that suppresses the cough are the standard treatment. Antibiotics should be used only if the infection is diagnosed as bacterial or if the patient is at high risk for pneumonia. Chronic bronchitis is a much more serious matter because the recurrent or persistent coughing and spitting up can lead to irreversible lung injury and an increased vulnerability to emphysema and heart disease. In chronic bronchitis, the victim coughs and spits up yellow mucus, especially in the morning and evening, and eventually the condition becomes irreversible. Too many patients wait until the disease approaches a disabling stage before seeing a doctor. The first and indispensable aspect of treatment is to stop smoking. In some cases rehabilitation may involve a change of job. In others the symptoms may gradually disappear after strict adherence to a wholesome regimen: proper diet, mild exercise, rest and relaxation, and avoidance of lung irritants.

Bronchodilators • Medications, usually delivered by inhalers, that relax the bronchial muscles, thereby counteracting the respiratory distress of an asthma attack.

Bruise • An injury in which small subcutaneous blood vessels are damaged but the skin surface remains intact; also called a contusion. When the skin is broken, the injury is called an abrasion or a laceration. In a bruise, the escape of blood into the surrounding tissues causes pain and swelling as well as the characteristic discoloration of the skin. The effects of a bruise may not be visible when a blow is sustained by a muscle, a bone, or an ear. Healing is usually hastened and pain reduced by the application of ice or of cold compresses just after the injury to slow down the bleeding. The application of heat to the bruised area the following day is likely to hasten the reabsorption of the blood. If symptoms increase rather than abate, a doctor should be consulted, especially where deeper internal bruises are suspected. Bruises resulting from spousal abuse should be called to the attention of the police. *See* BLACK EYE.

Bunion • A deformity of the foot that occurs when the big toe deviates from its natural position because of inflammation at the joint connecting the toe to the foot. Continuing pressure results in the hard swelling at the base of the toe and the development of the bunion. Discomfort is best relieved by correcting the footwear that causes the problem. In mild cases, with shoes that fit properly, the condition may be eliminated without further treatment. When the pain is severe enough to interfere with normal functioning even when wearing shoes with an orthopedic correction, surgery may be the only practical solution.

Burns • Injuries resulting from contact with dry heat (fire), moist heat (scalding by steam or liquid), electricity, chemicals, or the ultraviolet rays of the sun or a sunlamp. Whatever the cause, the injury is classified according to the extent of tissue damage. A first-degree burn is one in which the skin turns visibly red; a second-degree burn causes the skin to blister; a third-degree burn damages the deeper skin layers and may destroy the growth cells in the subcutaneous tissues. Even a first-degree burn is potentially dangerous if a large area of the body has been affected, especially if the victim is very young or very old. Until professional help is available a person who has sustained a serious burn should lie down and liquids should be administered but only if they can be consciously swallowed. Ice cold water can be gently applied to the burned area. *Do not* give any alcoholic beverage. *Do not* disturb blisters. *Do not* attempt to remove clothing adhering to burnt skin. *Do not* apply oily salves or ointments or antiseptic sprays except in cases of superficial burns involving a small area. Many hospitals are establishing special burn treatment centers where new techniques are applied to save lives and reduce suffering.

Bursitis • Inflammation of a bursa, one of the small fluid-filled sacs located at various joints throughout the body for the purpose of minimizing friction. Bursitis most commonly occurs at the joints receiving the most wear and tear: at the hip, shoulder, knee, and elbow. "Housemaid's knee" and "tennis elbow" are the result of bursa inflammation. A bunion is the result of inflammation of the bursa that lubricates the joint between the big toe and the foot. An acute, and acutely painful, attack of bursitis may occur after an accident, following unusual exertion connected with moving heavy objects, or as a job-related result of repetitive stress. Although such an attack may be self-healing within a week or ten days, the process can be eased and hastened by taking aspirin or some other analgesic and immobilizing the affected joint in a sling or a flexible bandage.

Calcitonin • A hormone that regulates the phosphorus and calcium levels in the blood and inhibits the degeneration of bone tissue.

BURSITIS OF THE SHOULDER

Bursa is swollen and filled with calcium deposits

Normal joint capsule

Scapula (shoulder blade)

Muscle   Humerus (upper arm)

Callus • An area of the skin that has thickened as a protection against repeated friction; also an irregular bump on a bone that has formed when the recalcification process closes a fracture. The calluses that form on the hands as a result of constant friction or repeated pressures can best be prevented by wearing protective gloves. Most of those that form on the soles of the feet or around the outer rim of the heels can be eliminated by wearing proper footwear. Calluses can be reduced by rubbing them with pumice or an emery board.

Cancer • The general term for a disease process in which the cells in a particular part of the body grow and reproduce with abnormal rapidity. This defect in the controls that govern normal cell growth characterizes about 200 different diseases known as cancers, most of which are also called malignancies or malignant tumors. Cancers that are created by disordered epithelial cells and arise on the surface of the lining of a tissue or within a duct are *carcinomas*. Malignancies that originate in bones and muscles are known as *sarcomas*. Those that originated in the blood-forming organs are called *leukemias*. Those that start in the lymphatics are called *lymphomas*. Malignancies created by the cells that carry the dark pigment melanin are called *melanomas*.

A cancer is said to be localized when the diseased cells remain clumped together even if the group of cells grows into a visible mass large enough to invade underlying or surrounding tissue. When some of the diseased cells break away and make their way into the bloodstream or the lymphatics eventually reaching other parts of the body, the cancer is said to have metastasized. *See* CARCINOGEN, CARCINOMA, SARCOMA, LEUKEMIA, MELANOMA, METASTASIS, "Breast Care," and "Gynecologic Problems and Treatment."

Canker Sore • An ulceration of the mucous membrane at the corner of the mouth or inside the lips or cheeks. While not attributable to a single cause, canker sores may result from a deficiency of vitamin B_{12} or iron, or their onset may be triggered by stress, viral infection, menstruation, sensitivity to particular foods, or mechanical irritation by a rough-edged tooth or filling or ill-fitting dentures. Most canker sores are occasional and self-healing. Recurrent canker sores so painful that they interfere with talking or eating should be treated by a physician.

Car Sickness • *See* MOTION SICKNESS.

Carcinogen • Any agent (tobacco smoke, X-rays, asbestos fibers, food additives, drugs, industrial pollutants, and so on) capable of causing changes in cell structure (mutagenesis) and therefore a potential cause of cancer.

Carcinoma • One of the two main groups of cancers; the other is sarcoma. A carcinoma originates in epithelial cells located in glandular structures, mucous membranes, and skin. Practically all malignancies of the skin, tongue, stomach, uterus, and breast come under this heading.

Cardiopulmonary   Resuscitation (CPR) • An emergency lifesaving technique in which oxygenated blood is sent to the brain and other tissues of the victim of cardiac arrest by the simultaneous administration of artificial respiration and external manipulation of the heart. CPR must be initiated at once following a heart attack, electric shock, or any other circumstance in which the lack of circulation has begun to deprive the brain of oxygen. Because of its proven effectiveness when administered by a properly trained individual, the Red Cross and the American Heart Association are encouraging ordinary citizens, including teenagers, to take the six- to twelve-hour CPR courses being offered under their auspices.

Carotene • A plant pigment especially plentiful in carrots and also found in yellow, orange, and red fruits and vegetables in smaller amounts. Carotene is essential in the diet because it is converted into vitamin A in the body. It is also one of the weaker pigments in human skin. Its yellowish tone is generally masked by the melanin pigment in dark-complexioned women, but a fair complexion will take on an orange hue if the diet contains an excessive amount of carrots. *See* "Nutrition, Weight, and General Well-Being."

Cartilage • The tough, whitish elastic tissue that, together with bone, forms the skeleton. There are three different types of cartilage. Hyaline cartilage forms the extremely strong slippery surface of the ends of the bones at the joints, acting as a shock absorber. It is also the material of which the nose and the rings of the trachea are made. Fibrocartilage is densely packed with fibers and forms the disks between the spinal vertebrae. Elastic cartilage is the most flexible, forming the external ear and the larynx. The stiffness in the joints that characterizes osteoarthritis is associated with a deterioration of cartilage.

CAT • *See* COMPUTERIZED AXIAL TOMOGRAPHY.

Catheterization • The procedure in which a tube is inserted through a passage in the body for the purpose of withdrawing or introducing fluids or other materials. Catheters have been used for centuries, but since the introduction of plastics they are less costly to manufacture and give minimal discomfort to the patient. In the more common applications, a catheter is introduced into the urethra for draining urine from the bladder; an intravenous catheter is used for "tube-feeding" following surgery; a nasogastric tube is used for withdrawing samples of material from the stomach as a diagnostic clue. Catheterization is essential in the administration of oxygen through the nose, and it can effectively remove stones lodged in the ureter, the passageway connecting the kidney and the bladder. Cardiac catheterization is routinely used to detect and measure critical abnormalities caused by circulatory disorders.

Cauterization • The burning away of infected, unwanted, or dead tissue by the application of caustic chemicals or electrically heated instruments. Cryosurgery used in the treatment of certain types of tumors is a form of cauterization; the removal of surface moles with an electrical needle is another. Cauterization of cervical tissue to prevent the spread of erosion is a common gynecological practice, and it is also used to remove a small, localized cervical cancer.

Cavities • *See* DENTAL CARIES.

Cell • The structural unit of which all body tissues are formed. The human body is composed of billions of cells differing in size and structure depending on their function. In spite of these differences every cell includes the same basic components: an outer limiting membrane that regulates the transport of chemical substances into and out of the cell, a mass of cytoplasm containing substances involved in metabolism and genetic transmission, a nucleus whose membrane contains the concentration of RNA and encloses the DNA that determines the hereditary transmission of genetic characteristics.

Cerebral Palsy • A neuromuscular disorder of unknown cause and varying degrees of severity whose symptoms usually appear by age 3. Cerebral palsy is characterized by an inability to control the muscles of the arms and legs, by mild or serious speech impairment, and by jerky movements of the head and torso. Intellectual disability is not necessarily associated with this disorder, but emotional problems are likely to become deep-rooted unless the child receives strong familial support and understanding treatment in school. Physical and speech therapy as well as medication to reduce spasticity are aspects of treatment. More than 25 percent of cerebral palsy cases occur every year among the 52,000 babies weighing less than 3.3 pounds at birth. However, there is some evidence that if mothers receive an injection of the natural

chemical magnesium sulfate when they go into premature labor, the likelihood of preventing cerebral palsy in the newborn is significantly increased. *See* "Pregnancy and Childbirth" and "Directory of Health Information."

ORIGINS OF CHEST PAINS

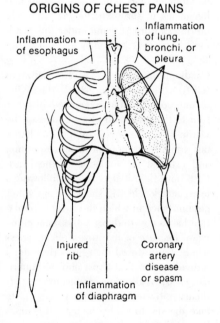

Chest Pains • Discomfort in any part of the thorax, usually caused by a disorder of one of the organs within the thoracic cavity enclosed by the rib cage, by an injury to a rib, or by a strained muscle. The site of a disorder may be the heart, lungs, large blood vessels, esophagus, or part of the trachea. Any viral or bacterial infection of the respiratory system may be accompanied by pain that may become acute when constant coughing is involved. Various allergies to mold, dust, animal dander, chemical pollutants may be another cause. Pain might be referred to the chest by the nervous system from areas outside the thoracic cavity. For example, certain types of indigestion produce a pain that may be mistaken for a heart attack. In most cases, however, the pain resulting from cardiovascular problems is the feeling of tightness and suffocation characteristic of angina pectoris. Almost all chest pains that originate in respiratory or circulatory disorders are intensified by smoking. Persistent chest pains should always be diagnosed and treated by a doctor. See ANGINA PECTORIS.

Chicken Pox • A common, highly contagious viral disease of childhood. Ninety percent of the four million cases occurring annually in the United States happen before age 15. When the disease occurs during adolescence or adulthood, there is a high risk of serious complications. A vaccine said to be 70 to 90 percent effective was approved by the FDA in 1995. Guidelines for its use have only recently been established. Women who have never had chicken pox should discuss immunization with their health care provider. It is not yet known whether the vaccine is strong enough to prevent eventual onset of shingles. See HERPES and "Immunization Guide."

Chilblains • Inflammation of the skin, accompanied by burning and itching, usually caused by exposure to cold. Special vulnerability to chilblains may result from poor circulation, inadequate diet, or an allergic response to low temperatures.

The condition is easier to prevent than to treat. Anyone sensitive to the cold should always wear warm clothes, especially woolen or partly woolen socks (never 100 percent synthetic), fleece-lined boots, and woolen gloves.

When chilblains have occurred, no attempts should be made to "stimulate" circulation by applying extreme heat or cold to the affected areas. In most cases a warm dry environment will bring about a return to normal. If the symptoms persist or if blisters form on the skin surface, a doctor should be consulted for further instructions.

Chiropractor • A specialist in the manipulation of the musculoskeletal system. See "You, Your Doctors, and the Health Care System" and "Alternative Therapies."

Chlorine • A chemical element widely used to purify public water supplies and disinfect swimming pools because it is cheap, easily manufactured, and effective against bacteria, viruses, and fungi. An excessively chlorinated swimming pool will cause temporary eye discomfort, and skin contact with chlorine in household bleaches will produce an itching and burning rash as an allergic reaction where sensitivity exists to this chemical.

Choking • Obstruction of the air passage in the throat by a swallowed object that has gone into the windpipe instead of into the esophagus. When food is being swallowed, an automatic mechanism closes the flap at the top of the trachea (windpipe). It is not unusual, however, for a morsel of food or, in the case of a small child, a foreign object such as a button to "go down the wrong way." This is apt to happen when a sudden intake of breath caused by laughing, talking, or coughing occurs while a person has food in her mouth. The immediate signs of choking are an inability to speak or breathe. In minutes the skin turns bluish, and unless emergency assistance is prompt, the results can be fatal. See HEIMLICH MANEUVER.

Chromosomes • Stringlike structures within the cell nucleus that contain the genetic information governing each person's inherited characteristics. Normal human body cells contain 46 paired chromosomes composed of DNA (deoxyribonucleic acid). An ovum contains 22 autosome and 1 sex (X) chromosomes. A sperm contains 22 autosome and 1 sex (X or Y) chromosomes so that when they combine during reproduction the offspring cell receives its full complement of 46 "message carriers."

The sex of an offspring is determined by the combination of the sex chromosomes designated as X and Y. If an egg is fertilized by a sperm carrying the X chromosome, the offspring will have two X chromosomes and will therefore be female (XX). If an egg is fertilized by a Y-bearing sperm, the offspring will have one of each and will be male (XY).

Chromosomal abnormalities vary in significance, the more serious ones being responsible for birth defects, mental retardation, and spontaneous abortion.

The possibility of abnormalities severe enough to warrant abortion can be determined through prenatal genetic counseling. Research in recent years indicates that environmental and occupational exposure to various chemicals can cause irreversible damage to chromosomes, leading to genetic mutations in the offspring. Possible effects of various drugs are discussed in the chapter "Substance Abuse." *See* SEX-LINKED ABNORMALITIES.

Chronic Fatigue Syndrome (CFS)   •
A condition defined by an international committee of medical experts in 1994 as one whose chief characteristic is severe, disabling fatigue of sudden onset that may last for months or even years. A distinctive aspect of this disorder is that the fatigue is not the result of physical activity, nor is it relieved by rest. A diagnosis of CFS is also based on at least four of the following symptoms: sore throat, muscle pain, muscle weakness, tender lymph nodes in the neck or underarm, head-

HEREDITY

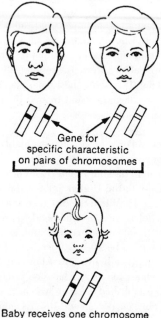

Gene for
specific characteristic
on pairs of chromosomes

Baby receives one chromosome
from each parent for each pair

aches, joint pains without swelling, memory loss, sleep disorders, and malaise lasting for a day or more after physical exertion.

This condition is debilitating but rarely fatal. It is not contagious, and there is no reliable test that can detect it. It is estimated that from 2 to 5 million people—mainly women—are stricken. Before arriving at a diagnosis of CFS, the patient should be evaluated for such conditions as multiple sclerosis, cancer, obesity, substance abuse, and depression.

Investigations have not been able to pinpoint a cause for CFS. Some researchers believe it to be a manifestation of the immune system in disarray; others believe that an imbalance in hormone production is responsible. In the meantime, many self-help and support groups have sprung up, several of which publish newsletters that keep patients and their families informed of developments. *See* "Directory of Health Information."

Chronic Symptom • Symptom of a disorder that lasts over a long period of time, sometimes for the remainder of the patient's life, such as the joint pains characteristic of rheumatoid arthritis or the cough associated with emphysema.

Cirrhosis • Degenerative disease especially of the liver in which the development of fibrous tissue with consequent hardening and scarring causes the loss of normal function. Cirrhosis of the liver is most frequently associated with chronic alcoholism, affecting 15 percent of all heavy drinkers. However, the condition may also occur after infectious hepatitis or, more rarely, as a consequence of toxic hepatitis in which liver cells are damaged because of sensitivity to such drugs as chlorpromazine (Thorazine) or chloramphenicol (Chloromycetin).

Cirrhosis is insidious because it may be asymptomatic until it has resulted in irreversible damage. When symptoms are manifest, they include abdominal swelling with fluid, soreness under the rib cage, swollen ankles, weight loss, and general fatigue. In advanced cases the signs are jaundice and possible vomiting of blood leading to collapse. When alcoholic cirrhosis is treated promptly at an early stage, the liver may repair and rehabilitate itself. Total abstention from alcohol and a diet rich in proteins and supplementary vitamins are essential to recovery. *See* LIVER and "You and Your Medications."

Claudication • *See* INTERMITTENT CLAUDICATION.

Claustrophobia • An irrational, persistent, and often insurmountable fear of enclosed places such as elevators, windowless rooms, and the like. *See* "Alternative Therapies."

Climacteric • The time in a woman's life when her childbearing capabilities come to an end; the menopause. *See* "Aging Healthfully."

Coagulation • *See* BLOOD CLOTTING.

Codeine • A mild narcotic drug derived from opium. *See* "Plain Talk About Medications."

Coffee • A beverage containing varying amounts of caffeine and producing such side effects as insomnia and heartburn and, in some people, withdrawal symptoms such as headaches, irritability, and fatigue. Decaffeinated coffee produces less of these side effects. *See* "Substance Abuse" and "Pregnancy and Childbirth."

Cognitive Therapy • A type of psychotherapy developed in the 1950s and now practiced in all major cities in the United States and around the world. Relatively short-term in achieving its results, it is based on the concept that depression is a consequence of distorted thinking and unrealistically negative views about oneself, one's place in the world, and future expectations. The goal is to change these views so that the patient learns to be as compassionate with herself as she would be with a good friend, and—briefly put—to see the cup as half full rather than half empty. Cognitive therapy is concerned not with probing and re-examining the past but rather with recognition of the patient's self-defeating views about the present in order to change them. *See* "Aging Healthfully" and "Alternative Therapies."

Coitus Interruptus • The withdrawal of the penis before ejaculation as a means of preventing pregnancy. As a contraceptive method its failure rate is high. *See* "Contraception and Abortion."

Cold Sores • *See* HERPES.

Colitis • Inflammation of the colon (large intestine). The type most frequently encountered is mucous colitis, also known as irritable bowel, a condition in which the lower bowel goes into spasms with or without cramps accompanied by an alteration of diarrhea and constipation. A far more serious condition is ulcerative colitis in which there is tissue impairment. A mucus and blood mixture is often found in the feces of persons with ulcerative colitis, the onset of which typically occurs among young adults of both sexes, eventually producing disabling attacks of diarrhea. Cancer of the colon or rectum develops in up to 10 percent of those who have had colitis for ten years or more.

Because patterns of remission and relapse are usual, ulcerative colitis must be treated with patience and care, including supervision of diet, bed rest, and elimination of as many tension-producing factors as possible. This is best accomplished through a combination of psychotherapy and a stress management program. *See* CROHN'S DISEASE and IRRITABLE BOWEL SYNDROME.

Colon Cancer • In terms of overall figures, colorectal cancer is the second biggest cancer killer in the United States following lung cancer. It has been calculated that 20 percent of all cases are traceable to an inherited predisposition, and 1991 marked the discovery of the gene now assumed to be responsible for initiating this cancer. Fortunately, there is a high success rate in curing it following early detection.

The American Cancer Society recommends the following procedures: after age 40, a digital rectal examination; after age 50, laboratory analysis of a stool sample every year, examinations every three years of the lower colon and rectum with a sigmoidoscope. People at high risk because of a history of rectal polyps, or because of a family history that includes cases of colorectal cancer, should schedule a colonoscopy every three years after age 40.

Colonoscopy • A diagnostic procedure that uses a long flexible instrument to examine the entire five-foot length of the large intestine. This procedure is done on an outpatient basis by a gastroenterologist. It requires special preparation by the patient involving a day of a liquid diet and the consumption of a gallon of a special liquid that thoroughly cleanses the entire bowel.

Colostomy • A surgical procedure by which an artificial anal opening is created in the abdominal wall. A colostomy may be performed as a temporary measure after bowel surgery or it may have to be a permanent procedure. Patients who have undergone a colostomy usually must regulate their diets to control the character of their stool. An important aspect of colostomy management is participation in a mutual support group where people who are experienced in coping with the physical, psychological, and social problems associated with this procedure help the new patient to adjust to it with a minimum of anxiety and embarrassment. *See* "Directory of Health Information."

Coma • Deep unconsciousness resulting from, among other circumstances, injury to the brain, stroke, poisoning by barbiturates or alcohol, overdose or under-

COLOSTOMY

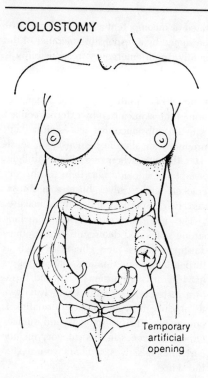

Temporary
artificial
opening

dose of insulin, coronary thrombosis, or shock.

Common Cold • The designation for any of a large number of brief and relatively mild virus infections of the upper respiratory tract that may produce uncomfortable symptoms in the nose (rhinitis), throat (pharyngitis), or voice box (laryngitis). Because allergies to grasses and pollens produce certain overlapping symptoms, they are often mistakenly labeled "summer colds." The development of a cold vaccine has so far proved impractical because the symptoms are caused by more than 200 different viruses.

An ordinary cold should *not* be treated with antibiotics. These medicines are ineffective against viruses and may cause undesired side effects such as changes in normal bacteria. However, a cold accom-

panied by a cough, a fever of over 100°, or a painful sore throat can be more than a common cold and should be diagnosed by a doctor. The ordinary upper respiratory viral infection may produce any or all of the following symptoms in combination: stuffed or running nose, mildly scratchy throat, teary eyes, heavy breathing, fits of sneezing, some impairment of the sense of taste and smell, mild headache, and a general feeling of lassitude. Many healthy adults do not bother to treat these symptoms and go about their business until the cold goes away, usually within three or four days. Some insist that regular doses of chicken soup are the most effective remedy. Others buy over-the-counter medicines containing antihistamines, often exchanging drowsiness for unclogged nostrils and dry eyes. While there is no unambiguous evidence that vitamin C can prevent or cure a cold, it is argued by some enthusiasts that its action is similar to that of interferon, a substance produced in the body that suppresses virus growth. It is this protein substance that scientists hope to synthesize eventually as the most generalized and effective method of fighting the many viruses that produce common cold symptoms. *See* PHARYNGITIS.

Computerized Axial Tomography (CAT scan) • A radiographic process in which a computer produces a three-dimensional image of an interior body structure from a series of cross-sectional images created along an axis. Since its introduction in the early 1970s, CAT scanning has become a reliable tool in the diagnosis of brain disorders, cancers, and other conditions previously inaccessible to conventional X-rays. A CAT scan is quick, painless, and can be accomplished in about half an hour on an outpatient basis.

Concussion, Cerebral • Impairment of brain function resulting from a blow to the cranium or jaw. Concussion is the mildest form of head injury causing a temporary loss of consciousness. Recovery may be accompanied by dizziness, headache, and amnesia about the events preceding the injury. Any head injury resulting in a loss of consciousness should be evaluated by a physician.

Conjunctivitis • Inflammation of the conjunctiva, the thin membrane that lines the eyelid and covers the front of the eye. The disorder is commonly called pink eye. Conjunctivitis may be caused by bacteria or a virus or it may be an allergic response to a new brand of eye makeup, a reaction to a chemical pollutant in the air or water or to radiation on the job or in the environment, or the result of irritation from an ingrown eyelash in the lower lid. An inflammation caused by bacteria or a virus is highly contagious, and precautions should be taken to prevent its spread to others and to minimize self-reinfection. In such cases, an ophthalmic antibiotic ointment is usually the effective treatment. When dandruff in the eyebrows and eyelashes is the cause of conjunctivitis, a non-prescription steroid ointment is the preferred treatment. An eye doctor should be consulted about the negative aspects of continued use.

Consent Laws • State legislation that covers the following circumstances. (1) *The age of consent:* the age of a woman before which sexual intercourse with her is considered statutory rape whether or not she has given her consent to the act. (2) *Treatment or diagnostic test consent:* a patient undergoing surgery or some other potentially hazardous procedure must sign a statement consenting to the operation. In the case of a child (defined differently in different states) or an incapaci-

tated or incompetent adult, the form must be signed by a responsible member of the family. In an emergency, responsibility is assumed by the physician.

Contact Dermatitis • An inflammation of the skin caused by external contact with any substance that acts as an irritant, produces an allergic response, or sensitizes the skin when exposed to sunlight. Symptoms include an itchy rash, dry cracked patches, hives, blisters, and in severe cases, soreness and general malaise.

The more common irritants include strong soaps and detergents that produce "dishpan hands" and chemicals such as turpentine, paint thinners, and strippers used by artists, housepainters, and furniture restorers. The culprit widely known to produce allergic contact dermatitis is poison ivy (also poison oak and sumac). Other substances in this category include certain metals, dyes, or fibers worn next to the skin.

Phototoxic substances include some sunscreening products and the fragrant oils and essences in certain lotions and cosmetics. Dermatologists increasingly report that they treat rashes caused by face makeup and hair preparations. Patients report that they suddenly develop allergic responses to topical medications they have been using over a long period to treat contact dermatitis, medications containing antibiotics or topical anesthetics.

Another self-defeating reaction occurs when the lanolin in skin softeners used to counteract the drying effect of exposure to cold or chemical irritants ends up by clogging the pores and causing a rash. *See* POISON IVY.

Contact Lenses • Plastic lenses that are measured so that they fit on the cornea and are ground to individual prescription so that they correct defects in vision. Contact lenses are worn by an estimated twenty-four million people, both young and old, and are especially popular with performers, athletes, and all those who associate eyeglasses with a negative self-image. In addition to their cosmetic advantages, contact lenses afford the wearer increased peripheral and side vision. Elderly people who have undergone cataract surgery are pleased to have contact lenses that provide almost perfect vision as an alternative to the thick-lensed glasses that used to be the only corrective for their visual impairment.

Anyone contemplating the switch to contact lenses or who needs vision correction for the first time and would prefer not to wear traditional eyeglasses should discuss the options with an ophthalmologist. Only an eye specialist can determine a person's suitability for contact lenses and which of the various types will provide the best visual correction with maximum comfort. This is determined not only by a thorough eye examination, including a glaucoma check, but also by a consideration of such conditions as diabetes, allergies, medications that dry the eyes, and working environments where dust and fumes are a problem.

Risks of damage to the eye can be avoided if care and cleaning instructions are followed to the letter. Frequent checkups are recommended, especially during the first year of use so that any problems of irritation and inflammation can be treated at once if the cornea is not to be scarred.

Convulsions • Violent and abnormal muscular contractions or spasms that seize the body suddenly and spontaneously, usually ending with unconsciousness. Convulsions are almost always a symptom of a serious disorder and they are the classic manifestation of the grand mal seizures of epilepsy. They are not uncommon among children during infections of the nervous system, during generalized infections that cause a very high fever, or as a sign of Reye's syndrome, which is associated with several viral diseases, especially with chicken pox. Convulsions are one of the critical consequences of withdrawal from barbiturates and alcohol following heavy and habitual use. They may also occur in adulthood from a tumor or from diseases that attack the brain and central nervous system, especially encephalitis and meningitis.

At first sign of seizure, the person should be placed lying down, with the head turned to one side. The mouth should be opened (forced open if necessary) and something (a knotted handkerchief, a wadded piece of sheet, or a smooth stick) put between the upper and lower teeth to keep the mouth open so that an airway can be maintained and to keep the patient from biting her tongue. If the tongue is swallowed, keep the mouth wide open and free the tongue with a finger. Then seek medical attention.

Cornea • The transparent tissue that forms the outer layer of the eyeball, covering the iris and the lens through which vision is achieved. The most serious disease that affects the cornea is herpes simplex keratitis; it causes more loss of vision in the Western world than any other corneal infection.

One of the hazards of wearing contact lenses is inflammation of the cornea, which must be treated promptly to avoid irreversible scarring. Any soreness or redness of the cornea, whether caused by the presence of a foreign particle or an infection should be called to an ophthalmologist's attention.

Corneal dystrophy is an inherited disease in which there is a progressive loss of vision resulting from an increasing cloudiness of the tissue. Corneal dystrophy as well as vision impairment caused by damage to the cornea can be corrected by a corneal transplant. *See* CONTACT LENSES, HERPES.

Corns • An area of thickened skin (callus) that occurs on or between the toes. There are two types of corns: hard corns usually located on the small toe or on the upper ridge of one of the other toes and soft and white corns that are likely to develop between the fourth and fifth toe. The hard core of both types of callus points inward and when pressed against the surrounding tissue causes pain. Corns are the result of wearing shoes that are too tight, and unless proper footwear is worn, they will recur.

Treating corns at home with razor blades or with strongly medicated "removers" can injure surrounding tissues, resulting in additional discomfort and sometimes in serious infection. The sensible course is a visit to a podiatrist.

Coronary Bypass Surgery • A procedure in which a healthy vein is removed from one part of the patient's body (usually the leg) and inserted between clogged and blocked coronary arteries and the aorta. By increasing the supply of blood to the heart, this type of surgery minimizes or eliminates severe angina attacks and other disabling coronary conditions. There is considerable controversy about the need for surgery in cases that can be effectively treated in less radical ways. Studies indicate that survival rate for patients who have undergone bypass surgery is not dramatically different from that of patients whose symptoms have been controlled with drug therapy.

While the operation is comparatively simple, it is not suitable for all cases of diseased coronary arteries. Anyone contemplating a bypass operation would be well advised to get more than one opinion

before proceeding. *See* ANGIOPLASTY and "Aging Healthfully."

Corticosteroids • *See* STEROIDS.

Cosmetic Surgery • *See* PLASTIC SURGERY and "Cosmetic Surgery."

Cosmetics • Most cosmetics are usually safe if proper precautions are taken to read label warnings, and they are less likely to produce problems if they are removed with mild soap and water and a washcloth rather than with a cleansing cream. Of recent concern are new antiaging products called "cosmeceuticals" that alter cell structures, thereby crossing the line between cosmetics and pharmaceuticals. Until the FDA can establish premarket control over safety of these products, women are advised to use them with caution. It should be kept in mind that the cosmetics industry is not legally obliged to supply the FDA with the results of product tests or specifications for quality control. The government is therefore in no position to provide information to consumers about the safety of a particular skin-bleaching cream or hair dye. Fortunately, negative reactions—redness, itching, general skin irritation—are relatively rare, and of these, only about 210 cases out of every million purchases require the attention of a doctor.

When any cosmetic produces a skin problem, the use of all cosmetics in the affected area should be discontinued. To relieve irritation, a 0.5 percent hydrocortisone cream can be applied several times a day. If the irritation persists after a week of home treatment, a dermatologist should be consulted. The problem should be brought to the attention of the manufacturer in a letter, and a copy of the letter should be sent to the local FDA office for a follow-up investigation.

Coughing • A reflex action for the purpose of clearing the lining of the air passages of an excessive accumulation of mucus or disturbing foreign matter. The air expulsed carries with it foreign irritants such as dust, industrial pollutants, particles of food, or abnormal secretions that are irritating the larynx, trachea, or bronchial tubes. A so-called "smoker's cough" is associated with chronic bronchitis. Persistent coughing and hoarseness may be a sign of cancer.

Medicines that loosen the secretions resulting from an inflammatory condition of the mucous membranes and make it easier to cough them up are called expectorants. The congestion may also be loosened and coughed up by a high fluid intake, especially hot tea or hot lemonade with honey. Steam inhalation is another helpful treatment. It is important to rid the air passages of the accumulated mucus by coughing it up, but if a "dry" cough interferes with sleep, the doctor may recommend a cough suppressant. Suppressant medicines may contain codeine or some other opiate that requires a prescription. Over-the-counter cough medicines that contain alcohol (and practically all of them do) should not be given to children, nor should they be used by anyone taking sleeping pills or tranquilizers.

Coughs associated with the flu may last two to three weeks after all other symptoms have disappeared. A cough that lasts longer or causes pain in the chest should be discussed with a doctor.

CPR • See CARDIOPULMONARY RESUSCITATION.

Crohn's Disease • Also called ulcerative colitis and regional ileitis because it is associated with chronic inflammation of the small intestine (ileitis) and/or parts of the large intestine. The two disorders are often grouped together as inflammatory bowel disease. No specific cause of Crohn's disease has been identified, although stress appears to be involved in all cases. Onset usually occurs in young adulthood and may be accompanied by such disorders as rashes, pains in the joints, and the formation of kidney stones. People with Crohn's disease have attacks of diarrhea, severe abdominal cramps, nausea, and fever. Weight loss is common and the consequences of malabsorption of vitamin B12 and calcium may also occur. The disease can be correctly diagnosed by barium X-rays of the upper and lower gastrointestinal tract and by inspection with a sigmoidoscope and colonoscope. Medical treatment on an outpatient basis consists of prescribing a drug in pill form that combines an aspirin derivative and a sulfa antibiotic. Steroids are available in suppository form as well as newer immunosuppressive drugs. Dietary supplements are part of ongoing treatment. Psychological support by family members, supplemented when necessary with therapy for the patient, makes a significant difference in the patient's morale. See "Plain Talk About Medications."

Cryosurgery • Operations in which tissues are destroyed by freezing them, usually with supercold liquid nitrogen or carbon dioxide. Cryosurgery is frequently used for the removal of hemorrhoids, warts, and moles and for treatment of cervical erosion. Cryosurgical instruments are also used successfully in certain types of delicate brain surgery, in correcting retinal detachments, and removing cataracts.

Cushing's Syndrome • A group of symptoms caused by the presence in the body of an excess of corticosteroid hormones. Formerly, Cushing's syndrome was a rare disorder resulting in most cases from overactivity of the adrenal cortex because of a glandular tumor or from hyperfunction of the pituitary gland. It has become more common because of the side effects of medication containing steroids prescribed as long-term therapy for chronic diseases of the kidneys, the joints, etc.

Early symptoms include weakness, facial puffiness ("moon" face), and fluid retention, followed by general obesity and an interruption of menstruation.

When Cushing's syndrome is attributable to glandular malfunction caused by a tumor, surgery is essential. If total removal of the gland is indicated, replacement therapy of the corticosteroid hormones is necessary for the remainder of one's life.

Cyanosis • A blue appearance of the blood and mucous membranes caused by an inadequate amount of oxygen in the arterial blood. A cyanotic appearance is one of the first signs of a number of respiratory diseases in which lung function is so impaired that the blood cannot take up a sufficient amount of oxygen. Cyanosis is also a characteristic of certain heart diseases characterized by abnormal shunting of blood. The cyanotic characteristic of the so-called blue baby is due to a congenital heart defect that leads to an excess of unoxygenated arterial blood. Surgery often is helpful in correcting such defects.

Cyst • An abnormal cavity filled with a fluid or semifluid substance. While some cysts do become malignant, most are harmless and are often reabsorbed by the surrounding tissues, leaving no trace of their existence.

There are several categories of cysts. Retention cysts occur when the opening of a secreting gland is blocked, causing the secretion to back up and form a swelling. In this category are several different types. Sebaceous cysts cause a lump to appear under the skin. Mucous cysts are commonly found in the mucous membranes of the mouth, nose, genitals, or inside the lips or cheeks. Breast cysts may result from a chronic mastitis that causes the ducts leading to the nipples to be blocked by the development of fibrous tissue. Kidney cysts are a congenital defect eventually proliferating to the point where they interfere with kidney function.

Ovarian, cervical, vaginal, and endometrial cysts are discussed in "Gynecologic Problems and Treatment."

Cystic Fibrosis • An inherited, disabling respiratory disease of early childhood. The disease is genetically transmitted to offspring when both parents are carriers; when only one parent is a carrier, some of the offspring may also be carriers. Although there is no known cure for cystic fibrosis, new treatments have increased the life expectancy of patients with the disease. A recent area of investigation is the long-term use of ibuprofen to decrease breathing difficulties. Thanks to developments in genetic engineering, the most promising treatment consists in introducing healthy copies of the defective disease-bearing gene into the bodies of patients who have inherited it. *See* "Directory of Health Information."

Cystocele • A hernia in which part of the bladder protrudes into the vagina. A cystocele causes a feeling of discomfort in the lower abdomen and may produce bladder incontinence. The abnormal position of the bladder results in an accumulation of residual urine that increases the possibility of bacterial infection. Surgical correction is therefore advisable.

Cystoscopy • A diagnostic procedure in which the inner surface of the bladder is examined by an optical instrument called a cystoscope. The procedure, usually performed by a urologist, consists of passing the cystoscope through the opening of the urethra into the bladder. Inflammation, tumors, or stones can be detected by means of an illuminated system of mirrors and lenses and tissue samples can be obtained. If diagnostic X-rays are to be taken during a cystoscopy, a catheter may be passed through the hollow tube of the instrument in order to inject radiopaque substances into the bladder.

Dandruff • A scalp disorder characterized by the abnormal flaking of dead skin. The underlying cause of the condition is not known, but it is directly related to the way in which the sebaceous glands function. There is no evidence that dandruff is triggered by an infectious organism, nor is it the result of poor hygiene. In fact, too-frequent shampoos are likely to worsen the condition.

Normal skin constantly renews itself as dead skin cells are shed. Oily dandruff is the result of overactivity of the tiny oil glands at the base of the hair roots, accelerating the shedding process. The hair becomes greasy and the skin flakings are yellowish and crusty, similar to the flakings that characterize "cradle cap" in infants. This condition can be especially troublesome when it affects the eyelashes.

A dry type of dandruff occurs when the sebaceous glands are plugged, causing the hair to lose its natural gloss and the flaking to be dry and grayish. In either type of dandruff it is important not to scratch the scalp, as broken skin may lead to infection.

If over-the-counter shampoos prove ineffective, treatment by prescribed medications may be necessary.

Death • Traditionally, the end of life was presumed to have occurred when breathing ceased and the heart was still. However, the increasing technological means for prolonging life and the concern of the medical profession as to precisely when a donor's organs should be removed for transplantation created a compelling need for a "redefinition" of death in terms acceptable to both the legal and medical professions. State legislatures now have statutes in which death is equated with the irreversible cessation of brain function. The criteria for brain-death are generally accepted by the medical profession throughout the world.

Following the lead of California in 1976, all 50 states and the District of Columbia have enacted laws empowering patients with the right to provide some type of advance directive prohibiting the use of unusual or artificial devices to prolong their lives if they become terminally ill. Massachusetts, Michigan, and New York have passed laws enabling people to appoint proxies to make similar decisions for them. Under the provisions of a federal law passed in 1991, hospitals are required to ask all patients if they want to fill out a "living will" or name someone as their health care proxy when they are terminally ill.

Most medical schools have introduced courses in dying and death as part of the curriculum, and doctors now discuss these previously taboo subjects not only among themselves but also with their patients and the families of those who are terminally ill. Also, a new respect for the natural and essential process of grieving has resulted in an increase in the number of therapists who specialize in bereavement counseling. Such counseling can provide supportive understanding following the death of a family member or a beloved friend.

Deficiency Disease • A disorder caused by the absence of an essential nutrient in the diet. Not until the twentieth-century discovery of the vital role of vitamins was this category of disease understood, although before that time people had discovered through trial and error what foods or extracts appeared to prevent particular disabilities such as the control of rickets with cod liver oil (rich in vitamin D) and the control of scurvy with citrus juice (rich in vitamin C). Pellagra was once prevalent in areas where meat, eggs, or other foods containing niacin were not part of the diet because of poverty. Through the use of synthesized niacin as an additive in commercially processed foods, this deficiency disease has practically disappeared.

Certain types of blindness and skin ulcers, once thought to be infectious ailments, were discovered to be the result of diets deficient in liver, eggs, and other foods rich in vitamin A. Margarine and many other widely used items are now fortified with this vitamin. Beriberi, a deficiency disease that produces gastrointestinal and neurological disturbances, is caused by a lack of fresh vegetables, whole grains, and certain meats, all of which contain vitamin B^1 (thiamine). Mild beriberi symptoms are likely to appear among people on restricted diets, among alcoholics, and among crash dieters who fail to take supplementary doses of this essential nutriment. *See* "Nutrition, Weight, and General Well-Being."

Dehydration • An abnormal loss of body fluids. Deprivation of water and essential electrolytes (sodium and potassium) for a prolonged period can lead to shock, acidosis, acute uremia, and, especially in the case of infants and the aged, to death. Under normal circumstances water accounts for well over half the total body weight. The adult woman loses about 3 pints of fluid a day in urine; the amount of water in feces is variable but

may account for another 3 or 4 ounces; vaporization through the skin (perspiration) and the lungs (breath expiration) account for another 2 pints. Normal consumption of food and water generally replaces this loss. A temporary increase in the loss of body fluid due to heat, exertion, or mild diarrhea is usually accompanied by extreme thirst or a dry tongue and can be rectified simply by drinking an additional amount of liquid.

Delusions • False and persistent beliefs contrary to or unsubstantiated by facts or objective circumstance; one of the symptoms of severe mental illness and also associated with overdoses of certain addictive drugs. Delusions are false beliefs, as differentiated from hallucinations, which are false sense impressions. As an example, an individual suffering from paranoid schizophrenia may have delusions of being destroyed by people who are thought to be enemies. In true paranoia the delusion becomes the focus of all activity. Some delusions are difficult to recognize and the person is merely thought of as an eccentric. When a delusion takes the form of ordering the individual to commit an illegal act or one destructive to himself or others, hospitalization is mandatory.

Dental Care • The strength or weakness of one's teeth begins with one's genetic inheritance combined with the prenatal health and diet of one's mother. (Pregnant women please note.) However, fluoridation of drinking water, good health, good habits of oral hygiene, and periodic dental checkups are the most important factors in preventing the decay of teeth. Tooth decay is incurable and irreversible, and prompt treatment of cavities is essential.

The most effective means of preventing dental caries is through regular visits to the dentist for checkups and cleanings and proper home hygiene. X-rays should be taken only when absolutely necessary.

Because dental fees vary considerably, not only in different parts of the country but in the same city or town, it is wise to discuss fees with the dentist prior to treatment. Health insurance coverage varies widely. Medicaid covers a major part of dental bills, but Medicare provides no dental coverage at all. *See* PLAQUE.

Dental Caries • Tooth decay, in particular cavities caused by bacteria. *Streptococcus mutans,* a microorganism that induces cavities, is related to the bacterial agent that causes strep throat. Some people appear to inherit an immunity to caries. The decay results from bacteria feeding on sugar and producing a corrosive acid. There are billions of bacteria in the saliva, but only S. *mutans* appears capable of creating an adhesive out of sucrose that adheres to the enamel tooth surface gradually destroying it. *See* DENTAL CARE.

Dentin • The hard calcified tissue that forms the body of a tooth under the enamel surface. When bacterial decay spreads from the enamel into the dentin, a toothache is likely to occur. If this symptom is ignored, the bacteria will eventually invade the pulp and increase the probability of the death of the tooth.

Dentures • Artificial teeth used to replace some or all natural teeth. Dentures may be removable or permanently attached to adjacent teeth. While preventive dentistry has reduced the number of women who need dentures at an early age, the loss of some teeth is almost inevitable with advancing age. Teeth should be replaced promptly to avoid the possibility of a chewing impairment, which can lead to a digestion problem, speech impedi-

ment, or the collapse of facial structure caused by the empty spaces. In addition, missing teeth imperil the health of the adjacent natural ones. Dental materials and techniques used today make it virtually impossible to distinguish between a person's artificial and natural teeth.

Dental implantation has become increasingly popular with those who can afford it or whose medical insurance provides partial coverage. In this procedure, artificial teeth are permanently attached to the jaw. Several different techniques are used, but it is not yet known how well any of them will withstand the test of time. *See* "Directory of Health Information."

Deodorants • *See* ANTIPERSPIRANT DEODORANTS.

Depilatory • *See* HAIR REMOVAL.

Depressant • A category of drugs (also called sedative-hypnotic drugs) that produce a calming, sedative effect by reducing the functional activity of the central nervous system. The two main groups are the barbiturates and the minor tranquilizers. See "Substance Abuse" and "Plain Talk About Medications."

Dermatitis • Inflammation of the skin, often accompanied by redness, itching, swelling, and a rash. Inflammation caused by direct contact with an irritant is called contact dermatitis; inflammation caused by psychological stress is called neurodermatitis. Types caused by viruses, bacteria, fungi, or parasites are called infectious dermatitis; they are discussed under entries entitled BOIL, FUNGAL INFECTIONS, and HIVES. Other forms appear under the headings CHILBLAINS, FROSTBITE, and HIVES. *See also* CONTACT DERMATITIS and RASH.

Desensitization • A process whereby an individual allergic to a particular substance is periodically injected with a diluted extract of the allergen in order to build up a tolerance to it. *See* ALLERGY.

Detoxification • A form of therapy, usually conducted in a hospital, whereby the patient is deprived of an addictive drug and given a substitute one in diminishing doses. Alcohol, heroin, and barbiturate detoxification produces severe withdrawal symptoms that can be eased by the use of sedatives on a transitional basis. When detoxification has been accomplished, a program of physical and psychological rehabilitation is essential. *See* "Substance Abuse."

Dextrose • A variant of glucose. *See* GLUCOSE.

Diabetes • A chronic disease characterized by the presence of an excess of glucose in the blood and urine. In juvenile diabetes, this condition prevails as a result of an insufficient production of insulin by the pancreas. In most cases of adult onset diabetes the amount of insulin produced is normal, but the body's ability to use it is not. Insulin is the hormone essential for converting carbohydrates (sugars and starches) into glucose, the body's most important fuel.

Although the basic cause of diabetes is still unknown, the condition can be controlled if treated correctly. The full name of the disease is diabetes mellitus, roughly translatable from the Greek and Latin as "a passing through of honey." At risk of developing the disorder are people over 40 who are overweight, rarely exercise, or have a family history of diabetes.

According to the American Diabetes Association, the number of people with diabetes is increasing, with approximately 14 million Americans being affected at this time. Of this number, seven million are aware of having the disease and are under treatment; seven million are unaware of their diabetic condition or are not being treated for it. There are 160,000 deaths each year from diabetes and its complications, making it the fourth highest cause of death from disease in the United States.

Symptoms are easily recognized, and once the diagnosis has been confirmed, most people with diabetes, given the proper treatment, are able to live normal lives. The increased life expectancy of people with diabetes, particularly in the case of women over 30, is largely due to the discovery of insulin by two Canadian scientists in 1921–22. This hormone, produced by the pancreas, regulates the body's use of sugar by metabolizing glucose and turning it into energy or into glycogen for storage for future use. An insufficiency of insulin or other abnormalities not fully understood results in the diabetic person's inability to metabolize or store glucose, thus leading to its accumulation in the bloodstream in amounts large enough to spill over into the urine. This metabolic aberration causes the characteristic symptoms of diabetes: frequent urination due to the abnormal amount of urine produced to accommodate the excess glucose that the kidneys filter out of the blood, chronic thirst, an excessive hunger. Dramatic weight loss occurs because, being unable to use glucose, the person with diabetes must use body fat and protein as a source of energy. In order to reach the proper balance of insulin production and glucose conversion, which is constantly being regulated by the normal body, each person with diabetes must be individually stabilized through a controlled regimen of medication, diet, and energy output.

In addition to the previously mentioned symptoms, other symptoms that indicate the possibility of diabetes are drowsiness and fatigue; changes in vision; repeated infections of the kidneys, gums, or skin; intense itching without a known cause; and cramps in the extremities. Any woman with symptoms suggesting diabetes should have a fasting plasma glucose test.

When medication is essential to maintain normal blood sugar levels, the amount of insulin needed is determined initially by the level of glucose in the blood. Thereafter it usually can be determined by the level of glucose in the urine, which is tested regularly by the patient. Variations in the results of the urine tests are the guide to necessary adjustments in diet, medication, and exercise. The use of oral drugs that stimulate the pancreas to produce its own insulin may be recommended with or without an insulin supplement. This procedure requires constant monitoring by the physician.

With the combined efforts of patient and doctor, satisfactory control can be attained and is reflected in the patient's general feeling of well-being, the maintenance of normal blood sugar and negative urine tests, and a minimal fluctuation of weight. Less severe cases of diabetes can be controlled successfully by diet and exercise alone.

Control is essential in order to avoid two specific reactions: hypoglycemia, a condition in which the blood sugar level is too low, and hyperglycemia, in which it is too high.

Hypoglycemia is likely to occur if the patient does not eat additional food to compensate for physical exertion, skips a meal, or takes too much insulin. Onset is sudden, the symptoms being nervous irritability, moist skin, and a tingling tongue. The situation can be corrected quickly by promptly eating or drinking anything containing sugar—a spoonful of honey, a glass of orange juice, a piece of candy, or a lump of sugar.

Hyperglycemia accompanied by acidosis and diabetic coma was the chief cause of early death from diabetes before the discovery of insulin. While rare today, hyperglycemic reaction does occur when the person with diabetes fails to take the necessary amount of insulin. Blood sugar builds up to a point at which the body begins to burn proteins and fats, a process that ends in the formation of chemicals known as ketones. When the accumulation of ketones leads to a critical imbalance in the body's acid concentration, the result can be a diabetic coma. This condition is characterized by a hot dry skin, labored breathing, abdominal pain, and drowsiness. The patient should be hospitalized immediately so that the correct doses of insulin can be administered. A person with diabetes should carry cubes of sugar and wear a diabetic identification tag or bracelet at all times. *See* MEDIC ALERT.

A woman with diabetes should use a contraceptive method other than the pill, because the pill can increase the already existing hormonal imbalance. Should she wish to become pregnant, her chronic condition will not affect her fertility, but once conception occurs, the blood sugar level of a diabetic woman may rise precipitously and behave erratically throughout the pregnancy. It is therefore essential that urine tests be made three or four times a day and that the blood sugar level be checked during prenatal visits as a guide to adjusting the dose of insulin. If the mother-to-be takes proper care of herself, there is every reason to expect a normal, healthy baby.

Most people with diabetes lead a productive and fulfilling life, both on a personal and professional level. Women applying for jobs are protected by a federal law that prevents employers from discriminating against applicants solely on the basis of this disorder. They should be in touch with their local chapter of the American Diabetes Association. This organization provides information on current research, job options, travel possibilities, summer camps, and international affiliations. It publishes a magazine that contains practical material on menu planning and medical equipment and provides a forum for an exchange of ideas on living with diabetes or with someone who has the disease. See DIABETIC RETINOPATHY and "Directory of Health Information."

Diabetic Retinopathy • An abnormal condition in the retina occurring among people with diabetes who have had the disease for a prolonged period of time. Leakage of blood and fluid from the retina's tiny blood vessels is the cause of the condition and the degree of vision impairment depends on the extent of the leakage. If the retinal hemorrhage is extensive and leads to a proliferation of "new" vessels and obstructive fibrous tissue, surgery is essential to prevent sight deterioration. Photocoagulation is the treatment in which a laser beam is directed at the diseased retinal tissue in an attempt to destroy it and prevent it from activating new obstructive tissue growth.

Dialysis • The separation of waste matter and water from the bloodstream by mechanical means, usually used in cases of loss of kidney function through temporary or permanent impairment.

Kidney dialysis may be essential for a limited period following complications caused by bacterial (streptococcus) infection or a viral disease such as hepatitis. However, permanent dialysis is a lifetime support for many Americans. They may have to cope with other conditions because of their dependence on this process,

but none is as life-threatening as the loss of kidney function.

Diaphragm • The large muscle that lies across the middle of the body, separating the thoracic and abdominal cavities. The diaphragm is convex in shape when relaxed. Approximately 20 times a minute, on receiving signals from the area of the brain that controls the respiratory process, it tenses and flattens so that the thoracic cavity enlarges, thus enabling the lungs to expand each time a breath is taken.

Many nerves pass through this muscle and it also contains large openings to accommodate the aorta, the thoracic duct, and the esophagus. When there is a weakening of the muscle structure that surrounds the esophagus, the stomach may push upward into the hole, causing the disorder known as a diaphragmatic or hiatus hernia. Involuntary spasms of the diaphragm are the cause of hiccups.

Diarrhea • Abnormally frequent and watery bowel movements usually related to an inflammation of the intestinal wall. The inflammation may follow infection caused by microorganisms that produce food poisoning or dysentery. Causes of diarrhea may be a particular food, caffeine, alcohol, a new medication, the regular use of certain antacids, too strong a cathartic, an allergy, excitement, or emotional stress. Diarrhea is also associated with toxic shock syndrome. Some women have mild diarrhea with the onset of menopause, and practically all women have diarrhea before the onset of labor. At times it is accompanied by stomach cramps, nausea, vomiting, and a feeling of debility due to loss of body fluids and salt.

Chronic diarrhea may be a symptom of any of the following: thyroid disturbance especially hyperthyroidism, nonspecific ulcerative colitis, a cyst or tumor of the bowel, low level chemical poisoning, and alcoholism. Diarrhea alternating with constipation is characteristic of ileitis and Crohn's disease.

The weakening effects of a brief siege of diarrhea can be remedied by the replacement of lost fluids and a bland diet. If the condition persists, the doctor may request a stool sample for laboratory analysis. If no infectious agent is discovered, diagnosis may involve internal examination with a proctoscope (a lighted tube that is passed into the rectum) or sigmoidoscope (a similar device for examining the sigmoid colon), blood tests, a barium test, or a CAT scan.

What has come to be known as traveler's diarrhea is the sudden onset of cramps and loose stools caused by infection with a strain of the bacterium *E. coli,* which produces a toxin that damages the colon's fluid-absorbing function. Mild cases may respond well to over-the-counter medicines. If the cramps and diarrhea continue in spite of this treatment, a doctor should be consulted.

Digitalis (Digoxin) • A substance derived from the dried leaves of the foxglove flower *(Digitalis purpurea)* and used in the treatment of heart disease. For several hundred years digitalis has been used effectively as a means of stimulating the action of the failing heart muscle while at the same time slowing down the heartbeat. *See* "Plain Talk About Medications."

Dislocation • Specifically, the displacement of a bone from its normal position in the joint; also called subluxation by chiropractors. Dislocations most commonly occur in the fingers and shoulder and less frequently in the elbow, knee, hip, and jaw. A dislocation does not necessarily involve a break in the bone, but it almost always involves some damage, either slight or serious, to the sur-

rounding ligaments and muscles. Anyone may experience a dislocation as a result of a fall or a blow, but it is a routine hazard among dancers and athletes.

Once the displacement occurs, particularly if the site is the shoulder or elbow, it is likely to recur because of the stretching of the sac and the ligaments that hold the joint in place. After several recurrences surgery is usually recommended to tighten the tissues.

A sudden dislocation can be extremely painful, and because the possibility of fracture as well as injury to surrounding nerves and blood vessels must be taken into consideration, prompt medical attention is essential to ensure restoring normal function. To minimize pain and swelling, cold compresses should be applied to the injured area. The injured joint should be immobilized while transporting the victim to the doctor or hospital.

Diuretic • Any drug that increases urinary output, thereby decreasing the body's sodium and water volume. Diuretics, also called water pills, are indispensable in the treatment of heart failure, and they are often used in treating high blood pressure and certain kidney and liver disorders.

Diverticulosis • The presence of diverticula, an abnormal mucous membrane pouch, in any part of the gastrointestinal tract but especially in the colon. Diverticulosis may be entirely without symptoms and is most commonly found in middle-aged and elderly women with a history of chronic constipation.

Diverticulitis is the inflammation of diverticula and it may produce cramps and muscle spasms in the lower left side of the abdomen. Treatment should be prompt to prevent the serious consequences of fistula development or complete intestinal obstruction. Bed rest, a bland low-residue diet, and antibiotics are usually successful therapy. In severe cases of diverticulitis, where a rupture of the colon may lead to peritonitis, surgery should be performed without delay.

Dizziness • *See* VERTIGO.

Dog Bites • *See* ANIMAL BITES.

Dopamine • A substance in the brain essential for the normal functioning of the nervous system. A decreased concentration of dopamine is assumed to be the underlying cause of Parkinsonism. *See* "Aging Healthfully."

Down Syndrome (previously called Down's Syndrome) • This most common form of inherited mental retardation is caused by defective chromosomal development in the embryo. About 5,000 babies are born every year with Down syndrome, formerly referred to as mongolism because of the downward curve of the affected offspring's inner eyelids. In addition to retardation, these children may suffer eye disorders and have a tendency to develop leukemia. However, as a result of the recent and ongoing reassessment of the capabilities of Down syndrome children, expectations have expanded to the point where language skills are being taught with computers. Institutionalization, which offered minimal stimulation, is no longer the prevailing option. It is increasingly ruled out in favor of home care and enrollment in special programs.

See "Pregnancy and Childbirth" and "Directory of Health Information."

Duodenal Ulcer • An open sore in the mucous membrane lining of the duodenum, the portion of the small intestine nearest to the stomach. *See* ULCER.

Dysentery • An infectious inflammation of the lining of the large intestine characterized by diarrhea, the passage of mucus and blood, and severe abdominal cramps and fever. There are two types: bacillary dysentery is caused by several different types of bacterial strains; amebic dysentery is caused by amebae. Both types are endemic in parts of the world where public sanitation is primitive. Dysentery is spread from person to person by food or water contaminated by infected human feces and by houseflies that feed on human excrement containing the infectious agent. It may also be spread by food handlers who transmit the disease by way of unwashed hands.

When bacillary dysentery is diagnosed in the very young or very old or in anyone with diabetes or some other chronic condition, hospitalization is usually recommended so that dehydration can be prevented or treated. In milder forms of dysentery, rest combined with a prescribed dose of an antibiotic or other medication is a common course of treatment. Close supervision is important in the case of amebic dysentery because the infection can become chronic if amebic abscesses are formed in the liver.

Travelers to parts of the world where infection is an ever-present hazard should take the necessary precautions against dysentery by drinking only bottled water or other bottled beverages (*never* with ice) and avoiding raw fruit and vegetables. *See* DIARRHEA.

Dyspnea • Labored breathing; the feeling of being "out of breath." Dyspnea is a symptom or sign of insufficiently oxygenated blood resulting from an obstruction in the air passages such as occurs in chronic respiratory diseases; a reduction in the capacity of the lungs to carry on the normal oxygen-carbon dioxide exchange because of areas of scar tissue; certain forms of heart failure in which the lungs fill with fluid; chronic anemia. An acute breathlessness may accompany asthma, bronchial pneumonia, the sudden onset of an allergic response that causes the swelling of the windpipe, and myocardial infarction. It is also one of the most distressing manifestations of an anxiety attack. Shortness of breath that often accompanies obesity can be rectified by loss of weight. When dyspnea is accompanied by chest pain or when it is chronic, medical evaluation is indicated.

MIDDLE AND INNER EAR

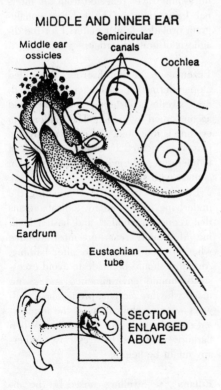

Ear • The organ of hearing and equilibrium. The ear is divided into three parts: the outer ear consists of the visible fleshy auricle that collects the sound waves, which are then transmitted through the ear canal; the middle ear contains the three bones of hearing; the inner ear is the site of the organ of hearing and the organ of balance. The thin layer of tissue known as the eardrum, also called the tympanus or tympanic membrane, forms the barrier between the outer ear and the middle ear. The bones of hearing in the middle ear, called the ossicles, are named for their respective shapes—the hammer, anvil, and stirrup. They are connected to the bone surrounding the middle ear by ligaments. When loud noises strike the eardrum, tiny muscles attached to the ossicles limit the vibrations of the eardrum by contracting, thus protecting it and the inner ear from damage. Equal pressure is maintained on both sides of the eardrum because the eustachian tube connects the middle ear to the upper rear part of the throat. The organ of hearing within the inner ear is called the cochlea, a spiral-shaped organ whose name means "snail" in Latin. The cochlea covers the nerves that sort out various sound messages and sends them on to the auditory center of the brain. The organ of balance, made up of the three semicircular canals situated in three different planes of space within the inner ear, maintains the body's equilibrium in relation to gravitational forces. Any disturbance or infection of the semicircular canals results in vertigo and imbalance.

The hearing process works in the following way. Any vibrating object that pushes air molecules at a rate ranging from 15 to 15,000 vibrations per second (the range of human audibility) causes waves to enter the ear canal and strike the eardrum. The vibrations are transmitted by the eardrum to the middle ear where their intensity is magnified by the ossicles. The waves are then sent through a membranous window behind the third bone and are transmitted through the fluid within the cochlea. Hairlike structures within the cochlea communicate with the auditory nerves in such a way that a sound of a particular pitch and volume is perceived by the brain.

Ear Disorders • Discomfort within the ear may range from irritation due to dermatitis of the outer ear to a feeling of pressure caused by congestion in the eustachian tube to acute pain resulting from bacterial infection of the middle ear. Any sharp pain in the ear, an earache that lasts more than a day, an earache accompanied by a discharge, or chronic pain resulting from exposure to dangerous sound levels should be investigated by a doctor immediately. The irreversible effects of exposure to occupational, recreational, or environmental sound that is excessively loud are discussed under NOISE.

Because the ears are directly connected to the nose and throat by the eustachian tube, a head cold is likely to cause the ears to feel "stuffed." The symptom may be remedied by the supervised use of nosedrops. Nostrils should not be held closed when blowing the nose, because closing both at once may force infectious material into the ear. Similar precautions should be taken while swimming. Air should be breathed in through the mouth and exhaled through the nose; if the mouth or nose fills with water, it should not be swallowed but rather sniffed into the back of the throat and spat out. Earplugs may be worn. If water enters the ear, it can usually be drained by the force of gravity when lying down with the ear to the ground.

Otomycosis, a fungus infection of the outer ear, results from swimming in polluted waters and causes itching, swelling, and pain. It is often accompanied by crusted sores that must be kept dry in order to cure the condition. Fungicidal oint-ments and antibiotic salves are usually effective treatment.

Infections of the middle ear, more common in childhood than in later years, can be brought under control by antibiotics. Changing the contour of the ear for esthetic reasons is discussed in "Cosmetic Surgery."

Echogram • A recording produced on an oscilloscopic screen that shows the difference between the wave patterns of healthy and diseased tissue, a difference that cannot be distinguished by X-rays. Echocardiograms provide tracings of the ultrasonic waves reflected from the internal heart tissues. The echo-encephalogram provides similar material for the diagnosis of brain disorders.

Eczema • A skin disorder, also called atopic dermatitis, characterized by redness, swelling, blistering, and scaling and accompanied by itching. The tendency to eczema is inherited, and onset at any age may be triggered by stress, extremes of temperature, allergy, medication, or skin contact with silk or wool.

Eczema is treated by eliminating the underlying cause and by topical creams that reduce discomfort and hasten healing. Medicated creams are most effective when applied immediately after bathing. An effort should be made to avoid excessively humid environments, and swimmers who are eczema-prone should always wear earplugs to avert the unpleasant consequences of ear infections. When flareups are traced to stress, psychotherapy might be helpful.

Edema • Swelling caused by the abnormal accumulation of fluid in the tissues. The archaic term for edema is dropsy, derived from the Greek word *hydrops* from *hydros,* meaning "water." Edema is a symptom of various disorders, many of which require immediate treatment. The edema that accompanies heart failure or circulatory impairments usually takes the form of swollen ankles, but it may occur in the more serious form of accumulation of fluid in the lungs. Edema may also be caused by impairment of kidney and liver function.

Puffy eyelids and ankles are among the symptoms of pre-eclampsia, a condition that afflicts pregnant women. Fluid retention and a bloated feeling are associated with premenstrual syndrome. Under normal circumstances, the edema and other discomforts vanish with the onset of menstrual flow. If the edema persists between periods, it should be checked by a doctor.

EEG • *See* ELECTROENCEPHALOGRAM.

Ejaculation • The reflex action by which semen is expelled during the male orgasm. Premature ejaculation, the most widespread sexual dysfunction, occurs because the male cannot control his level of sexual arousal and therefore reaches orgasm sooner than he or his partner desires.

The disorder is not associated with any physical abnormalities, and sex therapy techniques have a high success rate when both partners participate in a series of prescribed exercises over a period of several weeks. *See* "Sexual Health."

EKG • *See* ELECTROCARDIOGRAM.

Elavil • A tricyclic antidepressant (amitriptyline) prescribed to reinforce the effect of pain-killing drugs. Elavil has been found to be effective in reducing discomfort from ailments involving nerve inflammation, such as shingles (postherpetic neuralgia) and low back pain (sciatica). *See* "Plain Talk About Medications."

Elective Surgery • *See* "You, Your Doctors, and the Health Care System."

Electrocardiogram (EKG) • A tracing that represents the electrical impulses generated by the heart as measured by an electrocardiograph. The resulting pattern indicates the rate of the heart rhythm, tissue damage that may have occurred following a heart attack, the effect of various medications on the heart muscle, and other valuable information for the diagnosis of coronary disorders.

Electroencephalogram (EEG) • A tracing by an electroencephalograph of the electrical potential produced by the brain. Electrical impulses picked up by electrodes attached to the scalp are amplified so that they are strong enough to move an electromagnetic pen to make a record of brain wave patterns. This procedure is quick and painless. It is used routinely to diagnose tumors, brain damage resulting from an accident or injury to the head, and neurological disorders such as epilepsy. In recent years the EEG has been replaced for diagnostic purposes by a CAT scan or MRI.

Electrolysis • *See* HAIR REMOVAL.

Electroshock Therapy • Also called electroconvulsive therapy (ECT) and generally referred to as "shock treatment." A procedure in which a controlled amount of electric current is passed through the frontal area of the brain of a mentally ill patient. The physical response is convulsions and unconsciousness. The treatments may be administered on an outpatient basis, or, if a suicide attempt has been made or is anticipated, during hospitalization. Some specialists believe that ECT may yield insights into the relationship between the brain's biochemical and electrochemical behavior and the patient's severe depression; others agree with the patient advocacy movement that wants to outlaw the procedure altogether.

Electroshock is not a cure for any form of mental illness, but when treatments are given in series, they may temporarily relieve some of the more anguishing emotional symptoms and thereby make the patient accessible to other forms of psychotherapy. While it has largely been replaced by antidepressant drugs and tranquilizers, it may be the therapy of last resort for those mentally ill patients categorized as "treatment resistant" to all medication.

Encephalitis • Inflammation of the tissues covering the brain associated with such viral infections as measles, herpes simplex, chicken pox, and AIDS. In comparatively rare cases, it may also occur following vaccination against polio and other forms of immunization against viral disease. It may be produced by lead poisoning, or it may follow the infectious bite of certain ticks and mosquitos. The disease may occur at any age. Typical symptoms are fever, vomiting, headache, and in some cases convulsions. Correct diagnosis is made by laboratory tests of the blood, spinal fluid, and stools and by an electroencephalogram, and in some cases by examination of a sample of brain tissue. Where the cause is the herpes simplex Type I virus, specific medicines can be effective. In other cases, treatment consists of bed rest and medication to keep the fever down.

Endoscopy • Examination of a hollow cavity or an internal organ with an illuminated optical instrument (endoscope). Among the more commonly used instruments are the cystoscope for examining the bladder, the colonoscope and the proctoscope for examining the upper and lower portion of the intestine and rectum, and the bronchoscope for locating the origin and extent of respiratory disorders. Beyond all these, the arthroscope has inaugurated a new era of rehabilitative surgery for knees and hips previously immobilized by joint disease or injury.

Enema • The injection of a fluid into the lower bowel by means of a tube inserted into the rectum; also, the fluid injected. A barium enema is administered prior to X-rays of the lower gastrointestinal tract, a sedative enema may be used for a calming effect, and a warm water or special solution enema may be recommended in special cases of constipation. The habitual use of enemas as a means of bowel evacuation is not recommended because they are apt to impair the natural responses involved in the normal process of elimination. Disposable enema units are a convenient substitute for the more traditional equipment that must be washed and stored.

Enterocele • A hernia in which a loop of the small intestine protrudes into the vaginal wall. The condition may reveal itself when X-rays are taken to diagnose pain. Surgical correction is the usual treatment.

Enzyme • An organic substance, usually protein, manufactured by the cells of all living things and acting as a catalyst in the transformation of a complex chemical compound into a simple or different one. The human body produces hundreds of different enzymes, each with a specific function: some ward off invasive microbes; some are related to the chemistry of muscle function; three main groups of digestive enzymes are essential for the normal metabolic processing of proteins, fats, and carbohydrates; and particular enzymes are involved in maintaining normal respiratory function.

An inherited liver enzyme disease has been identified as the underlying cause of phenylketonuria (PKU disease), which can result in mental retardation unless diagnosed early and treated through special diet.

Epiglottis • The leaf-shaped flap of cartilage covered with mucous membrane that lies between the back of the tongue and the entrance to the larynx and the trachea (windpipe). In the act of swallowing, the epiglottis folds back over the opening of the larynx, which contains the vocal apparatus (in the glottis), and channels the food from the back of the tongue to the esophagus. The disruption of this mechanism, such as by a person's laughing while eating, may allow food to enter the windpipe, leading to a coughing spell and, in more serious cases, to choking.

Epilepsy • The general term for a category of symptoms characterized by overactive electrical discharge of the brain cells. This imbalance leads to seizures that vary in magnitude and duration. Petit mal seizures are brief, may recur many times a day, and are scarcely perceptible to the onlooker. They involve a sudden and short loss of consciousness and may be accompanied by twitching eye and face muscles. Grand mal seizures involve convulsive spasms, loss of consciousness, stiffening of the arms and legs, and sometimes, a loss of bowel control. The unconscious state may last for several minutes. On regaining consciousness, the person who has had the seizure may be disorientated for as long as a few minutes or a few hours.

There are as many as 4 million people in the United States who suffer from one or another form of epilepsy; in half these cases, the cause is unknown. The others can be explained by an injury to the brain, a stroke, tumor, or hereditary predisposition.

The seizures can be controlled in approximately 80 percent of all cases with anticonvulsant medicines. For some cases resistant to medication, surgery has proved an effective solution. Only a limited number of medical centers are equipped to evaluate and handle epileptic surgery.

An unambiguous diagnosis of epilepsy is based on an electroencephalogram, a CAT scan, as well as a complete physical examination, a medical history, and a family history.

Because some anticonvulsant medications are thought to reduce the effectiveness of birth control pills, women with epilepsy who are using this form of contraception should investigate alternative methods. See "Contraception and Abortion."

Epinephrine • See ADRENALIN.

Epstein-Barr Virus • See MONONUCLEOSIS.

Erection • The swelling and stiffening of the penis or increase in length, diameter, and firmness of the clitoris resulting from sexual arousal. The stimulus may be psychological (sexual fantasies), visual (the sight of a sexually appealing person), or physical (touch).

There is no correlation between the size of the flaccid penis and the same penis in erection, which may range on the average from 5 to 7 inches. There is no correlation between body size and the size of the erect penis nor between the size of the erect penis and sexual prowess. Inability to have an erection is called impotence. See "Sexual Health."

Erogenous Zone • Any area of the body, especially the oral, genital, and anal, that is the source of sexual arousal when stimulated by touch. *See* "Sexual Health."

Erythromycin • Generic name for an antibiotic commonly prescribed to patients with a penicillin allergy and to pregnant women and young children when tetracycline antibiotics are considered inadvisable. *See* "Plain Talk About Medications."

Esophagus • The muscular tube that transmits food from the mouth to the stomach; the gullet. This portion of the alimentary canal is approximately 10 inches long; it extends from the pharynx through the chest and connects with the stomach just below the diaphragm. Between the esophagus and the stomach is a muscular ring, the esophageal sphincter, that opens to permit food to leave the esophagus and descend into the stomach. Weakening of this sphincter muscle to the point where it does not close properly results in the back flow or reflux of some of the acid contents of the stomach. When this esophageal reflux occurs, the result is the sensation of "heartburn" or acid indigestion. Conditions that contribute to the malfunctioning of the esophageal sphincter include overweight and pregnancy.

Eustachian Tube • The canal that connects the middle ear with the back of the throat and equalizes the pressure on either side of the eardrum. Swallowing is the mechanism by which air is forced into the tube, correcting the stuffy sensation in the ears produced by a change in air pressure as occurs in an elevator or airplane. The eustachian tube is also the pathway through which infection may travel from the nasal passages into the middle ear.

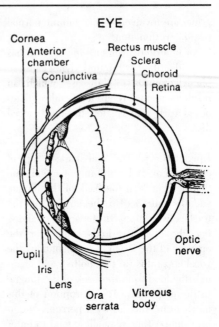

EYE

Cornea
Anterior chamber
Conjunctiva
Rectus muscle
Sclera
Choroid
Retina
Pupil
Iris
Lens
Ora serrata
Vitreous body
Optic nerve

Eye • The organ of vision. The eyes are contained in bony sockets of the skull. The extent of their movements depends on six delicate muscles attached to the top, sides, and bottom of each eyeball. The movements of the lids, which serve to protect the eyes, are controlled by other muscles that are both voluntary and involuntary.

The front of the eyeball is covered by the translucent tissue called the cornea. It is a continuation of the tough fibrous sclera, the white of the eye that protects the delicate structures within. Under the cornea is a middle pigmented layer that forms the iris, which is responsible for the color of the eyes and which is densely supplied with blood vessels. The iris functions in much the same way as the diaphragm of a camera, narrowing or widening in response to varying light conditions to expand or contract the pupil, the opening through which light enters the eye. The dilation of the pupil is influenced by various chemicals as well as by light intensity.

The light that passes through the pupil is focused on the retina, the expanded end of the optic nerve extending into the middle of the brain. Within the retina are the nerve cells, the light- and color-sensitive rods and cones, and the many connections that supply information to the occipital lobes of the brain where stimuli are transformed into the images called "seeing." The information the eyes continuously send to the brain may be acted on immediately or may be stored away as memory for future recall.

The main part of the eyeball is filled with a transparent jelly called the vitreous humor, and the area in front of the lens is filled with a watery substance called the aqueous humor. The eyes are constantly lubricated, cleansed, and protected from infection by the tears secreted through the lacrimal ducts.

Among the more common disorders of vision are astigmatism, farsightedness, and nearsightedness, all of which can be corrected by prescribed lenses.

Because many disorders of the eye progress slowly and insidiously, regular examinations should be scheduled *before* dramatic changes in vision occur. See DIABETIC RETINOPATHY and "Aging Healthfully."

Eyes that burn and itch may be reacting to an allergy or to indoor on-the-job pollution. Unpleasant eye symptoms may develop because of constant use of video display terminals. *(See* "Health on the Job.")

Foreign objects in the eye should be dealt with by an eye doctor. Eye makeup and especially the brushes used to apply it should never be borrowed or lent as a precaution against the spread of infection. Women engaged in racquet sports should *always* wear protective glasses. See SUNGLASSES.

Eye Examination • Any variation of vision, no matter how minor, should be evaluated. An ophthalmologist, a physician specializing in the eye, can diagnose or treat any disorder that might be affecting vision. Optometrists can check visual acuity and prescribe corrective lenses but cannot diagnose organic eye disease. (An optician makes the prescription lens.) Women over forty should schedule a routine checkup for glaucoma once a year. Anyone whose diabetes is insulin-regulated should have regularly scheduled examinations by an ophthalmologist familiar with the problem of diabetic retinopathy.

Eyeglasses • Lenses, made of glass or plastic, ground to individual prescription for the correction of defects in vision, such as nearsightedness, farsightedness, and astigmatism. Bifocals are worn when both short-range and long-range vision require correction. If vision is impaired at the middle distance as well, a second pair of glasses or trifocals may be necessary. For women whose distance vision is normal but who need reading glasses, half-lenses are often a satisfactory solution. Tinted glasses or sunglasses ground to individual prescription are both practical and useful for outdoor purposes. Women engaged in active sports should wear shatterproof glasses, and those who travel should carry an extra pair of glasses or the prescription for their corrective lenses. As changes in vision occur, the eyes should be checked for a new prescription. In order to decide whether to wear conventional glasses or contact lenses it is wise to consult an ophthalmologist. See CONTACT LENSES and SUNGLASSES.

Facial Tic • *See* TIC.

Fainting • A brief loss of consciousness caused by a temporary lack of oxygen to the brain. (Fainting should not be confused with shock, which is an emergency situation resulting from a critical loss of body fluids.) Fainting is usually preceded by lightheadedness, weakness, pallor, and a cold sweat. Circumstances that may reduce the brain's oxygen supply are a sudden emotional trauma, an excess intake of alcohol, and standing up for the first time after an illness. Standing still increases the chances of fainting because the blood supply to the brain is temporarily diminished. When one feels faint it is best to lie down or sit down with one's head lowered between the knees until the dizziness subsides. To help someone who has fainted, loosen all clothing and make certain that there is an adequate amount of fresh air to be breathed. Alcohol should not be administered as a means of reviving someone who has fainted. If consciousness is not regained within a minute or two, a doctor should be summoned.

Family History • Facts concerning the health conditions, both mental and physical, of a patient's blood relatives. Some diseases are clearly inherited; others that do not necessarily have a genetic foundation may run in the family. With the increasing recognition of inheritance and predisposition as determinants of many diseases, every woman should be aware of her family's past and present medical history and should give this information to her doctor in detail. It can be useful to collect the family's medical history while the older members are still living even though they may be geographically scattered. Especially relevant is information about asthma and allergies, breast cancer, glaucoma, severe mental illness, Alzheimer's disease, alcoholism, and carriers of recessive genes related to inherited diseases. In describing a grandfather's diabetes or another relative's Duchenne muscular dystrophy, for example, the patient is providing the doctor with information that may be a clue for the early diagnosis of a condition. See HEREDITY, MEDICAL RECORDS, GENETIC COUNSELING, and "You, Your Doctors, and The Health Care System."

Farsightedness • A disorder of vision in which only distant objects are seen clearly. Farsightedness occurs when the lens of the eye focuses the image behind the retina rather than directly on it because the eyeball is shorter than normal from front to back. This disorder is corrected by wearing a convex lens that bends the light rays to the center of the retina.

Fasting • See "Nutrition, Weight, and General Well-Being."

Feet • The underlying cause of most foot problems is often improperly fitted shoes. Shoes and hosiery should be selected carefully for proper fit, comfort, and support. Natural leather is preferred over other shoe materials because it allows the feet to "breathe" and has flexibility. Extremely high heels are inadvisable for those who walk a great deal because they place a strain on the foot and calf muscles and often cause posture problems that result in back pain. Support hosiery is helpful in cases where constant standing places extra pressure on the blood vessels of the feet and legs. When a blister occurs, it must be given prompt attention to avoid the possibility of infection.

Feet can be pampered by elevating them for short periods; circulation problems can be helped by immersing the feet in hot water and then rinsing with cold water. Exercises may keep feet limber and counteract the effects of poor circulation. These exercises may be simple ones such as wriggling the toes or picking up small objects with the toes. Walking barefoot on lawns or beaches is also helpful in keeping feet in good condition.

Runners and long distance walkers should have their footwear checked to find out about the advisability of installing a custom-made orthotic device in one or both shoes to compensate for bone or muscle irregularities.

For chronic foot problems, consult a podiatrist (formerly called a chiropodist). *See* ORTHOTICS and "Fitness."

Fever • Body temperature that rises significantly above 98.6°F or 37°C, presumably due to a change in metabolic processes. A one-degree variation is well within the normal range because temperature rises this much after exercise, after a heavy meal, during hot weather when the body must work harder to rid itself of heat, or during ovulation when the increase in the secretion of progesterone affects the body processes.

A high fever usually results from a bacterial infection. Any high fever accompanied by vomiting and/or diarrhea, by pains in the neck, throat, muscles, joints, and by severe headaches, requires a doctor's prompt attention. Some other circumstances that should receive professional diagnosis include onset of fever and abdominal cramps during pregnancy, and a persistent low-grade fever accompanied by a cough or general malaise.

Chills often precede or alternate with a high fever. As the temperature rises, the patient feels achy and thirsty, skin becomes hot and dry, urine is scant, and, depending on the cause, vomiting may take place. Until a doctor is consulted, a person with a high fever should stay in bed, drink lots of liquids, and take two aspirin or Tylenol tablets every four hours while awake.

Note that the temperature reading on a rectal thermometer is usually one degree higher than the reading on a mouth thermometer. It should also be kept in mind that the seriousness of an illness cannot be judged by the presence or absence of fever. *See* ROCKY MOUNTAIN SPOTTED FEVER, TYPHOID FEVER, and UNDULANT FEVER.

Fever Sores • *See* HERPES.

Fibrillation • A condition in which the fibers of a muscle contract in groups or singly rather than in unison, thus causing parts of the muscle to twitch in rapid succession. When fibrillation occurs in the ventricles of the heart, the muscle cannot contract in a coordinated way, and the heart stops beating. A patient in the intensive coronary care unit of a hospital who experiences ventricular fibrillation after a heart attack has a 90 percent chance of survival if treatment begins within one minute. Treatment consists of the use of a machine called a defibrillator, which attempts to jolt the heart back into its proper rhythmic pattern by means of electric current. Monitoring equipment in coronary care units can anticipate the onset of fibrillation by the characteristic EKG pattern of skipped ventricular beats. This monitoring system enables the doctor to prescribe medication that helps to prevent impending danger. Ventricular fibrillation is thought to be a major cause of sudden cardiac death in nonhospitalized women with no previous history of heart disease. Attempts are therefore being made to identify women likely to experience fibrillation *before* onset.

Fibromyalgia • Inflammation of the connective tissue, also known as fibrositis. This condition affects mainly women, especially those between the ages of 20 and 50. It is characterized by a broad spectrum of symptoms, many of which also characterize chronic fatigue syndrome:

exhaustion, generalized aches and pains, anxiety, depression, sensitivity to temperature changes, and sleep disturbances. Fibromyalgia may also be confused with rheumatoid arthritis because it is also characterized by morning stiffness and swelling in some joints. The procedure for establishing a firm diagnosis of fibromyalgia is to test 18 specific points of the body for tenderness to the touch. These points are located at the back and front of the neck, at the shoulders and chest, and the elbows, hips, and knees.

Although the cause of fibromyalgia is unknown, it usually follows a physical or psychological trauma—a car accident, a fall, the loss of a job, or the death of a loved one. These distressing events seem to change the body's chemical components, and the change appears to produce the symptoms. Treatment ranges from medications to reduce pain and those that ensure uninterrupted sleep, thus providing relief from fatigue. Aerobic exercises, posture improvement, and a course in stress management can also cause symptoms to abate. Anti-inflammatory drugs are not a suitable treatment for this condition. See "Plain Talk About Medications" and "Alternative Therapies."

First Aid • Emergency treatment administered to the victim of an accident or unexpected illness prior to the arrival of medical assistance. Instruction in the fundamentals of first aid are available under the auspices of local Red Cross chapters, hospitals, or community organizations. Such instruction enables the potential rescuer to provide emergency treatment in the event of a crisis. First aid can be effectively and promptly administered if the proper supplies are on hand. Every home should have the following first aid supplies available:

roll of 2-inch-wide sterile gauze
individually packaged gauze squares
cotton-tipped swabs
aspirin or Tylenol tablets
antihistamine tablets
oral and rectal thermometers
adhesive strip bandages, assorted sizes
sterile absorbent cotton
roll of adhesive bandage tape
paper tissues
tongue depressors
hydrogen peroxide
antiseptic spray
Betadine solution
Pepto-Bismol
rubbing alcohol
surgical scissors and tweezers

A first aid kit and a blanket should always be available in the car trunk for emergency use.

Fissure • A crack in a mucous membrane. Fissures at the corner of the mouth may result from a riboflavin (vitamin) deficiency. An anal fissure caused by chronic constipation may lead to the further inhibition of bowel movements due to the severity of pain accompanying the passage of stools. Another type of fissure, cracked nipples, is often found in nursing mothers. It can best be prevented by the use of lubricating cream. Because fissures may be a source of infection, a doctor should be consulted for proper treatment.

Fistula • An abnormal opening leading from a cavity or a hollow organ within the body to an adjacent part of the body or to the skin surface. Anal fistulas that occur because of a lesion or abscess in the anal canal or the rectum eventually become painful enough to require surgical removal. A fistula between the urethra and the vagina that results from damage to the organs during childbirth or during surgery may cause incomplete bladder control and urinary incontinence. A fistula between the vagina and the rectum may also occur after an operation. Both conditions should be evaluated for surgical correction.

Flu • *See* INFLUENZA.

Fluoridation • The addition of a fluoride (a chemical salt containing fluorine) to public drinking water. There are still some pockets of resistance to this practice, but health authorities, including the U.S. Public Health Service, the American Dental Association, the American Medical Association, and the World Health Organization, have found no compelling evidence of harmful effects and have found that fluoridation is responsible for a significant decrease in dental decay among children. There is no question that the incidence of cavities is much lower where fluorides occur naturally in the water supply than elsewhere.

The benefits of fluoridation are increased by the use of a toothpaste containing fluoride, and many dentists recommend the added protection of applying fluoride directly to the teeth of young children.

Studies have produced evidence that older people profit from the benefits of fluoridated water by having less fragile bones and thereby sustaining fewer fractures. This advantage appears to be especially significant for older women.

Food Poisoning (Food-Borne Illness) • The general term for any acute illness, usually gastrointestinal, which is caused by the ingestion of contaminated food or of uncontaminated food that is poisonous in and of itself. The term "ptomaine poisoning" is incorrect. The most common symptoms include nausea, vomiting, abdominal cramps, and diarrhea. These symptoms are often attributed (mistakenly) to "intestinal flu." Food can be contaminated by bacteria (salmonella, staphylococci, *Escherichia coli*, which is also the cause of "travelers' diarrhea," and *Clostridium botulinum*, which causes botulism, among others), viruses (hepatitis and the virus carried mainly by uncooked shellfish taken from waters contaminated by raw sewage), chemicals (such as sodium fluoride, monosodium glutamate), parasites, plankton, and poisonous plants eaten by milk-producing cows. Salmonella and staphylococci are the most common contaminants. Salmonella are the usual contaminants of meat, poultry, and especially of uncooked or undercooked eggs. It is in fact the raw egg in homemade mayonnaise and not the mayonnaise itself that is responsible for so many incidents of "picnic poisoning." When not killed and if present in sufficient numbers, salmonella infect the eater and cause abdominal cramps and diarrhea some eight or more hours after ingestion. Staphylococci, if present, produce a toxin that multiplies rapidly in high protein foods, especially those containing eggs, such as salads, mayonnaise, and custards, when exposed to warm temperatures for several hours. This toxin causes nausea and vomiting three to six hours after the foods containing it are eaten.

One important way to reduce the incidence of food poisoning is through improved government inspection of meat and poultry. It is also important to pay particular attention to how raw poultry is handled in the kitchen so that other foods are not in danger of contamination from an unwashed cutting board, knife, or one's hands. Fortunately, most victims recover quickly and spontaneously from food poisoning, although for infants and elderly people they can be life-threatening because of the danger of dehydration.

Poisonous foods include certain mushrooms, berries, nuts, and fish. Many authorities recommend that raw fish in any form, whether shellfish or sushi, should be avoided, especially by those who have liver problems, diabetes, or gastrointestinal disorders. Some practitioners of herbal medicine may not be sufficiently cautious or well informed about the poison potential of their recommended treatments. Indiscriminate use of "herbal cures" is therefore ill advised.

Food poisoning can produce serious illness and death especially if the central nervous system is affected as happens in botulism and mushroom poisoning. Anyone believed to be ill from food poisoning (usually recognized because several people become ill simultaneously), who has symptoms other than mild nausea, vomiting, abdominal cramps, and diarrhea, should seek medical attention promptly as should those who possibly have been exposed to botulism or poisonous plants. *See* BOTULISM and "Alternative Therapies."

Fracture • A crack or complete break in a bone. A closed or simple fracture is one in which the skin remains intact. An open or compound fracture is one in which the skin is ruptured because the broken bone has penetrated it or because whatever caused the fracture also opened the skin. A complex or comminuted fracture is one in which the bone has been broken into many pieces or part of it has been shattered. Fractures often involve damage to surrounding ligaments and blood vessels. Immobilization, preferably by splinting, is the safest way to manage a fracture until professional treatment is available. In many cases a simple fracture may be indistinguishable from a sprain except by X-ray.

Frigidity • The term, now considered scientifically inaccurate and unacceptable,

was previously used to describe a form of female sexual dysfunction characterized by the absence or inhibition of erotic pleasure and sexual responsiveness. *See* "Sexual Health."

Frostbite • Injury to a part of the body resulting from exposure to subfreezing temperature or wind-chill factor. Because the affected tissue can be irreversibly destroyed, frostbite is an emergency condition. The first signs are a tingling sensation and then numbness and a bluish-red appearance of the skin. If countermeasures are not taken at this stage, the affected areas begin to burn and itch as in chilblains, there is a total loss of sensation, and the skin turns dead white. Because the frostbitten area is extremely vulnerable to further injury, any clothing that may be an additional constraint to circulation, such as boots, socks, or tight gloves, should be removed as gently as possible. If circumstances permit, the injured parts of the body should be immersed quickly in warm—not hot—water. If this is not practical, the patient should be wrapped in blankets. If the feet are involved, walking should be forbidden. If an arm or a leg is involved, the person should be encouraged to elevate it. Absolutely no attempt should be made to massage the affected parts, rub them with snow, or apply heat. Hot beverages, a sedative, and a painkiller may be offered. Smoking is forbidden because the nicotine will constrict the already impaired circulation. A dry sterile dressing should be used to prevent infection. If there is no visible return of circulation after these measures have been taken and the person's condition appears to be deteriorating, medical care should be obtained without further delay.

Fungal Infections • Diseases caused by fungi and their spores that invade the skin, finger and toenails, mucous membranes, and lungs and may even attack the bones and the brain. These diseases are known as mycoses. Fungi are parasites that may feed on dead organic matter or on live organisms.

The more common fungal disorders are those confined to the skin, such as ringworm that results in red, scaly patches that itch and may form into blisters. Ringworm is highly contagious and can be passed on by household pets as well as by contaminated towels and bed linens. To prevent its spread from person to person and from one part of the body to another, ringworm should be treated promptly with suitable antifungicides. Athlete's foot (tinea pedis) is a form of ringworm that can be difficult to cure once it takes hold. The fungus usually lodges between the toes, multiplying rapidly in the warm, damp, dark environment and eventually causing the skin to crack and blister. To control a chronic case, feet should be kept meticulously clean and as dry as possible, a fungicidal powder should be sprinkled in the shoes, and a medicated ointment should be spread between the toes. If athlete's foot persists despite these measures, professional attention should be sought. The same fungus sometimes affects the nails (onychomycosis) and usually requires professional care.

Thrush is an oral fungus infection that attacks the mucous membranes of the mouth and tongue, and where resistance to infection is low, especially in the presence of the AIDS virus, or where the diet is deficient in vitamin B, it may spread into the pharynx. It is characterized by the formation of white patches that feel highly sensitive. Similar patches may also appear in the vagina and rectum (moniliasis or candidiasis). Where only the mouth is involved, mouthwashes containing gentian violet may be recommended. In cases of moniliasis, medicated suppositories are usually prescribed.

A regimen of certain antibiotics increases vulnerability to various fungus infections, because the medicines kill off not only the bacteria causing a particular disease but also the benign ones whose presence guards against the growth of fungi. In recent years the medical profession and public health authorities have been concerned with a group of fungus infections that attack the lungs and can eventually invade other organs. Of these, histoplasmosis and "cocci" or coccidioidomycosis (also known as desert fever) are the result of breathing in certain spores that float freely in clouds of dust. The spores are harmless if swallowed, but those that find their way into the air sacs of the lungs begin to grow and multiply, spreading inflammation through the respiratory system and eventually into other parts of the body. Typical symptoms include a chronic cough, fever, and other manifestations that may be confused with pneumonia or tuberculosis. When tests produce the correct diagnosis, hospitalization may be required.

Gallbladder • A membranous sac, approximately 3 inches long, situated below the liver. The gallbladder drains bile from the liver, stores and concentrates it, and eventually sends it on to the duodenum.

When the gallbladder has been surgically removed because of infection or blockage, bile goes directly from the liver to the intestine without any ill effects on digestion.

In some cases the concentrated bile in the gallbladder forms into gallstones. Inflammation of the gallbladder, technically called cholecystitis, may be acute or chronic. In its acute form it usually follows bacterial infection or a sudden blockage of one of the ducts by a tumor or a large stone. Symptoms of an attack are nausea, vomiting, sweating, and sharp pain in the upper right part of the abdo-

GALLBLADDER

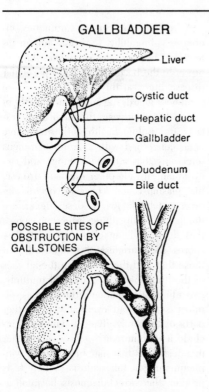

Liver

Cystic duct

Hepatic duct

Gallbladder

Duodenum

Bile duct

POSSIBLE SITES OF
OBSTRUCTION BY
GALLSTONES

men under the ribs, possibly extending to the shoulder. The gallbladder should not be removed unless X-rays indicate that the condition cannot be cured by routine medical treatment. A recent advance in gallbladder surgery has been made possible through the use of laparoscopy. This procedure involves only a very small incision in the neighborhood of the navel, and although the removal of the gallbladder is accomplished under general anesthesia, the patient is usually discharged a day after the operation.

Chronic gallbladder disease may cause gassiness and discomfort following a meal containing fatty foods. Abdominal pain may be brief but recurrent. In many cases the condition can be alleviated by a low-fat diet. When a low-grade infection of the bile ducts is the source of the discomfort,

antibiotics may be prescribed. *See* GALL-STONES.

Gallstones • Solid masses that form within the gallbladder or bile ducts. The stone-forming tendency of bile results in three different types of stones: those composed of a combination of calcium, bile pigments, and cholesterol; those that are pure cholesterol; and those rare formations that are made of bile pigments only. Gallstones of the first two types are especially prevalent following pregnancy and estrogen replacement. Overweight is another possible factor. Obese people are likely to have bile with a high cholesterol content, and when they go on a highly restrictive diet, the liver's production of bile acid decreases, thereby increasing the likelihood of stone formation. Bile acid supplements are recommended for anyone on a low-calorie diet, especially for dieters with a tendency toward or a family history of gallstone formation.

Cholesterol gallstones can be dissolved medically, but this method is not widely used because of limited success and unpleasant side effects. When surgery is indicated, the laparoscopic procedure is the preferred method.

Gamma Globulin • The portion of the blood richest in antibodies. It is produced mainly by the lymphocytes in the lymphoid tissues and is one of the body's strongest defenses against infectious disease. Gamma globulin in one of two forms may be injected to confer passive (temporary) immunity to certain diseases such as hepatitis. Immune serum globulin is derived from blood taken from donors who have an immunity to a specific disease either naturally or subsequent to active immunization. A specific preparation, such as measles immune globulin, is derived from donors who are convalescing from the disease or who have been recently immunized against it. Gamma globulin shots are also recommended for visitors to countries where attention to public sanitation is dangerously inadequate. *See* "Immunization Guide."

Gangrene • A condition in which tissue dies primarily due to loss of blood supply. Gangrene usually involves the extremities but may occur in any part of the body where circulation has been cut off or in which massive infection has caused the affected tissue to putrefy. Among the circumstances leading to most gangrene are severe burns, frostbite, accidents involving contact with corrosive chemicals, untreated ulcerated bedsores, a carelessly applied and improperly attended tourniquet, or any other condition that cuts off circulation.

It is now possible to prevent the spread of gangrene with antibiotics and surgery.

Generic Drugs • *See* "Plain Talk About Medications."

Gene Splicing • *See* GENETIC ENGINEERING.

Genetic Counseling • The National Institute of General Medical Sciences estimates that some 12 million Americans bear the risk of transmitting hereditary disorders. For this group of people genetic counseling has become a vital medical service. According to the National Society of Genetic Counselors, there are only about 1,000 of these specialists nationwide. The greater majority are attached to university hospitals that can administer the tests for genetic abnormalities. In addition to Down syndrome detectable by amniocentesis, there are upward of 2,000 diseases known to be caused by one or another single faulty gene. For those parents-to-be who are

alert to a family history of such disorders as Tay-Sachs disease, muscular dystrophy, or cystic fibrosis (among others), genetic counseling provides information about the factors associated with the particular disease, including diagnosis, the usual course of the disorder, and the risk of its occurrence or recurrence. Counseling also explores alternatives that take these factors into account and at the same time conform with the individuals' ethical principles and religious convictions. *See* HEREDITY, "Pregnancy and Childbirth," and "Directory of Health Information."

Genetic Diseases • *See* HEREDITY.

Genetic Engineering (Gene Splicing) • Since the genetic code was discovered in 1953 and deciphered in 1966, genetic engineering has become a major area of biotechnical advance. By splicing genes, the genetic structure of micro-organisms, yeasts, foods, and potentially any biologic entity including humans, can be altered to produce changes in structure and function. By now, recombinant DNA methods applied to bacteria and yeasts have yielded insulin and other hormones, human serum albumin, various toxins, vaccines, and interferon. These techniques have tremendous implications for treating disease, repairing genetic defects, and improving nutrition. However, there are definite possibilities of abuses. Several countries have moved in the direction of banning research on modifying human genes in ways that could be transmitted from generation to generation. In the United States, while universities and research organizations that receive money from federal sources are regulated by guidelines established by the Recombinant DNA Committee of the National Institutes of Health, regulatory constraints on private industry are difficult to achieve. Biotechnical manufacturers have been competing in the race that takes advantage of advances in genetic engineering to produce vaccines and other highly profitable products, and, as with many previous advances in science and technology, regulatory laws will eventually evolve through courtroom battles.

A milestone was marked in gene therapy in February 1992, when federal review granted permission for the first time to a commercial organization for this procedure. Clinical trials of gene implantation had already been conducted by individual researchers connected with one or another of the U.S. National Institutes of Health. It is expected that widespread commercialization of gene therapy for cancer patients and AIDS patients will occur well before the end of the century.

Gingivitis • Inflammation of the gums caused by an enzyme released by the bacteria that flourish in the plaque that accumulates on improperly cleaned teeth. This same circumstance is also the cause of cavity formation. Inflammation usually starts in the gingival crevice, a groove between the gum and the tooth.

Gingivitis is most prevalent in women who smoke, whose diet is deficient in a particular nutrient, and who have been negligent in practicing proper oral hygiene methods. When gingivitis is associated with pregnancy, it is usually temporary and associated with hormonal changes.

Because untreated gingivitis results in the destruction of bone tissue and the loosening or loss of teeth, gum inflammation should be treated promptly by a periodontist. *See* PLAQUE.

Gland • Any organ that produces and secretes a specific chemical substance. There are two categories of glands: the ductless or endocrine glands, whose se-

cretions are delivered directly into the bloodstream, and the exocrine glands, whose ducts transport their secretions to a precise location. The major endocrine glands are discussed and illustrated in the "The Healthy Woman."

The structures sometimes referred to as lymph glands are not glands and are properly called lymph nodes.

Glomerulonephritis • A kidney disease that affects the coiled clusters of capillary vessels, the glomeruli, through which the fluid content of the blood is partially filtered before it turns into urine. Each kidney consists of approximately a million of these filters. The capillaries may become inflamed following several varieties of bacterial infection, especially following a strep infection in the throat or elsewhere. Because acute nephritis may develop if the initial infection is not successfully treated with antibiotics, it is extremely important to consult a doctor immediately about any painful sore throat accompanied by a high fever. Postinfectious glomerulonephritis may also follow such viral infections as measles, mumps, chicken pox, hepatitis, and AIDS as well as syphilis and malaria. When glomerulonephritis occurs, the body retains fluid due to a collapse in the kidney's filtering capacity. Typical symptoms of the condition are puffy eyelids, swollen ankles, headaches, and decrease in urinary output.

Treatment for the underlying infection is combined with measures that prevent additional complications including limited salt and fluid intake followed by diuretics. If kidney failure is imminent, dialysis may be necessary for a short period. Practically all cases of postinfectious glomerulonephritis subside without further treatment when the underlying cause has been eliminated. *See* KIDNEYS.

Glucose • A sugar that occurs naturally in honey and in most fruit and the one into which starches and polysaccharide (complex) sugars are converted by the digestive process. Glucose is a major source of body fuel. Because it can be absorbed from the stomach, it is one of the quickest sources of energy. Glucose, or its variant dextrose, is also the nutrient usually administered intravenously when a patient cannot eat normally.

Glucose is normally not present in the urine; its presence there may indicate diabetes.

Goiter • An enlargement of the thyroid gland. This endocrine gland, located at the base of the neck, extracts the iodine absorbed by the blood from food and drinking water and uses it for the production of the hormone thyroxin. Thyroxin is stored in the glandular follicles and released into the bloodstream as needed for the regulation of the metabolic rate. The body's iodine requirements are no more than a few millionths of an ounce, and because iodine is generally present in the soil, in most areas the requisite amounts occur naturally in food and water.

Goiter is much more common among women than men because their bodies require considerably more thyroxin during puberty, the menstrual cycle, and pregnancy. A pregnant woman must be sure that her diet contains the iodine essential for the baby's healthy prenatal development.

Gold Treatments • Injectable gold in the form of water soluble salts or a gold compound taken orally as treatment for rheumatoid arthritis. *See* ARTHRITIS and "Plain Talk About Medications."

Gonads • The reproductive glands that in the female produce the ovum and in the male, the sperm cells.

Guillain-Barré Syndrome • A neurological illness that attacks the peripheral nerves, beginning with a loss of sensation in the extremities and, in severe cases, extending to the face, neck, and torso, thereby endangering the ability to swallow and to breathe. The syndrome may follow a virus infection of the throat or the flu, and, in rare cases, is triggered by a flu vaccination. Accurate diagnosis is based on analysis of cerebrospinal fluid (spinal tap) for differentiation from polio, Lyme disease, or from the consequences of ingesting poisonous substances that might produce similar symptoms. Severe cases require hospitalization and monitoring for failure of vital functions. In most instances, recovery is complete with few residual effects. In a small number of cases, rehabilitation therapy is necessary for restoration of muscle function.

Hair • A specialized body growth consisting of dead skin cells that are filled with a tough protein material called keratin, which is also the main constituent of the nails. Aside from the palms of the hand and the soles of the feet, hair covers almost the entire body surface to help to retain heat. Conservation of heat is accomplished by the reflex response whereby individual hairs stand erect and diminish the loss of body warmth ("goose flesh").

Color, texture, and distribution of hair are inherited. Color depends on the amount of the pigment melanin contained in the hair core: the less melanin, the lighter the color. Curly hair is oval in cross-section; straight hair is cylindrical. The average woman's head may contain as many as 125,000 hairs. Each hair root is encased and nourished by a follicle buried under the skin. The growing shaft is lubricated by the oily secretions from a sebaceous gland opening into each follicle.

Hair grows at an average rate of approximately half an inch a month.

Hair gradually turns gray as the melanin pigment is depleted. The age at which this occurs is a factor of inheritance. The growth and nourishment of hair are controlled by hormone secretions and the general state of one's health. The application of creams, lotions, vitamins or minerals does not affect the growth and thickness of hair in a healthy individual.

Products used on the hair should be selected carefully to avoid any which irritate the skin, contain chemicals that might damage hair or skin, or might clog the pores of the scalp. In 1994 a study by the American Cancer Society found that for more than 99 percent of women who use hair dye, there is no increased risk of fatal cancer, even with long-term use.

Hair Removal • Temporary or permanent elimination of unwanted hair, technically called depilation. The simplest and least expensive method for removal of unwanted hair from the legs and underarms is shaving after applying cream or a lather of soap. This method does not cause the hair to grow back in increasing amounts, as the number of hair follicles one is born with remains constant unless the hairs are removed by electrolysis. Sparse face hair or unwanted hair between the breasts can be removed with tweezers. While somewhat painful, waxing has become increasingly popular as a hair removal method and with proper training can be done at home. Hair may also be removed by a depilatory containing chemicals that dissolve the hair at the surface of the skin. A patch test should precede the use of a depilatory to rule out the possibility of an allergic response. Depilatories should be used with caution on the face and never applied immediately after a bath or shower while skin pores are still open. For the same reason they should be removed with cool rather than warm water.

Permanent hair removal is achieved when each hair bulb is destroyed electrically. The electrolysis procedure is expensive and time-consuming and must be performed by a trained licensed operator.

Hallucination • The perception of a sound, sight, smell, or other sensory experience without the presence of an external physical stimulus. Hallucinations are produced by certain drugs. Hallucinatory episodes may be associated with such organic conditions as hardening of the arteries of the brain (cerebral arteriosclerosis) or brain tumor and with exhaustion, sleep deprivation, or prolonged solitary confinement or isolation from normal stimuli. Such experiences are also characteristic of delirium tremens, some forms of mental illness, and psychotic interludes following sudden withdrawal from barbiturates.

Hangover • Symptoms of headache, queasiness, thirst, or nausea occurring the morning after drinking alcohol; also feelings of disorientation and befuddlement following the use of sleeping pills containing barbiturates. The amount of alcohol that will create a hangover varies from person to person and from time to time for the same person. It may result after having had very little to drink if one was tense, angry, tired, or hungry.

The physiological mechanisms that cause the symptoms originate in the disruptive effects of alcohol on body chemistry. Its diuretic properties result in thirst, irritation of the lining of the gastrointestinal tract causes nausea, and dilation of blood vessels leads to throbbing headache. If a remedy is necessary, aspirin will help a headache and an alkalizer may soothe the queasiness. *See* "Substance Abuse."

Hay Fever • *See* ALLERGY.

Headache • Any pain or discomfort in the head; one of the most common complaints and a symptom for which medical science has itemized upwards of 200 possible causes. While it may be difficult to pinpoint a cause in a particular case, it should be comforting to know that very few headaches are serious. Also, new medications in the form of inhalants and injections are now available for aborting and relieving the most severe symptoms.

Considering the complexity of the brain and the delicate mechanisms of pain perception and control, it is not difficult to imagine how many chemical, physical, psychological, neurological, bacteriological, viral, and other variables can lead to a headache. For example, swelling of the blood vessels, inflammation of the nerve endings, or muscular contractions at the base of the skull, will cause the head to pound, throb, or ache. The most recent explanation for head pain is the lowering of the level of serotonin, a neurotransmitter that also plays a critical role in depression and sleep disorders. It appears that serotonin levels are affected by factors ranging from anger and anxiety to the contents of certain foods such as chocolate, sour cream, and aged cheese.

Simple headaches occur at varying intervals and may be annoying or mildly disabling. Most simple recurring headaches are generally known as tension headaches. The usual reason is emotional stress. Such headaches may be mild or severe. If they occur only rarely and respond favorably to over-the-counter analgesics and/or massage of the tightened muscles in the back of the neck, they can be viewed as one of life's minor nuisances.

When headaches recur with debilitating frequency, further exploration into their cause is essential. They may be caused by chronic sinus infections; injuries to the head or neck; reactions to certain pharmacologic agents including alcohol; incorrect refraction of vision; a variety of diseases such as high blood pressure, diabetes mellitus, and hyper- or hypothyroidism; or temporomandibular joint problems. In trying to identify the cause of these headaches, women should not overlook the possibility that they might be triggered by a response to the chemicals in hairsprays, perfumes, room deodorizers, cleaning fluids, insecticides, and the like.

On-the-job headaches may occur not only because of tension but from exposure to noise, pollutants, the sick building syndrome, and because of eyestrain resulting from long hours in front of a video display terminal. Headaches may also be part of premenstrual syndrome. In the elderly, when a headache is accompanied by dizziness, it may be a sign of overmedication. And medication itself may cause a headache as a side effect or because it triggers an allergic response.

Nonsimple recurring headaches differ from simple ones in several ways. The most widely known of these headaches are the classic migraine headache and the common migraine headache. Migraines tend to run in families, affect about 10 percent of the population, and are more prevalent in women. (They may also occur in children as young as four years of age.) The classic migraine is pulsating in nature, affects only one side of the head at a time, may be preceded more or less immediately by loss of vision, flashing lights, or varying neurological symptoms, and is often accompanied by nausea and vomiting. The pain is most severe during the first hour and then subsides, but extreme sensitivity to light may last for several hours. Frequency tends to increase during stress and to decrease with age. Treatment varies and is varyingly successful. The common migraine headache is more widespread. Symptoms are less specific than those of classic migraine. Mood changes usually precede it and may last several hours or days before the headache starts. The headache, also on one side of the head, may last several days. Extreme sensitivity to light is a common symptom. Some women know precisely what triggers their migraine headaches: too little or too much coffee; too little or too much sleep; red wine, certain foods, MSG. Overmedication with painkillers is a special circumstance that produces a "rebound effect" in which the medication itself produces the symptoms. For those whose migraine trigger is stress, relaxation exercises and other alternative therapies can be very effective treatment.

There has been considerable progress in the medications available for migraine sufferers: those that can abort the headache if taken before it is full-blown; those that provide relief more quickly because they are available in nasal sprays that reach the neurological source of the pain almost at once; those that counteract nausea and prevent vomiting.

Severe recurrent headaches should never be dismissed as psychogenic in origin until *all* diagnostic tests, including a CAT scan, have ruled out the possibility of a brain tumor.

Headache treatment centers associated with hospitals and medical centers offer the latest diagnostic procedures and medications for headaches that seem to be treatment-resistant. *See* "Plain Talk About Medications," "Alternative Therapies," and "Directory of Health Information."

Heart-Lung Machine • A device that takes over the job of circulating and oxygenating the blood so that the heart can be bypassed and opened for surgical repair while it is relatively bloodless.

Heat Exhaustion • The accumulation of abnormally large amounts of blood close to the skin in an attempt to cool the surface of the body during exposure to high temperature and humidity. This disturbance of normal circulation deprives the vital organs of their necessary blood supply. The smaller vessels constrict, causing pallor and eventually, heavy perspiration. Pulse and breathing may be rapid, and dizziness and vomiting may follow, but the body temperature remains normal. Fainting may be forestalled by lowering the head to increase blood circulation to the brain. First aid consists of placing the individual in the shade if possible and providing sips of salt water in the amount of half a cup every quarter of an hour for an hour (the solution should consist of 1 teaspoon of salt per 1 cup of water or 0.25 grams salt per 8 ounces water). Feet should be elevated, clothing loosened, and as soon as it is practical to do so, cool wet compresses should be applied. If the condition does not improve or if the person is elderly, has diabetes, or has a heart condition, emergency hospital treatment is necessary.

Heat Stroke • A grave emergency in which there is a blockage of the sweating mechanism that results in extremely high body temperature; also known (mistakenly) as sunstroke and not to be confused with heat exhaustion. The person suffering from heat stroke is more likely to be male than female, old rather than young, and, not infrequently, an alcoholic. The condition is often precipitated by high humidity and may follow unusual physical exertion. Because fever may go as high as 106°F, irreversible damage may be done to the brain, kidneys, and other organs if treatment is not initiated immediately. The skin will be hot, red, and dry. If the face turns ashen, circulatory collapse is imminent. An ambulance must be summoned and in the meantime efforts must be made to bring the person's temperature down. All clothes should be removed, and the bare skin sponged with cool water. If possible, the person should be placed in a tub of cold (not iced) water until there are indications of recovery. No stimulants of any kind should be given. Drying off and further cooling with fans should follow the immersion. Because return to normal is likely to be slow and require close medical supervision, hospitalization after emergency treatment is usually recommended.

Height • The growth hormone of the pituitary gland controls growth during childhood and adolescence. When maximum adult height is reached during adolescence, at about age 16 for girls and 18 for boys, this mechanism stops. Although heredity and hormones determine body build, eventual height may be influenced to a degree by environmental factors such as diet, disease, and activity. *See* "Nutrition, Weight, and General Well-Being."

Heimlich Maneuver • A lifesaving technique used in cases of choking to dislodge whatever is blocking the air passages. An obstruction that cannot be loosened and coughed up following a few sharp blows on the back is likely to be ejected by the Heimlich maneuver. This is accomplished by squeezing the victim's body in such a way that the volume of air trapped in the lungs acts as a propulsive force against the obstruction, causing it to pop out of the throat. The rescuer stands behind the person who is choking and places both hands just above the abdomen. A fist made with one hand is grasped by the other hand and quickly and firmly pressed inward and upward against the victim's diaphragm. The pressure on the

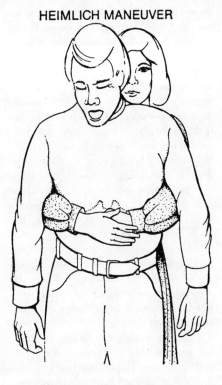

HEIMLICH MANEUVER

diaphragm compresses the lungs and expels the air. If you are choking and no one else is present, you may perform the maneuver on yourself by making a quick upward jab at the diaphragm with your fist or pushing forcefully under your rib cage against a table edge or chair back. *See* CHOKING.

Hemoglobin • The red pigment in red blood cells; a combination of the iron-containing *heme* and the protein-containing *globin*. This substance carries oxygen to the tissues and removes carbon dioxide from them. The amount of hemoglobin in the blood can be determined by a simple test. A less than normal amount indicates anemia.

Hemophilia • An inherited blood disorder characterized by a deficiency of those chemical factors in blood plasma involved in the clotting mechanism. It is a sex-linked genetic disorder; the gene is carried by the female, but only male offspring have the disease. The sons of men with hemophilia are normal (assuming marriage is with a noncarrying female). Transmission occurs through one of the mother's two sex chromosomes: 50 percent of her sons will have hemophilia, and 50 percent of her daughters will be carriers. Thus, while the disease runs in families, the pattern of transmission may cause it to skip several generations. Hemophilia varies in severity. It is not curable, but when bleeding occurs, it can be treated by the infusion of clotting components that are separated out from normal blood plasma. Such transfusions may also be used prior to surgery and may be administered regularly as a preventive measure against hemorrhaging.

Carrier screening and genetic counseling are available to those women who wish to be checked for the chromosomal defect that causes this hereditary disease. *See* GENETIC COUNSELING.

Hemorrhage • Abnormal bleeding following the rupture of a blood vessel. Hemorrhage may be internal or external; it may come from a vein, artery, or capillary. Subcutaneous hemorrhage follows a bruise or a fracture; blood may appear in the sputum, urine, stools, or vomit. When its source is arterial, it is bright red and spurts forth with the heartbeat; when it is venous, it is wine-colored and oozes out in a steady stream. Any untoward bleeding or signs of blood in the body's discharges should be called to a doctor's attention.

Hemorrhoids • Varicose veins in the area of the anus and the rectum; also called piles. External hemorrhoids are located outside the anus and are covered

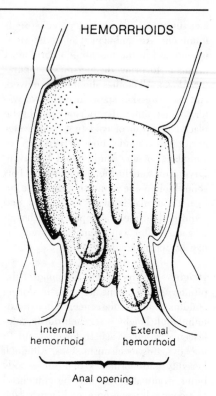

HEMORRHOIDS

Internal hemorrhoid   External hemorrhoid

Anal opening

with skin; internal hemorrhoids develop at the junction of the rectum and the anal canal and are covered with mucous membrane. Among the causes are chronic constipation, obesity, pregnancy, and less commonly, a rectal tumor. In most cases hemorrhoids are the result of constipation, for which the most effective treatment is a diet rich in fiber or roughage. Typical symptoms are intermittent bleeding during the passage of stools, itching, and when thrombosis (clotting) occurs, acute pain. Treatment depends on severity; warm sitz baths are soothing, medication can reduce itching, injections of chemicals can control bleeding and shrink the swollen veins, and, if necessary, an operation can remove the diseased veins by cryosurgery. Any frequent discharge of bright red blood from the anus, even when unaccompanied by pain, should be brought to a doctor's attention.

Heparin • An anticoagulant found in the mucosal linings of the liver and other tissues. In synthetic form it is used medically and surgically to prevent clotting and to treat clotting disorders.

Hepatitis • Inflammation of the liver which may be caused by various chemicals but is generally a viral infection. Several related but somewhat different viruses have been identified: A (hepatitis A virus, or HAV)—formerly referred to as infectious hepatitis); B (hepatitis B virus, or HBV)—formerly referred to as serum hepatitis; a third infectious agent, previously called non A non B and officially renamed hepatitis C in 1990; and hepatitis E, caused by a little-understood virus and very rare in the United States. In 1995 three new hepatitis viruses were discovered distinct from those causing hepatitis A through E. These newly identified viruses will (probably) be named hepatitis H through J and will be carefully investigated for the special problems they may cause.

Hepatitis A is transmitted to others from fecal bacteria entering the mouth either directly (via contaminated water) or indirectly by seafoods such as raw clams and oysters. It is a major problem in daycare centers and is also easily spread by restaurant kitchen workers and other food handlers with careless personal hygiene habits. Hepatitis A is also endemic in many parts of the Caribbean and Mexico. A recently licensed vaccine is now available for travelers who wish to be protected against infection, which produces symptoms of jaundice, fever, fatigue, and loss of appetite. Recovery is slow, and immunity is acquired through the infection.

Hepatitis B is the ninth leading cause of death worldwide. It continues to spread because many people who carry the virus have no symptoms and unwittingly pass it on. Hepatitis B is spread through contact with blood and body fluids, the most common route being sexual intercourse. It is 100 times as contagious as HIV and may be contracted by sharing a contaminated toothbrush, not to mention needles contaminated by intravenous drug users. Vaccination against hepatitis B infection is recommended by the Centers for Disease Control not only for health care and emergency workers, intravenous drug users, and sexually active teenagers and adults with multiple or serial sexual partners, but also for all babies. Three doses of hepatitis B vaccine provide better than 95 percent protection against infection.

Genetic engineering methods have devised a test that identifies hepatitis C antibodies. There is no vaccine for this virus, but alpha interferon, previously approved by the FDA for treating genital warts and some forms of cancer, has also been approved as a treatment for hepatitis C.

See "Sexually Transmissible Diseases" and "Immunization Guide."

Heredity • The transmission of characteristics from one generation to another, from parents to offspring, through the genetic information carried in the chromosomes. Geneticists are providing medical researchers with the tools for exploring the role of heredity in sickness and in resistance to disease. It is hoped that the dissemination of information about genetic disorders and the availability of genetic counseling will bring about a dramatic reduction in the medical, psychological, and economic problems created by hereditary diseases.

Among the more prevalent inherited diseases are: Tay-Sachs, Niemann-Pick, and Gaucher's disease, all three caused by faulty enzyme function and commonly associated with families of middle European Jewish ancestry; sickle-cell anemia, a blood disorder most common among blacks; Cooley's anemia, a more acute blood disease formerly called thalassemia; Huntington's chorea, a degenerative disorder of the central nervous system; hemophilia; several types of muscular dystrophy; galactosemia; phenylketonuria (PKU); cystic fibrosis, the most common genetic disease among Anglo-Saxons, carried by 1 in 20 whites or approximately 10 million Americans. Research on inherited immunities that seem to make some families immune to certain diseases is expected to yield information about resistance to disease in general. This research is still in an early stage of development. *See* CHROMOSOMES, GENETIC COUNSELING, and FAMILY HISTORY.

Hernia • The protrusion of all or part of an organ, most commonly, an intestinal loop or abdominal organ, through a weak spot in the wall of the surrounding structure. A hernia, which may be acquired or congenital, is classified according to the part of the body in which it occurs. The *inguinal hernia*, occurring in the groin, accounts for about 75 percent of all hernias and is much more common among men than women. The *umbilical hernia* is more common among infants than among adults; some cases are self-correcting and some require surgery. *Incisional* or *ventral hernias* may develop after abdominal surgery in cases of unsatisfactory healing or because a chronic cough or obesity subjects the weakened tissue to extra strain. The *esophageal* or *hiatus hernia* is more common among the middle-aged than the young. In this condition a portion of the stomach protrudes through the opening for the esophagus in the diaphragm, producing symptoms that range from mild indigestion and heartburn to serious breathing difficulties. Most her-

nias can be corrected by surgical repair of the weakened tissue.

Herpes • Any of a group of related virus diseases characterized by the eruption of blisters and ranging from mild to life-threatening. The herpes viruses share the capability of lying dormant in the body unless or until they are triggered into causing reinfection. There is no specific cure for any herpes disease, but drugs do exist that, when used early in the infection, can limit its course. The following are the herpes virus types and the diseases they cause:

Herpes simplex virus (HSV) belongs to the family of viruses that cause chicken pox, shingles, and infectious mononucleosis.

Herpes simplex type 1 (HSV1) causes "cold sores" or "fever blisters" that erupt on or inside the mouth. HSV1 also causes ulceration of the cornea (herpes keratitis), which can result in irreversible damage to vision unless controlled from the outset with the hourly use of antiviral drops.

Herpes simplex type 2 (HSV2) causes genital herpes, a sexually transmitted infection of the mucous membranes of the genital and anal area. No cure is available, but there are several drugs that can be taken to speed healing and limit recurrent attacks. *See* "Sexually Transmissible Diseases" and "Pregnancy and Childbirth."

Herpes zoster, the cause of chicken pox, is also the virus that causes shingles, a painful infection of the sensory nerves that results in inflammation of the skin along the pathway of the nerve. Herpes zoster, which means "blister girdle," is not contagious in this form. What activates the virus is not clearly understood. Inflammation typically occurs above the abdomen and less often along the path of the cranial nerve on the face and near the eye, with a potential for damage to the cornea. Sensitivity of the involved nerves

THREE COMMON TYPES OF HERNIAS IN WOMEN

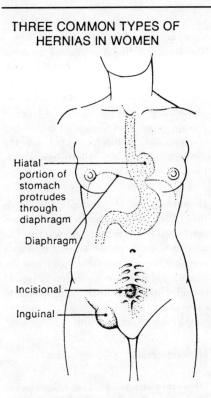

Hiatal portion of stomach protrudes through diaphragm

Diaphragm

Incisional

Inguinal

(neuritis) and blisters may take several weeks to disappear, and in stubborn cases the patient may be left with acute neuralgia, called post-herpetic neuralgia. There is no specific cure, but various medicines are available to reduce pain. Acupuncture is known to reduce pain or eliminate it altogether in about 60 percent of all cases. *See* CHICKEN POX.

Related to the herpes zoster virus are the Epstein-Barr virus that causes infectious mononucleosis and the cytomegalovirus (CMV) that causes a type of pneumonia in patients with AIDS.

High Altitude Sickness • A condition associated with the ascent to altitudes of 8,000 feet above sea level or higher, where the reduced concentration of oxygen in the air leads to oxygen deprivation in the blood. When the red blood cells are unable to absorb a full supply of oxygen as they pass through the lungs, breathing becomes increasingly quick and labored. Giddiness, headache, nausea, and disorientation are among the warning signals of high altitude sickness. Tourists who plan to visit high altitudes and mountain climbers or skiers who intend to reach higher altitudes than customary should have a medical checkup to make sure that their heart and lungs can tolerate the stress. Tourists in high altitudes should eliminate smoking and drinking for the first two days and keep physical exertion to a minimum until the body has adjusted to the environment.

Histamine • A chemical compound found in all body tissues, normally released as a stimulant for the production of the gastric juices during digestion and for the dilation of the smaller blood vessels in response to the body's adaptive needs. Under certain conditions some people produce excessive amounts of histamine as an allergic reaction, causing the surrounding tissues to become swollen and inflamed. For such allergic responses, antihistamine medicines are available. *See* ALLERGY and "Plain Talk About Medications."

Hives • Irregularly shaped red or white elevations of the skin accompanied by itching and burning, usually caused by an allergic response involving the release of histamine. Hives are most often triggered by such foods as shellfish, nuts, and eggs and by such medications as penicillin, sulfa, and anticonvulsants. They may occur on any part of the body or in the gastrointestinal tract, and in some cases the weals may be as large as an inch in diameter. A topical anesthetic ointment or lotion may provide relief, but an antihistamine drug is usually prescribed to prevent additional eruptions. When hives occur for the first time, an effort should be made to identify the cause, especially if a medication is suspected so that a more serious recurrence can be avoided. *See* "Plain Talk About Medications."

Hodgkin's Disease • A disorder of the lymphatic system characterized by the progressive enlargement of the lymph nodes throughout the body, especially of the spleen. It is a type of cancer that typically attacks young adults; men are twice as vulnerable as women. Some specialists believe the disease is genetically determined; others think that an environmental factor or a virus is responsible. If the disease is localized, a 95 percent cure rate can be achieved by radiation treatment. If the disease spreads to the point where vital organs are endangered, various types of chemotherapy have proved effective.

Holistic Medicine • An approach to health and healing that views each patient as a psychobiological unit in a particular physical and psychosocial environment. This approach has been an attempt to counteract the dehumanizing results of medical specialization—one doctor for the heart, another for the skin, yet another for the psyche. The term *holistic* conveys the sense that each individual has a reality that is more important than and independent of the sum of his or her parts. Similar views have been propounded in the past, especially by doctors who focus on psychosomatic medicine on the assumption that the mental and physical aspects of a patient are inextricably bound together. The holistic attitude also takes into account the role played by the person's environment, family history, interpersonal situation, occupational factors, exposure to potential carcinogens, and the like.

Practitioners of holistic medicine stress the importance of patient involvement in the healing process, pointing out that passivity on the part of the patient encourages the view that "medicine is magic." The form that this involvement takes includes self-help wherever possible, self-awareness in recognizing messages from one's feelings and one's body, and open-mindedness about the validity of types of therapy other than those that are part of conventional medical practice in the Western world. *See* "Alternative Therapies."

Homosexuality • Sexual and emotional attraction to a member of one's own sex; called lesbianism among women. Extensive research on the subject of homosexuality has not provided a concrete explanation of its cause. Today, many people consider homosexuality to be as natural to some people as heterosexuality is to most people. *See* "Sexual Health."

Hyperglycemia • *See* DIABETES.

Hyperventilation • Loss of carbon dioxide from the blood caused by abnormally rapid or deep breathing. Hyperventilation produces symptoms of dizziness, muscle spasms, and chest pains and is one of the most common signs of an anxiety attack. Because the symptoms are an additional cause of anxiety, the condition may worsen to the point where it appears to be an emergency. Effective treatment consists of breathing into and out of a paper or plastic bag so that the exhaled carbon dioxide is reinhaled until the proper blood level is achieved, at which point the symptoms vanish. Breathing exercises recommended for stress management are also helpful. *See* "Alternative Therapies."

Hypochondria • An obsessive preoccupation with the symptoms of illness and supposed ill health. Any suggestion that physical checkups indicate normal organic health is greeted with resentment and disbelief. It is a malady in itself because it is usually an expression of psychic distress. Hypochondria can sometimes be relieved by psychotherapy.

Hysteria • In the psychiatric sense, a condition of uncontrolled excitability and intense anxiety sometimes accompanied by sensory disturbances (such as hallucinations) and general disorientation.

Iatrogenic Disease • Any disorder or disease caused by a physician's medical treatment or by hospital mismanagement. It has been estimated that approximately 300,000 people are hospitalized each year in the United States because of an adverse drug reaction. Women can partially protect themselves by questioning the doctor about the possible side effects of any prescribed medication and by keeping records of any unusual responses. Where a particular treatment carries with it a risk potentially equal to the condition being treated, the patient has a right to have this explained so that she can make a responsible choice. See "Plain Talk About Medications."

Ibuprofen • The generic name of the analgesic drug marketed in prescription strength as Motrin and Rufen and in over-the-counter lower dosage as Nuprin and Advil. These medicines are widely used as painkillers by people who cannot tolerate aspirin and who find them more effective than Tylenol for certain conditions such as menstrual cramps and arthritis. However, since their introduction in 1984, complaints have been accumulating about gastric complications when they are used in large amounts for their anti-inflammatory properties. Ibuprofen medication is also reported as a trigger of asthma attacks. It should not be taken with diuretics because the combination can lead to kidney

damage. See "Plain Talk About Medications."

Ileitis • Inflammation of the lower portion of the small intestine. See CROHN'S DISEASE.

Ileostomy • A surgical procedure to create an artificial anus to bypass the colon by bringing the ileum (the lowest part of the small intestine) through an opening made in the abdominal wall. An ileostomy is performed when ulcerative colitis, cancer, or other disease requires the removal of the colon (large intestine). It may also be performed as a temporary measure so that an obstruction in the colon can be removed without removing the colon itself.

Immunity and Immunization • Immunity is a biologic state of being resistant to or not susceptible to a disease or condition, usually, and here specifically, due to the presence of antibodies against the causative agent (antigen). The immunity may be congenital (acquired from the mother and present at birth but not long lasting), natural (resulting from an infectious disease that produces antibodies), or induced by immunization (vaccination).

Active immunization against some diseases may require periodic boosters to maintain the immunity; against others, the initial immunization may last a lifetime.

Passive immunization is achieved by introducing antibodies rather than antigens into the body. Antibodies are introduced by the injection of blood serum obtained from humans who have a natural immunity, have been actively immunized, or are convalescing from a particular disease. Individuals differ greatly in the efficiency of their immune responses depending on genetic inheritance and exposure to antibody formation. Some women may have a single experience with a genital herpes infection and never another because the virus is kept dormant. In other cases, the immune system is incapable of fighting off the recurrent attacks of infection. It is thought that a damaged immune system is responsible for some types of cancer, and in AIDS the immune system has been undermined to the point where the body is mortally vulnerable to infection and disease. *See* "Immunization Guide."

Impotence • Inability of the male to achieve and maintain an erection (erectile impotence); also, inability to achieve orgasm following erection (ejaculating impotence). Almost all men experience impotence at some time in their lives. It may be occasional and temporary or it may be chronic. It may be psychological, resulting from conflicts that arise from guilt, unacknowledged homosexuality, anxiety, distrust of women, or self-punishment. It may also be related to physical causes of fatigue, general poor health, and organic conditions such as diabetes, hormonal aberration, or inherited disorders of the genitals. Occupational exposure to radiation or certain chemicals, alcoholism, drug addiction, and certain prescribed drugs and tranquilizers are other causes. When impotence exists, psychiatric counseling or a professionally accredited sex therapy clinic should be considered only after a complete physical checkup has been conducted. *See* "Sexual Health" and "Infertility."

Infantile Paralysis • *See* POLIO.

Influenza • A contagious respiratory disease caused by a Type A or B virus; generally known as the flu and previously called the grippe. All strains of the flu virus are airborne, and the infection is spread in the coughs, sneezes, and exhaled breath of the affected person. The disease may reach epidemic proportions rapidly, especially because natural or artificially acquired immunity against one particular strain of the virus provides no guaranteed protection against another strain.

Symptoms may range from mild to severe. Typical manifestations are inflammation of the membranes that line the respiratory tract causing a running nose, scratchy throat, and mucous congestion that results in coughing. Fever may not be present or temperature may go as high as 104°F. Aching joints, appetite loss, and general malaise characterize even the mildest cases. When symptoms clear up, usually within ten days, the flu patient may feel weak and tired for some time. The cough may be persistent, and relapses may occur as a result of lowered resistance and premature resumption of normal activities. Lowered resistance to bacterial infection is the most serious complication of the flu. When a healthy adult has the illness, the usual treatment is bed rest, aspirin or Tylenol, lots of fluids, and as much sleep as possible. A cough medicine containing an expectorant may be prescribed to facilitate the hawking up of the accumulated phlegm. For flu patients over 65, a person with diabetes, or anyone with a heart, lung, or kidney disorder, antibiotics may be prescribed in addition.

People susceptible to serious complications should be vaccinated each year with a vaccine made from the killed viruses of the current strains responsible for the disease. *See* "Immunization Guide."

Inguinal Glands • A group of lymph nodes located in the groin. Any painful swelling or persistent soreness in this area should be brought to a doctor's attention.

Inner Ear • *See* EAR.

Insect Stings and Bites • While usually no more than a nuisance, the bite of an insect can at times cause disease or life-threatening emergencies. The stinging insects—hornets, wasps, yellow jackets, and bees—do not transmit disease, but the venom they inject may cause a severe allergic response known as anaphylactic shock. Ordinarily, however, the sting results in no more than swelling, redness, and localized pain. In the case of a bee sting the skin should never be squeezed in order to extricate the stinger, because this only forces the venom farther into the tissues. Instead, the stinger should be removed with a pair of tweezers held flat against the skin. Any sign of a systemic response to a sting, such as body swelling or respiratory distress, indicates the need for immediate professional attention. Women who are extremely hypersensitive to the venom should be desensitized by an allergist and continue the maintenance treatments usually necessary four or five times a year. Even after desensitization emergency adrenalin should be carried when there is the threat of a sting. A device no larger than a fountain pen and containing adrenalin for self-administration in an emergency is recommended.

Biting and bloodsucking flies and mosquitos can transmit serious diseases. The common housefly does not bite but may be a carrier of infection. Aside from diseases endemic to the tropics, such as yellow fever and malaria, encephalitis can be transmitted by certain local mosquitos. Horseflies are also harmful because they can transmit rabbit fever (tularemia). Among dangerous parasites found in several parts of the world are fleas that transmit bubonic plague and typhus. It should be noted that the ticks that cause Rocky Mountain spotted fever are not indigenous to the West and may be found in other parts of the country. Immunization is available against all the above infections and should be taken into consideration by anyone planning a trip to an area of high-risk exposure. A parasite common in the rural South, known as the chigger, is the larval stage of the mite that causes scabies. While chiggers are not disease-bearing, their bite irritates the skin thereby leading the way toward a secondary infection. Once bitten, the victim can be relieved of the itching by the application of a paste of baking soda and water or calamine lotion.

Lyme disease, also called Lyme arthritis, is the most recently identified disease known to be caused by a tick bite.

While most spiders and other arachnids are harmless, there are three or four that inflict bites that must receive prompt attention: the scorpion found in the Southwest, the black widow spider (identifiable by its shiny black body whose underside is marked with a red hourglass shape), and a species of hairy tarantula found near the Mexican border. The aggressive fire ant is a more recent menace spreading its way through the Southern states. Its attack can be easily identified because it inflicts multiple stings around the original bite. The bite of a fire ant can cause severe systemic response in certain people. Anyone living in an area where fire ants exist should consider the advisability of desensitization.

Certain practical measures can reduce the hazards and discomforts of bites and stings without the use of insecticides that pollute the environment with dangerous chemicals. A few suggestions are the application of insect-repellent lotions containing such effective chemicals as diethylmetatoluamide, dimethyl phthalate, or dimethylearbate on exposed parts of the body several times a day; wearing protective clothing during walks in the country; avoiding the use of perfumes, lotions, sprays, and jewelry because scents and colors attract stinging insects; burning insect-repellent candles or incense sticks at picnics when food is exposed; keeping foods covered; and using screens for indoor protection. Women who own or rent vacation houses should heed the warnings of local health authorities about insect-borne diseases and the precautions one can take to combat them. *See* ALLERGY, LYME DISEASE, and "Plain Talk About Medications."

Insomnia • Sleeplessness, either chronic or occasional. Because it is generally believed that dependence on sleeping pills will only intensify insomnia, anyone trying to cope with the problem should find another solution for it. Consultation with a sleep disorder specialist may be helpful.

Sleeplessness may be caused by any one of many factors easily corrected, such as eating rich food or drinking beverages containing caffeine within two hours of bedtime, watching overly exciting television programs, sleeping in a poorly ventilated room or on an uncomfortable mattress. When snoring and other noises interfere with sleep, ear plugs can often relieve the problem. Daytime exercise, a hot bath in the evening, and a glass of warm milk before retiring are often as effective as pills. Scientists have found that an amino acid, L-triptophane, contained in certain foods, including milk, seems to act as a sedative. When insomnia is a result of depression or anxiety, the cause of the emotional distress should be explored before resorting to medication. *See* SLEEP, "Substance Abuse," and "Alternative Therapies."

Insulin • The hormone secreted by the groups of cells in the pancreas called the islets of Langerhans. Insulin performs several vital functions and is especially critical in stabilizing the body's metabolism of sugars and starches. The isolation of insulin by Canadian scientists in 1921–22 inaugurated the successful treatment of diabetes using insulin derived from the pancreas of pigs and cows. Most recently, insulin is supplied by genetically engineered bacteria. *See* GENETIC ENGINEERING.

Interferon • A cellular protein produced by white blood cells and fibroblasts that suppresses viral DNA reproduction. This antiviral substance is available as a genetically engineered drug, but it remains too expensive for widespread use. Promising experimental results have been achieved in the use of interferon for treatment of some cancers and to counteract the effects of hepatitis C and HIV, the virus that causes AIDS.

Intermittent Claudication • In simple language, occasional limping caused by an inadequate supply of blood to the lower leg during exercise because of partial blockage of a major artery in the upper leg by fatty deposits. This causative condition is called arteriosclerosis obliterans. The pain in the lower leg that causes limping subsides after a period of rest. The condition is not life-threatening, but the unexpected and sudden onset of pain can be immobilizing. Short of surgery to bypass or clean out the diseased artery, other measures that can be effective are total abstention from smoking, weight loss as necessary, and participation in a walking-for-exercise program.

Irritable Bowel Syndrome • A common condition in which an abnormal pattern of bowel contractions results in diarrhea alternating with constipation, bloat, and pain. Irritable bowel syndrome, also called spastic colon, is experienced by an estimated 22 million people, two-thirds of whom are women. A significant number of these are young adults who avoid seeking medical advice for the condition, which is likely to be more responsive to a course in stress management than to medication. A diet high in fiber and, if necessary, a high-fiber dietary supplement usually minimize the symptoms. Because many of the symptoms are similar to those of Crohn's disease and because the likelihood of cancer is an overriding fear of those who do seek a physician's advice, tests are usually given to rule out these more serious possibilities. See CROHN'S DISEASE, "Nutrition, Weight, and General Well-Being," and "Alternative Therapies."

Itching • An irritation of the skin; technically called pruritis. Among the most common causes are insect bites, fungus infections, allergies, or contact dermatitis. Itching in the anal region may be caused by worms or hemorrhoids; in the vaginal area it may occur spontaneously or follow the use of certain antibiotics. Severe itching around the pubic hair may indicate the presence of crabs. Among other causes are an accumulation of dried body secretions under the arms, in the crotch, on the scalp, or between the toes; vaginal discharges; the drying out of the vaginal mucous membranes that occurs during menopause; exposure to cold temperatures; new skin growth following sunburn or scar healing; chafing by one body surface against another (e.g., under the breasts) or by tight clothing; emotional stress. A doctor may refer to local or generalized itching as neurodermatitis if no specific cause can be found. Certain serious disorders are accompanied by itching: diabetes, anemia, leukemia, jaundice, gout, liver malfunction, and cancer.

The impulse to relieve itching by energetic scratching should be controlled because the irritation will only become more intense and the nails may cause breaks in the skin leading to secondary bacterial infection. Sometimes it is necessary to wear gloves. If topical medication provides no relief, medication taken orally or by injection may be necessary to relieve the itching until the underlying cause can be diagnosed and eliminated. The disorder that has the distinction of being called "the itch" is discussed under scabies. See "Sexually Transmissible Diseases."

Jaundice • A yellowish appearance of the skin and the whites of the eyes resulting from an excessive amount of bile in the blood. As a sign of a disorder of the liver or the biliary tract, jaundice may be accompanied by diarrhea, abdominal pain caused by liver enlargement, bitter-tasting greenish vomit, and itching in various parts of the body. Among the usual underlying causes, the most common is infectious hepatitis; others are gallstones, cirrhosis, hemolytic anemia, and tumors that obstruct the normal circulation of bile. The treatment of jaundice depends on the diagnosis of the condition.

Kaposi's Sarcoma • A malignant disease, primarily of the skin, which has a high prevalence in people with AIDS. See ACQUIRED IMMUNE DEFICIENCY SYNDROME.

Kegel Exercises • To benefit women with mild stress incontinence, Dr. Arnold Kegel devised exercises for strengthening the muscles between the vagina and the anus that support the base of the bladder. The procedure begins with identifying the musculature in question by trying to stop the flow of urine when seated on the toilet. Another way of identifying the muscles is to put a finger into the vagina and tighten up until the finger feels squeezed. The exercises consist of tightening these muscles from front to back and holding the contraction for a slow count of 10. Repeat this exercise 10 times each time. It should be done about 20 times a day to be effective. Kegel exercises can be done no matter what position the body is in—standing, sitting, or lying down.

Kidneys and Kidney Disorders • The kidneys are twin organs, each about 4 inches long, located on either side of the spinal column at the back wall of the abdomen approximately at waist level. Examined in cross-section under a microscope, the functional units of the organ—the nephrons—are seen to consist of clusters of blood vessels, the glomeruli, that act as filters. The vital process in which the kidneys are indispensable is the continuous filtering of the blood to remove wastes and excess fluid while retaining or reabsorbing other materials. The kidneys also secrete hormones involved in the regulation of blood pressure and the red blood cell count. In order to understand how certain disorders originate, it is helpful to have some idea of how the kidneys work. As arterial blood enters the kidneys from the heart, it passes through the millions of nephrons. The waste materials go by way of the ureter into the bladder for eventual elimination through the urethra in the form of urine. The cleansed and filtered blood goes back into circulation through the veins, returning to the heart for recirculation. With a combined weight of only about 2/3 pound, the kidneys process more than 18 gallons of blood every hour and filter about 60 percent of all the fluid taken into the body, excreting as much as 2 quarts of urine each day.

The kidneys are subject to a number of disorders, some merely temporary, others potentially fatal. The most common problem is infection and the most common infection is pyelonephritis, an infection of the kidney's urine-collecting ducts. It may occur with no significant symptoms or it may be accompanied by back pain, fever, and chills. An acute attack of pyelonephritis occurs in about 5 percent of all pregnancies and usually requires antibiotic

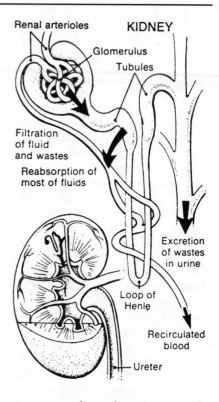

treatment. Kidney obstructions in the form of stones (usually calcium), cysts, or other abnormalities can lead to improper drainage, inflammation, and damage to surrounding tissues. Nephrosis, also known as the nephrotic syndrome, is a group of symptoms frequently accompanying some other condition. It is characterized by the leakage of large amounts of protein into the urine and leads to generalized swelling, especially a marked puffiness under the eyes. Kidney disease may also result from untreated hypertension, gout, and diabetes or as a consequence of chemical poisoning or prolonged shock. Chemical poisoning by certain drugs, individually or in combination, results in acute interstitial nephritis. This toxic reaction occurs especially when a combination of drugs doubles the negative side effects of each one. For example, anyone on a regular regimen of diuretics for hypertension should be aware of the potential hazard of taking some other medication in addition prescribed by a different doctor for a different condition. When any disorder reaches the point where the kidneys can no longer function, uremia (accumulation of urea nitrogen in the blood) occurs. Acute kidney failure may be helped by short-term dialysis. When irreversible damage to both kidneys has occurred, long-term dialysis or tissue transplant can prevent fatal consequences.

Any signs of kidney disease should be taken seriously, especially during pregnancy. Symptoms may include back pain below the rib cage, a change in the color or composition of urine or discomfort during urination, puffiness of any part of the body especially the area around the eye. Treatment depends on the specific diagnoses and may only require changes in the diet and the use of diuretics. Antibiotics are often prescribed for bacterial infection. In the case of an obstruction, surgery may be necessary. *See* DIALYSIS, GLOMERULONEPHRITIS, "Plain Talk About Medications," and "Directory of Health Information."

Knee Disorders • The knee is one of the largest and strongest joints in the body, formed by the junction of the tibia (shinbone), the femur (thighbone), and the patella (kneecap). The bones are bound by ligaments and tendons and cushioned by cartilage and fluid-filled sacs called bursas. "Housemaid's knee," so called because it usually results from frequent kneeling on hard surfaces, is a form of bursitis. "Water on the knee" is a condition in which there is an excessive accumulation of the lubricating fluid secreted by the membranous lining of the ligaments that bind the knee joints together. This oversecretion, which may fol-

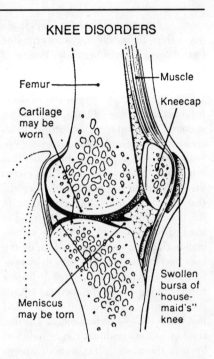

KNEE DISORDERS

Femur —
Muscle
Kneecap
Cartilage may be worn
Meniscus may be torn
Swollen bursa of "housemaid's" knee

low an injury or infection or may accompany arthritis, causes the kneecap to be raised and the surrounding tissue to become painful. Keeping the knee raised and rested is usually sufficient treatment. Chronic inflammation of the joint that occurs during arthritis can be relieved by therapeutic doses of aspirin or other nonsteroidal anti-inflammatory drugs. In severe cases, injections of steroids into the joint may be recommended for short-term therapy. Damage to the knee joint by rheumatic disease or athletic injury resulting in torn cartilage can be restored by a type of surgery made possible by the use of an arthroscope. This instrument can "see" disorders in the joint not easily made visible by X-ray or more traditional means. Other instruments attached to the arthroscope are manipulated by the surgeon in order to remove the damaged cartilage.

With the advancement in prosthetic devices, replacement of knee (and hip) joints has enabled those suffering from crippling joint disease to enjoy a greater degree of mobility than previously possible.

Lacrimal Ducts • Three sets of ducts involved in the flow of tears: 6 to 12 tiny openings that lead from the lacrimal (tear) gland at the upper, outside rim of the eye to the lacrimal sac; the lacrimal duct that leads from the inner corner of the eye to the conjunctival sac; and the nasolacrimal duct that leads from the lacrimal sac to the nose. When the duct in the nose is blocked or swollen by allergy or inflammation during a respiratory infection, the eyes become watery. The dry, itchy eyes that may afflict the elderly result from a partial drying up of the lacrimal glands and a consequent decrease in the fluid that keeps the eye surface moist. The discomfort of this condition can be relieved by over-the-counter preparations known as artificial tears.

Lactose Intolerance • An inability to metabolize milk and milk products without discomfort because of low levels of the enzyme lactase in the surface of the small intestines. Lactase is the enzyme essential for the proper absorption of the major sugar in milk, lactose. This malabsorption problem, estimated to affect between 30 and 50 million Americans, results in symptoms similar to those of spastic colon or colitis: diarrhea, cramps, and gassiness. When these discomforts occur after eating any and all dairy products, a simple blood test can diagnose the problem correctly so that suitable changes can be made in the diet. Lactaid pills, a product containing lactase, are recommended as an alternative to eliminating dairy products from the diet.

Laryngitis • Inflammation of the mucous lining of the larynx, affecting both breathing and voice production. The condition may be chronic or acute; occurring because of a virus or bacterial infection; an allergic response; an irritation of the membrane by chemicals, dusts, or pollens; or recurrent misuse of the voice. The symptoms of milder cases usually include a dry cough, a tickling sensation in the throat, and hoarseness or a complete loss of voice, all of which result from swelling of the vocal cords. Fever may be present when laryngitis is produced by bacterial infection. The most effective treatment is silence. Whispering is inadvisable since it puts additional stress on already irritated tissues. Laryngitis is also helped by a day or so of bed rest in a room where the temperature is warm and the humidity is high enough to prevent irritating dryness, if necessary through the use of a humidifier or a vaporizer. Spicy foods, hot soups, smoking, or any other irritants should be eliminated. Chronic laryngitis may be the result of longtime exposure to such irritants as alcohol, smoking, or industrial fumes. Because hoarseness may also accompany the development of tuberculosis or cancer, it should be investigated by a doctor if it persists for more than a few weeks.

Larynx • The cartilaginous structure that contains the vocal cords and is held together by ligaments and moved by attached muscles; also called the voice box. Obstruction of the larynx may occur because of an abscess in the cartilage lining or because of an injury. Tumors are not uncommon and are removed surgically, even if benign. Singers and politicians are more likely to develop nodes on their vocal cords than other people. Such growths may also be eliminated by surgery. Cancer of the larynx, which is more common in men than women, is associated with smoking. Smokers are six times more likely to develop cancer of the larynx than

CROSS-SECTION OF MOUTH AND LARYNX

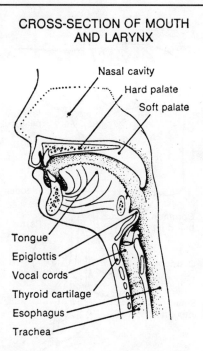

Nasal cavity
Hard palate
Soft palate

Tongue
Epiglottis
Vocal cords
Thyroid cartilage
Esophagus
Trachea

nonsmokers, and the risk is greater still for heavy drinkers.

If examination with a laryngoscope and various laboratory tests including a biopsy verify the presence of an obstructive malignancy unresponsive to radiation treatment, a laryngectomy (the surgical removal of part or all of the larynx) is performed. The surgery itself is not complicated, but because it involves removal of the voice box, the patient must undergo postoperative rehabilitation in order to learn a new speech process.

Laser • A device containing a gas such as carbon dioxide or other substance that amplifies and concentrates light waves into a tiny beam of immense heat and power. Called a "bloodless scalpel," the laser permits pinpoint (¹/₁₀₀ of a human hair's width) surgery by vaporizing tissue layer by layer without affecting adjacent tissue only a few cell widths away.

Laxative • Preparation that increases the bulk and water content of the bowel, thereby loosening the stool and encouraging evacuation. A dependence on laxatives for the treatment of constipation is likely to worsen the condition because it deprives the colon of its natural muscle tone. There are, however, bulk-forming agents that have a laxative effect and can be taken every day indefinitely. *See* "Nutrition, Weight, and General Well-Being" and "Aging Healthfully."

Legionnaire's Disease • A form of pneumonia ranging from mild to life-threatening caused by the bacterium *Legionella pneumophila*. This microorganism may be found in soil and especially in the stagnant water that accumulates in the air ducts of air conditioning systems in public buildings, in the workplace, and in hotels. The disease is airborne (person-to-person contamination is not known to occur) and is characterized by severe general malaise followed by high fever, chills, and a cough. When untreated at this stage, Legionnaire's disease has been fatal in more than 15 percent of all cases. There have also been many instances when symptoms are so mild as to go unnoticed and unidentified. When this occurs, the infection runs a course similar to that of a cold. *See* "Plain Talk About Medications."

Leukemia • A group of diseases characterized by a proliferation in the bone marrow and lymphoid tissue of white blood cells whose excessive production interferes with the manufacturing of normal red cells. Different types of white cells are involved in the various forms taken by the disease. While there is no accepted theory about the cause of leukemia, it is assumed that its rising incidence results from increased exposure to radioactivity in its many manifestations: industrial pollution, food contamination, too many diagnostic X-rays over too short a period, or radiation therapy for some other disease. It is also a likely concomitant of a breakdown in the body's immune defenses as occurs in AIDS.

Diagnosis of all leukemias is based on microscopic examination of blood samples, bone marrow, or lymph tissue. Treatment consists of a combination of anticancer drugs, corticosteroids, radiation, antibiotics, and transfusions of hemoglobin and platelets. Several of the leukemias that were formerly fatal have gone into remission as a result of the effectiveness of the new drugs, the use of generalized radiation, and the transplanting of healthy bone marrow.

Ligament • Band of tough fibrous tissue that connects and stabilizes bones at the joints. An injury resulting in the stretching or tearing of ligaments is called a sprain.

Light Therapy • *See* "Alternative Therapies."

Liver • The body's largest internal organ, dark red, wedge-shaped, weighing from 3 to 4 pounds, and located underneath the lower right side of the rib cage. Among its many vital functions are: the production of bile essential for fat digestion; the production and storage of glycogen for conversion to glucose; the synthesis of protein and the formation of urea; the storage of vitamins A, D, E, and K; the production of several blood components including the clotting factors; the inactivation of nicotine ingested during smoking before it can reach the stomach; the neutralization of poisons such as carbon tetrachloride, arsenic, and others that may enter the body from without as well as of those created from within. Inflammation of the liver (hepatitis) may be

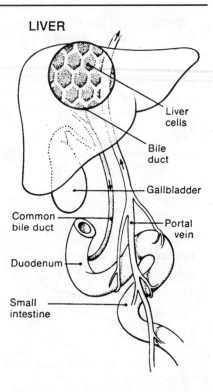

LIVER

Liver cells

Bile duct

Gallbladder

Common bile duct

Portal vein

Duodenum

Small intestine

caused by chemical poisons, by sensitivity to certain medications, and by disease agents, especially the viruses that cause the several types of hepatitis. If the infection is severe, the cells that are affected may be replaced by scar tissue, causing cirrhosis of the liver.

A nourished liver that contains stored amounts of vitamins, proteins, and other nutrients is less likely to suffer irreversible harm from alcohol than a liver that is undernourished. The liver may also be adversely affected by disorders of the gallbladder, especially by gallstones. The signs and symptoms of liver disorder may include the following depending on the severity of the disease: a gradual swelling of the abdomen and sensitivity to pressure below the rib cage, clay colored stools, dark urine, and vomiting of blood. When disorders are treated promptly and a wholesome regimen is followed, recovery is usually complete. *See* CIRRHOSIS and HEPATITIS.

Liver Spots • Irregularly shaped reddish brown skin blemishes once mistakenly attributed to malfunctioning of the liver. The spots, which are concentrations of melanin pigment similar to but larger than freckles, are not due to aging as such but rather to long exposure to sun and wind, to minor metabolic disturbances, and in some women to systemic changes that occur during pregnancy. The spots are generally harmless and can be covered with a special cosmetic preparation. If such a blemish suddenly thickens and hardens or if the surrounding tissue feels sore, a dermatologist should be consulted.

Lou Gehrig's Disease • *See* AMYOTROPHIC LATERAL SCLEROSIS.

Lower Back Pain • *See* BACKACHE.

Lupus (also known as Systemic Lupus Erythematosus or SLE) • An inflammatory disease that may involve various parts of the body and cause permanent tissue damage. Typical cases are women of childbearing age. In its milder discoid form it affects the skin only, producing a butterfly-shaped rash that spreads across the nose to both sides of the face. The rash may be accompanied by fever and weight loss as well as by arthritic pains in the joints. In its more serious form lupus involves the kidneys and the blood vessels. Lupus is classified as a disorder of the immune system. It is usually diagnosed through blood tests or a skin biopsy. The cause is unknown and the disease may flare up unexpectedly, leaving the patient exhausted and weak. Recent research indicates that the disorder may occur or worsen when a latent virus is ac-

tivated by overexposure to sunlight, emotional stress, or an unrelated infection.

Lupus is a condition requiring long-term supervision. Medications that control the disorder, especially heavy therapeutic doses of anti-inflammatory drugs, corticosteroids, and other drugs, may produce adverse side effects. The prescribed regimen must be carefully followed and readjusted from time to time depending on individual reactions. Patients with this disease should use a contraceptive other than the pill. If they do become pregnant, special management is needed. In all cases including the mildest, exposure to extreme sunlight should be avoided. *See* "Directory of Health Information."

Lyme Disease (also called Lyme Arthritis) • This disease, named for the town in Connecticut where it made its first known appearance in 1975, is caused by the bite of a tick usually found on deer in wooded areas. Since that time the disease has spread to the Midwest, and cases have been reported on the West Coast as well. It has been so heavily publicized that most primary care doctors know how to recognize and treat it or, if necessary, make a referral to a rheumatologist.

The tick transmits a disease-bearing organism called a spirochete. The first stage of the disease occurs when a characteristic rash appears at the site of the bite. Red spots may appear elsewhere on the body, combined with symptoms similar to those of the flu: fatigue, headache, aching joints, sore throat, and fever. These symptoms may disappear on their own (as they do with the flu), but about 50 percent of the cases eventually develop arthritis with attacks ranging from mild to immobilizing that occur at unpredictable intervals. Even these complications vanish, but some few people are left with flare-ups of pain and inflammation similar to those of rheumatoid arthritis. In the most serious cases, the spirochete invades the brain and spinal cord, producing meningitis and encephalitis. Lyme disease is effectively treated at early onset with antibiotics. The earlier the treatment, the less likely the eventual complications.

In the event of chronic and debilitating symptoms similar to fibromyalgia and chronic fatigue syndrome, it is advisable to seek treatment at a reputable Lyme disease treatment center connected with a teaching hospital.

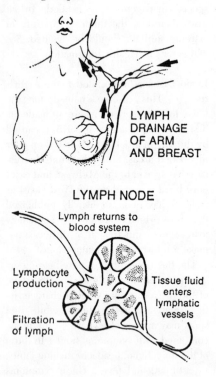

LYMPH
DRAINAGE
OF ARM
AND BREAST

LYMPH NODE

Lymph returns to
blood system

Lymphocyte
production

Tissue fluid
enters
lymphatic
vessels

Filtration
of lymph

Lymph Nodes • Glandlike organs located throughout the body that manufacture the disease-fighting cells known as lymphocytes. These cells are collected in the lymphatic vessels and delivered to the circulatory system in the fluid called lymph. Lymph is part of the blood's plasma. Among the most important lymph nodes and the ones that are superficially located are those found behind the ears, at the angle of the jaw in the neck, in the armpit, and in the groin. When reference is made to "swollen glands," a condition characteristic of such diseases as infectious mononucleosis, it is the nodes that are involved, because in addition to providing the system with protective lymphocytes, they also filter foreign bodies and bacteria out of the lymphatic fluid. Other masses of lymphatic tissue that produce specialized white cells for counteracting infection are the tonsils, thymus gland, and spleen. The general term for inflammation of lymphatic tissue, of which tonsillitis is an example, is lymphadenitis: a tumor of this tissue is a lymphoma, and a malignancy of the lymph nodes is a lymphosarcoma. Hodgkin's disease is a cancer of the lymphatic system, and in lymphocytic leukemia, the proliferation of defective lymphocytes leads to invasion of the bone marrow.

Magnetic Resonance Imaging • This diagnostic procedure, usually referred to as MRI, subjects the body to radio waves in the presence of a magnetic field, thereby providing finely detailed images of body tissue without the use of potentially dangerous ionizing radiation. Not only is MRI scanning safer than X-ray imaging, but its results are greatly superior because it can see through soft tissue, measure blood flow, depict cerebrospinal fluid, detect brain tumors, and show the abnormal deposits on brain cells that indicate the presence of multiple sclerosis— all without the injection of contrast dyes. *See* "You, Your Doctors, and the Health Care System."

Malignant • A term used to describe a tumor or growth that spreads to surrounding tissues or migrates through the lymphatics or bloodstream to more distant tissues. In common parlance, a malignancy is synonymous with cancer.

Malnutrition • Inadequate nourishment resulting from a substandard diet or a metabolic defect. Among common causes unrelated to the availability of adequate food are alcoholism, unnecessary vitamins substituted for essential foods, metabolic disorders, and crash dieting. *See* DEFICIENCY DISEASE, ANEMIA, and "Nutrition, Weight, and General Well-Being."

Malocclusion • Failure of the teeth of the upper and lower jaw to come together properly when the jaws are closed. A bite that is out of alignment should be corrected not only for esthetic reasons but also because, by achieving an even distribution of the pressures on the teeth, orthodontic correction contributes to the health of the gums. Maloccluded teeth are much more difficult to clean, and the faulty condition also subjects facial muscles to an abnormal stress that may lead to earaches and headaches. Even though orthodontia is a slow and costly process, an increasing number of adult women are finding the time and money well spent in terms of improvements in appearance and oral health. *See* ORTHODONTIA and "Cosmetic Surgery."

Manic-Depressive Illness • A mental disturbance characterized by periods of overenergized and overconfident elation followed by profound depression; also known as bipolar depression. Attacks may be severe and cyclic, with varying periods of normalcy occurring between onsets of the illness. Lithium carbonate administered at the beginning of the manic phase has a stabilizing effect on many people suffering from this disorder. *See* "Plain Talk About Medications."

Marfan Syndrome • A genetically transmitted degenerative disease of the body's connective tissue that can lead to death from cardiovascular complications. About one in 10,000 people have inherited this disorder, with symptoms of varying severity. Typically they have elongated fingers and limbs and an abnormal chest contour. More than half have some type of heart trouble involving an enlarged aorta. The disorder is best known for its role in the deaths of the Olympic volleyball player Flo Hyman and the University of Maryland star Chris Patten. Having isolated the gene responsible for Marfan syndrome, researchers hope to be able to determine through DNA testing of dried blood left on Abraham Lincoln's clothing following his assassination whether the President had this disease, a conclusion held by many specialists in the disorder.

Medic Alert • A three-part system for emergency medical protection consisting of a metal emblem worn on the wrist or around the neck that identifies otherwise hidden medical problems, a wallet card with additional information, and an emergency, 24-hour, toll-free telephone answering service to provide still further information about the wearer's physical condition and medical needs in the event of collapse. For women with diabetes, a life-threatening allergy to insect stings, or other problems that could lead to the need for prompt professional attention, the Medic Alert identification can prevent potential disaster. Further information is available from the Medic Alert Foundation (a voluntary nonprofit organization). *See* "Directory of Health Information."

Medical Records • While it is assumed that physicians keep detailed records about their patients and that these records are made available when requested by another physician, every

MEDIC ALERT

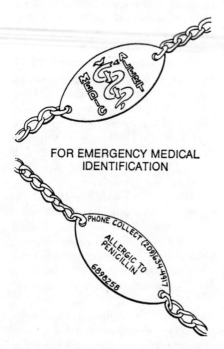

FOR EMERGENCY MEDICAL IDENTIFICATION

woman should keep her own medical records, and they should be kept up-to-date. Information should be compiled in a notebook set aside for the purpose and should consist of relevant family history, immunization shots and dates, pertinent facts about hospitalization, X-ray and other test reports when results are other than normal, allergies, and current medications. Side effects should also be noted. The records should be cumulative, and past pages should not be discarded. Entries about surgery ten years before or a siege of pneumonia years before that may turn out to be unexpectedly helpful to the physician of the moment. *See* FAMILY HISTORYand "You, Your Doctors, and the Health Care System."

Melanin • The pigment that determines the color of a person's skin, hair,

and eyes. The main function of melanin is to provide protection against the sun's ultraviolet rays. It is produced by specialized cells called melanocytes whose number is the same in all races. Color differences are caused by the quantity of melanin produced and how it is distributed. *See* HAIR.

Melanoma • A tumor composed of cells heavily pigmented with melanin. A malignant melanoma has the appearance of a mole, but it is the rarest and most treacherous type of skin cancer and the leading cause of death from skin disease. Melanomas, which do not usually develop before middle age, are more prevalent among women than among men, especially among blondes who are blue eyed and fair skinned. It is assumed that the increase in this cancer in the last few decades is due to overexposure to the sun. Researchers suggest that the use of sunscreens might increase the risk of melanoma by providing a false sense of security. Because melanomas can develop on any skin surface, changes in the size or appearance of a mole or any bleeding or itching in the tissues that surround it should be diagnosed by a doctor immediately. The sudden appearance of a black spot on the white portion of the eyeball should be checked promptly as well.

Melatonin • A natural hormone produced by the pineal gland deep within the brain. With melatonin levels in the bloodstream ten times higher at night than in the daytime, one of its most important functions is known to be the promotion of sleep. Especially significant is that the levels of melatonin vary dramatically with the seasons: in the winter when days are short, the amount secreted in the female brain increases; with the arrival of summer, nocturnal melatonin drops dramatically. These seasonal changes do not occur in men, which may explain why women's greater sensitivity to the absence of natural light causes them to suffer in much greater numbers than men from seasonal affective disorder (SAD). The fact that melatonin levels decrease with age is thought to account for the insomnia problems of the elderly.

Melatonin in synthetic form has not yet been approved by the FDA. Studies are still trying to determine the amounts that will be suitable for various therapeutic purposes. Although melatonin capsules have been available in health food stores for several years, they may be sold in doses that are unsafe. Melatonin is a powerful substance that in excessive amounts is likely to interfere with the normal function of other hormones, thereby causing infertility, depression, and other disorders. See "Plain Talk About Medications" and "Alternative Therapies."

Ménière's Disease • A disturbance of the labyrinth of the inner ear resulting in vertigo, nausea, hearing loss, and tinnitus (ringing in the ears). While the basic cause is not known, the symptoms arise because an increase in the amount of fluid in the labyrinth creates an abnormal pressure on the membrane of the labyrinth wall leading to loss of hearing and impairment of the sense of balance. An attack may be mild and last for only a few minutes, or it may be severe, with disabling vomiting and dizziness lasting for several hours. Ménière's disease, which characteristically affects one ear, is more common among women than among men. Treatment is varied and includes the use of diuretics, antihistamines, tranquilizers, drugs that dilate the blood vessels, and a low-salt diet. See "Plain Talk About Medications."

Meningitis • Inflammation of the meninges, the membranes that surround the brain and spinal cord; also known as cerebrospinal meningitis. The inflammation may be caused by a virus or bacteria. Bacterial meningitis moves quickly and is fatal in about 12 percent of cases. It can be transmitted by kissing, sneezing, or sharing food, or the bacteria can reach the meninges by way of the bloodstream from some other systemic infection.

Viral meningitis, also called aseptic, may accompany other virus infections, especially mumps, measles, herpes simplex, and AIDS. Whatever the source of the inflammation, the symptoms are the same: severe and persistent headaches accompanied by vomiting, high fever, sensitivity to light, and confusion.

It is characteristic for the patient to hold the neck stiff, because movements of the head intensify the already acute pain. Any signs that indicate the onset of meningitis should be checked immediately by a doctor who can make a definitive diagnosis following laboratory examination of a sample of cerebrospinal fluid. Prompt treatment with one of the newer antibiotics usually brings about recovery in bacterial meningitis if the diagnosis is made early. The outcome of viral meningitis varies depending on the underlying cause.

Mental Illness • Any of a group of psychobiological disturbances, generally categorized as psychoses (as distinct from neuroses) and characterized by such symptoms as severe and pervasive mood alterations, disorganization of thought, withdrawal from social interaction into fantasy, personality deterioration, hallucinations and delusions, bizarre behavior often without a loss of intellectual competence. While there is disagreement about the basic causes and mechanisms of severe mental disorders, one of the greatest advances in treating them has been the use of drugs that make seriously disturbed patients more accessible to other forms of therapy. *See* MANIC-DEPRESSIVE ILLNESS, PSYCHOSIS, SCHIZOPHRENIA, SENILE DEMENTIA, "Aging Healthfully," and "Plain Talk About Medications."

Mercury • A silver-white metallic element that remains fluid at ordinary temperatures; also called quicksilver. It is used as the medium of measurement in fever thermometers because of its response to heat and in sphygmomanometers, the instruments that measure blood pressure, because of its weight.

The dumping of industrial wastes containing mercury has irreversibly polluted many bodies of water in the United States and has so contaminated the fish in them that they are dangerous to eat. Occupational exposure to industrial fumes containing mercury is responsible for irreversible damage to kidneys, lungs, and the nervous system. According to the U.S. Environmental Protection Agency, *any* exposure to mercury is a health hazard.

Metabolism • The combined processes involved in the production and maintenance of the substances essential for carrying on the body's vital functions. Metabolism occurs within each cell where groups of enzymes catalyze and control the chemical reactions that must occur during the normal absorption of oxygen and nutrients and their transformation into energy. The basal metabolic rate is an important diagnostic aid that measures the rapidity of the metabolic processes when the body is at rest. The rate is abnormally high or abnormally low in certain glandular disorders. Many diseases, previously mysterious, are now known to be caused by genetically determined enzymatic aberrations in the metabolic process.

With the realization that drugs are metabolized at different rates depending on sex and age, manufacturers are adjusting recommended doses to conform with these variables, especially for patients over 60 who may have to take a maintenance medication for the next 20 years of their lives. *See* ENZYME and "Plain Talk About Medications."

Metastasis • The spreading of a cancerous growth by extension to surrounding tissue (direct metastasis) or by the breaking away of clumps of diseased cells that invade other parts of the body (blood borne or lymphatic metastasis) where they settle and form secondary tumors. The invasive tumors are called metastatic growths.

Microsurgery • Meticulous surgery done under magnification using a special microscope. It is done when operating on small organs such as eyes, fallopian tubes, and ovaries; when reconnecting tiny blood vessels; and to minimize scarring.

Migraine • *See* HEADACHE.

Mole • A raised pigmented spot on the upper layers of the skin, usually brown and sometimes hairy. Moles may also have a blue appearance when buried more deeply, although the pigmentation is still brown. Yellowish rough-textured bumps produced by an abnormally active oil-secreting gland are called sebaceous moles. Any of these may be present from birth or they may appear early and disappear spontaneously. When such a blemish suddenly begins to change shape, itch, grow, or to bleed, it should be examined by a dermatologist. *See* MELANOMA.

Mononucleosis, Infectious • A virus infection that causes an abnormality of and increase in the number of white blood cells containing a single nucleus. The symptoms are somewhat similar to those of the flu: fever, very sore throat, general malaise, and swollen lymph nodes. The infection is diagnosed by simple blood tests. Because the infectious agent, the EB virus (Epstein-Barr), is present in the throat and saliva, it is perhaps transmitted by mouth-to-mouth contact, explaining why younger people call mononucleosis the "kissing disease." The swelling of the lymph nodes is caused by the fact that the virus stimulates the number and size of the white blood cells (lymphocytes) which then become ineffective in carrying out their disease-fighting function. While the patient may suffer from extreme fatigue and complications such as a jaundiced liver, enlargement of the spleen, inflammation of the joints, or a secondary infection of the throat, hospitalization generally is not necessary.

The treatment is usually no more than bed rest, but it is important that a doctor be in charge of the patient so that medication can be prescribed if secondary conditions develop. While most patients fully recover, a small percentage are plagued with a lingering form of the illness, with general malaise, low fever, and fatigue persisting intermittently over a period of years. Instead of assuming that the patient is malingering, the continuing presence of high levels of Epstein-Barr antibodies in a blood sample can verify the fact that the virus, and not the patient's imagination, is producing the symptoms.

Monosodium Glutamate • A flavor enhancer, also known as MSG, that in many people produces a complex of reactions often referred to as the Chinese restaurant syndrome: dizziness, sweating, faintness, ringing in the ears, and mood changes. It has been especially implicated as a headache trigger, especially for those who suffer from migraine. It is estimated that 20,000 tons of MSG are added to processed foods each year: to soups, meats, frozen dinners, potato chips, seasonings, and tenderizers. Accent and Lawry's seasoned salt contain MSG in large amounts. Anyone sensitive to its effects should learn which foods to avoid and request that the food they order in Asian restaurants be prepared without it.

Morphine • The active constituent in opium and the basis of the painkilling effects of all opiates, of which codeine (methyl morphine) is the weakest. The application of morphine is no longer restricted to terminal patients and severe accident cases. Many hospitals now conform to recent recommendations that all patients in severe pain be provided with the necessary amounts for alleviating it. *See* PAIN.

Motion Sickness • Nausea and vomiting resulting from a disturbance in the balancing mechanism of the inner ear. The discomfort may occur in a car, train, airplane, or elevator, but it is most common on a ship that is simultaneously pitching and rolling. There are various antinauseant medications that can be taken in advance of a trip. A doctor can advise on which medicine might be most suitable for the particular circumstance and what the possible side effects might be. Car sickness is rarely experienced by the driver and is less likely to occur to a passenger sitting in the front seat with the window open.

MSG • *See* MONOSODIUM GLUTAMATE.

Mucous Membrane • Thin layers of tissue that line a body cavity, separate adjacent cavities, or envelop an organ and contain glands that secrete mucus. Mucus, a watery exudate or slimy secretion, keeps the tissue moist. It may change in quantity and quality with disease, especially infections.

Multiple Sclerosis • A chronic degenerative disease of the central nervous system and the brain. The cause is not known, although evidence indicates that a factor such as an allergy or a virus triggers an autoimmune response in which the body's defense system turns against its own tissues. In this disease, disease-fighting cells called lymphocytes bring about the progressive destruction of the fatty material known as myelin that sheathes the nerves. The designation "multiple" is used because, while the disease attacks mainly the nerves of the spinal cord and the brain, there is no special order or pattern to the destruction. In some people the first symptom may be eye dysfunction; in others a coronary disorder or a locomotion problem. When the nerve endings of the brain are attacked, symptoms include speech changes and emotional swings.

Multiple sclerosis is prevalent mainly in temperate climates: an estimated 1 in 5,000 persons living in northern United States and 1 in 20,000 living in southern United States are affected by it. The disease commonly appears between the ages of 20 and 40, with women twice as susceptible as men. Because the symptoms are easily confused with other disorders, multiple sclerosis is often very difficult to diagnose. Research has therefore been directed not only toward finding the specific cause but to developing an accurate blood test that would unequivocally identify the disease and rule out all other possibilities. Treatment must be adjusted to individual cases and continually supervised because one of the characteristics of multiple sclerosis is that it may subside for months or even years and then flare up suddenly

with serious effects. Relief is usually provided by anti-inflammatory medication, corticosteroids, antispasmodics, and muscle relaxant drugs. Physical therapy, bed rest, and special diets are other forms of treatment. *See* "Directory of Health Information."

Muscular Dystrophy • Any of a group of chronic genetic diseases characterized by the progressive deterioration of the muscles. The particular designation of the dystrophy is based on the muscle groups first affected, the age of the patient at the onset of symptoms, and the rate at which the degeneration proceeds. While a dystrophic disease may affect anyone at any time, it occurs five times more often among males than females. No form of the disorder is contagious, and while no cure has yet been found, various types of treatment, including special orthopedic devices, can relieve the debilitating symptoms.

The most common and most crippling of the dystrophic diseases is Duchenne muscular dystrophy, the only one known to be transmitted entirely by female carriers, with sons having a 50 percent likelihood of being affected by the disease and daughters a 50 percent chance of becoming carriers. Fortunately for women who are aware of the presence of the disease in their family, there is a blood test for the detection of carriers of Duchenne MD. *See* GENETIC COUNSELING and "Directory of Health Information."

Myasthenia Gravis • A comparatively rare neuromuscular disease characterized by abnormal weakness and fatigue following normal exertion. Depending on the muscles affected, symptoms include drooping eyelids, double vision, difficulty in locomotion, incapacity in chewing and swallowing, and, in the most threatening cases, inability of the muscles controlling respiration to function. The disease may be triggered by an infection, pregnancy, or a tumor of the thymus gland or it may be due to an inherited fault in the body's autoimmune system. Whatever the basic reason for the disturbance, the immediate cause appears to be an aberration in the neuromuscular production of the chemical acetylcholine, essential for stimulating the muscle fibers to contract. Successful treatment for some patients has consisted of medicines that help transmit nerve impulses to the muscles.

Mycoses • *See* FUNGAL INFECTIONS.

Myelography • A procedure that produces X-ray images of the area between the spinal cord and the membrane covering it, thereby providing the basis for diagnosing an injury to the spinal nerve, a tumor, or a herniated (slipped) disk.

Myopia • *See* NEARSIGHTEDNESS.

Nail • Extension of the outermost skin layer of the fingers and toes. Nails are formed from the fibrous protein substance called keratin that also forms the hair that grows outward from the scalp. This elastic horny tissue (actually made up of dead cells) is pushed upward from the softer living matrix of the nail below the cuticle. It takes about six months for a nail to be replaced from the base of the cuticle to the tip of the finger. The general well-being of nails is best maintained by good hygiene and diet. No special supplement is necessary, nor does eating gelatin toughen the nails.

Healthy nails should be pale pink, smooth, and shiny. Variations in their appearance may be indications not only of local disorders but of serious diseases. When nails are bluish and the fingertips clubbed, they are a sign of a circulatory or respiratory disorder; spoon-shaped nails are a sign of anemia; split or deformed nails may occur when there is arthritic inflammation of the finger joints; bitten nails indicate a response to emotional stress or simply a habit. White spots on the nails may develop after a nail has been bruised or injured or when too much pressure is exerted at the cuticle during manicuring. A more serious injury may lead to severe pain and the loss of the nail. Unless the nail bed from which the nail grows has been crushed, the new nail that grows back will be normal in all ways.

Fingernails and toenails are vulnerable to fungal infections, particularly to ringworm that can spread quickly into the nails from their free edge, causing discoloration and deformity. Peeling or splitting may be a sign of poor nutrition or a reaction to a particular brand of detergent or nail polish; the use of nail-hardening preparations may have an adverse effect, especially in chronic or extreme cases. Brittle nails that split often are a common problem of aging related to poor circulation. Splitting is also the result of constant immersion in water. Because nails swell when they are wet and shrink when they are dry, the repeated change in their condition makes them vulnerable at the tips.

Ingrown toenails are common among women whose shoes are too tight. It is usually the nail of the big toe that is forced to grow forward into the toe's nail bed at one or both corners. This distorted growth can be extremely painful, and it can also lead to infection. Self-treatment is possible, if undertaken early, by inserting a tiny cotton swab under the nail edge, thus lifting up the nail so that it is less painful and can grow forward more easily. During treatment comfortable low-heeled shoes should be worn because high heels throw body weight against the toes. If there is any sign of redness or pain in the area, a podiatrist or medical doctor should be consulted without further delay. Ingrown toenails are best prevented by cutting the nails straight across rather than in an oval arch and by wearing shoes that fit properly.

Manicuring and pedicuring too often are likely to be damaging, and if nail lacquer is regularly used, it should not extend to the base of the nail because the live tissue in this area should be exposed rather than constantly covered. Costly salon treatments that extend the nails by building them up with acrylic powders use solvents and glues that can produce allergic reactions or fungal and bacterial infections leading to the loss of the entire nail. Dermatologists also advise against the use of plastic press-on nails because of problems resulting from the application of instant-type glues.

Among the more common diseases associated with the nails are infections of the fingers or toes resulting from cuts, hangnails, or any lesions that permit bacterial invasion. The application of a softening cream will decrease the likelihood of cracked cuticles and hangnails. Such infections can be extremely painful because of the pus and inflammation at the side of the nail. When soaking does not lead to drainage, it may be necessary to have the infected area lanced.

Narcolepsy • A neurological abnormality characterized by four symptoms that may occur singly or in any combination. The most common symptom is constant fatigue combined with attacks of sleep at inappropriate times. The second is a loss of muscle tone (catalepsy) triggered by a strong emotional response such as anger, laughter, or astonishment. The onset of catalepsy causes total body paralysis even though the mind is alert and awake. The other symptoms are the occurrence of frighteningly real hallucinations immediately before falling asleep or immediately after arising and the experi-

ence of complete momentary paralysis at the same times. Anyone who suspects she has the illness should arrange for a simple and accurate laboratory test in which brain wave patterns and eye movements are monitored during sleep. While narcolepsy is not yet curable, various treatments are available for the different symptoms. The disease is under continuing study at sleep disorder clinics that are a part of hospital research centers. *See* "Alternative Therapies" and "Directory of Health Information."

Nausea • The feeling that signals the possible onset of vomiting. Nausea occurs when the nerve endings in the stomach and in various other parts of the body are irritated. This irritation is transmitted to the part of the brain that controls the vomiting reflex, and when the signals are strong enough, vomiting does occur. Nausea may be triggered by psychological as well as physical conditions. Many women are nauseated by the sight of blood, unattractive sights and smells, strong feelings of fear or excitement, severe pain, or nervous tension. Nausea may accompany physical problems such as infectious disease, gallbladder inflammation, ulcer, appendicitis, the early months of pregnancy, and, most typically, indigestion, motion sickness, and irritation of the inner ear. The nausea caused by anticancer drugs may be treated by the active chemical (THC) in marijuana, available through the National Cancer Institute. In some women nausea is a side effect of contraceptive pills. The symptom may be relieved by taking the pill at bedtime rather than in the morning.

Nearsightedness (Myopia) • A structural defect of the eye in which the lens brings the image into focus in front of rather than directly on the retina so that objects at a distance are not seen clearly.

This aberration of vision is usually inherited and occurs when the eyeball is deeper than normal from front to back. Nearsightedness manifests itself in childhood, becoming worse until adulthood, when it stabilizes at approximately age 40. Corrective glasses or contact lenses prescribed by an ophthalmologist or an optometrist should therefore be checked regularly for necessary adjustments.

Correction by a surgical procedure called radial keratomy was introduced in 1980, and although some patients are satisfied with the results, the long-term effects of this expensive operation have yet to be definitively evaluated. In 1994 the results of a 10-year study indicated that although serious complications following the surgery were rare, close-up vision declined and became fuzzier in two out of five of the patients in the long-term study.

Neoplasm • The general term for any new and abnormal tissue growth; a tumor, either malignant or benign.

Nephritis • *See* GLOMERULONEPHRITIS.

Nephrosis • *See* KIDNEYS AND KIDNEY DISORDERS.

Neuralgia • Pain in the form of a sharp intermittent spasm along the path of a nerve. The term is considered imprecise except when it designates the disorder trigeminal neuralgia or the condition known as post-herpetic neuralgia that may follow a case of herpes zoster or shingles.

Neuritis • Inflammation of a nerve or a group of nerves. The symptoms vary widely from decreased sensitivity or paralysis of a particular part of the body to excruciating pain. Treatment varies with the cause of the inflammation. Among the disorders caused by neuritis in a particu-

lar group of nerves are Bell's palsy, herpes zoster, sciatica, and trigeminal neuralgia.

Neuromuscular Diseases • A category of disorders affecting those parts of the nervous system that control muscle function. *See* CEREBRAL PALSY, BELL'S PALSY, MULTIPLE SCLEROSIS, and MYASTHENIA GRAVIS.

Neurosis • A form of maladjustment in relationship to oneself and to others; usually a manifestation of anxiety that may or may not be expressed in chronic or occasional physical symptoms; also called psychoneurosis. One defining trait of a person who is neurotic is that she alternates between believing that she is better than other people or worse and cannot accept the fact that she is more like most people than she thinks she is.

Noise • Strictly speaking, any unwanted sound. The unit that expresses the relative intensity of sound is the decibel. On the decibel scale 0 represents absolute silence and 130 is the sound level that causes physical pain to the ear. A civilized two-way conversation measures about 50 decibels. The background noises in major American cities measure more than 70 decibels. Rock and disco music are usually played at about 110 decibels.

High intensity sounds cause physiological damage. The cells that make up the organ of Corti in the cochlea, which transmits sound vibrations to the auditory nerve, are hairlike structures that break down either partially or totally when subjected to abnormally strong sound vibrations. In the cochlea of retired steelworkers, for example, these hair cells are almost totally collapsed, and it is estimated that 60 percent of workers exposed to high intensity on-the-job noise will have suffered significant hearing loss by age 65 in spite of such safety precautions as ear plugs, ear muffs, "sound-proofed" enclosures, and the like.

The Environmental Protection Agency estimates that more than 16 million people in the United States suffer from hearing loss caused by sonic pollution and another 40 million are exposed to potential health hazards without knowing it. The dangers to the emotional and physical well-being of individuals, families, and communities are in many cases obvious, but in even more instances they are insidious and cumulative. Here are some facts that trouble environmentalists and health experts. According to the National Institute for Occupational Safety and Health, two or three years of daily exposure to 90 decibel sounds will result in some loss of hearing. Constant exposure to moderately loud noise (over 75 decibels) increases the pulse rate and respiration and may eventually cause tinnitus, ulcers, high blood pressure, and mental problems associated with stress. A daylong ride in a snowmobile can irreversibly damage the organ of hearing. Many young people who regularly attend rock concerts where the sound is amplified to ear-splitting levels and who wear earphones when they listen to loud music have already sustained some permanent hearing loss; according to an extensive survey of students entering college, 60 percent have some impairment of hearing. Steady, moderately loud noise (power mowers, dishwashers, washing machines, vacuum cleaners, power tools, garbage disposal units) can cause the equivalent in housewives of battle fatigue in soldiers: constricted blood vessels, increased activity of the adrenal glands, irritability, dizziness, and distorted vision. People who are subjected to or subject themselves to high intensity sound are nastier and more aggressive than those who live and work in quiet surroundings. Children who live within earshot of the acoustical overload produced by the traffic on a superhighway are found to have more learning problems than a similar sampling of children whose nervous systems do not have to cope with constant background noise.

If exposure to noise is occasionally unavoidable, the use of ear plugs is recommended. If these are not available in an unexpected situation imperiling one's hearing, the ears should be covered with one's hands or fingers. Elements in the immediate environment that make unnecessary noise should be eliminated or toned down wherever possible. In addition, the Environmental Protection Agency encourages local community groups to establish noise complaint centers empowered to investigate and eliminate all sources of unnecessary noise.

Nonsteroidal Anti-inflammatory Drugs (NSAIDs) • A category of drugs that are as powerful as aspirin in controlling inflammation of the joints but do not irritate the stomach or potentially cause internal bleeding when taken in the large doses necessary for long-term treatment of arthritis. See "Plain Talk About Medications."

Nosebleed • Bleeding, either mild or profuse, from the rupture of blood vessels inside the nose. Nosebleeds may be caused by injury, disease, blowing one's nose too energetically, strenuous exercise, sudden ascent to high altitudes, or constantly breathing in dry air that causes the mucous membranes to crack. Many women experience nosebleeds during pregnancy. They may also occur for no discernible reason and with no ill effect. Bleeding can usually be controlled by sitting up (not standing or lying down), tilting the head forward (tilting the head back can cause the blood to obstruct the windpipe), and pressing the soft flesh directly above the nostril against the bone for a few minutes. If this method is ineffective, the nostril may be packed with sterile cotton gauze that should remain in place for several hours. If the bleeding cannot be stopped promptly, emergency hospital treatment is advisable. If nosebleeds occur so frequently that they interfere with normal routines, it may be necessary to tie or cauterize the bleeding vessel. Any bleeding from the nose or mouth following an accident or a bad fall requires immediate medical attention.

Nuclear Medicine • A special branch of radiology that applies the advances in nuclear physics to the diagnosis and treatment of disease. One of the most important applications is the use of radioactive isotopes to irradiate abnormalities within the body so that they become visible on scanning machines. Radioactive chemicals are widely used in nuclear cardiology to diagnose abnormalities in coronary arteries and heart function and in treating certain cancers and hyperthyroidism. Radioactive needles have made delicate nerve surgery possible.

Occupational Therapy • Formerly associated only with the use of arts and crafts for the rehabilitation of the mentally ill or the psychological well-being of the elderly, occupational therapy is now an indispensable aspect of the team approach to patients who have to learn new ways of coping with the mechanics and logistics of daily living as a result of temporary or permanent impairment. An occupational therapist teaches the victim of a stroke how to get dressed and undressed and how to get things done in the kitchen. A patient progressively crippled by arthritis is taught new ways of getting into and out of an automobile. When irreversible disablement occurs because of a spinal injury, an occupational therapist trains the patient to accomplish essential tasks in al-

ternative ways so that the greatest degree of independence can be achieved. Professionals in this category are licensed and usually work in a hospital or rehabilitation center under the supervision of an attending doctor, most often a physiatrist. Services are provided on an inpatient or outpatient basis, or, following a hospital stay, in the patient's home. See PHYSICAL THERAPY.

Orthodontia • The branch of dentistry that specializes in the correction of irregularities in the way upper and lower teeth come together when the jaw is closed.

Although orthodontia is often undertaken for cosmetic reasons, dentists agree that gross malocclusions should be corrected for reasons of health: chewing is improved, cleaning is simplified, and gum disease is less likely to occur.

Before embarking on extensive orthodontia, a prospective patient should, in discussion with the family dentist and the orthodontist, compare the relative benefits of the treatment with any disadvantages, such as adverse effects on teeth, discomfort, time, and expense. See MALOCCLUSION and TEMPOROMANDIBULAR JOINT.

Orthotics • A specialty of medical science and mechanics that deals with the support of weak muscles and/or joints. "Orthotics" is also the term used to describe the custom-made devices to insert into shoes in cases where correction increases efficiency and reduces pain during walking or when running or participating in other athletic activities. Orthotists also provide specially fitted braces and other supports made of molded plastic or lightweight metal to be worn as recommended by doctors for patients with potentially deforming diseases of the joints or spine.

Ostomy • An operation in which an artificial opening is formed between two hollow organs or between a hollow organ and the abdominal wall, enabling a diseased organ to be "bypassed." Examples are: ileostomy (between ileum and abdominal wall) and ureterostomy (between ureter[s] and abdominal wall). *See* COLOSTOMY and "Directory of Health Information."

Pacemaker, Artificial • A transistorized device implanted under the skin in the area of the shoulder and connected by wires to electrodes implanted in heart tissue for the purpose of supplying a normal beat when the natural pacemaker has been irreversibly damaged or destroyed by disease. The device with all its components weighs less than 2 ounces, and recent models last about 10 years. Pacemakers are tested regularly by telemetry so that operational defects can be corrected. Studies conducted at two major medical centers in 1995 indicated that digital phones held next to the chest disrupt the pulse generator of pacemakers. Individuals using this type of phone who are fitted with a pacemaker are therefore advised to switch to an analog phone or to discuss this problem with their cardiologist.

Pain • A distress signal from some part of the body, usually of brief duration and originating in the largest number of cases in a traceable disorder. Pain—throbbing, aching, pulsating, stabbing—arises in two different ways. Peripheral pain resulting from a cut finger or an abscessed tooth begins in nerve fibers located in the extremities or around the body organs; central pain, usually caused by injuries or disorders affecting the brain or central nervous system such as a tumor, stroke, or slipped disk, originates in the spinal cord or the brain itself. When this type of pain is chronic, it is the most difficult to re-

lieve. Both types of impulses eventually reach the brain stem and thalamus where pain perception takes place.

It is known that the brain produces chemical substances that are the body's own opiates against pain perception. These are known as endorphins and include the recently isolated dynorphin, which is 200 times more powerful than morphine in its action and 50 times more powerful than any previously known substance of its kind. It is hoped that with greater understanding of how these chemicals work, they will be used as powerful nonaddictive drugs for the control of pain as well as to produce other important effects on the brain for those suffering from mental illness and seizure disorders.

In the meantime, where pain is chronic and severe or where the perception of pain has become a problem in itself separated from its possible source, treatment is available in pain clinics that have made this problem their specialty. Among the methods that provide relief, separately or in combination, are acupuncture, electrical stimulation, biofeedback, and hypnosis. The chief dangers connected with the use of chemicals for minimizing severe or persistent pain are serious adverse effects of a particular chemical itself or in combination with other drugs. The possibility of drug addiction is no longer a consideration in supplying post-surgical hospital patients with morphine and other opiates in order to speed recovery by minimizing their pain. *See* "Alternative Therapies" and "Plain Talk About Medications."

Palpitations • *See* ARRHYTHMIAS.

Pancreas • The large, mixed gland situated below and in back of the stomach and the liver. The pancreas is about 6 inches long. Its function is two-fold. One is the secretion of pancreatic juice, which contains the enzymes that flow into the digestive tract and are essential for the continuing breakdown in the duodenum and small intestine of fats, carbohydrates, and proteins. The second function is the secretion of insulin produced by almost a million clusters of specialized cells called the islets of Langerhans.

When these cells produce insufficient insulin for the body's needs, the result is diabetes. Other disorders of the pancreas include the formation of stones and of benign and malignant tumors, both treated surgically. Inflammation of the pancreas, pancreatitis, may be acute or chronic. Acute pancreatitis is a grave condition in which one of the enzymes begins to devour the tissue itself, leading to hemorrhage, vomiting, severe abdominal pain, and collapse. It may be associated with overdrinking, gallbladder infection, gallstones, or trauma. Chronic pancreatitis may be the result of recurrent acute pancreatitis. It is characterized by abdominal and back pain, diarrhea, and jaundice. When these symptoms exist, exploratory surgery is usually recommended to rule out the possibility of cancer. Smokers are five to six times more likely than nonsmokers to develop pancreatic cancer, which is the second deadliest cancer, superseded only by a rare brain tumor. *See* "Substance Abuse."

Panic Attack • *See* ANXIETY ATTACK.

Paranoia • A mental disturbance characterized by delusions of persecution and sometimes accompanied by feelings of power and grandeur. A clinically paranoid person may not suffer from personality disintegration and may appear to be living a normal life, but it is not unusual for the disturbance to erupt into psychotic behavior. Antipsychotic drugs are often prescribed for clinical paranoia. The term "paranoid" may also be used to describe a general mental state that is not psychotic but is characterized by distrustfulness, suspiciousness, and a tendency toward persecution of others. This mental state frequently accompanies amphetamine and cocaine abuse and may also result from the intermittent use of marijuana. *See* "Substance Abuse" and "Plain Talk About Medications."

Peptic Ulcer • *See* ULCER.

Periodontal Disease • The deteriorative process in which the tissues surrounding a tooth are destroyed by bacteria to the point where erosion of the bone results in the loosening and eventual loss of the tooth itself. While assiduous cleaning and flossing of teeth can keep cavities at a minimum and contribute to the health of the gums, periodontal disease is caused by a particular type of bacteria that thrive in the tartar that forms when some kinds of dental plaque become hardened. Pockets of infection gradually surround the tooth, and if they are not cleaned out by a periodontal specialist either by deep scaling or surgery (or a combination of both) they will eventually undermine the tooth. *See* GINGIVITIS.

Peritonitis • Inflammation of the peritoneum, the membrane that lines the abdominal cavity and covers the organs within it. The cause of acute peritonitis is usually the perforation or rupture of the appendix with a consequent spread of bacteria and interference of circulation. The condition is an emergency requiring prompt hospitalization. Surgery is almost always inevitable.

Perspiration • The process by which the salty fluid (99 percent water and 1 percent urea and other wastes) is excreted by the sweat glands of the skin; also the fluid itself. The body has approximately 2 million sweat glands located in the lowest layers of the skin. They are connected with the outer skin layer, the epidermis, by tiny spiral-shaped tubes. The largest sweat glands are located in the groin and the armpit. The sweat glands normally produce about 1½ pints of sweat a day in a temperate climate. The chief function of perspiration is to maintain constant body temperature despite variation in environmental conditions or energy output. Thus, when the internal or external temperature goes up, sweat can be seen on the skin surface where it cools the body by evaporation. The sweating process is controlled by the hypothalamus at the base of the brain. Because this gland is also responsive to emotional stress, fear and excitement will cause an increase in perspiration. "Breaking out in a cold sweat" is a common phenomenon.

Any disturbance in the functioning of the sweat glands is likely to be a symptom of some other disorder. Excessive perspiration may be due to a disease that also produces a high fever such as malaria or one that produces a chronic rise in temperature such as tuberculosis. Excessive sweating and urinating are possible symptoms of untreated diabetes. The hot flashes of the menopause are often accompanied by heavy sweating. Excessive sweating of the palms or soles of the feet is usually psychogenic in origin. Cold sweats accompany withdrawal from some addictive drugs, especially heroin. *See* AN-TIPERSPIRANT DEODORANTS.

pH • A measure of the degree of alkalinity or acidity of a given solution; the letters derive from *pouvoir Hydrogène* ("hydrogen power" in French), because the concentration of the hydrogen ion determines the pH number. Acidity is indicated by pH values from 0 to 7; pH 7.0 is neutral, and pH values above 7 indicate alkalinity.

Pharyngitis • Inflammation, either acute or chronic, of the pharynx, the tube of muscles and membranes that forms the throat cavity extending from the back of the mouth to the esophagus. Infection is most commonly viral, occurring as a minor sore throat. This type of infection usually runs its course in a few days and does not require treatment with antibiotics. Chronic pharyngitis and hoarseness are usually the result of the misuse of the voice, regular exposure to irritating vapors or fumes, or heavy intake of alcohol. Even mild pharyngitis is aggravated by smoking.

Phenobarbital • An addictive drug of the barbiturate family prescribed in supervised doses as an anticonvulsant. Combinations with other medications must be carefully monitored. *See* "Substance Abuse" and "Plain Talk About Medications."

Pheromones • Odorless chemicals exuded by practically all mammals that send meaningful signals to members of their own species, usually of the opposite sex. Research is being conducted on pheromone perception in humans, especially on how this perception might influence feelings and behavior.

Phlebitis • Inflammation of the vein walls, most commonly of the legs, and especially where varicosities exist. Phlebitis in a superficially located vein is usually accompanied by tenderness, redness, and swelling. Simple phlebitis may be caused by overweight, progressive arterio- or atherosclerosis, or it may follow an extended convalescence requiring bed rest. Phlebitis may also accompany pregnancy. Under these circumstances, the condition is not too serious and can be treated by elevating the leg, applying heat, and taking aspirin or some other anti-inflammatory medication to reduce pain and discomfort. Support stockings may be helpful if normal activities are to be pursued.

Phobia • An irrational and exaggerated fear of an object or situation usually related to an anxiety neurosis. Phobic response may be so encompassing as to be immobilizing. In severe anxiety or panic attacks the victim may experience dizziness, palpitations, profuse sweating, and in some cases a tendency toward suicide. Although almost any object or situation may elicit phobia in different individuals, several have been identified as common sources of phobic response: agoraphobia, the fear of being in open places; acrophobia, the fear of heights; ailurophobia, the fear of cats; and claustrophobia, the fear of being confined in small areas.

Phobias are a form of mental illness difficult to cure. In some cases the phobia may decrease as a result of life experiences that resolve the underlying conflict; in other cases, when the phobia is immobilizing (as in agoraphobia) or seriously interferes with one's career (as in fear of flying or of using an elevator), anti-anxiety medication combined with psychotherapy and such alternate therapies as hypnosis, visualization, and breathing exercises may produce positive results. Group therapy should be considered for mutual support in dealing with the same problem. See "Alternative Therapies" and "Directory of Health Information."

Physiatrist • A doctor who specializes in physical medicine and rehabilitation. Most pain treatment centers and rehabilitation centers are directed by physiatrists (pronounced fiz-e-*at*-rist). See PAIN and "Alternative Therapies."

Physical Therapy • Treatment of disease or disability by physical means, exercises, water, heat, massage, and electricity. Physical therapists trained in schools approved by the American Medical Association usually work under the supervision of doctors in hospitals and clinics that have rehabilitation programs for both inpatients and outpatients. See OCCUPATIONAL THERAPY and "Alternative Therapies."

Pineal Gland • A small pine coneshaped structure (pineal body) near the center of the brain but not a part of it. It secretes the hormone melatonin. See MELATONIN.

Placebo • A preparation or procedure without pharmacologic or physiologic properties, which is administered for psychological benefit. Although placebos are no more than inert concoctions, they are known to cause a measurable difference in how some patients feel. Called "the placebo effect," this result is thought to be connected in some way with the brain's release of endorphins.

Placebos play an indispensable role in evaluating the effectiveness of new drugs. In a procedure known as the double-blind test, half the participants are given the coded drug and the other half a coded placebo similar in appearance. When the test is completed, the code is deciphered and the results are tabulated and compared for assessment of the drug.

Plantar Wart • A wart that develops in the sole of the foot. Such growths often are especially painful because they grow inward and thus interfere with walking. All warts are technically called verrucae and are caused by a virus. Treatment is surgical. Post-operative care involves several days of immobility to permit the tissue to heal before pressure is put on it.

Plaque • A flat patch; most commonly, dental plaque, which refers to a film of mucoid-like substance that adheres to tooth surfaces and provides the medium in which bacteria that liberate destructive acids thrive on the various forms of sugar entering the mouth. The acids eventually destroy tooth enamel. Thus dental plaque is largely responsible for cavities. It can be effectively removed by brushing the teeth, using unwaxed floss according to the dentist's instructions, and having a professional cleaning twice a year. There is evidence that some mouthwashes may provide additional protection against plaque formation. *See* GINGIVITIS and PERIODONTAL DISEASE.

Plastic Surgery • Operations in which damaged or abnormal tissue is repaired and rebuilt. Such damages or abnormalities may be congenital, as a hare lip, or they may be acquired, as disfiguring scars caused by burns or other injuries. Plastic surgeons also remove growths extensive enough to require skin grafting following the operation and they also specialize in the reconstruction of missing tissue with a prosthesis, a substitute manufactured of metals and plastics rather than of organic materials taken from another part of the body. Artificial limbs, jaws, breasts, and ears are some of the more customary prosthetic replacements. Change in appearance for esthetic reasons is called cosmetic surgery. *See* "Cosmetic Surgery."

Platelets • Round or oval discs in the blood that contain no hemoglobin and are essential to the clotting process; also called thrombocytes. This blood component is manufactured in the bone marrow. Platelet deficiencies occur in a number of diseases (leukemia, myeloma, lymphoma), as a result of certain drugs, and spontaneously. Platelets can be transferred fresh or frozen for transfusion as needed.

Pleurisy • Inflammation of the pleura, the double membrane that lines the chest cavity and encloses the lungs. Pleurisy may be a consequence of pneumonia or a complication of tuberculosis. Pleurisy may or may not be acutely painful, but it always requires prompt treatment. Thanks to antibiotics, this disease has almost disappeared in the United States.

Pneumocystis Pneumonia • A lung disease caused by *Pneumocystis carinii*, an especially virulent protozoan. It is one of the complications, usually fatal, of AIDS and is considered an "opportunistic infection" because it primarily affects people, such as leukemia patients, whose immunity is compromised. *See* ACQUIRED IMMUNE DEFICIENCY SYNDROME.

Pneumonia • An acute infection or inflammation of one or both lungs, causing the lung tissues and spaces to be filled with liquid matter. Pneumonia, which may be a primary infection or a complication of another disorder, has three main causes: bacteria, viruses, and mycoplasmas. Inflammation may also be caused by fungus infections or by the aspiration of certain chemicals or irritant dusts. Among the bacteria, the pneumococci are by far the most common cause; there are over 80 different types responsible for approximately 500,000 cases of the disease each year. The most deadly of the bacterial pneumonias is caused by Group A streptococcus. The pneumonias that are viral in origin account for about half of all cases. While in some cases recovery may be spontaneous without treatment or special precautions (many people have had "walking pneumonia" without realizing it), the disease known as primary influenza virus pneumonia is extremely serious, especially because the infectious organism multiplies with practically no accompanying sign of disease in the lung.

Mycoplasmas are microorganisms smaller than bacteria and larger than viruses that share characteristics of both. Mycoplasma pneumonia typically involves older children and young adults and is usually mild in its symptoms and brief in duration. Pneumonia that involves a major part or an entire lobe of a lung is known as lobar pneumonia, and when both lungs are involved, double pneumonia. Bronchopneumonia, which affects a smaller area, is slower to develop and is localized in the bronchial tubes with patches of infection reaching the lungs. While rarely fatal, bronchopneumonia is insidious because it may recur and resist conventional treatment.

In all cases of bacterial pneumonia, but especially in cases where resistance is low because of age, debility, or alcoholism, treatment with antibiotics must be initiated at once. Some cases may require hospitalization, while others may be supervised at home. According to the American Lung Association, early detection is critical for full recovery from bacterial and mycoplasma pneumonia. While there is as yet no effective treatment for viral pneumonia, adequate rest, proper diet, and sufficient time devoted to convalescence usually result in full recovery. Since 1977 an immunizing vaccine has been available that offers protection against some types of pneumococci. It is administered to those considered especially vulnerable to infection—people over 50, anyone in a nursing home, and anyone of any age suffering from chronic diseases of the heart, lungs, and kidneys and from diabetes and other metabolic disorders. The use of the vaccine is especially important because many strains of pneumococci have developed a resistance to previously effective antibiotics. *See* "Plain Talk About Medications" and "Immunization Guide."

Poison • Any substance that can severely damage or destroy living tissue. Certain substances are harmful in any amount, while others, which are harmless or even beneficial in supervised doses, are poisonous in excessive amounts. Most poisonings result from swallowing dangerous substances in small amounts or taking medications in overdoses. The most frequent victims are children under 5.

Because prompt action can make the difference between life and death, every member of the family, including children from the earliest possible age, should know that the number of the local poison control agency is posted next to the telephone with other emergency numbers. Local telephone directories usually list the number under Poison Control. When no such listing appears, efforts should be made *before* a crisis occurs to locate the closest agency by consulting the telephone operator, the nearest hospital, or the local Red Cross chapter. *See* "Directory of Health Services."

Poison Ivy, Oak, and Sumac • Plants containing a poisonous chemical, urushiol, to which a majority of people in the United States eventually become sensitive. It is extremely unwise to assume that insensitivity to these plants is permanent. The chemical, which is contained in all parts of the plants—leaves, berries, roots, and bark—produces contact dermatitis in those allergic to it. In cases of hypersensitivity, the itching and blistering rash may develop not only when the skin has touched the plant directly but also when a part of the body touches a piece of contaminated clothing or a dog or cat whose coat is contaminated by the allergen. Because the chemical can be spread by smoke from burning the plant, it should never be burned but destroyed by a suitable herbicide. When exposure does occur, contaminated clothing should be removed at once for laundering, and the potentially affected parts of the body washed with a strong, alkaline laundry soap. These preventive measures should be undertaken as soon as possible to limit the spread of the poison. When the rash appears, the discomfort can be reduced by the application of topical medications. The best way to prevent contact is to make a serious effort to learn what the plants look like so that they can be scrupulously avoided.

Polio • This acute infectious disease also known as poliomyelitis and infantile paralysis has been virtually eliminated thanks to effective immunization introduced in 1954. Because polio epidemics are not uncommon where sanitation is primitive and public health measures practically nonexistent, travelers who plan to venture into the rural areas of Third World countries are advised by the U.S. Quarantine and Immunization Service to be reimmunized against the disease.

A phenomenon known as the "post polio" syndrome has been experienced by a significant number of the survivors of the disease. Progressive weakening of certain muscles occurs very slowly; if the original polio attack was a virulent one, the syndrome that sets in 40 or 50 years later may cause considerable discomfort. Doctors who know the history of these patients have been able to differentiate this muscle disability from the onset of other neuromuscular diseases.

Polyp • A smooth, tubelike growth, almost always benign, that projects from mucous membrane. Such growths are of two main types: pedunculate polyps that are attached to the membrane by a thin stalk and sessile polyps that have a broad base.

While polyps may occur in any body cavity with a membranous lining, they are most commonly found in the nose, uterus, cervix, and rectum. Those that develop in the nasal canal or sinuses may result from such irritations as frequent colds or allergies. While rarely dangerous, they can interfere with breathing and with the sense of smell; they may also be the cause of chronic headaches. Surgical removal is recommended in such cases, but there is no guarantee that the underlying irritation will not produce them again. Uterine polyps may cause irregular or excessive menstrual flow and may also be one of the causes of sterility. They can usually be removed without the need for hospitalization. The presence of cervical polyps may be manifested by bleeding between menstrual periods, after menopause, or with intercourse, or they may be "silent," only discovered during a routine gynecological checkup. Removal is considered advisable, with a biopsy to rule out the possibility of cancer. Polyps in the colon or the rectum are likely to cause discomfort in the lower abdomen and diarrhea as well as blood and mucus in the stools. A rectal polyp is usually removed as an office procedure by a proctologist. Annual postoperative checkups are recommended.

Posttraumatic Stress Syndrome • A psychological disorder resulting from experiencing a major disaster or a deeply distressing emotional trauma. The disorder may be the immediate consequence of a rape or mugging, or it may occur within weeks or months after witnessing the death and destruction caused by an earthquake, a terrorist attack, or some other cataclysmic event affecting one's family, friends, or the entire community. The syndrome was first defined and diagnosed as a problem affecting many of the men and women who participated in the Vietnam War. It is widespread among people of all ages who experienced the devastation and disruption following the Oklahoma City bombing.

Symptoms of posttraumatic stress syndrome vary from person to person and from time to time in the same person. They include nightmares, anxiety attacks, survivor guilt, withdrawal from interpersonal relationships, inexplicable outbursts of anger, insomnia, loss of interest in daily routines, and a total suppression of feelings or thoughts about the event. These symptoms may be immobilizing for a short while, or they may come and go with unpredictable irregularity.

Coping with posttraumatic stress syndrome depends on whether the precipitating event was personal or one that involved the well-being of many other people. Where family members or neighbors and an entire community have been affected, group counseling and mutual support are the foundation for recovery. In cases of rape, suicide of a child or spouse, or some other circumstance with a long-term emotional aftermath, one-to-one psychotherapy may be the only effective treatment.

In all cases of posttraumatic syndrome, a major aspect of overcoming the damaging consequences of the trauma is the determination to talk honestly and openly about one's deepest feelings to loved ones and, if necessary, to a professional therapist.

Posture • The natural position or carriage of the body when sitting or standing. Good posture is the unconscious result of mental and physical health. While a rigidly held neck or a sunken chest may be second nature by the time adulthood arrives, poor posture can be improved by suitable exercise. *See* "Fitness," "Health Safeguards for Working Women," and "Alternative Therapies."

Premature Ejaculation • *See* EJACULATION.

Premature Infant • An infant born before the completion of 37 weeks' (starting from the date of its mother's last normal menstrual period) gestation. Infants weighing less than 2,500 grams (five and a half pounds) at birth generally are also considered to be premature infants. *See* "Pregnancy and Childbirth."

Proctoscopy • An internal examination with an instrument called a proctoscope, which enables the physician to see the rectum and the lower portion of the large intestine. The procedure may be performed by a proctologist or by one's prime care doctor. It is used in diagnosing hemorrhoids, in detecting polyps and cysts, and in routine screening for cancer in patients over 40.

Prostaglandin • A hormonelike substance composed of unsaturated fatty acids and found in almost every tissue and body fluid. Prostaglandins are being identified in increasing numbers as indispensable for normalizing blood pressure, kidney processes, the reproductive system, gastrointestinal activity, and the release of sex hormones. Of those specifically isolated, the prostaglandins manufactured by the endometrium increase considerably just before the onset of the menstrual period. Because they cause strong uterine contractions, they are responsible for the premenstrual cramps suffered by some women. Antiprostaglandin drugs previously used only for treating arthritis because of their anti-inflammatory action are proving to be an effective treatment for painful menstrual periods. *See* "Gynecologic Problems and Treatment."

Pruritis • *See* ITCHING.

Psoriasis • A common skin disease of unknown cause, characterized by excessive production of cells of the outermost skin layer, which produces scaly red patches. As the new cells proliferate, they cover the patches with a silvery scale, and as the scales drop off, the area below is revealed as tiny red dots. Psoriasis is neither contagious nor dangerous, but it can damage a woman's self-esteem and impair her romantic involvements. It can also limit her employability. Symptoms may appear for the first time in early childhood, in adolescence, or not until later in life. The condition may be chronic or intermittent; it may be triggered by injury, illness, emotional stress, or exposure to excessive cold. The red patches may or may not be accompanied by itching. The parts of the body most often affected are the scalp, chest, elbows, knees, abdomen, palms, finger nails, and soles of the feet. About 10 percent of patients have an associated arthritis or gout.

In spite of advertising claims to the contrary, there is no cure for psoriasis. Professionally prescribed treatments that have been somewhat effective have had unfortunate side effects in many instances or have required weeks of hospitalization. A treatment that shows promising results is known as photochemotherapy. It combines oral medication with a photoactive drug followed by exposure to ultraviolet radiation. Recently, some patients treated with the anticancer drug methotrexate have experienced a reduction of psoriasis symptoms, but the negative side effects may be considered worse than the disease.

Psoriasis patients almost always benefit from participation in a support group and from seeking out a doctor who is patient and who treats not only the disease but the many consequences of living with it. *See* "Directory of Health Information."

Psychiatry • The medical specialty that deals with the diagnosis and treat-

ment of disorders of the mind and the emotions. *See* "Health Care Personnel."

Psychoanalysis • A method originated by Dr. Sigmund Freud for treating mental illness and emotional disturbances. The method is based on certain assumptions about the development from infancy onward of the human psyche or the mind as an entity with a life of its own that governs the total organism in all its relationships with others and with the environment. Psychoanalysts may be psychiatrists as Freud himself was, or they may be lay practitioners.

Psychoneurosis • *See* NEUROSIS.

Psychosis • Any mental illness characterized by disorganization of personality and a disordered contact with reality combined with bizarre behavior consisting of unpredictable mood swings and garbled speech and accompanied by hallucinations, delusions, and disconnected thoughts. Psychotic episodes may occur as a result of the use of addictive drugs, including the delusional episodes experienced by alcoholics. *See* "Substance Abuse" and "Plain Talk About Medications."

Psychosomatic Illness • Any disorder that is functional in nature and that may be ascribed wholly or partly to emotional stress.

Psyllium • A plant whose seeds are the chief ingredient of Metamucil and similar commercial products effective in preventing constipation.

Puerperal • Relating to childbirth. *See* "Pregnancy and Childbirth."

Pus • The thick yellowish or greenish liquid that develops during certain infections. Pus is composed of white blood cells, tissue decomposed by bacteria or other microorganism, and the destroyed organism that caused the infection. It is often contained in an inflamed swelling called an abscess.

Quickening • The stage of pregnancy in which the mother becomes aware of fetal movements within the womb; also, the fetal movements themselves. *See* "Pregnancy and Childbirth."

Rabies • A disease of the central nervous system that affects all mammals, including humans. Rabies is found throughout the United States, except in Hawaii, as well as in Canada, Mexico, and many countries worldwide. People and animals become infected by the rabies virus if they are scratched or bitten by a rabid animal. As many as 18,000 people are treated for the disease in this country every year. Since contact with wild animals is the usual way that people and their pets are exposed to infection, any such contact, especially with skunks, raccoons, and bats, should be avoided. Dogs and cats should be vaccinated, especially if they are permitted to roam free in rural areas.

If you suspect that an animal is rabid because it is drooling or foaming at the mouth, is seen in the daytime when normally it is active only at night, or appears to be nervous or aggressive, *do not attempt to catch the animal yourself.* Notify the local animal warden or the health department.

If you are bitten or deeply scratched by any animal, cause the wound to bleed, wash it thoroughly with soap and water, and call your doctor without delay for further instructions. If your doctor is unavailable, go to the emergency room of the nearest hospital. Also notify your local or state health department.

Although rabies vaccination is not a re-quirement for entry into any foreign country, the recommendation of the U.S. Centers for Disease Control is that in places where rabies is endemic, any animal bite or scratch should be cleansed promptly and evaluated by a local doctor or health authority. Pre-exposure vaccination is recommended for persons living in (or visiting for more than 30 days) countries in Central and South America, the Indian subcontinent, Southeast Asia, and most of Africa. *See* "Immunization Guide."

Radiation Therapy • The treatment of disease with X-rays and with rays from such radioactive substances as cobalt, iodine, and radium; also called irradiation. The effectiveness of this therapy, which is the special province of the radiologist, is constantly being increased by the invention of new machines and techniques that minimize the dangers of radiation exposure to healthy tissues at the same time that enough irradiation can be provided to benefit tissue already diseased. *See* X-RAY.

Radium • A highly radioactive metal that spontaneously gives off rays affecting the growth of organic tissue. Body exposure, inhalation, or ingestion of radium may produce burns as well as several kinds of cancer, especially of the lungs, blood, and bones.

Rash • A skin eruption often accompanied by discoloration and itching and in most cases a temporary symptom of a particular infectious disease, allergy, or parasitic infestation. Rashes may be flat or raised, some run together into large blotches, and others turn into blisters. Prickly heat, contact dermatitis, hives, and allergic responses to food, animals, plants, chemicals, and other substances are common causes of rashes. Rashlike symptoms usually accompany infections caused by funguses, parasites, and rickettsial organisms such as ticks. Virus diseases (mononucleosis) and sexually transmissible diseases, especially secondary stage syphilis, are characterized by rashes. Any skin eruption accompanied by fever or other acute symptoms such as a sore throat or tender swollen glands should be examined by a doctor. See "Plain Talk About Medications."

Remission • The decrease or disappearance of signs and symptoms during the course of a disease or a chronic disorder. The term "spontaneous remission" is used when there appears to be no therapeutic explanation for the abatement of the symptoms.

Resistance • The body's ability to ward off or minimize disease either through genetic capability, the presence of antibodies produced by immunization or environmental exposure, or a high enough level of physical and psychological health to combat infection without succumbing to it. The most efficient way to produce resistance to an increasing number of infectious diseases is by immunization. See "Immunization Guide."

Relaxation Therapy • See "Alternative Therapies."

Retina • The innermost layer of cells at the rear of the eyeball; a membrane consisting of the light-sensitive rods and cones that receive the image formed by the lens and transmit it through the optic nerve to the brain. Retinal disease of one kind or another is the chief cause of blindness in the United States.

When a hole or tear develops in the retina or when an eye infection or tumor forces an excess of the vitreous fluid to seep between the retinal layers, the result can be a retinal detachment that can end up in a permanent loss of eyesight. Thanks to photocoagulation and new microsurgical techniques, restoration of vision is accomplished in a large number of cases. See EYE and DIABETIC RETINOPATHY.

Retinoic Acid (Retin-A) • This substance is not only prescribed for the treatment of acne. It is also promoted as an ingredient in cosmetic creams that cause wrinkles to "disappear" if applied regularly. The Retin-A peels away the aging skin layer, revealing a new, smoother skin surface. Since the long-term effect of the constant use of these creams is not known, they have not yet received FDA approval.

Retrovirus • A member of a class of viruses that implant themselves in cells and eventually cause full-blown disease—for example, HIV, which eventually causes AIDS. Disorders such as lupus and rheumatoid arthritis, in which the immune system attacks not only foreign invaders but also its own cells, are thought to be triggered by retroviruses not yet identified. See HIV.

Rheumatism • A nonscientific designation for any painful disorder or disease of the joints, muscles, bones, ligaments, or nerves. See "Aging Healthfully" and "Plain Talk About Medications."

Rheumatoid Arthritis • See ARTHRITIS.

Rhinitis • Inflammation of the mucous membranes that line the nasal passages caused by viral or bacterial infection, allergy, or inhalation of irritants. Acute rhinitis, the technical medical term for the nasal disturbance of the common cold, is its most common form. In some cases viral rhinitis is complicated by bacterial invasion that may reach the ears and the throat. When streptococcus, staphylococcus, or pneumococcus bacteria are involved, the nasal discharge will be thick and yellowish with pus instead of being practically colorless, loose, and runny. Another form of inflammation is caused by an allergic reaction to grass, trees, dog hair, or other substances.

Obvious symptoms of chronic rhinitis should be treated by a doctor. When rhinitis is associated with fever or other manifestation of bacterial infection, antibiotic therapy may be advisable. However, the typical stuffed or runny nose characteristic of an ordinary cold is likely to clear up as the cold runs its course. It has been observed that thousands of Americans abuse nasal sprays, especially those containing long-lasting vasoconstrictors that shrink the blood vessels in the nose and eliminate the symptom of "stuffed nose" associated with colds, allergies, and some sinus conditions. This dependence produces a "rebound" phenomenon in which the "cure" causes the symptoms to return in more acute form, so that more and stronger nasal decongestants are needed. Specialists therefore advise a careful reading of label warnings about dosage and continued application of all such medications.

Ribonucleic Acid • *See* RNA.

Rickettsial Diseases • A category of infectious diseases caused by microorganisms larger than viruses, smaller than bacteria but with characteristics of both, called rickettsiae after their discoverer, the pathologist H. T. Ricketts (1871–1910). Rickettsiae inhabit certain rodents as parasites and are transmitted to humans and animals by the bites of ticks, mites, fleas, and lice. (This group of diseases should not be confused with rickets, a vitamin D deficiency disease.) *See* ROCKY MOUNTAIN SPOTTED FEVER and TYPHUS.

Ringworm • *See* FUNGAL INFECTIONS.

RNA • Ribonucleic Acid, the chemical compound contained in the cytoplasm of all cells and the carrier of genetic information provided by DNA to the ribosomes, the structures that synthesize amino acids into proteins. Through the information transmitted by RNA, inherited characteristics make their way from one generation to the next.

Rocky Mountain Spotted Fever • An infectious disease transmitted to humans by the bite of the American dog tick in the Eastern states and from rodents to humans by the wood tick in Western states; also called tick fever or Eastern spotted fever. In addition to a headache, fever, and aching muscles, one of the distinguishing characteristics is a rash that begins on the palms of the hands and the soles of the feet, spreading upward during the course of the illness. Other symptoms include sensitivity to light, abdominal cramps, and vomiting. Early diagnosis and prompt treatment with antibiotics ensure complete recovery. Vacationers should find out if warnings of tick infestation have been issued in their location. Dogs should not be permitted to roam in tick-infested surroundings; where, in an attempt to eliminate ticks, areas have been sprayed with chemicals harmful to people and their pets, precautions should be taken against potentially dangerous contact. Another precaution is protective clothing. Anyone whose vacation plans or job requirements necessitate a prolonged stay in a tick-infested area should investigate the advisability of vaccination. *See* "Immunization Guide."

Root Canal • The passageway through the root of a tooth for the nerve. When tooth decay has proceeded unchecked from the enamel into the dentin that surrounds the pulp chamber and the root canal, the only treatment that can prevent the loss of the tooth by extraction is known as root canal therapy. This consists in removing the nerve and the diseased pulp, sterilizing the chamber, and filling the area with an inert substance. The specialist who performs this type of treatment is called an endodontist.

Rubella • An acute virus infection accompanied by fever and a rash, a common contagious disease of childhood; also known as German measles. In spite of the fact that long-lasting immunization against this disease is available, many young women reach childbearing age without vaccination against it and without natural immunization from infection during childhood. Rubella immunity precludes the potentially harmful consequences to the fetus from exposure to the disease during the early months of pregnancy. Such consequences include brain damage, heart defects, blindness, and other deformities in as many as 50 percent of the affected offspring. If rubella is contracted during the first trimester of pregnancy, it is considered a valid reason for an abortion. Women of childbearing age who have never been vaccinated against German measles and who test antibody negative should receive a one-shot immunization against the disease. A three-month wait following the immunization should be scheduled before initiating a pregnancy so that the embryo's safety from contamination is ensured.

Rupture • A popular term for a hernia. *See* HERNIA.

Sacroiliac • The cartilaginous joint that connects the sacrum at the base of the spinal column to the ilium, the open section on either side of the hipbone. Low

back pain can sometimes be ascribed to arthritis in this joint.

SAD (Seasonal Affective Disorder) • *See* "Alternative Therapies."

Salmonella • A group of rod-shaped bacteria especially irritating to the intestinal tract and responsible for most cases of acute food poisoning as well as for paratyphoid and typhoid fever. Abdominal cramps and diarrhea are the typical symptoms of salmonella infection. *See* FOOD POISONING.

Sarcoma • A malignant tumor composed of connective tissue such as bone or of muscle, lymph, or blood vessel tissue; one of the two main groups of cancer, the more common being carcinoma (cancer of epithelial or gland cells). A sarcoma usually metastasizes rapidly, either through the bloodstream or through the lymphatics. While treatment is difficult, a combination of chemotherapy, radiation, and surgery can be effective in halting the progress of different types of sarcoma.

Schizophrenia • A category of psychosis, in which the victim suffers from severely disturbed patterns of thinking and feeling that lead to bizarre behavior. The schizophrenic syndrome, for which there is no known direct cause and no specific cure, is most likely to occur in early adulthood, although no age is immune. Common parlance has given the term the sense of a split personality, but this popular definition has nothing to do with the psychiatric diagnosis of mental illness. As with the manic-depressive psychosis, schizophrenic symptoms may be periodic and sometimes so immobilizing that hospitalization is necessary and at other times mild enough to liberate the patient for a comparatively normal life. Among the most striking symptoms of the condition are auditory hallucinations, delusions usually of grandeur or of persecution (paranoia), obsessive-compulsive behavior, distinct personality changes and mood swings without visible cause, and, above all, loss of control over fantasies. While there are many theories about the cause of the illness, circumstances that trigger its onset, and reasons for its remission, no single explanation is definitively convincing. Among the areas of ongoing research are constitutional predisposition in the form of an inherited recessive gene or a combination of genes; constitutional predisposition associated with oxygen deprivation of the brain during birth triggered by a metabolic aberration or related to a prenatal protein deficiency; environmental circumstances that create an atmosphere of anxiety and hostility and especially a conflict between parents or extreme parental disapproval and criticism.

When the disease is suspected, diagnosis is usually based on a complete physical examination, a series of psychiatric interviews, an electroencephalogram, and standard psychological tests. Conventional treatment may begin with one of the major psychotropic drugs combined with psychotherapy, which may involve the family. Environmental therapy, involving residence in a halfway house rather than a hospital, is used in less severe cases, in those where symptoms have abated, or in those where living at home is out of the question because the family situation appears to be part of the problem rather than a possible solution. This form of therapy conditions or reconditions the schizophrenic for participation in the normal world even though some symptoms are ineradicable. Megavitamin therapy is used by some doctors, but conclusive evidence of its effectiveness has not yet been provided. In cases where the more immobilizing symptoms cannot be alleviated in any other way, electroshock may be used

as a last resort. *See* "Plain Talk About Medications."

Sciatica • Pain extending along the sciatic nerve, which is the largest nerve in the body and which supplies sensation from the back of the thigh, along the outer side of the leg, and into the foot and toes. The most common cause of sciatica is a slipped or herniated disk of the lower spine. Relief may be provided by physical therapy, a girdle, and the application of wet heat combined with as much bed rest as possible.

Recent evidence suggests that one in five cases of sciatica occurs when a muscle deep in the buttocks presses on the sciatic nerve. This muscle, known as the piriformis muscle, helps turn the hip out and raise the leg to the side. The entrapment of the sciatic nerve by this muscle is called the piriformis syndrome and is often incorrectly diagnosed and improperly treated. Scanning procedures are useless. The problem can be discovered through a series of postural tests or tests involving electrical nerve signals. When this syndrome is discovered to be the cause of the immobilizing pain, the best treatment is a combination of special exercises and the application of deep heat.

Scoliosis • A sideways curvature of the spine, usually accompanied by an asymmetrical rib cage and protrusion of one shoulder blade. Although poor posture accounts for some cases, scoliosis may begin in infancy, but it may not become apparent until adolescence. Because the asymmetry of the spine leads to widely separated ribs on one side of the body and compressed ribs on the other, respiratory problems may develop. Scoliosis is easily recognized, and milder cases can be corrected by exercises that improve posture and strengthen muscles of the spine. More severe cases may require a corrective brace to prevent further spinal curvature.

Scrotum • *See* SEX ORGANS, MALE.

Sebaceous Glands • The oil-secreting glands situated in the epidermal layer of the skin, lubricating the surface and protecting it from the harmful effects of absorbing too much or too little moisture. The number of these glands, which may be as many as 12 to the square inch, varies from person to person and from one part of the body to another. The sebaceous glands secrete sebum that constantly seeps upward through the pores. Too little sebum production results in dry skin; too much in oily skin. During adolescence and pregnancy hormonal changes may affect the activity of the glands, leading to acne. Other conditions resulting from sebaceous disorders are dandruff and cysts. *See* ACNE, SKIN, and SKIN CARE.

Senile Dementia • Manifest and abnormal deterioration of mental function associated with aging and caused by physical or mental disease or a combination of both. While damage to brain function by arteriosclerosis and stroke are among the conspicuous causes of senility, psychological and social factors that lead to personality deterioration may be equally responsible. Among the most prominent of these factors are withdrawal from normal life, lack of interpersonal relationships, feelings of worthlessness aggravated by familial and social neglect, unrelieved anxieties about disease and death. From the diagnostic point of view, the correct designation of Alzheimer's disease is senile dementia of the Alzheimer type.

Symptoms that mimic senile dementia in the form of forgetfulness and wild mood swings have, in a significant number of cases, been traced to overmedication of older patients in hospitals and nursing homes. In all cases of seeming mental impairment, it is essential that a complete physical checkup, especially of vision and hearing be completed before assuming that the cause of the dementia is irreversible deterioration of brain/mind function. The cumulative effect of alcoholism should also be investigated. "Senile" is a clinical term and should never be used to describe anyone who is going through the normal aging process that may involve a slower rate of activity and response. *See* "Aging Healthfully."

Serotonin • A chemical neurotransmitter that performs vital brain/mind functions. Low levels of serotonin are associated with migraine headaches, depression, and sleep disorders.

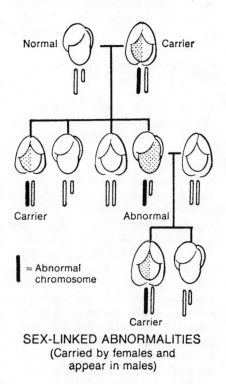

SEX-LINKED ABNORMALITIES
(Carried by females and
appear in males)

Sex-Linked Abnormalities • Inherited disorders transmitted by a genetic defect in the X chromosome. Women have two X chromosomes and men have one X chromosome paired with a Y chromosome. Because the presence of a Y chromosome determines maleness, fathers always transmit their X chromosome to their daughters and their Y chromosome to their sons. Because of these factors, defective genes in the X chromosome follow a particular pattern of heredity. If in a female an inherited disordered X chromosome is balanced by a normal X chromosome, she will carry the disease trait without having the disease itself. If a male offspring of the female carrier inherits her genetically abnormal X chromosome, because it is his only X chromosome, he will have the disease. When a mother is a carrier, there is therefore a fifty-fifty chance that her male offspring will inherit her abnormal X chromosome and have the disease. Female offspring have a fifty-fifty chance of inheriting the abnormal chromosome and therefore a fifty-fifty chance of being carriers. Among the most common sex-linked abnormalities are hemophilia and Duchenne muscular dystrophy. *See* GENETIC COUNSELING.

Sex Organs, Male • The male reproductive organs. One of the most obvious differences between the reproductive organs of the male and the female is that whereas the scrotum and penis are visible, the female counterparts are hidden from view. Another major difference is that for the male, an erotic response in the form of an erection is generally essential for the reproductive role of the penis, but no such psychophysiological requirement exists for the procreative function of the female. The male sex organs consist of the penis, scrotum, testicles, and several glands, including the prostate. Within the testicles, which are loosely contained in

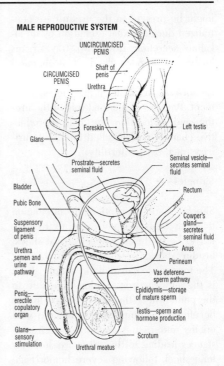

MALE REPRODUCTIVE SYSTEM

UNCIRCUMCISED PENIS

CIRCUMCISED PENIS

Shaft of penis

Urethra

Foreskin

Glans

Left testis

Prostrate—secretes seminal fluid

Seminal vesicle—secretes seminal fluid

Bladder

Rectum

Pubic Bone

Cowper's gland—secretes seminal fluid

Suspensory ligament of penis

Anus

Urethra semen and urine pathway

Perineum

Vas deferens—sperm pathway

Penis—erectile copulatory organ

Epididymis—storage of mature sperm

Glans—sensory stimulation

Testis—sperm and hormone production

Scrotum

Urethral meatus

the scrotum, are structures called the seminiferous tubules in which sperm cells are manufactured from puberty onward. The spermatozoa are conveyed from the tubules into the epididymis, part of the sperm conduction system, where they are stored temporarily until they make their way into the seminal duct (vas deferens) and from this duct into the seminal vesicles, which secrete a viscous material that keeps them viable. The urethra, which also carries urine from the bladder, is enveloped by the prostate gland. The prostate manufactures another fluid that mixes with the sperm and the seminal fluid to form the combination known as semen. The urethra passes through the length of the penis. When the penis is in a state of erection, muscular spasms send the semen through the urethra in the act of ejaculation that immediately follows the male orgasm. Any traces of urine that might be present in the urethra are neutralized during sexual excitation by an alkaline secretion from two tiny organs known as Cowper's glands. This chemical process is critical because spermatozoa cannot remain viable in an acid environment. Because of the dual role of the urethra and its location, the male reproductive channel is also called the genito-urinary tract. *See* "Infertility."

Shingles • *See* HERPES.

Shock • A disruption of circulation that may be fatal if not promptly treated; not to be confused with electrical shock, insulin shock, or electroshock therapy. The immediate cause of circulatory shock is the sudden drop in blood pressure to the point where the blood can no longer be effectively pumped through the vital organs and tissues. Among the circumstances leading to this crisis are: low-volume shock following severe hemorrhage as occurs in multiple fractures, bleeding ulcers, major burns, or any accidents in which so much blood and plasma are lost that there is an insufficiency for satisfying vital needs; neurogenic shock in which the nervous system is traumatized by acute pain, fear, or other strong stimulus that deprives the brain of oxygen and results in a temporary loss of consciousness; allergic shock, also called anaphylactic shock, following the injection into the bloodstream of a substance to which the recipient may be fatally hypersensitive such as bee venom or penicillin; cardiac shock in which the pumping action of the heart is impeded by an infarction or by fibrillation; septic shock resulting from the toxins introduced into the circulatory system by various harmful bacteria as in toxic shock syndrome. Whatever the circumstances, shock produces similar symptoms in different degrees of swiftness: extreme pallor, profuse sweating combined

with a feeling of chill, thirst, faint speedy pulse, and, as the condition intensifies, increasing weakness and labored breathing. Immediate hospitalization is mandatory. If shock is the result of a serious accident or of a heart attack, the patient should not be moved except by people professionally trained to do so.

Shock Treatment • *See* ELECTROSHOCK THERAPY.

Sigmoidoscopy • A diagnostic procedure for detecting precancerous lesions in the descending colon. It is performed on an outpatient basis and should be scheduled every three to five years for people over 50.

Sinuses • Cavities within bones or other tissues; in ordinary usage, the paranasal sinuses, the eight hollow spaces within the skull that open into the nose. These cavities are symmetrically located in pairs. The maxillary sinuses are in the cheekbones, the frontal sinuses are above the eyebrows in the part of the skull that forms the forehead, the ethmoid sinuses are behind and below these, and the sphenoid sinuses are behind the nasal cavity. The sinuses act as resonating chambers for the voice, they help to filter dust and foreign materials from the air before it reaches the lower airway passages, and they lighten the weight of the skull on the vertebral bones of the neck that balance and support the head. Because all the sinuses are lined with mucous membrane, they are vulnerable to infection, to inflammation by allergens, and to the formation of polyps.

Sinusitis • Inflammation of the mucous membranes that line the sinuses. The passageway that connects the sinuses to the nasal cavity is narrow and therefore susceptible to obstruction because of colds, allergies, or the presence of polyps. Such obstruction prevents free drainage of the sinuses, causes an entrapment of air that cannot escape through the nostrils, and leads to an accumulation of mucus that can become a locus of viral or bacterial infection. Infectious organisms may be transported into the sinuses through the nose when an individual is swimming in contaminated water or may invade the maxillary sinuses by way of an abscessed tooth in the upper jaw. The characteristic symptom of sinusitis is a severe headache and face pain in the location of the affected sinus. Fever, swelling, discomfort in the neck, earache, and a stuffed nose are other symptoms.

Acute sinusitis usually clears up in a few days of bed rest; aspirin or other analgesic, limited use of nosedrops, steam inhalation, and air filters can make the recovery period more comfortable. If secondary bacterial infection develops in the sinuses the doctor may prescribe antibiotics.

When sinusitis becomes chronic, every effort should be made to find out the cause. If it can be traced to nasal polyps, consideration should be given to having them removed. When an allergy is responsible, precautions may require the use of an antihistamine combined with other medications that will keep the nasal passages clear. Heavy smoking is another cause as well as a contributing factor when other causes already exist. Irritation by the chlorinated water in swimming pools is yet another cause. Because surgical drainage is advisable only in extreme cases, chronic sufferers should do what they can for themselves: smoking should be eliminated, air conditioners and humidifiers installed, and the environment indoors kept as free of dusts and pollens as possible by using air filters.

Skin • The body's outer surface and its largest organ, covering an area of approximately 25 square feet and weighing about 6 pounds. The skin envelops the body completely and is also a continuation of the mucous membranes of the mouth, nose, urethra, vagina, and anus. Among its many vital functions are the following: it provides a barrier against invasion by infectious agents; offers the delicate tissues beneath it a large measure of protection against injury from the outside; regulates body temperature by the expansion and contraction of its supply of capillaries and by the activities of the sweat glands; participates in the excretion of some of the body's wastes. Through its production of melanin, it wards off some of the damage of the sun's ultraviolet rays, and it also helps transform sunshine into essential vitamin D. In addition, the skin is one of the body's most delicate sense organs: through its vast network of nerve fibers, it transmits messages of pain, pleasure, pressure, and temperature.

What is commonly identified as "the skin" is merely its visible portion or the outermost layer of the epidermis. The epidermis is made of several layers of living cells and an outer horny layer of dead cells constantly being shed and requiring no nourishing blood supply from below. This is the comparatively tough layer that provides a shield against germs as long as it remains unbroken: the same non-living skin cells form the hair and nails. Beneath the epidermis lies the dermis or true skin, bright red in appearance and containing the nerve endings and nerve fibers, sweat and sebaceous glands, and hair follicles. Beneath the dermis is a layer of fatty tissue, called subcutaneous tissue, which helps to insulate the body against heat and cold and which contains the fat globules that through a pattern of distribution give individuality to the features of the face and determine the contours of the body. Also within the subcutaneous tissue are the muscle fibers responsible for the subtle changes of facial expression.

Skin Care • For a healthy woman skin care need consist of rituals no more complicated or costly than cleansing with soap and water to remove accumulated grease, perspiration, dirt, and dead cells and maintaining a proper balance of the protective oils on the skin surface to prevent drying, scaling, and chapping. Medicated soaps are inadvisable unless recommended by a doctor, and when dryness is a chronic problem, detergent preparations may be less dehydrating and less irritating than true soap. Cleansing lotions, cleansing creams, or cold creams removed with

tissues will never leave the skin as clean as rubbing a lather over it with a soft washcloth and removing the suds with warm water. All makeup should be removed before going to bed. The least expensive cleansing cream will do, followed by washing with soap and water.

Whether or not the skin is naturally oily or dry is an inherited factor. A vaporizer or humidifier is the best aid to counteracting the drying effects of central heating or air conditioning. Animal fat, especially lanolin that comes from sheep wool, is the oil closest to human sebum and is, therefore, the best thing to use when skin begins to flake or crack at the knees, elbows, or fingers. It is preferred to mineral oil or vegetable oil for the purpose of lubrication. A sensible regimen of diet, rest, exercise, and good habits of personal hy-

CROSS-SECTION OF SKIN

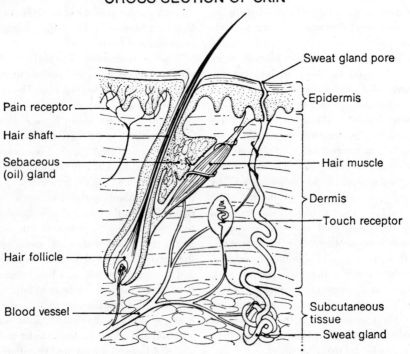

Pain receptor

Hair shaft

Sebaceous (oil) gland

Hair follicle

Blood vessel

Sweat gland pore

Epidermis

Hair muscle

Dermis

Touch receptor

Subcutaneous tissue

Sweat gland

giene are all the care that the average woman's skin should require.

Skin Diseases • It cannot be repeated too often that most skin cancers are caused by overexposure to the sun. They are also the most common type of cancer, but fortunately, with the exception of malignant melanoma, fatal in one out of three cases, skin cancers are treatable with topical medication and/or surgery. Other skin diseases are discussed under individual headings. See ACNE, CONTACT DERMATITIS, ECZEMA, MELANOMA, PSORIASIS, ETC.

Sleep • The period during which the body withdraws from wakeful participation in the environment but is by no means in a continuous state of rest and repose. Sleep and dream research has yielded the information that there are alternating stages of sleep during which the activities of body and brain vary greatly. Of special interest is the recurring stage known as REM (Rapid Eye Movement) sleep during which dreaming occurs. In the four stages of sleep leading up to the REM stage, the body becomes progressively more inert. With the onset of REM, the brain suddenly becomes alert and active, while the body, except for the perceptible movement of the eyes under the closed lids, is deeply "asleep." The brain chemistry of REM sleep can now be duplicated experimentally with drugs, and it is hoped that investigations of dreaming will provide information about the brain chemistry of mental illness.

What has been known for several decades is that all the phases of sleep are essential for well-being and that one of the dangers of barbiturate and alcohol addiction is that these drugs suppress REM sleep and thereby suppress dreaming.

Different individuals have different sleep needs, and these needs differ at various times in the same individual's life.

Some women never need more than six hours; others need at least nine to function well. While it is true that older people need less sleep, they are also likely to take brief naps during the day.

A normal state of health is characterized by, as well as promoted by, good sleeping patterns, and when sleeping problems exist over a considerable period or when they arise suddenly without visible explanation, they should be investigated. Immediate recourse to hypnotics or barbiturates is no solution to the problem; rather, it creates a new problem in and of itself. A promising alternative to sleep-inducing drugs is the recent application of light therapy for sleep disorders.

Unaccustomed sleepiness or drowsiness may be a temporary phenomenon resulting from a wide variety of causes: overexposure to the sun; too much alcohol, especially in an overheated room; poor ventilation; too many tranquilizers; antihistamines; hangover effects of sedatives, tranquilizers, or sleeping pills; and low-grade infection. Chronic sleepiness may be due to thyroid deficiency, anemia, sleep apnea, hardening of the arteries of the brain, or in rare cases the disorder known as narcolepsy. See INSOMNIA, NARCOLEPSY, SLEEP APNEA, "Substance Abuse," and "Alternative Therapies."

Sleep Apnea • A sleep disorder characterized by an interruption in breathing, causing the sleeper to wake up frightened and gasping for air. In typical cases, fitful sleep results in chronic daytime drowsiness. Since the disorder is typically related to obesity, weight loss can usually correct it. Special breathing equipment and medication are other treatments. If these measures are ineffective, surgical enlargement of the airway may be the only solution. Before embarking on this procedure, evaluation by a sleep-wake disorder facility is advisable. These facilities are usually directed by the oto-laryngologists.

Slipped Disc • The dislocation or herniation of one of the cartilaginous rings

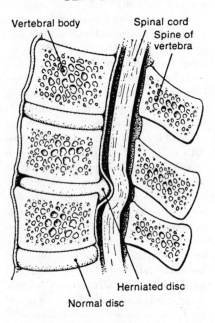

SLIPPED DISC

Vertebral body

Spinal cord

Spine of vertebra

Herniated disc

Normal disc

that separate the spinal vertebrae from each other. The column of 33 bones that make up the spine bears much of the body's weight above the hips. The vertebrae themselves are constantly being subjected to stress and sudden shock due to lifting, bending, and performing other activities that are part of one's daily routine. The discs between the vertebrae are the built-in shock absorbers held in place by rings of tough, fibrous tissue.

As the tissue degenerates with age, it compresses more and more, resulting in the feeling of occasional stiffness. When a disc slips out of position because of this compression, it presses on a spinal nerve—most commonly the sciatic

nerve—causing pain to radiate along its path. In severe cases, the pain radiates from the lower back into the buttocks, through the thighs and calves, and into the feet. When the pressure on the nerve is not so intense, discomfort may be restricted to the lower back. In either case, whether mild or immobilizing, the condition is called sciatica. If the pain is thought to originate along the path of a nerve higher up, an X-ray of the spine may be necessary.

Before more radical measures are taken, treatment consists of bed rest on a firm mattress, aspirin or equivalent painkillers, and for people who want to remain as active as possible, a back support. Some patients are helped by acupuncture followed by a program of exercises that strengthen the back muscles. Most cases of slipped disc recover without surgery.

A recent nonsurgical treatment whose long term benefits have yet to be evaluated is the injection of an enzyme (chymopapain) that dissolves the central portion of the disc. The procedure, called chemonucleolysis, is performed under local or general anesthesia in only a few hospitals.

Prevention of the slipped disc problem is best achieved by: participating in an exercise program directed towards strengthening the muscles that support the back, maintaining proper body weight, wearing high heels only for special occasions, and lifting heavy objects (including one's children) not by bending from the waist but by bending the knees.

Smegma • A sebaceous secretion of a cheeselike consistency that accumulates near the clitoris and under the foreskin of the penis. Unless scrupulously washed off, it is likely to be retained and cause irritation under the foreskin of the uncircumcised male, leading to inflammation and pain.

Spastic Colon • *See* IRRITABLE BOWEL SYNDROME.

Speech Disorders • Abnormalities in spoken word formation that may be the result of organic anomalies, trauma to the brain, medication, disease, or emotional stress. For example, disordered speech may be caused by a cleft palate or severe malocclusion; overmedication with tranquilizers or an addictive use of barbiturates; diseases such as parkinsonism or cerebral palsy; conditions such as the aftermath of a stroke, and cumulative hearing loss, and normal occasions of emotional tension resulting in "stammering with embarrassment" or "sputtering with rage." Mild speech defects, such as a lisp or an inability to articulate the *r* or *l* sound correctly, may be a sufficient source of self-consciousness to require concentrated corrective therapy, especially if the defect causes a curtailment of such activities as speaking in public or produces difficulties during job interviews. Biofeedback techniques are being used in some speech therapy clinics with varying success depending on the seriousness of the disability. For adult stutterers corrective procedure may combine psychotherapy, medication, and disciplined reeducation of the tempo of word production as well as counseling for family members in how to help the stutterer. *See* "Alternative Therapies."

Spleen • The flattened, oblong organ located behind the stomach in the lower left area of the rib cage. It is purplish red in color and weighs approximately 6 ounces. The spleen acts as a reservoir for red blood cells, and through a network of white cells called phagocytes, it also cleanses the blood of parasites, foreign substances, and damaged red cells. In its paler lymphatic tissue it manufactures the white cells known as lymphocytes that ward off infection.

Spotting • Irregular or recurrent nonmenstrual bleeding from the uterus, cervix, or vagina. The most common cause of spotting prior to menopause is hormonal imbalance, either natural or resulting from taking oral contraceptives. Causes after menopause are fibroids, endometrial cancer, excess synthetic estrogen. Spotting that occurs after strenuous exercise or sexual intercourse may indicate the presence of cervical polyps or erosions or small vaginal tears. Spotting should be investigated promptly with a pelvic examination, pap smear, and perhaps a D&C. When it occurs during pregnancy, it may signal the onset of a spontaneous abortion. *See* "Pregnancy and Childbirth" and "Gynecologic Problems and Treatment."

Sprain • An injury to the soft tissues around a joint. Ligaments can be torn or stretched, with damage to associated tendons, blood vessels, and nerves. The severity of a sprain depends on how badly the joint was twisted or wrenched. In some cases the pain is immobilizing and there is considerable swelling accompanied by a large area of discoloration. Because the symptoms are practically indistinguishable from those of a simple fracture, it is sensible to have the injured part X-rayed. If this procedure must be delayed, the first-aid measures known as the RICE treatment should be observed: *R*est, *I*ce application, *C*ompression with an elasticized bandage, and *E*levation. If the site of the sprain (or possible fracture) is in the wrist or elbow, the arm should be supported by a neck sling improvised from a large scarf or a torn sheet. In milder injuries the healing process may be hastened by the application of heat the next day and the intermittent application of heat for short periods of time thereafter.

Staphylococcus Infection • A category of diseases caused by various strains of staphylococcus bacteria, so named for their tendency to grow in grapelike clusters (staphylo) and their round shape (coccus). They are responsible for toxic shock syndrome and for a life-threatening pneumonia that can follow an attack of viral flu; they cause some types of food poisoning; they produce skin disorders such as impetigo, boils, and sties; and they are also a cause of osteomyelitis, an inflammation of the bones, and of bacterial endocarditis, an inflammation of the inner lining of the heart. While many of these bacteria have developed strains resistant to penicillin and the older antibiotics, newer broad spectrum antibiotics are able to combat them effectively. *See* "Plain Talk About Medications."

Sterility • *See* "Infertility."

Steroids • A group of hormones, also called corticosteroids, produced from cholesterol by the adrenal cortex and also available in synthesized form. At least 30 of these substances have been identified, of which the best-known and most widely used is cortisone.

The fact that steroids suppress inflammation has provided helpful treatment for a large number of disorders formerly unresponsive to drug therapy such as lupus erythematosus, nephritis, and contact dermatitis as well as asthma, arthritis, and allergies. However, steroid therapy is usually scheduled on a short-term basis not only because of the unpleasant side effects but also because of the threat it poses to the immune system. Monitoring is also required because of the dangers of

sudden withdrawal after protracted use. *See* "Plain Talk About Medications."

Stethoscope • A diagnostic instrument that amplifies the sounds produced by the lungs, heart, and other organs; used by doctors during the listening part of an examination known as auscultation.

Strain • A mild injury to a muscle, usually caused by subjecting it to unaccustomed tension, as occurs through overexertion or an accident; also called a pulled muscle. (A sprain is more serious, involving stretched or torn ligaments.) Among the most common are twisted ankles caused by a misstep and strained back muscles caused by lifting a heavy weight incorrectly. Wrist muscles may also be strained in various athletic endeavors. For treatment, *see* SPRAIN.

Streptococcus Infection • A category of diseases caused by strains of streptococcus bacteria, so named for their chainlike arrangement (strepto) and their round shape (coccus). Among the strep-caused disorders are pharyngitis (strep throat), scarlet fever, puerperal fever, and some pneumonias. Rheumatic fever or glomerulonephritis may follow a strep infection if it has not been definitively controlled by a full course of antibiotics.

Group A streptococcus, which ordinarily causes such manageable diseases as strep throat and impetigo, has evolved into a virulent form. At its most deadly it causes the "flesh-eating" disease technically known as necrotizing fasciitis. This variant strep infection may occur when the immune system is impaired or as an aftermath of surgery or a deep bruise or cut. Symptoms are a sudden high fever, a dramatic drop in blood pressure, swollen lymph nodes, dizziness, and severe pain at the sight of the infection. In up to half of all cases, the bacteria actually begin to eat away the flesh. Of the approximately 5,000 cases that occur in the United States every year, 2,000 are fatal. Antibiotics administered within the first three days can halt the progress of the infection and bring about a complete recovery.

The species *Streptococcus viridans*, which is normally present in the mouth and harmless for most people, is a cause of subacute bacterial endocarditis in people who have damaged heart valves. Because this species also surrounds the roots of abscessed teeth and because they may enter the bloodstream following the extraction of the tooth, a prophylactic dose of antibiotic medicine before a tooth is pulled is mandatory. The American Heart Association is the authority for the dosage.

Stress • Physical, chemical, or emotional factors that constrain or exert pressure on body organs or processes and on mental processes; in popular usage, psychological pressures. *See* "Alternative Therapies."

Stuttering • *See* SPEECH DISORDERS.

Sty • A bacterial infection of a sebaceous gland at the rim of the eyelid, usually at the root of an eyelash. If the infection does not respond to home treatment of hot compresses applied for about fifteen minutes every two hours and the use of ophthalmic ointment that can be bought without prescription, a doctor should be consulted.

Sulfonamides • A group of medicines, known as sulfa drugs, that inhibit the growth and reproduction of various bacteria. Because many of these drugs have negative side effects, they have largely been replaced by antibiotics. However, some sulfa drugs, especially sulfadiazine, may be prescribed, often in combination with other sulfa drugs, for meningococcal, *E. Coli*, and other infections.

Because sulfa drugs may reduce the effectiveness of the contraceptive pill, a temporary shift to another form of birth control is advisable during the period of sulfa therapy. *See* "Plain Talk About Medications."

Sunburn • Inflammation of the skin caused by overexposure to the ultraviolet rays of the sun or a sunlamp. The lighter the skin, the more quickly it burns. The condition may be limited to a reddening or it may be equivalent to a second-degree burn with blisters and a fever. The best treatment for a mild burn is to avoid the sun for a while and to leave the burned area alone or apply cold, wet dressings to reduce swelling and discomfort. A severe burn may require professional medical attention.

Irrefutable conclusions of medical research indicate that prolonged exposure is the main cause of skin cancer and that constant exposure to the sun during childhood increases the risk of skin cancer in adulthood. For the elderly and anyone with a heart condition, lupus erythematosus, or high blood pressure, the sun can be downright dangerous, especially if there is any possibility of the onset of heat stroke. Women taking certain medicines either for indefinite or short-term therapy should be aware of the fact that overexposure to the sun may produce skin eruptions. *See* SUNSCREEN.

Sunglasses • Eyeglasses whose main purpose has become to protect the eyes from the damaging effects of ultraviolet radiation. Until recently most women wore sunglasses for two main reasons: to diminish the discomfort of the sun's glare at the beach, on the slopes, or during sailing, tennis, and golf, and to make a fashion statement. Today, however, sunglasses are taken much more seriously because of compelling evidence of the irreversible damage to sight caused by long-term exposure to the sun. In the same insidious and painless way that the sun's ultraviolet rays can eventually cause skin cancer, they can also cause cataracts when eyes are unprotected.

The sunglasses that afford the best protection are those to which ultraviolet-absorbing chemicals have been added. These chemicals are usually colorless, and the lenses are tinted for style and comfort rather than for safety. Specialists recommend sunglasses carrying labels that indicate they block 99 percent of the most destructive ultraviolet rays and 60 percent of .the less powerful ones. Other recommendations: plastic lenses are safer and lighter than glass; gray-tinted lenses provide the best color perception, and wraparound glasses that fit the face snugly are the best style choice. Don't be misled by higher prices. Some of the most expensive sunglasses are made with the worst lenses. In general, a good pair should cost less than $25. (This price does not take into account lenses that have to be ground to an individual's corrective prescription.)

Sunscreen • A light-absorbing chemical that protects the skin from the harmful effects of exposure to the sun. Most cosmetics contain one or another sunscreen, and it may be this very ingredient that causes the user to develop an allergic rash. As such, however, sunscreens are indispensable in reducing the likelihood of sunburn and the eventual possibility of ordinary skin cancer.

The number by which the sun protection factor (SPF) is rated indicates its ability to prevent the skin from reddening after measured exposure to intense artificial ultraviolet light. Dermatologists currently recommend a sunscreen with SPF 15. La-

bel information about "waterproof" and "water-resistant" effectiveness should also be closely followed. Vulnerability to the sun because of complexion and skin color should be considered in determining one's length of time of exposure even with a sunscreen. Also available are special sunscreens for women who work in the sun or who perspire heavily when playing tennis or golf. These products are said to be sweat-resistant and therefore won't end up in one's eyes.

Since there is evidence that sunscreens may not provide protection against melanoma, skin cancer experts recommend that when the sun is at its peak, from late morning to early afternoon, people should also wear protective clothing and stay in the shade. *See* MELANOMA.

Syndrome • A group of signs and symptoms that occur together and characterize a particular disease or abnormal condition.

TB • *See* TUBERCULOSIS.

Tear Glands • *See* LACRIMAL DUCTS.

Telemetry • The long-distance transmission by electronic signals of measurement data and other information. Telemetric devices, originally developed for rocketry and space science, have been adapted for attachment to telephones so that, for example, a doctor in a rural hospital can transmit a patient's electrocardiogram or electroencephalogram to medical specialists thousands of miles away for further evaluation. The technique is also widely used for testing artificial pacemaker competence by telephone.

Temperature • *See* FEVER.

Temporomandibular Joint (TMJ) • The joint in front of each ear where the skull connects with the lower jaw. The action of the joint, which is always bilateral, is controlled by a group of large muscles that enable the lower jaw to move up and down, and more rarely, sideways. When the jaw muscles are tensed unconsciously in tooth grinding, or consciously in clenching the teeth, or when they cannot function smoothly because of malocclusion, pains of seemingly mysterious origin are the result, especially pains in the ear or headache. A dentist who specializes in the diagnosis and treatment of the TMJ syndrome should be consulted when there is reason to believe that this irregularity is the source of chronic discomfort.

TENS • *See* TRANSCUTANEOUS ELECTRIC NERVE STIMULATION.

Tetanus • An acute infectious disease caused by the entrance into the body through a break in the skin of the microorganism *Clostridium tetani.* A tetanus-prone wound is one which is deep, has much tissue damage and necrosis (destruction), is uncleaned for four or more hours, and is contaminated by soil, manure, or street dirt. The exotoxin produced by the *C. tetani* bacteria affects the nervous system in such a way as to cause paralyzing muscle spasms, hence the term lockjaw to describe one of the early symptoms. The tetanus bacilli grow in the intestines of all mammals and are found in soil and dust contaminated by the feces of the carriers. It is not spread from one person to another. Once a widespread and fatal disease, it affects fewer than 500 people a year in this country, thanks to routine immunization of infants and booster shots for children and adults. Any injury that might be a tetanus-prone wound is sufficient reason for consulting the closest doctor within 24 hours about proper immunization and antibiotic administration. *See* "Immunization Guide."

Tic • Involuntary and repeated spasmodic contractions of a muscle or group of muscles; also called habit spasms or nervous tics. Such movements usually develop in childhood in response to emotional stress, and while they may subside from time to time during adulthood, they almost inevitably return during periods of fatigue or tension. Among the more common tics are blinking, clearing the throat, jerking the head, twitching the lips. Psychotherapy and tranquilizers can sometimes eliminate a tic, but the former treatment may be too time-consuming and too expensive and the latter may lead to problems more unpleasant than the tic itself. The specific instance in which involuntary spasms of facial muscles originate in a physical disorder is the symptom known as tic douloureux discussed under TRIGEMINAL NEURALGIA.

Ticks • Blood-sucking parasites. Some ticks are comparatively harmless, but others transmit disease. *See* LYME DISEASE, RICKETTSIAL DISEASES, ROCKY MOUNTAIN SPOTTED FEVER, and TYPHUS.

Tinnitus • The sensation of hearing sounds—humming, buzzing, ringing—that originate within the ear rather than as a result of an outside stimulus. The buzzing and ringing may be the temporary result of a blocked eustachian tube such as occurs during an upper respiratory infection or an allergic response. It may also occur after a head injury, following exposure to an extraordinarily loud noise, or as a side effect of certain medications. The diseases with which it is associated are Ménière's disease, otosclerosis, and brain tumor, but most cases are of mysterious origin. If the noises can be ignored, so much the better. When they are disturbingly intrusive at bedtime, they can be masked by soft music from a nearby radio. In recent years, ultrasonic irradiation of the inner ear has achieved some success. Where a hearing problem is also present, an electronic device that produces a sound that masks the noise of tinnitus can be fitted inside the casing of the ordinary hearing aid. *See* "Plain Talk About Medications."

Tobacco • The three major components of tobacco smoking that cause medical concern are tars, nicotine, and carbon monoxide. Tars are not absorbed by the body, but because they are deposited in the cells lining the respiratory tract and lung air spaces, they act as cell irritants.

Nicotine is the powerful drug to which smokers become addicted. The carbon monoxide in inhaled smoke is absorbed into the blood where it impairs the red blood cells and prevents them from transporting oxygen from the lungs to the body tissues. *See* "Substance Abuse."

Tonsils • Two clumps of spongy lymphoid tissue lying one on each side of the throat, visible behind the back of the tongue between the folded membranes that lead to the soft palate. Together with the adenoids, which are located behind the nose at the opening of the eustachian tube, the tonsils function somewhat like filters, guarding the respiratory tract against foreign invasion. When they become infected, inflamed, or enlarged, they are the source of complications leading to difficulties in swallowing and to the spread of the infectious agents to surrounding tissues. When the infection is streptococcal (strep throat), antibiotic treatment must be prompt to prevent the further complication of kidney infection or heart involvement. When enlarged tonsils are a chronic cause of respiratory difficulties over several years or when the adenoids constantly transmit infection to the sinuses or the middle ear, removal by surgery should be considered. However, a tonsillectomy or adenoidectomy should not be undertaken without substantial indication that the operation is justifiable as a health measure.

Toxemia • A condition in which the bloodstream has been invaded by toxic substances; similar to septicemia, and also called blood poisoning. The condition once known as the toxemia of pregnancy is now called eclampsia. *See* "Pregnancy and Childbirth."

Toxoplasmosis • A systemic infectious protozoal disease that may be serious and occasionally is fatal. A fetus whose mother is infected during pregnancy may become severely infected. The infectious organism is most commonly found in raw meat and the feces of infected cats. Pregnant cat owners should therefore wear protective gloves when changing cat litter and when gardening. Uncooked and very rare meat should be scrupulously avoided. If the likelihood of infection exists, a blood test should be scheduled as soon as pregnancy is verified.

Transcutaneous Electric Nerve Stimulation (TENS) • A pocket-size device that can suppress certain types of pain by the application of weak electrical current to the affected area. *See* "Alternative Therapies."

Transvestite • An individual (usually male) whose emotional and sexual gratification is achieved by dressing and behaving like a member of the opposite sex.

Traveler's Diarrhea • *See* DIARRHEA.

Tremor • Involuntary shaking or quivering, usually of the hands, but also of the head or other parts of the body. Tremors may be coarse or fine, depending on the amplitude of the oscillation. They may occur when the body is at rest, ceasing when intentional movement occurs, or they may occur only during acts of volition. The latter are called "intention tremors." Tremors may also accompany a chill or fever or may be one of the symptoms of withdrawal from alcohol, cocaine, barbiturates, and other drugs. Among the diseases with which tremor is associated are cerebral palsy, multiple sclerosis, parkinsonism, hyperthyroidism, arteriosclerosis of the brain, and late syphilis. The trembling that accompanies an anxiety attack or the onset of hysteria may be controlled by sedatives. When an organic disorder is the cause, the tremor usually diminishes with proper treatment of the disease.

Trench Mouth • *See* GUMS.

Trigeminal Neuralgia • Intermittent and acute sensitivity of the fifth cranial nerve (the sensory nerve of the face); also known as tic douloureux. The condition is characterized by the sudden and unpredictable onset of paroxysms of extreme pain seemingly unaccompanied by any change in the nerve itself. The disorder is of unknown origin. It is more common among women than men and rarely occurs before middle age. The spasms of pain may be triggered by such random circumstances as a draft of cold air, blowing the nose, or an anxiety attack. Spontaneous remission may occur after a month of attacks, with recurrence months or years later. Drug therapy provides some pain relief. Acupuncture may bring about a cure. If these methods are unsuccessful and recurrent attacks become so frequent and so painful that they interfere with eating and interrupt sleep, neurosurgery is recommended. *See* "Alternative Therapies."

Tuberculosis • A major infectious disease caused by the tubercle bacillus that usually attacks the lungs and less frequently the bones, joints, kidneys, or other parts of the body; once called phthisis and consumption, now commonly referred to as TB. The disease continues to flourish wherever poverty, poor diet, and crowded substandard living conditions prevail. The infectious organisms are spread through the air from person to person from the coughs and sneezes of anyone with the disease in an active stage. People whose immune system has been compromised by HIV infection, diabetes, Hodgkin's disease, etc., are especially vulnerable.

In recent years, contrary to optimistic expectations about its eventual elimination by the year 2000, the disease has been on the rise as a public health threat, reaching epidemic proportions in some inner cities. In some parts of the country, many cases have become resistant to treatment with one or the other of the two drugs (isoniazid and rifampin) previously effective for all TB patients.

Many people have gone through an active TB episode, mistaking the symptoms, if any, for those of a heavy cold: a cough, chest pains, and feelings of fatigue. Such an occurrence usually leaves a small area of scar tissue in the affected part of the lungs. It is not at all uncommon for a woman between the ages of 20 and 40 to take a tuberculin skin test as part of a thorough physical checkup and to be told that the results are positive. Under these circumstances a chest X-ray is suggested to find out if the lungs show any active disease. If the patient does not have active disease, prophylactic medication is often prescribed to suppress the possibility of later activation of the dormant bacilli. Anyone suffering from a chronic cough, chest pains, breathing difficulties, chronic feelings of fatigue, weight loss, heavy sweating at night, and irregularity in the menstrual cycle is advised to have these symptoms checked to rule out the possibility of TB.

Tumor • A swelling in or on a particular area of the body, usually created by the development of a mass of new tissue cells having no function. The presence of a tumor within the body may be unsuspected until it grows large enough to produce symptoms of pain or to interfere with the normal function of an adjacent organ or nerve. Diagnosis by biopsy determines whether the growth is cancerous or not. A malignant tumor may be treated surgically or with radiotherapy and chemotherapy. A benign growth may or may not be removed surgically, depending on its location and its potential for becoming cancerous. *See* "Breast Care" and "Gynecologic Problems and Treatment."

Typhoid Fever • An acute and highly contagious disease caused by the bacterial bacillus *Salmonella typhi* (related to the bacteria that cause food poisoning); also called enteric fever. Typhoid and paratyphoid infections are endemic wherever the laxity of public health measures results in the contamination of the food and water supplies by urine and feces containing the disease-bearing organisms. Flies may transmit the disease; restaurant workers or food handlers who have had the disease may be carriers who spread the disease unless they are scrupulous in matters of personal hygiene. The infection may also be transmitted by shellfish from contaminated waters. In a case of typhoid fever, the bacteria attack the mucous membranes of the small intestine, producing stools and occasionally urine containing the typhoid bacteria. Symptoms begin after an incubation period of about two weeks and include fever, headache, vomiting, stomach cramps, fatigue, and mental disorientation. A rash of a few days' duration may erupt on the chest and abdomen. Milder cases subside spontaneously within a week or so. Antibiotics with or without corticosteroids will effect a complete cure when administered before major complications occur. Immunization against typhoid fever in adulthood is considerably less trouble than the infection and is at least moderately effective. Travelers to those parts of the world where the disease is endemic are therefore advised to get the necessary shots against it. Because three successive inoculations are necessary over a three-week period, the immunization or the booster shots should be planned well in advance of departure. *See* "Immunization Guide."

Typhus • An infectious rickettsial disease transmitted by the body louse. The disease is endemic in parts of Asia, Africa, and on the shores of the Mediterranean. In another form known as flea typhus it is common in the Far East and the Southwest Pacific. Typhus is not related to typhoid fever in any way. The onset of the disease begins with a headache, acute pains in the legs and back, and sieges of uncontrollable shivering. Within a few days a rash spreads from the torso to the arms and legs, and high fever may cause delirium. Antibiotic treatment is usually effective. Travelers to places where the disease is prevalent should have an anti-typhus vaccination, which provides immunity for about one year. *See* "Immunization Guide."

Ulcer • A chronic lesion in the epithelial tissue either on the visible surface of the body or on the lining of an interior cavity such that the tissues below the skin or mucous membrane may be exposed. Ulcers may occur for many reasons: poor circulation (bedsores, ulcerated varicose veins), infections by microorganisms (ulcerated gums, syphilitic sores), and dam-

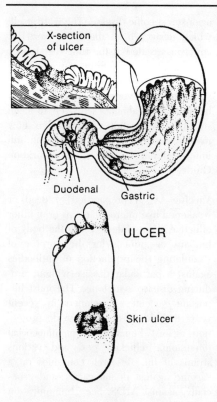

X-section
of ulcer

Duodenal   Gastric

ULCER

Skin ulcer

tion is a burning pain that recurs a few hours after eating. When the condition worsens to the point where the acid that has been burning a hole in the mucous membrane eventually eats into a blood vessel and causes a hemorrhage, the condition (bleeding ulcer) requires hospitalization and emergency treatment.

Considerable progress has been made in the diagnosis and treatment of ulcers thanks to the use of fiberoptic devices that look directly at the ulcer surface. It is now accepted that antimicrobial drugs rather than diet play the crucial role in treatment. These drugs are currently prescribed together with the more traditional ones that suppress acid and those that provide a protective gel covering for sensitive tissue.

While there is no doubt that stress plays some part in the ulcer problem, the one variable that postpones healing more than any other—more than coffee or spicy food—is smoking.

age caused by extremes of heat, cold, malignant growths, or chemicals.

Peptic ulcers include gastric ulcers, which occur in the stomach itself, and duodenal ulcers, which occur in the upper portion of the small intestines and are ten times more common than gastric ulcers. Although it has long been assumed that the immediate cause of peptic ulcers is the secretion of hydrochloric acid when there is no food in the alimentary canal to neutralize its corrosive effects, there is now compelling evidence that some duodenal ulcers are caused by a bacterial agent (campylobacter).

An ulcer diagnosed and treated when the symptoms first appear is more likely to heal quickly and less likely to recur than if it is ignored or treated with home remedies for indigestion. The first indica-

Undulant Fever • A disease caused by drinking unpasteurized milk taken from cows (also from sheep or goats) infected with Brucella microorganisms; also called brucellosis or Malta fever. In rare cases, improperly cooked meat contaminated with these microorganisms also can be a source of the disease. Characteristic symptoms are pains in the joints, fatigue, chills, and a fever that may rise and fall at various times of the day or be low in the morning and rise slowly to 104°F by evening. These fluctuations in temperature account for the name of the disorder. If the disease goes untreated, the liver, spleen, and lymph nodes become swollen and sore. Because the symptoms may be confused with those of mononucleosis or rheumatic fever, a blood test should be made so that the nature of the infectious agent can be identified. The disease is curable with antibiotics.

Uremia • *See* KIDNEYS AND KIDNEY DISORDERS.

Urine Tests • The examination of a urine specimen by various laboratory procedures; also called urinalysis. Because normal urine is of constant composition within definite limits, changes in the color, consistency, clarity, or specific gravity are usually, but not always, a sign of disorder. Thus, every complete physical checkup, whether during health or illness and especially at frequent intervals during pregnancy, should always include a urine test as well as questions about urination. Any visible changes in the color of urine, which is normally a pale amber, might suggest disease. Laboratory tests check for several abnormalities. Albuminuria (proteinuria) is the presence in the urine of certain proteins (albumins) indicating the possibility of kidney disease, inflammations such as cystitis or urethritis, or, during pregnancy, preeclampsia. Albuminuria may also be a response to certain drugs. Glucosuria is the consistent presence in the urine of glucose (not the occasional presence of one of the other sugars) and is usually the indication of diabetes. Hematuria, or blood in the urine, warrants further examination by instruments (cystoscopy) or X-ray if the hematuria persists in order to discover what part of the urinary tract is the source of the bleeding. Among the more common causes are the presence of a kidney stone, a tumor, or some degree of kidney failure. Pyuria, or white blood cells in the urine, is an indication of an infection of the urinary tract, in most cases cystitis or urethritis.

Vaccination • Inoculation with a preparation of dead or attenuated live germs for purposes of immunization

against a specific disease. The word itself, which derives from the Latin word for cow, was created at the time that Jenner developed vaccine from cowpox as a method of immunizing humans against smallpox. Until very recently, vaccination has been used almost exclusively to mean smallpox vaccination. The word is now used synonymously with inoculation and immunization. *See* "Immunization Guide."

Vaccine • A preparation of dead or weakened live microorganisms or of other effective agents injected into the body of humans or animals for the purpose of stimulating the production of antibodies against a particular disease without producing disease symptoms. The most important vaccines developed in recent years include those that provide protection against hepatitis B, pneumococcal pneumonia, chicken pox, and various strains of flu. Research continues on a vaccine against dental caries, and especially, against AIDS. *See* "Immunization Guide."

Vertebra • Any of the bones of the spine. The vertebrae are separated from each other by fibrous tissue and cartilage discs that act as shock absorbers. When the displacement of one of these discs causes pressure on a nerve, the result may be acute pain. Osteoarthritis of the vertebral bones is one of the chronic diseases of aging responsible for backaches. Back discomfort may also originate in poor posture that affects vertebral position in relation to surrounding musculature. Tuberculosis of the spine is also a cause of vertebral collapse and deformity. *See* BACKACHE and "Aging Healthfully."

Vertigo • A sensation of irregular or whirling motion, either of oneself or of nearby objects; also called dizziness, although this latter term often is used incorrectly to describe a sensation of lightheadedness or feeling faint. There are many possible causes of vertigo. It can be brought on by rapid, continuous, whirling motion, such as riding a merry-go-round, or by watching objects in apparent rapid motion, such as telephone poles observed from a fast-moving car. It can be caused by various diseases that affect, directly or indirectly, the labyrinthine canals in the middle ear. *See* MÉNIÈRE'S DISEASE.

Virus • A submicroscopic disease-causing agent capable of reproducing only in the living cells of plants, animals, and humans. Among humans, viruses are responsible for a long list of otherwise unrelated communicable infections, including AIDS, and ranging from the common cold to a very rare and fatal brain disease (Creutzfeld-Jakob). When a viral strain responsible for a particular disease can be isolated and transformed into an effective immunizing vaccine, the disease itself can eventually be controlled. This has been the case with smallpox and to a large extent with such virus-caused infections as polio, measles, and rubella. Antibiotics are ineffective, and usually inappropriate, therapy for virus diseases except in cases where the patient might be critically vulnerable to secondary bacterial infection. Interferon, an antiviral substance naturally produced by the body, is being investigated as a possible treatment for colds and other viral infections. Widespread application depends on the ability to produce a genetically engineered substance at a practical price. *See* INTERFERON, HEPATITIS, INFLUENZA, HERPES, RETROVIRUS, *etc.*

Vocal Cords • The two ligaments within the larynx that vibrate to create the extraordinary range of human sounds. Each reedlike cord is attached at one end

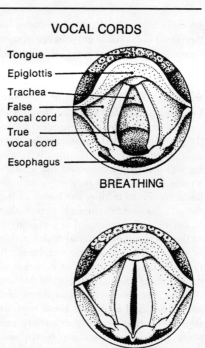

VOCAL CORDS

Tongue
Epiglottis
Trachea
False vocal cord
True vocal cord
Esophagus

BREATHING

TALKING

to the front wall of the larynx (voice box) with the ends placed closely together. The other ends are connected to small rotating cartilage rings near the back wall of the larynx. These rotations cause the cords to separate or to close, thus controlling the amount of air that passes through the larynx. When the cords are open, the air passes through without producing sounds. When the cords are close together, the air that is forced through them causes them to vibrate like the reeds in a musical instrument. These vibrations create sound waves in the form of a voice, and when the sound waves are articulated and controlled in a particular way, they produce speech and song. The pitch of the voice depends on the tension in the cords, and its depth depends on their length. Men's voices are deeper than women's because their vocal cords are longer. A common occurrence among singers and public speakers is the development of nodes on the vocal cords. These growths are usually removed by surgery. *See* LARYNGITIS and LARYNX.

Vomiting • The mechanism whereby the sudden contraction of the muscles of the stomach and the small intestine forces the partially digested contents of these organs upward and out of the mouth. Vomiting and the feeling of nausea that characteristically precedes it may occur as a reflex response to tickling the inside of the throat, to an overfull stomach, to ingesting an emetic such as mustard or a poison, or to the presence of bacterial toxins acting as an irritant on the gastric membrane. It may also occur because of stimulation of the vomiting center of the brain. Motion sickness, overdoses of certain drugs and anesthetics, and emotional stress, such as strong feelings of revulsion or anxiety, can cause a reaction of vomiting. It may also occur because of obstructions in the intestines, uncontrolled paroxysms of coughing, the hormonal changes associated with pregnancy, and migraine headaches. Any recurrent or uncontrollable attacks of vomiting should be diagnosed by a doctor. In coming to the aid of someone who is vomiting following an accident, the person's head should be held forward, not back so that the patient does not inhale the vomitus and fatally obstruct breathing.

Wart • An abnormal growth on the skin caused by a virus. Warts may occur at any age, but they appear less frequently as people grow older because an immunity to the virus may develop over the years. Because the virus can spread to lesions in the skin caused by scratching, shaving, or other factors, warts may appear in groups or in succession.

A wart on the sole of the foot is called a plantar wart. Because constant pressure causes it to grow inward, it may eventually press on a nerve and cause considerable pain. Because warts on other parts of the body are not sensitive or itchy, any sudden discomfort associated with them or any change in appearance or size should be called to a doctor's attention. Removal for cosmetic or other reasons is accomplished by various techniques including cauterization with chemicals or an electric needle, surgical incision, or by cryosurgery, a painless procedure that freezes the wart with liquid nitrogen. Genital warts are discussed in "Sexually Transmissible Diseases." *See also* PLANTAR WART.

Water Retention • *See* EDEMA and DIURETIC.

Withdrawal Method • *See* COITUS INTERRUPTUS.

Wrinkles • The lines and furrows that mark the skin as it ages and loses elasticity. Heredity, hormonal interplay, emotional and physical health, and exposure to sun and wind are the chief factors that determine the age at which skin begins to wrinkle. Also, the skin of women who smoke seems to wrinkle earlier and more than of those who do not. Wrinkles cannot be removed or permanently delayed by creams or lotions; cosmetics can mask them, but those that claim to contain "magic" ingredients may do more harm than good. The technique of dermabrasion can temporarily erase the more superficial lines, but they will inevitably reappear as the sagging skin continues to move away from the supporting structures beneath. Cosmetic surgery can eliminate wrinkles for several years, but the decision to undergo such a procedure should be carefully considered. *See* RETINOIC ACID and "Cosmetic Surgery."

X-ray • Radiation of extremely short electromagnetic waves capable of penetrating certain matter opaque to ordinary light and producing images on photosensitive surfaces; also the image produced. Under ordinary circumstances, X-rays are more easily absorbed by bone than by flesh. By placing a fluorescent screen behind the body, the bones are delineated as shadows. This technique is called fluoroscopy. When permanent records are wanted, photographic plates that are sensitive to X-rays are used to produce images that can be dated and preserved as part of a patient's medical history. From its original application to injuries or disorders of the skeletal system, X-ray technology has been broadened by the technique of introducing radiopaque substances into the patient's body to provide information about nonskeletal disorders. For information about gastrointestinal problems, barium is introduced into the body either by mouth or by enema. Contrast dyes are administered intravenously to help in the location of kidney stones.

Within recent years, newer techniques have increasingly replaced X-ray imaging. Scanning machines, magnetic resonance imaging, ultrasonography, and fiberoptic instruments enable the diagnostician to get information previously inaccessible by X-ray imaging. There is also a movement away from unnecessary "routine" X-rays of the chest and teeth. X-ray photos of the chest do not give any indication of the early phases of emphysema or bronchitis. However, breast X-rays (mammography) are considered a useful tool for discovering breast cancer as soon as signs appear in cellular anomalies.

Whether for diagnostic purposes or, more likely, as treatment (*see* RADIATION THERAPY), the danger of overexposure to X-rays has become a widespread problem. Among the consequences of overexposure are destruction of skin, loss of hair and nails, development of certain cancers, and damage to the genes, the reproductive organs, and fetuses. Pregnant women should avoid exposure to X-rays except in the greatest emergency. When a medical doctor suggests X-rays, ask what their purpose is, whether other tests do the same thing, whether the lowest possible radiation is being used to achieve the necessary result, and when the equipment was last inspected. Many states have no laws requiring that X-ray equipment be checked every year to make sure that it does, in fact, deliver intended doses rather than perilously higher ones and that it in no way exposes the patient to unnecessary hazards because it is incorrectly operated or outmoded. If X-ray pictures must be taken, it is advisable to have them done by a radiologist. While specialists are more expensive than general practitioners, they are more likely to have the most up-to-date equipment and the best-trained technicians operating it. Anyone who has undergone a series of X-rays and is changing doctors or moving to another city should ask the doctor or dentist for the films so that they can be turned over to whoever will be in charge of medical care in the new location.

Yogurt • A food of custardlike consistency created by heating milk to produce the beneficial bacillus *Streptococcus thermophilus* and then fermenting the milk with an additional beneficial bacterial strain (*Lactobacillus bulgaricus*). In the process of fermentation the milk sugar lactose is transformed into lactic acid, giving yogurt its characteristically tart flavor. In addition to its nutritional assets, yogurt is more easily digested than milk, and its bacteria have a beneficial effect on the intestinal tract, fighting off infectious bacteria and adding benign ones, especially those that might have been destroyed by antibiotics. Yogurt sold as a frozen solid may be a less fattening dessert than ice cream, but its beneficial bacteria are presumed to have been destroyed in the freezing process.

APPENDIXES

SUGGESTED HEALTH EXAMINATION SCHEDULES FOR WOMEN AT NORMAL RISK*

	Age 18–40	Age 41–60	Age 61+
General physical examination and life-style counseling	2 years	1 year	1 year
Dental examination	6 months	6 months	6 months
Eye examination including glaucoma test	2 years	1 year	1 year
Breast examination	3 years	1 year	1 year
Breast self-examination	1 month	1 month	1 month
Pap smear	1 year	1 year	1 year
Pelvic examination	1 year	1 year	1 year
Tests for sexually transmissible diseases	6–12 months**	6–12 months**	6–12 months**

	Age 35–49	Age 50+
Mammography	Initial at age 35–39; thereafter yearly or every other year	1 year

Endometrial tissue sample	At menopause and periodically thereafter for women taking estrogens

	Age 40+	Age 50+
Finger rectal examination	1 year	1 year
Test for blood in stool		1 year
Proctosigmoidoscopy		3–5 years

* Different intervals may be recommended for some women by their physicians.

** Frequency depends on life-style and potential risk. The Centers for Disease Control estimates that one in approximately 800 women is HIV-positive. Sexually active women and women in the health professions are especially vulnerable and should therefore schedule HIV tests on a regular basis. The test for chlamydia should be a routine part of a Pap smear procedure.

IMMUNIZATION GUIDE

- *Tetanus-diphtheria toxoid booster:* After age 18, every 10 years, and after exposure.
- *Influenza (flu) inactivated vaccine:* Beginning at age 60, every year. High-risk individuals with chronic conditions such as asthma, heart disease, or diabetes should ask their doctor about when to begin getting flu shots.
- *Rubella live virus vaccine:* Because the rubella (German measles) virus can cause birth defects if infection occurs during the first three months of pregnancy, all women of childbearing age who lack proof of having been vaccinated against this disease during childhood, and who test antibody negative, should receive one dose of vaccine *if not already pregnant* and should wait at least three months following vaccination before planning a pregnancy.
- *Pneumococcal vaccine for bacterial pneumonia:* All people age 65+ should receive one dose of vaccine. This immunization is also recommended for individuals at high risk, including those with disorders of the liver, kidneys, or spleen; alcoholics; and individuals with heart disease, diabetes, or organ transplants.
- *Hepatitis B inactivated virus vaccine:* For health care workers, dentists, and doctors likely to be in contact with needles contaminated with this virus; for people with hemophilia who receive frequent blood transfusions; also for women who are sexually active and whose partners may be intravenous drug users. The vaccine is administered in three separate doses that confer almost 100 percent immunity.

INTERNATIONAL TRAVELERS

The Centers for Disease Control maintains a free Fax Information Service that supplies frequently updated material on immunizations recommended for travelers to specific parts of the Caribbean, Asia (including India), Africa, and Central and South America. If you (or your doctor) has a fax machine, you can receive the CDC information by dialing 1-404-332-4565 and following the prompts. If you know which country you are traveling to but are not certain of the region to ask for, request document #220000. This service operates on a round-the-clock schedule, so your requests can be made at any time of the day or night on any day of the week.

COMMON MEDICAL TERMS

Most of the words used by doctors are made up of two or three parts (prefixes, roots, suffixes) that come from Greek or Latin. Knowing the meaning of these word parts makes it easier to understand and use medical terminology.

PREFIXES

a-, an-	without (anesthesia)	anti-	against (antiseptic; antihistamine)
ad-	toward or near (adhesions; adrenal)	bi-	two (biceps; bisexual)

co-, con-	with, together (concussion; constipation)	hypo-	under, below (hypothyroid; hypothermia)
cyano-	blue (cyanosis)		
dys-	impaired, abnormal (dysmenorrhea; dysfunction)	leuko-	white (leukocytes; leukorrhea)
		ortho-	straight, correct (orthodontia; orthopedist)
ecto-	outer, outside (ectopic)		
endo-	inner, within (endocardium; endometrium)	pre-, pro-	before (premenstrual; prophylaxis)
epi-	over, among (epiglottis; epidermis)	re-, retro-	back, again (regression; retroperitoneal)
eu-	good, well (euphoria; euthanasia)	sub-	beneath, under (subconscious; subcutaneous)
ex-	out, away from (expectorant)	super-	higher, above (superego)
hyper-	excessive (hyperacidity; hypertension)	sym-, syn-	together (symbiosis; synapse)
		trans-	across (transfusion)

ROOTS RELATING TO MEDICINE AND THE BODY

aden-	gland (adenoma; adenoid)	derma-	skin (dermatitis; epidermis)
angio-	blood vessel (angiography; hemangioma)	diaeta-	regimen (diet)
		emetos-	vomit (emetic)
arthro-	Joint (arthritis)	enterion	intestines, gut (enteritis; dysentery)
bronchos-	throat (bronchitis; bronchoscopy)	gastro-	stomach (gastric ulcer; gastritis)
cardi-,	heart (cardiogram;		
coro-	coronary)	haemo-	blood (hemangioma; hemoglobin)
cerebro-	brain (cerebral palsy)		
chole-	bile (cholesterol; cholelith)	hepato-	liver (hepatitis)
		metro-	uterus (endometritis)
colo-	colon (colostomy)	myo-	muscle (myocardial; myoma)
cyst-	sac; bladder (cystoscope)		
cyto-	cell (leukocyte)		

narce-	numbness (narcotic; narcolepsy)	proctos-	anus (proctoscope)
		rhinos-	nose (rhinitis)
nephros	kidney (nephritis)	sarcos-	flesh (sarcoma)
osteo-	bone (osteoarthritis)	sphygmos-	pulse (sphygmomanometer)
ophthalmos-	eye (ophthalmologist)		
otos-	ear (otitis)	soma-	body (psychosomatic medicine)
pepsis-	digestion (peptic ulcer; dyspepsia)	phlebs-	vein (phlebitis)
pneuma-	lungs (pneumonia)		

SUFFIXES RELATED TO SYMPTOMS, DIAGNOSIS, SURGERY

-algia	pain (neuralgia)	-osis	disease (tuberculosis)
-ectomy	cutting out (appendectomy)	-ostomy	opening (colostomy)
		-otomy	incision (episiotomy)
-genic	source (psychogenic)	-pathy	disease (psychopathic)
-graph	record, writing (electrocardiograph)	-rhagia	overflow (hemorrhage)
-itis	inflammation (laryngitis)	-rrhea	stream, discharge (dysmenorrhea; rhinorrhea)
-lysis	dissolving, separating (analysis; dialysis)	-scopy	inspection (cystoscopy; microscopy)
-oid	resembling (fibroid)		
-oma	tumor (lymphoma)		

HEALTH CARE PERSONNEL

PHYSICIAN

Doctor of Medicine (M.D.). Has received a degree from a school of medicine. Doctor of Osteopathic Medicine (D.O.). Has received a degree from a college of osteopathic medicine.

After graduating from one of the above schools or colleges, all physicians must complete one year of postgraduate training (internship or first year of postgraduate training—P.G. 1) in an approved hospital to be eligible for a permanent medical license anywhere in the United States. Thereafter they may take additional years of postgraduate training (residency) in an approved hospital to become specialists. They also may spend additional time as research or clinical fellows at a medical school.

To practice medicine in the United States, a physician must be licensed by the state in which he or she practices. When in practice, a physician will have a primary, and perhaps a secondary, field of practice or specialty and be referred to accordingly. He may be a family practitioner, internist, hematologist, surgeon, internist-cardiologist, etc.

Physicians are listed in the "Consumer Yellow Pages" of the telephone directory according to their specialty as well as by locality in the community in which they practice. Some of these specialties are:

ANESTHESIOLOGY. The anesthesiologist is responsible for choosing and administering the appropriate anesthesia for whatever surgery is planned. This choice is based on an assessment of the patient's medical history and present condition. *See* ANESTHESIA.

DERMATOLOGY. The dermatologist diagnoses and treats diseases of the skin, which is the largest body organ.

EMERGENCY MEDICINE. A physician who has specialized in this area is an expert in the split-second recognition, evaluation, stabilization, and care of trauma, acute illness, and emotional crisis. Most such physicians practice only in hospital or free-standing emergency departments.

FAMILY PRACTICE. The family practitioner (sometimes called general practitioner or primary care provider) offers basic and comprehensive medical care to any individual of any age. However, not all family practitioners do surgery or obstetrics.

INTERNAL MEDICINE. The internist (not to be confused with "intern") diagnoses most medical conditions but treats only those which do not require surgery. Many internists have a subspecialty, and some limit their practice to it. Among the better-known subspecialists are: allergist, endocrinologist (glandular and hormonal problems), hematologist (blood disorders), cardiologist (heart disease), and gastroenterologist (digestive disorders).

NEUROLOGY. The neurologist diagnoses and treats organic disorders and diseases of the nervous system which do not require surgery. *See* "Surgery" below.

OBSTETRICS AND GYNECOLOGY. The obstetrician is concerned with pregnancy and delivery; the gynecologist, with disorders and diseases of the female reproductive system and with birth control. Some obstetrician-gynecologists limit their practice to one of these two specialties. *See* "Contraception and Abortion," "Pregnancy and Childbirth," "Infertility," and "Gynecologic Problems and Treatment."

OPHTHALMOLOGY. The ophthalmologist diagnoses and treats diseases of the eye and disorders of the structure and function of the eye such as myopia and presbyopia. *See* EYE EXAMINATION.

ORTHOPEDICS. The orthopedist diagnoses and treats all diseases and injuries affecting the skeletal system, including joints, muscles, ligaments, tendons, and bones.

OTOLARYNGOLOGY. The otolaryngologist (ENT specialist) diagnoses and treats diseases of the ear, nose, and throat and hearing disorders.

PATHOLOGY. The pathologist is concerned with structural and functional changes in tissues and organs of the body which cause or are caused by disease. These changes are identified by examining, through various tests, blood, body fluids, tissue, feces, and other materials. *See* AUTOPSY, BLOOD TESTS, and URINE TESTS.

PEDIATRICS. The pediatrician diagnoses most medical conditions in children but treats only those which do not require surgery. Some pediatricians have a subspecialty to which they limit their practice. Among the better-known subspecialties are: cardiology, endocrinology, nephrology (kidney disease), and neonatology (care of premature or ill newborn infants).

PHYSICAL MEDICINE AND REHABILITATION. A physician specializing in this area is known as a physiatrist, and is concerned with minimizing the disabilities of people who have had a disease such as a stroke or an injury that affects function of one or more parts of the body. *See* PHYSICAL THERAPY.

PLASTIC SURGERY. The plastic surgeon deals with the repair, restoration, or replacement of malformed, damaged, or missing parts of the body resulting from injury or from congenital defect—for example, repair of cleft palate, skin grafting after major burns, reconstruction of facial bones damaged in an accident, and replacement of a joint or limb with a prosthesis. Cosmetic surgery is the branch of plastic surgery concerned with changing appearance solely for esthetic reasons. See "Cosmetic Surgery" and PLASTIC SURGERY.

PREVENTIVE MEDICINE. A physician who practices preventive medicine is usually associated with community health programs and public health measures that aim to anticipate and prevent disease and injuries.

PROCTOLOGY. The proctologist specializes in medical and surgical treatment of disorders of the anus and rectum.

PSYCHIATRY. The psychiatrist is a licensed physician who specializes in the diagnosis, treatment, and prevention of mental and emotional disorders.

RADIOLOGY. A radiologist uses X-rays, sonography, radioactive substances, and other forms of radiant energy in the diagnosis and treatment of disease. See RADIATION THERAPY and X-RAY.

SURGERY. A general surgeon performs any type of operation. Most surgeons specialize in a particular type of surgery. For example, the thoracic surgeon performs operations involving the lungs and heart. Neurosurgeons are called upon for the removal of brain tumors, repair of nerves following injury, and similar operations.

UROLOGY. A urologist specializes in medical and surgical treatment of disorders of the urinary tract.

In checking on the credentials of a recommended specialist, a reliable source available at most public libraries is the annual compendium published by the American Board of Medical Specialties. This source provides up-to-date professional and biographical profiles of physicians who have met the certification requirements of their respective medical specialty boards. The 1996 edition contains this information about the 466,354 American and Canadian physicians known as "Diplomates" after they have had from three to seven years of postgraduate medical training in an approved residency or fellowship program and have successfully completed an extensive certification examination in one (and in some cases more than one) of the following specialties:

Allergy and Immunology	Otolaryngology
Anesthesiology	Pathology
Colon and Rectal Surgery	Pediatrics
Dermatology	Physical Medicine and Rehabilita-
Emergency Medicine	tion
Family Practice	Plastic Surgery
Internal Medicine	Preventive Medicine
Medical Genetics	Psychiatry and Neurology
Neurological Surgery	Radiology
Nuclear Medicine	Surgery
Obstetrics and Gynecology	Thoracic Surgery
Ophthalmology	Urology
Orthopaedic Surgery	

There also exist various "colleges" of physicians whose members have additional credentials. A member becomes a Fellow of the American College of Cardiology

(F.A.C.C.), Gastroenterology (F.A.C.G.), Obstetrics and Gynecology (F.A.C.O.G.), Physicians (F.A.C.P.), Radiology (F.A.C.R.), or Surgeons (F.A.C.S.).

All physicians must devote a certain number of hours to graduate medical education activities each year to maintain their state medical licenses and hospital privileges. *See* "You, Your Doctors, and the Health Care System."

DENTIST

Doctor of Dental Medicine (D.M.D.) or of Dental Surgery (D.D.S.) has received one of these degrees (which are one and the same) from a school of dentistry.

After graduating from dental school and obtaining a license to practice dentistry from the state in which they intend to practice, dentists may begin immediately to practice general dentistry. They also may take additional training at a dental school or approved hospital to become specialists.

The American Dental Association recognizes nine dental specialties. They are: Endodontics (root canal therapy); General Practice (also called family dentistry); Oral Pathology (laboratory activities); Oral Surgery; Orthodontics (correction of tooth irregularities); Pedodontics (children's dentistry); Periodontics (treatment of diseases of the gums); Prosthodontics (replacement and reconstruction of teeth); and Public Health.

About 15 percent of dentists in the United States have been certified by a Specialty Board of the American Dental Association. There are eight such boards: Dental Public Health; Endodontics; Oral and Maxillofacial Surgery; Oral Pathology; Orthodontics; Pedodontics; Peridontology; and Prosthodontics.

All dentists must complete a certain number of hours of graduate dental education each year to maintain their state medical licenses.

CHIROPRACTOR

Doctor of Chiropractic (D.C.) has graduated from a chiropractic school or college.

After graduating from chiropractic school and obtaining a license to practice chiropractic from the state in which they intend to practice, chiropractors may begin to practice immediately. They use a therapeutic system based on the theory that disease is caused by subluxations—that is, partial dislocations—of the vertebral bones that cause pinching of the nerves emanating from them. The pinching of the nerves impairs the function of vital organs and is corrected by spinal adjustment. (*See* "Alternative Therapies.")

OPTOMETRIST

Doctor of Optometry (O.D.) has graduated from a school of optometry.

After graduating from optometry school and obtaining a license to practice optometry from the state in which they intend to practice, optometrists may begin to practice immediately. They do refractions to determine visual impairment and prescribe corrective lenses when indicated. They also do tests for glaucoma and certain other conditions but do not treat them.

PODIATRIST

Doctor of Podiatry Medicine (D.P.M.) has graduated from a college of podiatry.

After graduating from a college of podiatry and obtaining a license to practice podiatry from the state in which they intend to practice, podiatrists may begin to practice immediately. They specialize in treating problems of the feet such as corns, warts, bunions, calluses, ingrown toenails, heel pain, hammer toes, and painful arches. Podiatrists formerly were called chiropodists. *See* "Fitness."

HEALTH CARE WORKERS

There are many such professionals, and some of them work independently of doctors all or part of the time. A few have Ph.D. degrees and therefore are called "Doctor."

AUDIOLOGIST. A person with at least a master's degree who specializes in hearing testing and disorders.

CLINICAL PSYCHOLOGIST. A person with either a master's or a Ph.D. degree who administers psychologic tests and treats mental and emotional problems.

DENTAL ASSISTANT. A person who assists with the work in a dental office processing X-rays, preparing patients for examination, etc.

LAY MIDWIFE. A person with varying levels of training who delivers babies at home. The degree of state regulation of midwives is diverse. *See* "Pregnancy and Childbirth."

LICENSED PRACTICAL NURSE (L.P.N.). A person with brief training, usually a few weeks in a hospital program, in the nursing care of patients.

NURSE MIDWIFE. A registered nurse who has completed an organized program of study and clinical experience recognized by the American College of Nurse Midwives. This advanced study qualifies her to extend her practice to the care of pregnant women, to the supervision of labor and delivery, and to postnatal care in cases in which no abnormalities are present. *See* "Pregnancy and Childbirth." *See* REGISTERED NURSE below.

NURSE PRACTITIONER (N.P.). A registered nurse with advanced training in diagnosing and treating disease. Nurse practitioners take medical histories, do physical examinations, perform diagnostic tests, develop treatment programs, and counsel patients. State regulations regarding their duties vary greatly. Some nurse practitioners practice independently, others work in clinics, physicians' offices, or hospitals. *See* "Registered Nurse" below.

OCCUPATIONAL THERAPIST (O.T.). A person with at least a bachelor's degree and six months of specialized training. He or she teaches handicapped patients vocational and other necessary skills so that they may function as independently as possible.

OPTICIAN. A person who fits, supplies, and adjusts eyeglasses and contact lenses. Opticians are licensed in about half of the states.

PHYSICAL THERAPIST (P.T.). A person with at least a bachelor's degree and usually some specialized training in physical therapy. He or she provides special therapy for people who, because of disease or injury, have diminished strength, mobility, or range of motion. Exercise, heat, cold, and water are the major therapeutic methods. *See* PHYSICAL THERAPY.

PHYSICIAN ASSISTANT (P.A.). A person who, after at least two years of college, takes two years of specialized training to learn to do some of the things traditionally done by physicians. He or she takes medical histories, does physical examinations, performs diagnostic tests, and develops treatment plans. P.A.'s are always under the supervision of a physician either directly or, in some instances, by telephone. In some states they can prescribe certain medications.

REGISTERED DENTAL HYGIENIST (R.D.H.). A person with at least two years of formal training in examining, cleaning, and polishing teeth. Licensed by the state, he or she generally works under the direct supervision of a dentist.

REGISTERED DIETITIAN (R.D.). A person with at least a bachelor's degree and a dietetic internship or an approved coordinated undergraduate program in dietetics. He or she provides dietary counseling and nutritional care.

REGISTERED NURSE (R.N.). A person with a nursing diploma from a diploma school of nursing (hospital nursing school) or, as is more and more the trend, a bachelor's degree from a nursing school in a college. Nurses must be licensed by the state in which they practice. In addition to performing bedside nursing duties, R.N.'s often have administrative and teaching positions in hospitals and other health care facilities. This is particularly true of the degree nurses, some of whom also have master's degrees and Ph.D. degrees. Registered nurses also work in physicians' offices, clinics, and community health programs.

SOCIAL WORKER. A person with at least a bachelor's degree, but usually also a master's or Ph.D. degree in social work. Social workers in health care institutions help patients and their families in attempting to resolve various psycho-social-economic problems that are created by their illness.

SPEECH-LANGUAGE PATHOLOGIST. A person with at least a master's degree who assists persons whose speech is impaired by disease or injury to improve their verbal communication. *See* SPEECH DISORDERS.

DIRECTORY OF HEALTH INFORMATION

Note: Many of the organizations listed below maintain a local office in your community. Check your telephone directory for listings.

ABORTION

National Abortion Federation (202) 667-5881
    1436 U St. NW, Suite 103, Washington, DC 20009
    Fax (202) 667-5890
National Abortion Rights Action League (NARAL) (202) 973-3000
    1156 Fifteenth St. NW, Suite 700, Washington, DC 20005
National Right to Life Committee, Inc. (202) 626-8800
    419 Seventh St. NW, Suite 500, Washington, DC 20004

ADDICTION: ALCOHOLISM, DRUG ABUSE, SMOKING

Al-Anon Family Group Headquarters (212) 302-7240
    PO Box 862, Midtown Station, New York, NY 10018
Alcoholics Anonymous World Services (212) 870-3400
    475 Riverside Dr., New York, NY 10163
    Fax (212) 870-3003

Children of Alcoholics Foundation (212) 754-0656
    PO Box 4185, Grand Central Station, New York, NY 10163
    Fax (212) 754-0664
National Clearinghouse for Drug and Alcohol Abuse Information   (800) 729-6686
National Council on Alcoholism and Drug Dependence (212) 206-6700
    12 West 21st St., New York, NY 10010
Secular Organization for Sobriety (716) 834-2922
    PO Box 5, Buffalo, NY 14215
    Fax (716) 834-0841
Women for Sobriety (215) 536-8026   (800) 333-1606
    PO Box 618, Quakertown, PA 18951
Cocaine Anonymous World Services (310) 559-5833   (800) 347-8998
    3740 Overland Ave., Suite H, Los Angeles, CA 90034-6337
    Fax (310) 559-2554
Pills Anonymous (212) 874-0700
    PO Box 772, Bronx, NY 10451

Smoking

ACTION on Smoking and Health (ASH) (202) 659-4310
    2013 H St. NW, Washington, DC 20006
CDC Office on Smoking and Health (404) 639-3534
    Public Information, Mail Stop K 50, Atlanta, GA 30333
Smokenders   (800) 828-4357
    1430 E. Indian School Rd., Suite 102, Phoenix, AZ 85014
Stop Teenage Addiction to Smoking (413) 732-STAT
    511 E. Columbus Ave., Springfield, MA 01105
    Fax (413) 732-4219

Rehabilitation and Treatment

Hazelden Foundation (612) 257-4010   (800) 257-7800
    15245 Pleasant Valley Rd., PO Box 11, Center City, MN 55012

ADOPTION

Adoptee-Birth Parent Searches (310) 285-6786
    Jeannette, PA 15644
Adoptees in Search (301) 656-8555
    PO Box 41016, Bethesda, MD 20824
    Fax (301) 652-2106
Adoptive Families of America (612) 535-4829   (800) 372-3300
    3333 Highway 100 N, Minneapolis, MN 55422
    Fax (612) 535-7808
Committee for Single Adoptive Parents (202) 966-6367
    PO Box 15084, Chevy Chase, MD 20825

AGING

Older Women's League (OWL) (202) 783-6686
    666 Eleventh St. NW, Suite 700 Washington, DC 20001-4512
Administration on Aging (202) 401-4634
    Hubert H. Humphrey Bldg.
    200 Independence Ave. SW, Washington, DC 20201
American Association of Retired Persons (AARP) (202) 434-2277
    601 E Street NW, Washington, DC 20049
    Fax (202) 434-2320
American Society on Aging (415) 974-9600
    833 Market St., Suite 512, San Francisco, CA 94103
    Fax (415) 882-4280
Children of Aging Parents (CAPS) (215) 945-6900
    1609 Woodbourne Rd., Levittown, PA 19057
    Fax (215) 945-8720
Elderhostel (617) 426-8056
    75 Federal St., Boston, MA 02110
Foster Grandparents Program (202) 606-5000
    1201 New York Ave., Washington, DC 20520
Gray Panthers (202) 466-3132
    2025 Pennsylvania Ave. NW, Washington, DC 20006
    Fax (202) 466-3133
National Caucus and Center on Black Aged (202) 637-8400
    1424 K St. NW, Suite 500, Washington, DC 20004
    Fax (202) 347-0895
National Council on the Aging (202) 479-1200
    409 Third St. NW, Washington, DC 20024
    Fax (202) 479-0735
National Council of Senior Citizens (202) 347-8800
    1331 F St. NW, Washington, DC 20004
    Fax (202) 624-9595

AIDS

AIDS Clinical Trial Groups NIH (301) 496-8210
    6003 Executive Bldg., Rm. 2A47, Bethesda, MD 20892
CDC National AIDS Clearinghouse   (800) 458-5231
    PO Box 6003, Rockville, MD 20849-6003
    Fax (301) 738-6616
National Association of People with AIDS (202) 898-0414
    1413 K St. NW, Washington, DC 20005
People with AIDS Coalition (212) 647-1415
    50 W. 17th St., 8th fl., New York, NY 10011-1607

ALLERGY AND ASTHMA

Allergy Research Group   (800) 545-9960
    PO Box 480 400 Preda St., San Leandro, CA 94577
American Allergy Association (415) 322-1663
    PO Box 7273, Menlo Park, CA 94026
Asthma and Allergy Foundation (202) 466-7643   (800) 7-ASTHMA
    1125 Fifteenth St. NW, Suite 502, Washington, DC 20005
    Fax (202) 466-8940
National Asthma Education Program (301) 495-4484
    4733 Bethesda Ave., Suite 350, Bethesda, MD 20814
National Institute of Allergy and Infectious Diseases (301) 496-5717
    NIH, Bldg. 31, Rm. 7A32, Bethesda, MD 20892

ALZHEIMER'S DISEASE

Alzheimer's Association (312) 335-8700   (800) 272-3900
    919 N. Michigan Ave., Suite 1000, Chicago, IL 60611
    Fax (312) 335-1110
Alzheimer's Disease International (312) 335-5777
    12 S. Michigan Ave., Chicago, IL 60603
    Fax (312) 335-1122
Association for Alzheimer's and Related Diseases   (800) 621-0379
    919 N. Michigan Ave., Suite 1000, Chicago, IL 60611-1676
    Fax (312) 335-1110

ARTHRITIS

The Arthritis Foundation (404) 872-7100   (800) 283-7800
    1314 Spring St., Atlanta, GA 30309
National Institute of Arthritis (301) 495-4484
    Box AMS, Bethesda, MD 20814

BIRTH DEFECTS (See also GENETIC COUNSELING below.)

March of Dimes/Birth Defects Foundation   (800) 326-2229
    1275 Mamaroneck Ave., White Plains, NY 10605
    Fax (914) 428-8203

BIRTH CONTROL (See FAMILY PLANNING below.)

BLOOD DISEASES: HEMOPHILIA, LEUKEMIA, SICKLE CELL DISEASE

National Hemophilia Foundation (212) 219-8180
    110 Greene St., Suite 303, New York NY 10012
Leukemia Society of America (212) 573-8484
    600 Third Ave., New York, NY 10016

National Sickle Cell Disease Branch (301) 496-4868
  National Heart, Lung, and Blood Institute NIH
  Rm. 504 Federal Bldg., 7550 Wisconsin Ave., Bethesda, MD 20892
  Fax (301) 402-3203
Sickle Cell Disease Association (310) 216-6363
  200 Corporate Point, Suite 495, Culver City, CA 90230-7633
Sickle Cell Disease Foundation of Greater N.Y. (212) 865-1500
  127 W. 127th St., New York, NY 10027

BONE DISEASES: OSTEOPOROSIS, PAGET'S DISEASE, SCOLIOSIS

National Osteoporosis Foundation (202) 223-2226
  2100 M St. NW, Washington, DC 20037
Osteoporosis Center (415) 476-5549
  University of California, San Francisco, CA 94143
Foundation for Paget's Disease (212) 229-1582   (800) 237-2438
  200 Varick St., Suite 1004, New York, NY 10014-4810
  Fax (212) 229-1502
Scoliosis Association Inc.   (800) 800-0669
  Box 811705, Boca Raton, FL 33481-1705

CANCER

American Cancer Society (404) 320-3333   (800) ACS-2345
  1599 Clifton Rd. NE, Atlanta, GA 30329
  Fax (404) 325-0230
Chemotherapy Foundation (212) 213-9292
  183 Madison Ave., Rm. 403, New York, NY 10016
  Fax (212) 689-5164
National Cancer Information Service (301) 496-4000
  9000 Rockville Pike, Bethesda, MD 20892
National Cancer Institute   (800) 4-CANCER
  Cancer Information Clearinghouse
National Organization for Breast Cancer Information   (800) 221-2141
  18220 Harwood Ave., Harwood, IL 60430
Reach to Recovery (212) 586-8700
  19 W. 56th St., New York NY 10019
  Fax (212) 237-3855
Rose Kushner Breast Cancer Advisory Center
  PO Box 224, Kensington, MD 20895
  Fax (301) 949-1132

CEREBRAL PALSY

United Cerebral Palsy Association (212) 979-9700
  120 East 23rd St., New York, NY 10010
  Fax (212) 260-7469

CHRONIC FATIGUE SYNDROME

CFIDS Association   (800) 442-3437
    PO Box 220398, Charlotte, NC 28222

CYSTIC FIBROSIS

Cystic Fibrosis Foundation   (800) 344-4823
    6931 Arlington Rd., Bethesda, MD 20814

DENTAL HEALTH

American Dental Association (312) 440-2500
    Bureau of Health Education and Audiovisual Services
    211 E. Chicago Ave., Chicago, IL 60611

DES

DES ACTION   (800) 337-9288
    1616 Broadway, Suite 510, Oakland, CA 94612
    Fax (510) 465-4815
DES Department, National Cancer Information Service (301) 496-4000
    9000 Rockville Pike, Bethesda, MD 20892

DIABETES

American Diabetes Association   (800) 232-3472
    PO Box 363, Mount Morris, IL 61054
National Diabetes Information Clearinghouse (301) 565-4167
    Box NDIC, Bethesda, MD 20205

DIGESTIVE DISEASES

National Foundation for Ileitis and Colitis Inc.   (800) 243-3637
    368 Park Ave. S., 17th fl., New York, NY 10016
    Fax (212) 779-4098
National Digestive Disease Information Clearinghouse (301) 654-3810
    2 Information Way, Bethesda, MD 20892
    Fax (301) 907-8906

DISABILITIES

American Disability Association (205) 323-3030
    2121 Eighth Ave. N. Suite 1623, Birmingham, AL 35203
    Fax (205) 251-7417
Americans with Disabilities Act (ADA)
    PO Box 27067, Houston, TX 77227
Assistance Dogs of America (419) 825-3622
    8806 State Route 64, Swanton, OH 43558

Clearinghouse on Disability Information (202) 205-8241
    U.S. Dept. of Education
    Office of Special Education and Rehabilitative Services
    400 Maryland Ave. SW, Washington, DC 20202
    Fax (202) 205-9252
Intern Center for the Disabled (ICD) (212) 679-0100
    340 E. 24th St., New York, NY 10010
    Fax (212) 889-2440
Learning Disabilities Association of America (412) 341-1515
    4156 Library Rd., Pittsburgh, PA 15234

DOMESTIC VIOLENCE

Domestic Violence Hotline   (800) 333-7233
Domestic Abuse Intervention Project (218) 722-2781
    206 W. Fourth St., Duluth, MN 55806
National Association for Child Abuse and Family Violence   (800) 222-2000
    1155 Connecticut Ave. NW, Washington, DC 20036
National Coalition Against Domestic Violence
    National Office—Denver: (303) 838-1852
    Washington Office: (202) 638-6388
National Organization for Victim Assistance   (800) TRY-NOVA
    1757 Park Rd. NW, Washington, DC 20010 (202) 232-6682
    Fax (202) 462-2255

DYING

Choice in Dying (212) 366-5540   (800) 989-9455
Hospice Association of America (202) 546-4759
    519 C St. NE, Washington, DC 20002

EATING DISORDERS

American Anorexia/Bulimia Association (212) 891-8686
    425 E. 61st St., New York, NY 10021
    Fax (212) 891-8613
Anorexia Nervosa and Associated Disorders
    PO Box 7, Highland Park, IL 60035
    Fax (708) 433-4632
National Eating Disorders Organization
    445 Granville Rd., Worthington, OH 43085
    Fax (614) 785-7471

ENVIRONMENT

Environmental Protection Agency (202) 260-2090
    Public Information Center, 401 M St. SW, Washington, DC 20460

EPILEPSY

Epilepsy Foundation of America (301) 459-3700   (800) 332-1000
     4351 Garden City Dr., Suite 406, Landover, MD 20785
     Fax (301) 577-2684

EYE DISORDERS AND VISION IMPAIRMENT

American Council of the Blind (202) 467-5081   (800) 424-8666
     1155 Fifteenth St. NW, Suite 720, Washington, DC 20005
Association for Macular Diseases Inc. (212) 605-3719
     210 E. 64th St., New York, NY 10021
Fight for Sight (212) 751-1118
     160 E. 56th St., New York, NY 10022
     Fax (212) 688-9641
Guiding Eyes for the Blind (914) 245-4024 (914) 245-1609
     611 Granite Springs Rd., Yorktown Heights, New York 10598
The Lighthouse Inc.
     Products to Help People with Impaired Vision   (800) 829-0500
National Association for the Visually Handicapped (212) 889-3141
     22 W. 21st St., New York, NY 10010
     Fax (212) 727-2931
National Braille Association (716) 427-8260
     3 Townline Circle, Rochester, NY 14623
     Fax (716) 427-0263
National Eye Institute (301) 496-5248
     Bldg. 31, Rm. 6A32, Bethesda, MD 20892
National Library Service for the Blind and Visually Handicapped
     Library of Congress (202) 707-5100
     1291 Taylor St. NW, Washington, DC 20542
Prevent Blindness America (708) 843-2020   (800) 331-2020
     500 East Remington Rd., Schaumburg, IL 60173
     Fax (708) 843-8458
Recording for the Blind, Inc. (609) 452-0606
     20 Roszel Rd., Princeton, NJ 08540

FAMILY PLANNING AND SEX INFORMATION

The Alan Guttmacher Institute (212) 248-1111
     120 Wall St., 2nd fl., New York, NY 10005
     Fax (212) 248-1951
Planned Parenthood Federation of America, Inc. (212) 541-7800
     810 Seventh Ave., New York, NY 10019
     Fax (212) 245-1845

GENETIC COUNSELING

National Society of Genetic Counselors (610) 872-7608
     233 Canterbury Dr., Wallingford, PA 19086

HEADACHE

National Council for Headache Education   (800) 255-ACHE
    875 Kings Highway, Woodbury, NJ 08096
National Headache Foundation (312) 878-7715
    5252 N. Western Ave., Chicago, IL 60625

HEALTH AND SAFETY

American Public Health Association (202) 789-5600
    1015 Fifteenth St. NW, Washington, DC 20005
    Fax (202) 789-5681
Consumer Product Safety Commission (301) 504-0000   (800) 638-8270
    4330 E. West Highway, Bethesda, MD 20814
    Fax (301) 504-0124
Council on Family Health (212) 578-3617
    225 Park Ave. S., Suite 1700, New York, NY 10003
    Fax (212) 598-3665
MedicAlert (209) 668-0333   (800) 344-3226
    Turlock, CA 95380

HEARING

Alexander Graham Bell Association for the Deaf (202) 337-5220
    3417 Volta Pl. NW, Washington, DC 20007
American Speech, Language, Hearing Association   (800) 638-8255
    10801 Rockville Pike, Rockville, MD 20852
The Deafness Research Foundation (212) 768-1181
    15 W. 39th St., New York, NY 10018
    Fax (212) 768-1782
National Association of the Deaf (301) 587-1788
    814 Thayer Ave., Silver Spring, MD 20910
    Fax (301) 587-1791
National Information Center on Deafness (202) 651-5051, 5052 TDD
    Gallaudet University, 800 Florida Ave. NE, Washington, DC 20002
    Fax (202) 651-5054
Self-Help for Hard-of-Hearing People (301) 657-2248
    7910 Woodmont Ave., Suite 1200, Bethesda, MD 20814
    Fax (301) 913-9413
Service Dog Center (206) 226-7357
    PO Box 1080, Renton, WA 98057-9906

HEART DISEASE

American Heart Association Mended Hearts Club   (800) 242-8721
    7272 Greenville Ave., Dallas, TX 75231
Coronary Club Inc. (216) 444-3690
    9500 Euclid Ave., Rm. E4-15, Cleveland, OH 44195

National Heart, Blood, and Lung Institute (301) 496-4236
    Bldg. 31, Rm. 4A21, Bethesda, MD 20892

HYPERTENSION AND STROKE

Courage Stroke Network   (800) 553-6321
National High Blood Pressure Education Program (301) 951-3620
    Information Center NIH, 7200 Wisconsin Ave., Bethesda, MD 20814
National Institute of Neurological Diseases and Stroke   (800) 352-9424
National Stroke Association (303) 839-1992
    8480 E. Orchard Rd., Suite 1000, Inglewood, CO 80111

INCEST

Incest Survivors Anonymous
    PO Box 17245, Long Beach, CA 90807-7245
Incest Survivors Resource Network (505) 521-4260
    Las Cruces, NM 88006

INCONTINENCE

Continence Restored (212) 879-3131
    785 Park Ave., New York, NY 10021
National Association for Continence (864) 579-7000   (800) BLADDER
    PO Box 8310, Spartanburg, SC 29305
    Fax (864) 579-7902

INFERTILITY

American Society for Reproductive Medicine (205) 978-5000
    1209 Montgomery Hwy., Montgomery, AL 35216-2809
Resolve Inc. (617) 623-0744
    1310 Broadway, Somerville, MA 02144-1731
    Fax (617) 623-0252

KIDNEY DISEASE

National Kidney Foundation (212) 889-2210   (800) 622-9010
    30 East 33rd St., New York, NY 10016
    Fax (212) 779-0068
National Kidney and Urologic Diseases Clearinghouse
    PO Box NKUDIC, 900 Rockville Pike, Bethesda, MD 20892

LESBIAN ISSUES

Custody Action for Lesbian Mothers (CALM) (215) 667-7508
    PO Box 281, Narberth, PA 7508
Old Lesbians Organizing for Change (713) 661-1482; (510) 439-8003

LUPUS

Lupus Foundation of America (301) 670-9292   (800) 558-0121
    4 Research Pl., Suite 180, Rockville, MD 20850
Lupus Network (203) 372-5795
    230 Ranch Dr., Bridgeport, CT 06606

LYME DISEASE

Lyme Disease Foundation (203) 871-2900   (800) 886-LYME

MARRIAGE COUNSELING

American Association for Marriage and Family Counseling   (800) 374-AMFC
    1100 Seventeenth St. NW, Washington, DC 20036
    Fax (202) 223-2329
Contact USA (formerly Teleministries USA) (717) 232-3501
    Pouch A, Harrisburg, PA 17105
    Fax (717) 232-3505

MENTAL HEALTH

National Institute of Mental Health (301) 443-4513
    U.S. Dept. of Health and Human Services
    5600 Fishers Lane, Rockville, MD 20857
National Mental Health Association (703) 684-7722
    1021 Prince St., Alexandria, VA 22314

MULTIPLE SCLEROSIS

National Multiple Sclerosis Society (212) 986-3240   (800) 344-4867
    733 Third Ave., 6th fl., New York, NY 10017
    Fax (212) 986-7981

MUSCULAR DYSTROPHY

Muscular Dystrophy Association (602) 529-2000
    3300 Sunrise Dr., Tucson, AZ 85718
Muscular Dystrophy Society (718) 793-1100
    5 Dakota Dr., Suite 108, Lake Success, NY 11042

MYASTHENIA GRAVIS

Myasthenia Gravis Foundation (212) 533-7005   (800) 643-0808
    61 Gramercy Park N., New York, NY 10010
    Fax (212) 533-0178

NUTRITION

American Dietetic Association (312) 899-0040
    216 W. Jackson Blvd., Suite 800, Chicago, IL 60606-6995

Community Nutrition Institute (202) 462-4700
    2001 S St. NW, Washington, DC 20009
FDA Office of Consumer Affairs Public Inquiries (301) 443-3170
    5600 Fishers Lane (HFE 88), Rockville, MD 20857
Food Safety, Dept. of Agriculture   (800) 535-4555

OSTEOPOROSIS (See BONE DISEASES.**)**

PAIN

American Chronic Pain Association (916) 632-0922
    Box 850, Rocklin, CA 95677
    Fax (916) 632-3208
American Pain Society (708) 966-5595
    6700 Old Orchard Rd., Skokie, IL 60077
    Fax (708) 966-9418
Chronic Pain Outreach Support Group (714) 775-8402
    16699 Sequoia, Fountain Valley, CA 92708
Committee on Pain Therapy (708) 825-5586
    American Society of Anesthesiologists
    520 N. Northwest Hwy., Park Ridge, IL 60068-2573
    Fax (708) 825-5586
National Chronic Pain Outreach Association (301) 652-4948
    7979 Old Georgetown Rd., Bethesda, MD 20814
    Fax (301) 907-0745
Pain Treatment Program of Lenox Hill Hospital   (800) 474-1276
    130 E. 77th St., New York, NY 10021
    Fax (212) 535-6994

PARKINSONISM

American Parkinson Disease Foundation   (800) 223-2732
    1250 Hylan Blvd., Staten Island, NY 10305
    Fax (718) 981-4399
National Parkinson's Foundation (305) 547-6666   (800) 327-4545
    1501 NW Ninth Ave., Miami, FL 33136
    Fax (305) 547-6666
Parkinson Foundation, Columbia Presbyterian Hospital   (800) 457-6676
    710 W. 168th St., New York, NY 10032
    Fax (212) 923-4778

PLASTIC SURGERY

American Board of Plastic Surgery (215) 587-9322
    7 Penn Center, Suite 400
    1635 Market St., Philadelphia, PA 19103
American Society of Plastic and Reconstructive Surgery   (800) 635-0635
    444 E. Algonquin Rd., Arlington Heights, IL 60005
    Fax (708) 228-9131

POISON CONTROL

Poison Control Centers: For local referral— (800) 764-7661

PREGNANCY AND DELIVERY

American College of Nurse-Midwives (202) 728-9860
    1522 K St. NW, Suite 1000, Washington, DC 20005
    Fax (202) 289-4395
National Association of Childbearing Centers (215) 234-8068
    3123 Gotschall Rd., Perkiominville, PA 18074
    Fax (215) 234-8829

RAPE

Center for Women Policy Studies (202) 872-1770
    2000 P Street NW, Suite 508, Washington, DC 20036
    Fax (202) 296-8962
National Center for Prevention and Control of Rape (301) 443-3673
    National Rape Information Clearinghouse, NIMH
    5600 Fishers Lane, Parklawn Bldg., Rm. 13A-44
    Rockville, MD 20857

REHABILITATION

American Academy of Physical Medicine and Rehabilitation (312) 922-9366
    122 S. Michigan Ave., Chicago, IL 60603-6107
American Physical Therapy Association (703) 684-2782
    111 Fairfax St., Alexandria, VA 22314
National Rehabilitation Information Center (800) 346-2742
    8455 Colesville Rd., Suite 935, Silver Spring, MD 20910-3319

RESPIRATORY DISEASES

American Lung Association (212) 315-8700 (800) LUNG-USA
    1740 Broadway, New York, NY 10019
    Fax (212) 315-8872
Emphysema Anonymous (813) 391-9977
    726 N. Highland Ave., Clearwater, FL 34615-5463
National Heart, Lung, and Blood Institute (301) 594-7430
    5333 Westbard Ave., Bethesda, MD 20892
    Fax (301) 594-7487
National Jewish Center for Immunology and Respiratory Medicine
    1400 Jackson St., Denver, CO 80206 (800) 222-LUNG

SEX EDUCATION AND THERAPY

American Association of Sex Educators, Counselors, and Therapists
    435 N. Michigan Ave. #1717, Chicago, IL 60611 (312) 644-0828
    Fax (312) 644-8557

Sex Information and Education Council of the U.S. (SIECUS)
    Resource Center and Library (212) 819-9770
    130 W. 42nd St., Suite 350, New York, NY 10036

SEXUALLY TRANSMISSIBLE DISEASES

American Social Health Association (919) 361-8400
    PO Box 13827, Research Triangle Park, NC 27709
    Fax (919) 361-8425
CDC Herpes Resource Center   (800) 230-6039
CDC STD Hotline   (800) 227-8922

SLEEP DISORDERS

American Narcolepsy Association (415) 788-4793
    1255 Post St., Suite 201, San Francisco, CA 94109
American Sleep Apnea Association (617) 489-4441
    PO Box 66, Belmont, MA 02178
    Fax (617) 489-4761
American Sleep Disorders Association (507) 287-6006
    1610 Fourteenth St. NW, Suite 300, Rochester, MN 55901
    Fax (507) 287-6008
National Sleep Foundation (202) 785-2300
    1367 Connecticut Ave. NW, Suite 200, Washington, DC 20036
    Fax (202) 785-2880

STERILIZATION

Association for Voluntary Surgical Contraception (212) 561-8000
    79 Madison Ave., New York, NY 10016
    Fax (2112) 779-9489, 9439
Zero Population Growth (202) 332-2200
    1400 Sixteenth St. NW, Suite 320, Washington, DC 20036
    Fax (202) 332-2302

SUICIDE

The Samaritans (617) 247-0220
    500 Commonwealth Ave., Boston, MA 02215
Seasons: Suicide Bereavement (801) 649-8327
    PO Box 187, Park City, UT 84060

WEIGHT CONTROL

Weight Watchers International   (800) 221-2112

WOMEN'S HEALTH

Melpomene Institute for Women's Health Research (612) 642-1951
    1010 University Ave., St. Paul, MN 55104
    Fax (612) 642-1871

National Black Women's Health Project (404) 758-9590
    1237 Abernathy Blvd. SW, Atlanta, GA 30310
    Fax (404) 758-9661
National Women's Health Network (202) 347-1140
    1325 G St. NW, Washington, DC 20005
National Women's Health Resource Center (202) 293-6045
    2440 M St. NW, Washington, DC 20037
Office of Research on Women's Health, NIH (301) 402-1770
    9000 Rockville Pike, Bldg. 1, No. 201, Bethesda, MD 20892
    Fax (301) 402-1798

WOMEN AT WORK

National Institute for Occupational Safety and Health   (800) 356-4674
9 to 5 National Association of Working Women   (800) 522-0925
Women Work: National Network for Women's Employment (202) 467-6346
    (formerly National Displaced Homemakers Network)
    1625 K St. NW, Suite 300, Washington, DC 20006
    Fax (202) 467-5366

INDEX

Page references in italics refer to illustrations. Bold-faced references refer to the Encyclopedia of Health and Medical Terms.

795